Frontofacial Monobloc Advancement with Internal Distraction

Eric Arnaud • Giovanna Paternoster
Roman Hossein Khonsari • Samer E. Haber

Frontofacial Monobloc Advancement with Internal Distraction

Tactics and Strategy in Faciocraniosynostosis

Springer

Eric Arnaud
Craniofacial Unit
French Reference Center for Craniosynostoses
and Craniofacial Malformations (CRANIOST)
Hôpital Necker - Enfants Malades
Paris & Clinique Marcel Sembat
Boulogne-Billancourt, France

Giovanna Paternoster
Craniofacial Unit
Department of Pediatric Neurosurgery
French Reference Center for Craniosynostoses
and Craniofacial Malformations (CRANIOST)
Hôpital Necker - Enfants Malades
Paris, France

Roman Hossein Khonsari
Craniofacial Unit
Department of Maxillofacial Surgery
and Plastic Surgery
French Reference Center for Craniosynostoses
and Craniofacial Malformations (CRANIOST)
Hôpital Necker - Enfants Malades
Paris, France

Samer E. Haber
Craniofacial Unit
French Reference Center for Craniosynostoses
and Craniofacial Malformations (CRANIOST)
Hôpital Necker - Enfants Malades
Paris & Clinique Marcel Sembat
Boulogne-Billancourt, France

ISBN 978-3-031-07573-5 ISBN 978-3-031-07574-2 (eBook)
https://doi.org/10.1007/978-3-031-07574-2

This Springer imprint is published by the registered company Springer Nature Switzerland AG
The registered company address is: Gewerbestrasse 11, 6330 Cham, Switzerland

Honor those who go first, even if those
who come later go further (…).

- *To the memory of my father, remarkable by his lucidity and who supported me so much, to my mother who taught me the value of effort resulting in pleasure, and to my two beloved children Bianca and Henry, who are enlightening my life.*
- *To my craniofacial mentors Daniel Marchac and Dominique Renier.*
- *To the memory of Jean-Marie Servant, a Master in Plastic Surgery, and to Marc Revol, a noble teacher.*
- *To the memory of Fernando Ortiz Monasterio, the Maestro, who simplified complex problems.*
- *To Christian Sainte-Rose and Giuseppe Cinalli, supportive friends and talented neurosurgical leaders.*
- *To Patrick Diner, with whom we started the distraction Odyssey.*
- *To my sister Caroline, who is a very fine psychologist.*
- *To Yves, who is an atypical and skeptical author.*
- *To Sophie, who is a teammate, at sea as well as in life.*

Eric Arnaud, M.D.

Preface

Simple words may be wrong,
but complicated explanations are incomprehensible…
(Translated from French author Paul Valery)

As a resident in plastic surgery, a trauma case I was participating in involved the skull base, and dura-mater was exposed…. Later I discovered the fascinating field of craniofacial surgery with Daniel Marchac and Dominique Renier in Hôpital Necker—Enfants Malades.

My discovery in the late 1980s of the drawings of the so-called monobloc technique in the pioneer's publications (Tessier 1970, 1981, and Ortiz-Monasterio 1978) was a revelation of audacity and completeness. However, this procedure developed in the 1970s before the distraction era had been abandoned, because of severe or fatal complications…. Thirty years later, we reintroduced in September 2000 the frontofacial monobloc advancement (FFMBA) with internal distraction for a severe Pfeiffer patient aged 4 months who had recurrent eyeball luxation… Immediate improvement was obtained in a smooth manner. Since then, more than 175 FFMBA procedures have been performed at some point during the sequence of treatment of a cohort of more than 700 faciocraniosynostoses among 5500 craniosynostoses treated in the Craniofacial Unit of Hôpital Necker—Enfants Malades since 1976. In the management of those mainly *FGFR2*-related conditions, a strategy of treatment including various surgical procedures has to be elaborated based on each patient specificity.

I would like to thank Giovanna, Hossein, and Sam, with whom working on a daily basis is a pleasure and who have honored me of being one of their mentors. I would also like to thank Nathalie Marty and Salima Medini for organizing everything in our craniofacial unit. I am grateful to Cassandra Vion and Emma Blanc-Tailleur for illustrating this atlas. All co-contributors who participate in the genuine multidisciplinary management of our syndromic patients should be deeply thanked for their input in the quality of the care we provide to these complex patients.

This atlas tries to address the treatment of a complex condition in a simple manner.

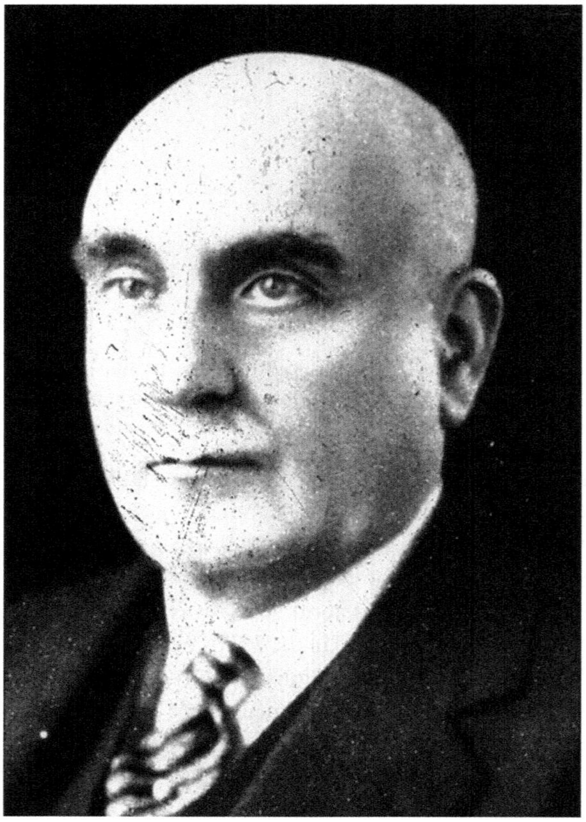

Fig. 1 Docteur Octave Crouzon, Paris, 1912

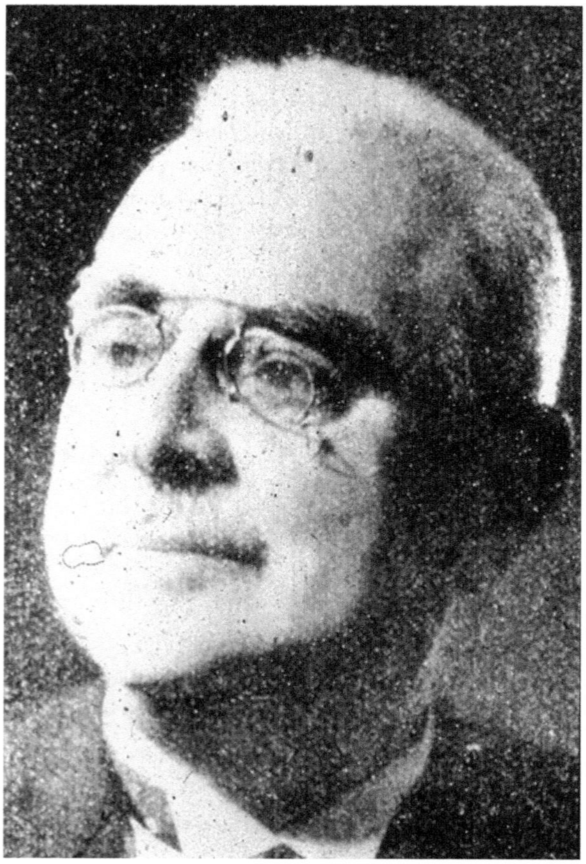

Fig. 2 Docteur Émile Apert, Hôpital Necker, Paris, 1906

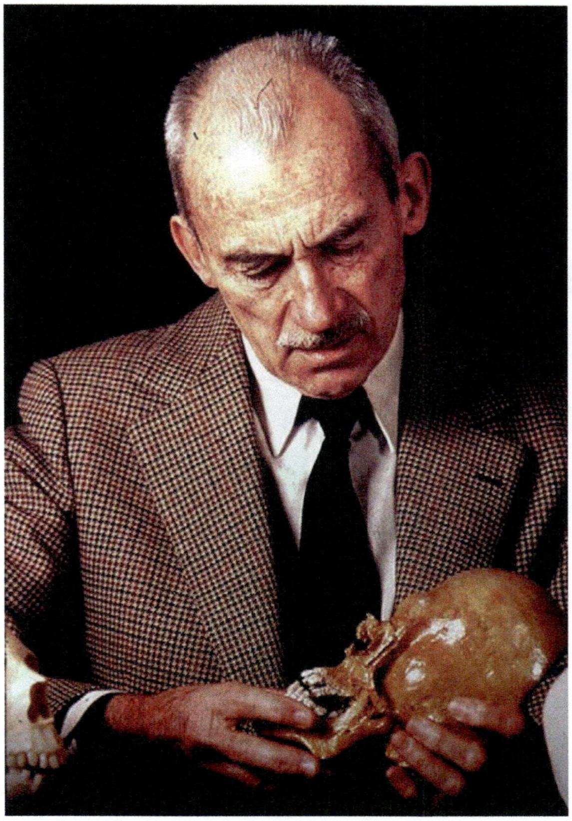

Fig. 3 Docteur Paul Tessier, plastic surgeon, Paris, 1967

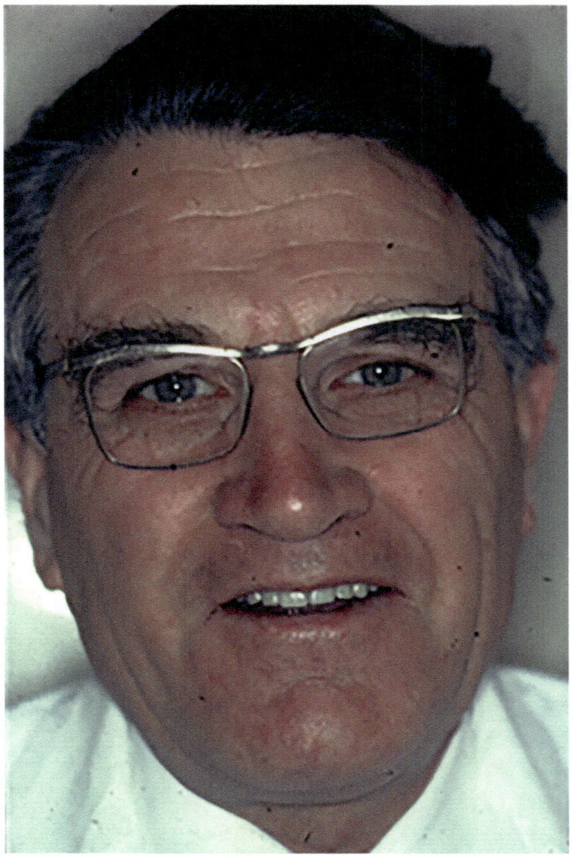

Fig. 4 Docteur Gérard Guyot, neurosurgeon, Hôpital Foch, Suresnes, 1967

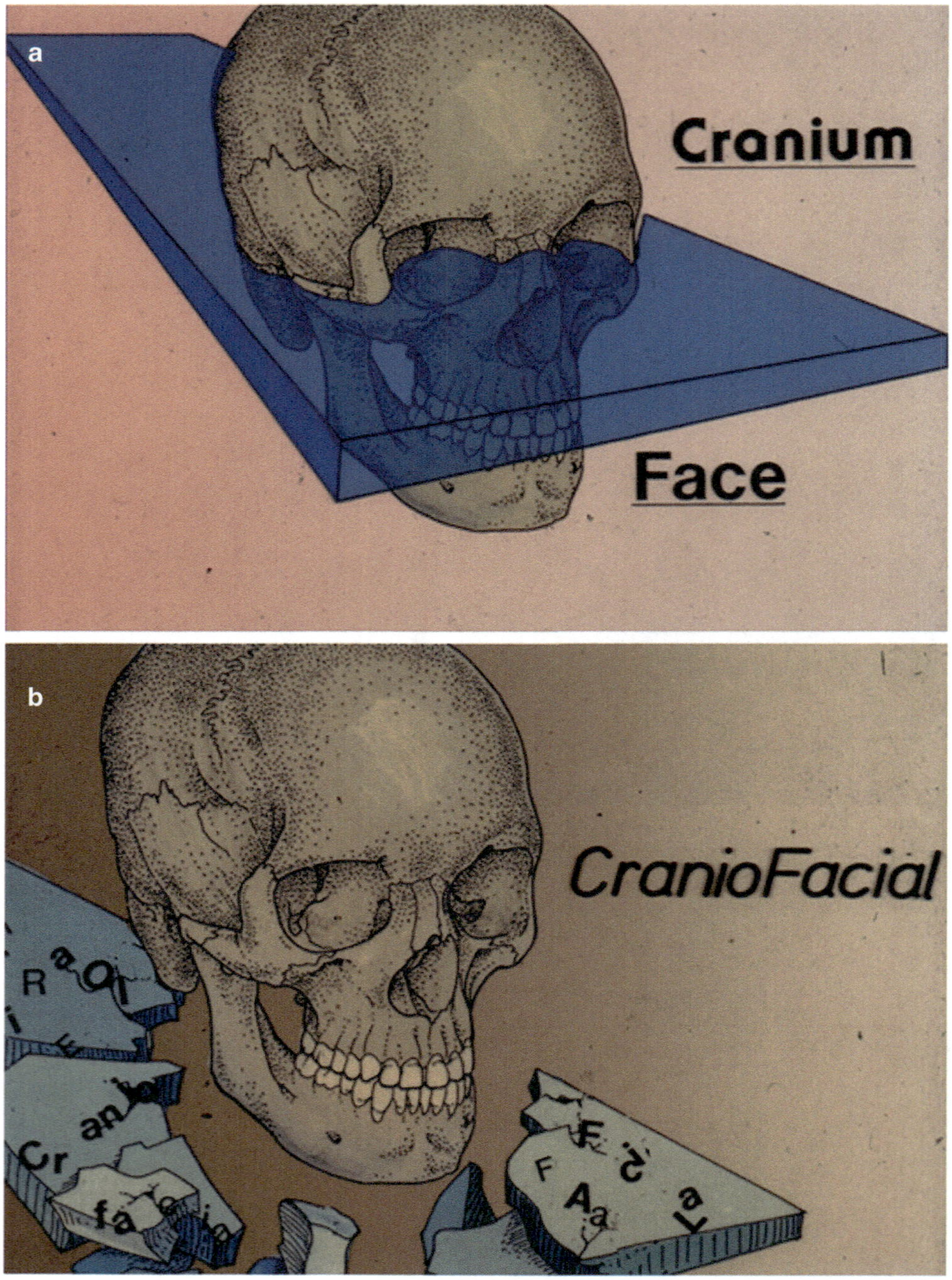

Fig. 5 (**a**) Before the craniofacial surgery era: the divided territories. (**b**) The craniofacial territory (adapted from Paul Tessier, oral conference material)

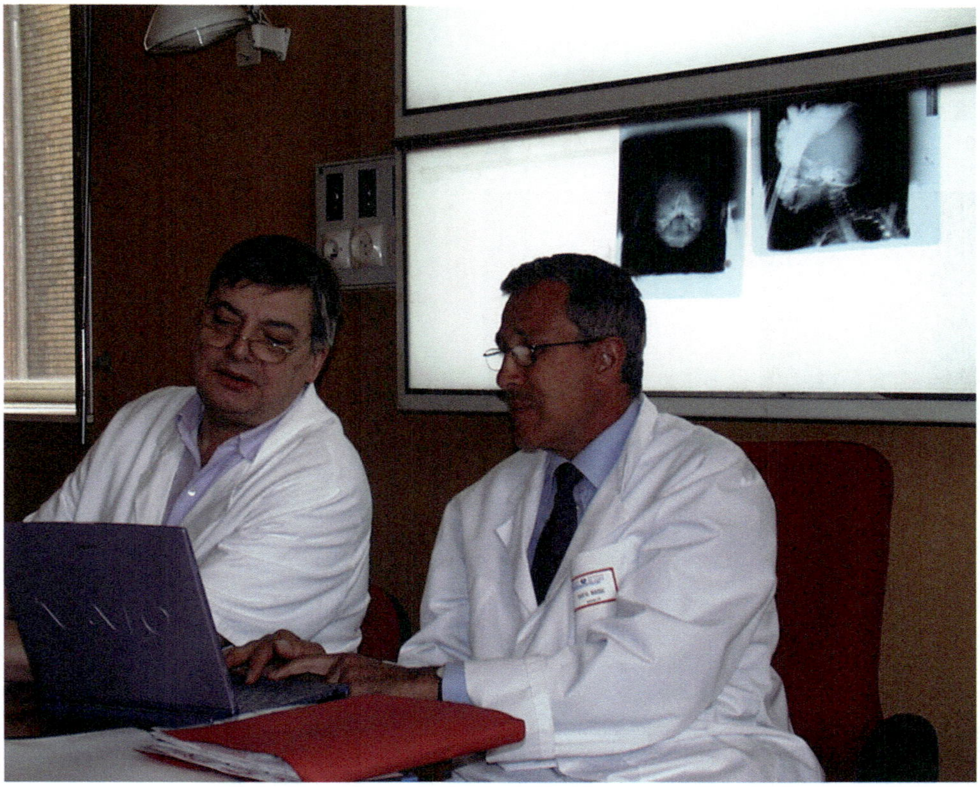

Fig. 6 Professor Dominique Renier (neurosurgeon, left) and Doctor Daniel Marchac (plastic surgeon, right) co-directed the craniofacial unit in Hopital Necker—Enfants Malades from 1976 to 2008

Contents

List of Contributors

Karine André Department of Pediatric Neurosurgery, Necker–Enfants Malades University Hospital, Paris, France

Thomas Baugnon Department of Anesthesia and Reanimation, Necker–Enfants Malades University Hospital, Paris, France

Geneviève Baujat Department of Genetics, Necker–Enfants Malades University Hospital, Paris, France

Emma Blanc-Tailleur Scientific Illustrator, Paris, France

Jebrane Bouaoud Department of Maxillofacial and Plastic Surgery, Pitié-Salpêtrière Hospital, Paris, France

Martin Catala Department of Neurology, Pitié-Salpêtrière Hospital, Paris, France

Corinne Collet Molecular Genetics Unit, Department of Genetics, Robert Debré Hospital, Paris, France

Valérie Cormier-Daire Department of Genetics, Necker–Enfants Malades Hospital, Paris, France

Raphaël Cornette Morphometrician, National Natural History Museum, Paris, France

Vincent Couloigner Department of Pediatric Otolaryngology, Necker–Enfants Malades Hospital, Paris, France

Patrick Diner Department of Maxillofacial Surgery and Plastic Surgery, Necker–Enfants Malades Hospital, Paris, France

Caroline Ea Department of Maxillofacial Surgery and Plastic Surgery, Necker–Enfants Malades Hospital, Paris, France

Brigitte Fauroux Pediatric Pneumologist, Pediatric Non-Invasive Ventilation and Sleep Unit, Necker–Enfants Malades Hospital, Paris, France

Eva Galliani Department of Maxillofacial Surgery and Plastic Surgery, Necker–Enfants Malades Hospital, Paris, France

Nicolas Garcelon Head of Data Science Platform, Imagine Institute, Paris, France

Quentin Hennocq Department of Maxillofacial Surgery, Pitié-Salpêtrière Hospital, Paris, France

Syril James Department of Pediatric Neurosurgery, Necker–Enfants Malades Hospital, Paris, France

Nicolas Kogane Department of Maxillofacial Surgery and Plastic Surgery, Necker–Enfants Malades Hospital, Paris, France

Nicolas Leboulanger Department of Pediatric Otolaryngology, Necker–Enfants Malades Hospital, Paris, France

Laurence Legeai-Mallet Developmental Biologist, Laboratory of Molecular and Physiopathological Bases of Osteochondrodysplasia, INSERM UMR 1163, Imagine Institute, Paris, France

Junnu Leikola Cleft Palate and Craniofacial Center, Department of Plastic Surgery, Töölö Hospital, Helsinki University Central Hospital, Helsinki, Finland

Romain Luscan Department of Pediatric Otolaryngology, Necker–Enfants Malades Hospital, Paris, France

Philippe Meyer Department of Anesthesia and Reanimation, Necker–Enfants Malades University Hospital, Paris, France

Mehran Moazen Department of Mechanical Engineering, University College London, London, UK

Anne Morice Department of Maxillofacial Surgery and Plastic Surgery, Necker–Enfants Malades Hospital, Paris, France

Marie-Paule Morisseau-Durand Department of Pediatric Otolaryngology, Necker–Enfants Malades Hospital, Paris, France

Daniel Nowinski Department of Surgical Sciences, Uppsala University, Department of Plastic and Maxillofacial Surgery, Uppsala University Hospital, Uppsala, Sweden

Johan Nysjö Department of Information Technology, Centre for Image Analysis, Uppsala University. Uppsala, Sweden

Leslie Pamphile-Tabuteau Department of Pediatric Neurosurgery, Necker–Enfants Malades University Hospital, Paris, France

Arnaud Picard Head of the Department of Maxillofacial Surgery and Plastic Surgery, Necker–Enfants Malades Hospital, Paris, France

Matthieu Robert Department of Ophthalmology, Necker-Enfants Malades Hospital, Paris, France

Ludovic Sicard Department of Maxillofacial Surgery and Plastic Surgery, Necker–Enfants Malades Hospital, Paris, France

François Simon Department of Pediatric Otolaryngology, Necker–Enfants Malades Hospital, Paris, France

Maxime Taverne Craniofacial Growth and Form laboratory, Necker-Enfants Malades University Hospital, Paris, France

Briac Thierry Department of Pediatric Otolaryngology, Necker–Enfants Malades Hospital, Paris, France

Catherine Tomat Department of Maxillofacial Surgery and Plastic Surgery, Necker–Enfants Malades Hospital, Paris, France

Romain Touzé Department of Ophthalmology, Necker-Enfants Malades Hospital, Paris, France

Estelle Vergnaud Department of Anesthesia and Reanimation, Necker–Enfants Malades University Hospital, Paris, France

Cassandra Vion Scientific Illustrator, Paris, France

Veronique Viot-Blanc Pneumologist, Sleep Clinic, Lariboisière Hospital, Paris, France

Abbreviations

CPAP:	Continuous Positive Airway Pressure
CSF:	Cerebrospinal Fluid
CT:	Computed Tomography
ETV:	Endoscopic Third Ventriculostomy
EVD:	External Ventricular Drain
FCST:	Faciocraniosynostosis
FFMBA:	Frontofacial Monobloc Advancement
FGFR:	Fibroblast Growth Factor Receptor
FM:	Foramen Magnum
GERD:	Gastro-Esophageal Reflux Disease
ICP:	Intracranial Pressure
LF3:	Le Fort III Facial Advancement
MRI:	Magnetic Resonance Imaging
OSA:	Obstructive Sleep Apnea
PVE:	Posterior Vault Expansion
RED:	Rigid External Distraction
VEM:	Very Early Monobloc

1 Introduction: A Simplified Strategy for Complex Craniosynostotic Conditions

Treatment Principles

1. PVE, tarsorrhaphy, and turbinectomy/tonsillectomy are the most common first treatment steps in FCST management.
2. They aim to decompress the brain and open the airway until FFMBA can be performed safely.
3. The ideal age for performing FFMBA is around 2.5 years (between 2 and 3 years of age).
4. Consider very early monobloc (FFMBA before 18 months of age) in severe forms of FCST.
5. Try to avoid shunting at any stage or at least delay shunting unless/until absolutely mandatory.
6. Most patients require a secondary LF3 after FFMBA during or after mixed dentition for respiratory or aesthetic indications.
7. Orthognathic surgery after the end of growth and ancillary aesthetic procedures allow optimal results during teenage years or early adulthood.

As it has been extensively debated, potential functional issues due to delayed, inappropriate, or even absent treatment in patients with FCST may be summarized as follows:

- Raised ICP with risk of cognitive impairment, tonsillar herniation, hydrocephalus, and optic nerve atrophy [1–7].
- Corneal exposure by exorbitism (the orbit is not deep enough) causes amblyopia, strabismus, and blindness [8–12].
- Sleep apnea syndrome, resulting in hypoxemia, raised ICP, cognitive decline, and global hypotrophy (delay in global development) [13–19] (Fig. 1.1).
- Occlusal anomalies in older patients [20–22].
- Aesthetic prejudice impairing social interactions and quality of life [23–25].

These consequences depend on the causal *FGFR* mutation (mainly *FGFR2*, and rarely *FGFR1* or *FGFR3*). The disease process and the phenotype are progressive since the prenatal period and throughout growth. At each step of development, the risks of surgical procedures need to be weighed against their benefits before a procedure can be decided and performed.

However, the following surgical sequence ends up being adopted in the vast majority of cases:

1. PVE with distraction between 3 and 12 months of age—with or without foramen magnum decompression (for tonsillar herniation or hydrocephalus)—avoid ventriculoperitoneal shunting if possible—discuss tracheostomy, which may be avoided by choanal surgery at an early stage.
2. FFMBA after 18 months (between 24 and 36 months if possible).
3. LF3 indicated in case of airway issues or aesthetic requests during childhood (discuss palatal transverse distraction before or after LF3).
4. Ancillary procedures until completion of growth (orthognathic surgery, genioplasty, canthopexy, fat grafting, rhinoplasty) to obtain a satisfactory morphological outcome.

The previous steps might be modified or repeated depending on the severity of the condition at a given moment and the various tools of the craniofacial armamentarium may be employed differently depending on each phenotype (Fig. 1.2).

Ancillary ENT procedures and neurosurgical shunts may be considered at various steps. Aesthetic refinements are usually carried out last, after orthognathic procedures.

Risks

1. Raised ICP, corneal exposure, and obstructive sleep apnea syndrome are the most common yet detrimental factors of severity in FCST.
2. The phenotype is variable according to the *FGFR* mutation.
3. Early brain decompression before 1 year of age is the rule.

E. Arnaud et al., *Frontofacial Monobloc Advancement with Internal Distraction*, https://doi.org/10.1007/978-3-031-07574-2_1

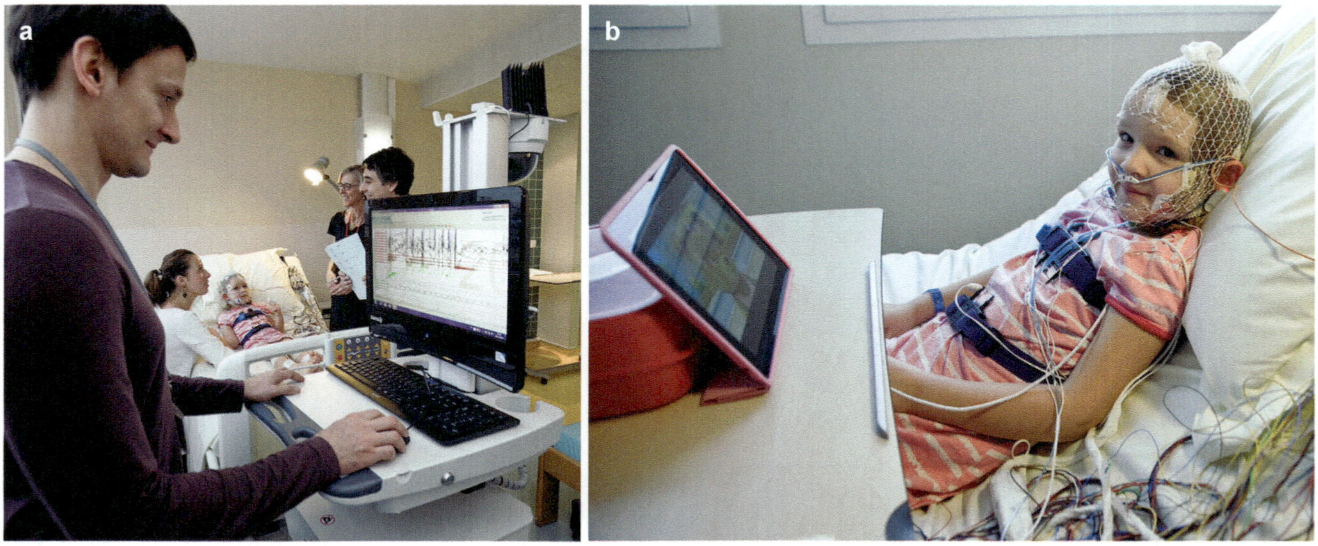

Fig. 1.1 (**a**, **b**) Sleep study (polysomnography, PSG)

One of the major decisions in the strategy of facial advancement is to choose between FFMBA or the combination of FOA followed by LF3 osteotomy (Fig. 1.3).

The main discussion is to determine whether FFMBA may provide a long period of time (>10 years) without any treatment and therefore delaying or avoiding LF3 (Fig. 1.4).

In the strategy with FOA followed by LF3, the age at facial osteotomy is critical: an early LF3 will probably lead to a secondary one later because of the underlying genetic growth deficiency and functional factors (Fig. 1.4).

Some examples of these various strategies are illustrated in chap. 11 with clinical examples.

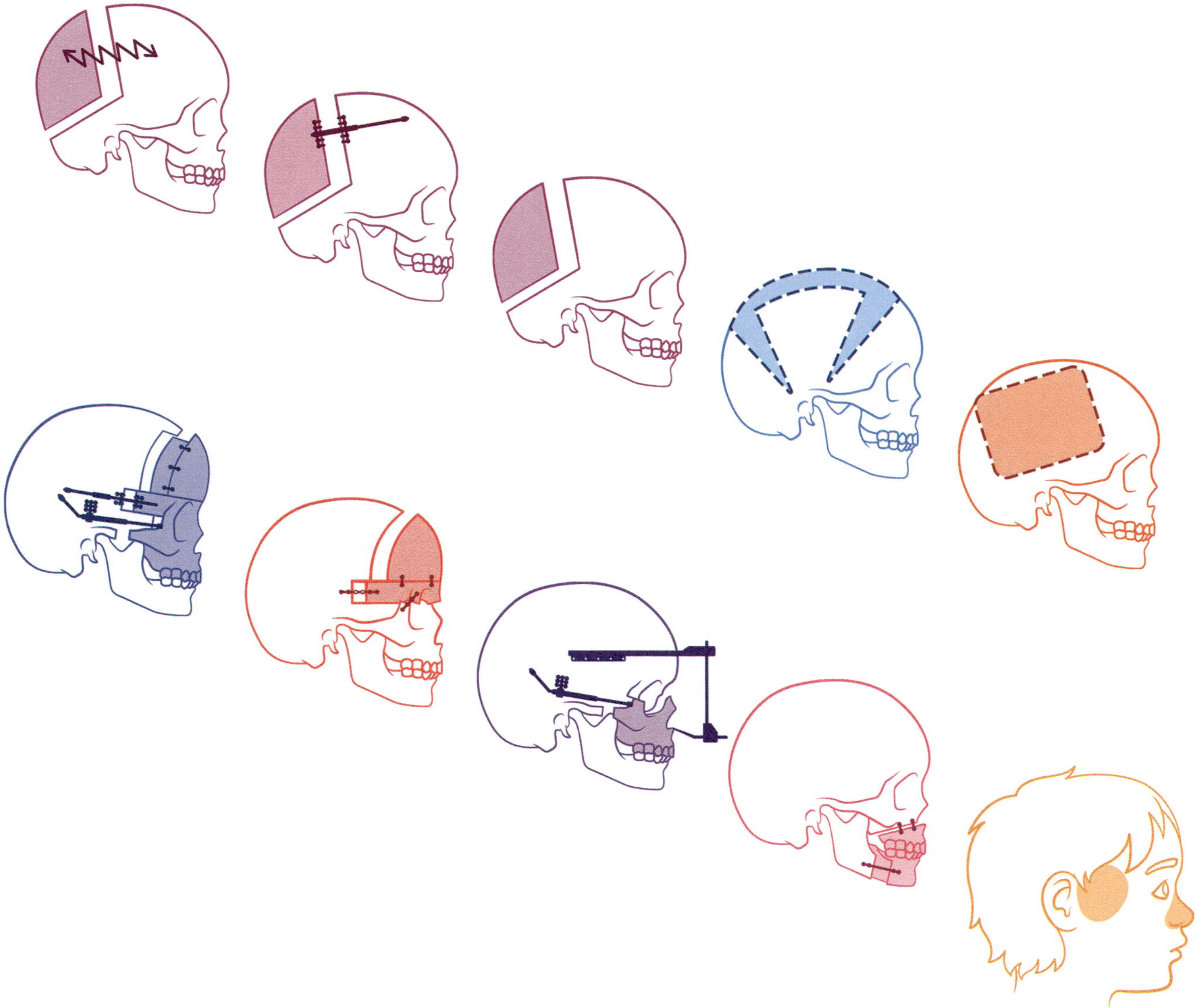

Fig. 1.2 The major craniofacial tools to treat faciocraniosynostoses. Upper diagonal (from left to right): spring-mediated PVE, distractor-mediated PVE, brain-mediated PVE, H craniectomies, and biparietal decompression. Lower diagonal (from left to right): FFMBA with double internal distraction, FOA without distraction, Le Fort 3 osteotomy (LF3), usually with internal and external distraction, orthognathic surgery, and ancillary aesthetic procedures (temporal and/or zygomatic fat grafting, rhinoplasty). © Cassandra Vion

Fig. 1.3 The basic algorithms: (**a**) FFMBA; (**b**) FOA followed by LF3. © Cassandra Vion

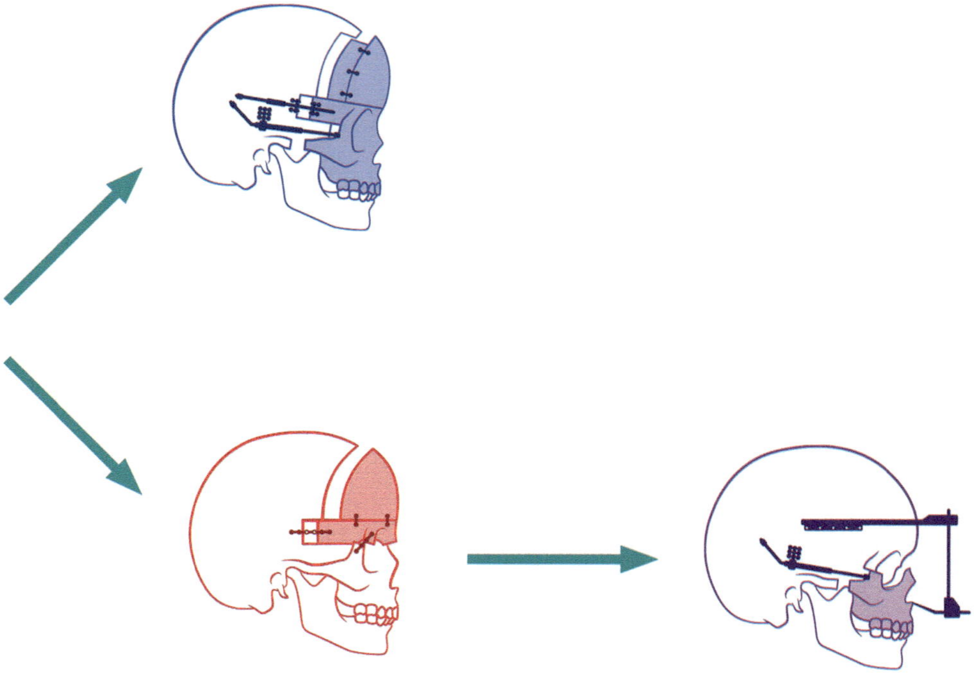

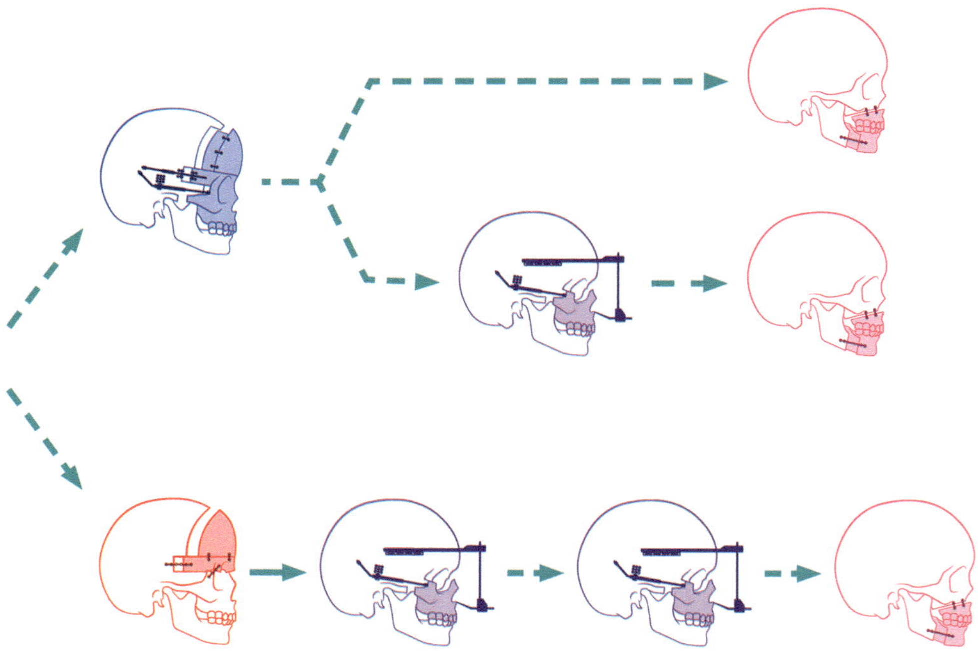

Fig. 1.4 Same algorithm as in Figure 1.3 with further details. After FFMBA, some patients do not require LF3 and go for orthognathic surgery in adolescence. Because an early LF3 around 6 years of age will deteriorate with time and necessitate another LF3 procedure around adolescence, patients with respiratory impairment would be preferably operated on with a FFMBA

References

1. Franceschetti A, Maeder G, Dolivo G, et al. Three cases of craniofacial dysostosis (Crouzon); the importance of changes of the optic nerve from the neurosurgical viewpoint. Confin Neurol. 1955;15(2):107–14.
2. Renier D, Sainte-Rose C, Marchac D, et al. Intracranial pressure in craniostenosis. J Neurosurg. 1982 Sep;57(3):370–7.
3. Renier D. Intracranial pressure in craniosynostosis: pre- and post-operative recordings-correlation with functional results. Scientific foundations and surgical treatment of Craniosynostosis Baltimore: Williams & Wilkins 1989; 263–269.
4. Francis PM, Beals S, Rekate HL, et al. Chronic tonsillar herniation and Crouzon's syndrome. Pediatr Neurosurg. 1992;18(4):202–6.
5. Cinalli G, Renier D, Sebag G, et al. Chronic tonsillar herniation in Crouzon's and Apert's syndromes: the role of premature synostosis of the lambdoid suture. J Neurosurg. 1995 Oct;83(4):575–82.
6. Cinalli G, Chumas P, Arnaud E, et al. Occipital remodeling and suboccipital decompression in severe craniosynostosis associated with tonsillar herniation. Neurosurgery. 1998;42(1):66–71. discussion 71–73
7. Doerga PN, Rijken BFM, Bredero-Boelhouwer H, et al. Neurological deficits are present in syndromic craniosynostosis patients with and without tonsillar herniation. Eur J Paediatr Neurol. 2020 Sep;28:120–5.
8. Khan SH, Nischal KK, Dean F, et al. Visual outcomes and amblyogenic risk factors in craniosynostotic syndromes: a review of 141 cases. Br J Ophthalmol. 2003 Aug;87(8):999–1003.
9. Gray TL, Casey T, Selva D, et al. Ophthalmic sequelae of Crouzon syndrome. Ophthalmology. 2005 Jun;112(6):1129–34.
10. Lehman S. Strabismus in craniosynostosis. Curr Opin Ophthalmol. 2006 Oct;17(5):432–4.
11. Rosenberg JB, Tepper OM, Medow NB. Strabismus in craniosynostosis. J Pediatr Ophthalmol Strabismus. 2013 Jun;50(3):140–8.
12. Touzé R, Bremond-Gignac D, Robert MP. Ophthalmological management in craniosynostosis. Neurochirurgie. 2019 Nov;65(5):310–7.
13. Hess CW, Sauter K, Bonfils P. Severe adult hypersomnia--sleep apnea syndrome in craniofacial dysostosis. Respiration. 1986;50(2):147–52.
14. Cohen SR, Suzman K, Simms C, et al. Sleep apnea surgery versus tracheostomy in children: an exploratory study of the comparative effects on quality of life. Plast Reconstr Surg. 1998 Nov;102(6):1855–64.
15. Gozal D. Morbidity of obstructive sleep apnea in children: facts and theory. Sleep Breath. 2001;5(1):35–42.
16. Bannink N, Nout E, Wolvius EB, et al. Obstructive sleep apnea in children with syndromic craniosynostosis: long-term respiratory outcome of midface advancement. Int J Oral Maxillofac Surg. 2010 Feb;39(2):115–21.
17. Driessen C, Mathijssen IMJ, De Groot MR, et al. Does central sleep apnea occur in children with syndromic craniosynostosis? Respir Physiol Neurobiol. 2012;181(3):321–5.
18. Driessen C, Joosten KFM, Florisson JMG, et al. Sleep apnoea in syndromic craniosynostosis occurs independent of hindbrain herniation. Childs Nerv Syst. 2013 Feb;29(2):289–96.
19. Khonsari RH, Haber S, Paternoster G, et al. The influence of fronto-facial monobloc advancement on obstructive sleep apnea: an assessment of 109 syndromic craniosynostoses cases. J Cranio-Maxillofac Surg. 2020;48(6):536–47.
20. Posnick JC, Craniofacial dysostosis. Staging of reconstruction and management of the midface deformity. Neurosurg Clin N Am. 1991 Jul;2(3):683–702.
21. Kahnberg K-E, Hagberg C. Orthognathic surgery in patients with craniofacial syndrome. I. a 5-year overview of combined orthodontic and surgical correction. J Plast Surg Hand Surg. 2010 Dec;44(6):282–8.
22. Nout E, Koudstaal MJ, Wolvius EB, et al. Additional orthognathic surgery following Le fort III and monobloc advancement. Int J Oral Maxillofac Surg. 2011;40(7):679–84.
23. Arnaud E, Haber SE, Paternoster G, et al. Secondary surgeries in craniosynostosis and faciocraniosynostosis. Ann Chir Plast Esthet. 2019 Nov;64(5–6):494–505.
24. Warschausky S, Kay JB, Buchman S, et al. Health-related quality of life in children with craniofacial anomalies. Plast Reconstr Surg. 2002;110(2):409–14. discussion 415–416
25. Park KM, Tripathi NV, Mufarrej FA. Quality of life in patients with craniosynostosis and deformational plagiocephaly: a systematic review. Int J Pediatr Otorhinolaryngol. 2021 Aug;6(149):110873.

Intracranial Pressure Management and Posterior Vault Distraction

2

1. PVE is usually the first craniofacial procedure in FCST.
2. Internal distractors are most commonly used to drive posterior expansion. Other options include springs and brain-mediated expansion.
3. PVE aims to increase intracranial volume in the posterior aspect of the skull (increasing the volume of posterior fossa) and delay FFMBA ("buying time").
4. FM decompression may be associated in a single stage to PVE, or performed separately.
5. In case of a normal posterior fossa, biparietal decompression may be considered as the first-line procedure before FFMBA.
6. Decompression techniques (PVE, biparietal decompression, and FM decompression) may be combined together or realized in chronologically different sequences.
7. Accurate management of vault expansion may prevent the need for ventricular shunting when stabilization of CSF flux is obtained.

FCST is characterized by multi-sutural fusions, often progressive, associated with the upper cervical spine and facial anomalies including maxillary hypoplasia, added to a wide spectrum of additional and variable anatomic anomalies. FCST presents a significant and early risk for restricted brain growth and increased ICP.

The management of ICP in these patients is one of the main issues to consider in defining an efficient and multistage surgical strategy.

Fronto-facial monobloc advancement (FFMBA) with distraction can be performed at very young ages, but results are best when this procedure is proposed after 2 years of age to avoid zygomaticomaxillary subluxation and to reach long-lasting maxillary advancement.

In the first months of life, the management strategy aims to address intracranial hypertension that results from constriction of the rapidly growing infant's brain by the fused sutures. The surgical technique should increase intracranial volume while avoiding osteotomies to the forehead and the temporal areas, to avoid burning bridges for the eventual FFMBA to come.

Considering the problems related to the small posterior fossa and to the cerebellar tonsillar herniation in many FCST patients, we adopted PVE, with internal distraction if possible, as the primary surgical procedure in FCST. Foramen magnum (FM) decompression may be added at any stage of this basic sequence.

Exceptions include, on the one hand, extremely severe cases where exorbitism threatens vision and imposes a very early FFMBA to contain the eyeballs inside the orbits, or, on the other hand, mild cases without posterior brain crowding, in which FFMBA could very well be the first and only step around age 2–3 years.

2.1 Historical Evolution of the Strategy of Care

Strategies and surgical schedules drastically changed over the past 40 years. FFMBA was initially developed without distraction and had been abandoned. It was later reintroduced in 2000 using distraction in our unit. PVE was rarely performed. Before 2004 (Fig. 2.1), FFMBA was either performed primarily or secondarily after FOA or a subtotal vault remodeling: In that initial period, many cases had to be reoperated because of insufficient results. It soon became apparent that the morbidity associated with secondary FFMBA was higher than that of primary FFMBA.

E. Arnaud et al., *Frontofacial Monobloc Advancement with Internal Distraction*, https://doi.org/10.1007/978-3-031-07574-2_2

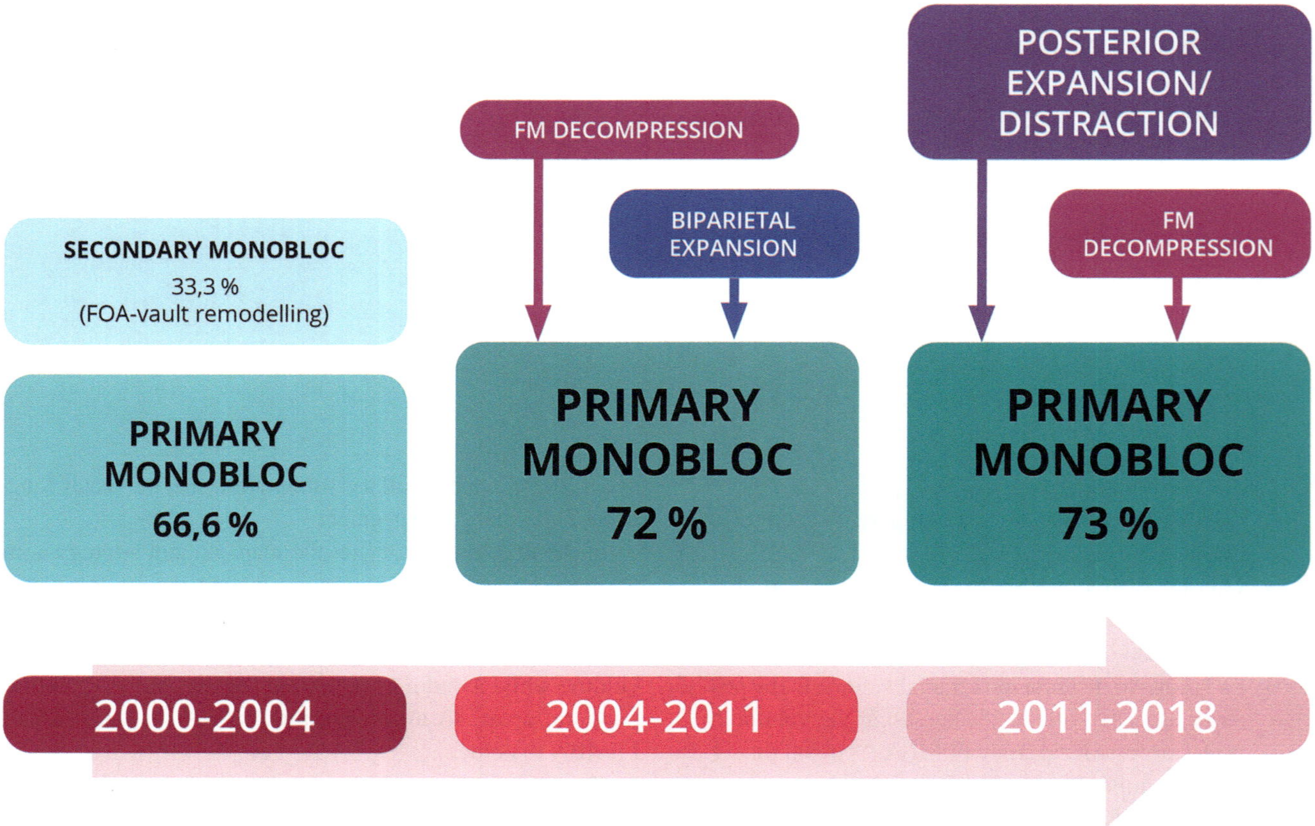

Fig. 2.1 Modifications of the early management of faciocraniosynostoses since 2000 at Necker-Enfants Malades

Between 2004 and 2011, given the morbidity of FFMBA in secondary cases, the intervention was reserved for primary cases without previous fronto-orbital interventions and whose intact pericranium could be pedicled anteriorly to seal the anterior cranial fossa from the underlying sinuses and nasal cavities.

During that period, biparietal expansion was considered the first-line intervention before FFMBA when urgent intracranial decompression was indicated. Foramen magnum decompression could also be indicated before FFMBA in the case of cerebellar tonsillar herniation.

As of 2011, we finally adopted our current protocol consisting of beginning with PVE with—whenever possible—internal distractors. Compared to biparietal expansion, PVE offers many advantages. It provides better morphological improvement of the brachycephaly as it directly corrects the anteroposterior shortening of the cranium. It is capable of more cranial expansion, especially when distraction osteogenesis can be performed. It directly augments posterior fossa volume with adequate cerebellar decompression and radiological improvement of cerebellar tonsillar hernia on the MRI. It also allows more posterior temporal osteotomy lines which clears the path for the upcoming FFMBA osteotomies several years later. When needed, it facilitates simultaneous foramen magnum decompression thanks to prone intraoperative positioning (Fig. 2.2).

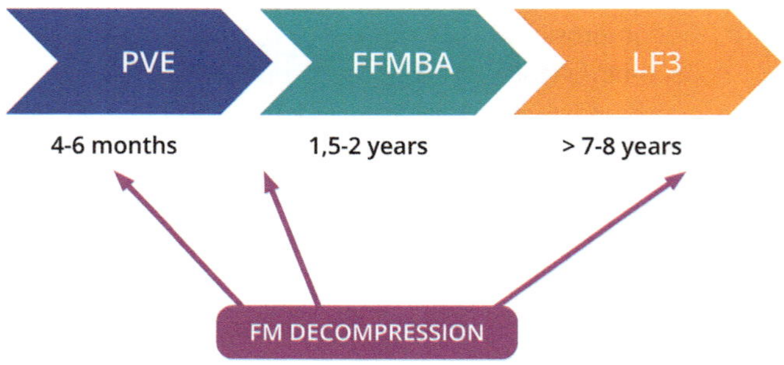

Fig. 2.2 Classical strategy for the management of faciocraniosynostosis. Foramen magnum decompression can be performed at any stage when necessary. *PVE* posterior vault distraction; *FFMBA* fronto-facial monobloc advancement; *LF3* Le Fort 3 osteotomy

Early PVE in the management sequence may be more important than mere intracranial volume optimization. Long-term follow-up has detected isolated cases of syringomyelia in young adults with FCST who had undergone the historical sequence without PVE (FFMBA followed by LF3) suggesting obstruction to CSF flow in the posterior fossa. The development of distraction techniques has lowered the morbidity of the tongue and groove PVE (Fig. 2.3) initially proposed by the Birmingham team in the 1980s. More precisely, PVE without distraction and with tongue and groove osteosynthesis carries increased morbidity linked to the complete undermining of the occipital pole and the risk of venous sinus injuries. Bone resorption is another risk due to devascularization. Distraction does not require bone undermining and hence avoids those risks. For more than a decade now, PVE with distraction has become the standard of care for first-line brain decompression of FCST in the craniofacial unit of Necker–Enfants Malades.

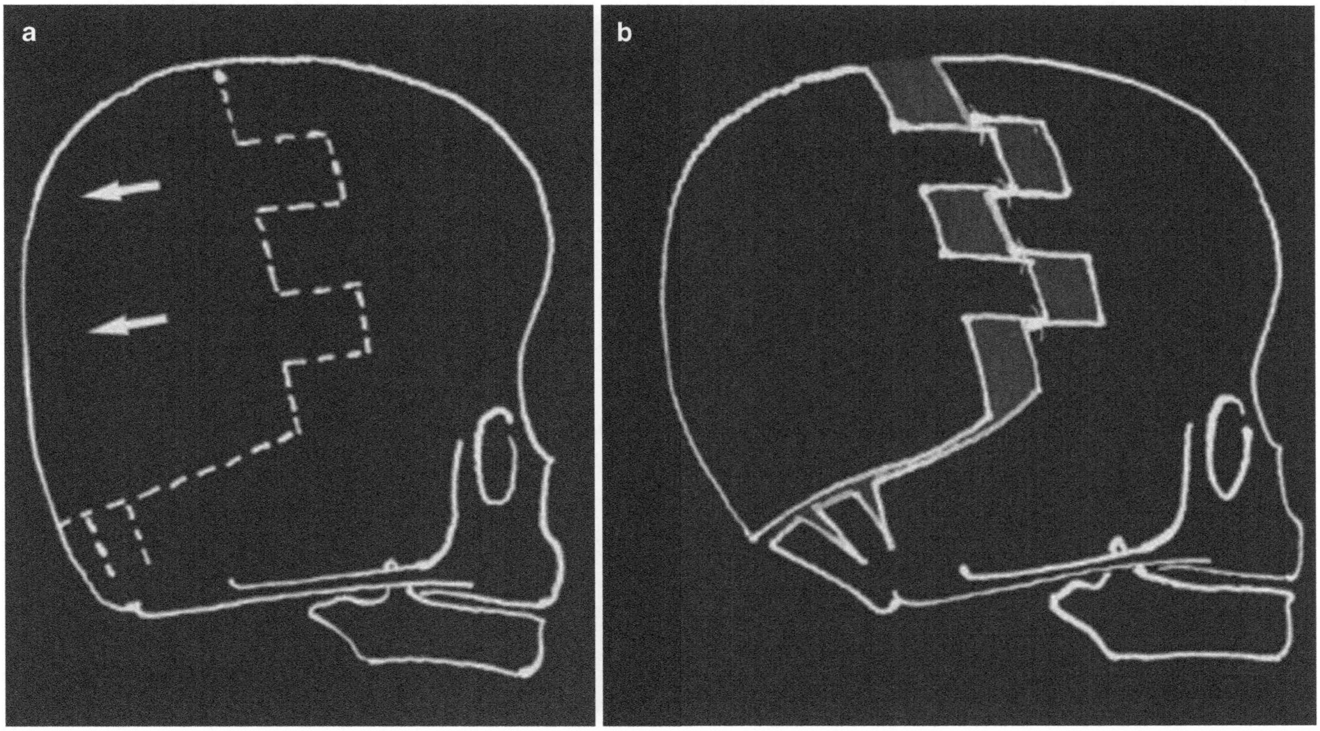

Fig. 2.3 (**a**, **b**) Schematic design of the conventional tongue and groove design of posterior expansion, allowing simple osteosynthesis but subjected to the risks of venous injuries and bone resorption secondary to devascularization. This technique is not applied anymore. (**c**) Conventional posterior expansion without distractions requires complete undermining. (**d**) Design of posterior calvarial cuts with 3 × 3 cm tongues & grooves. (**e**) Complete separation and elevation of the bony flap, which may be reinforced by absorbable osteosynthesis plates (ultrasonic welding type). (**f**) Advancement is maintained with simple wires and reinforced with absorbable osteosynthesis. (**g**) Brachycephalic aspect before posterior expansion. (**h**) Normalization of the preexisting skull deformation. Again, this technique is not applied anymore

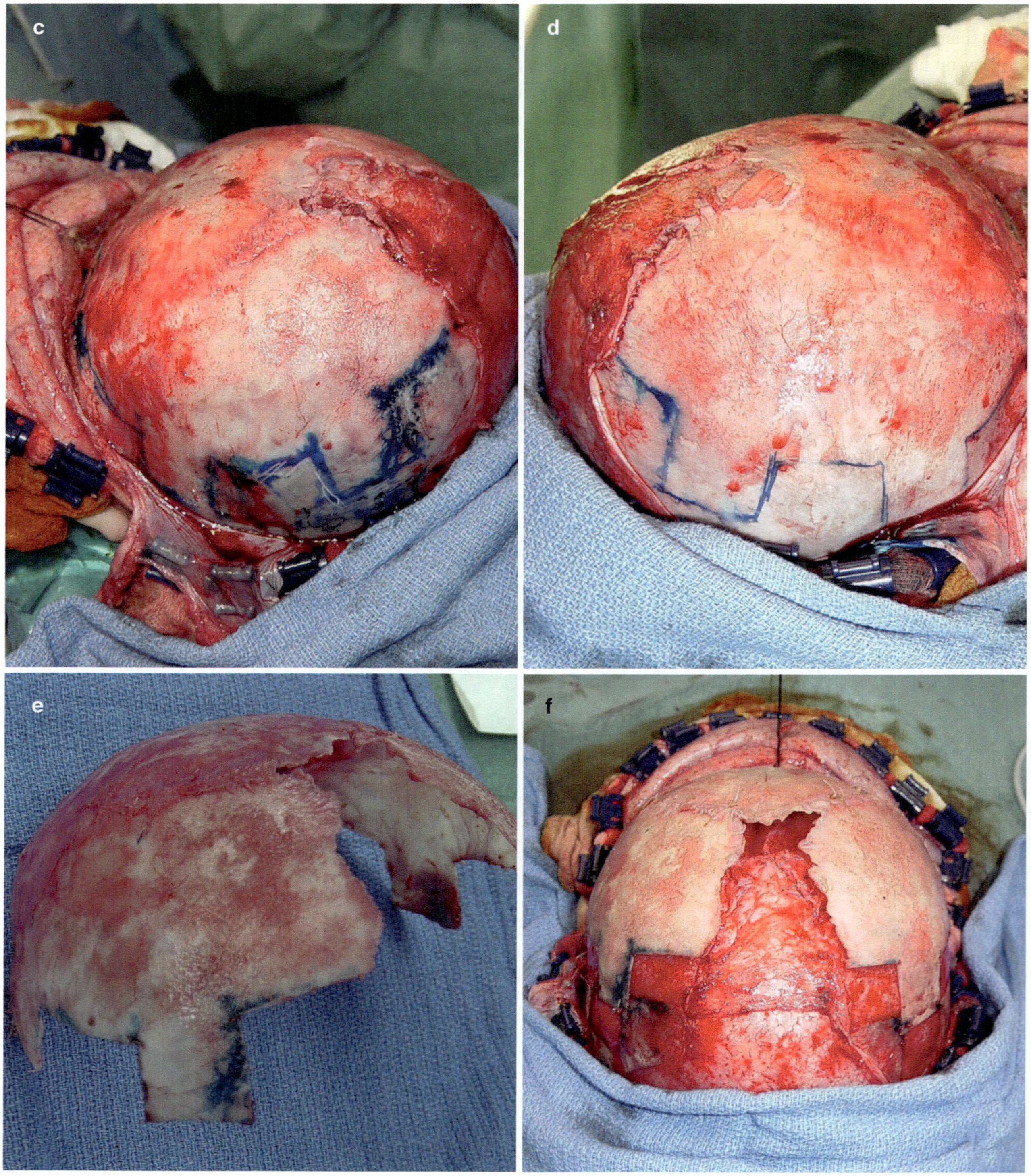

Fig. 2.3 (continued)

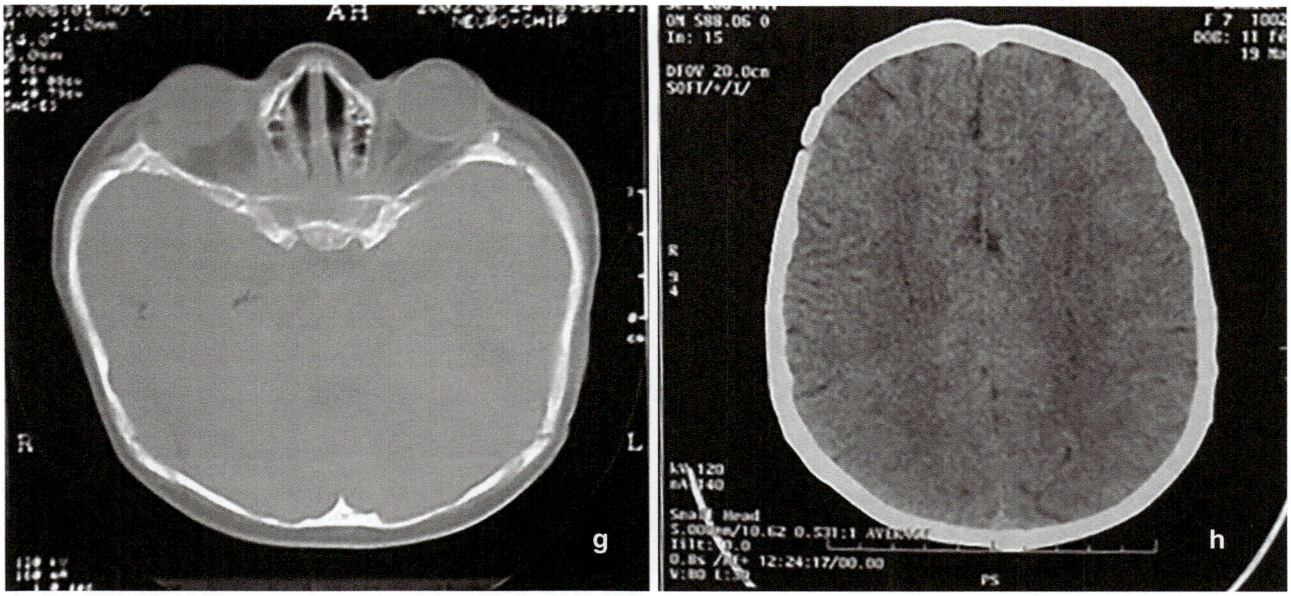

Fig. 2.3 (continued)

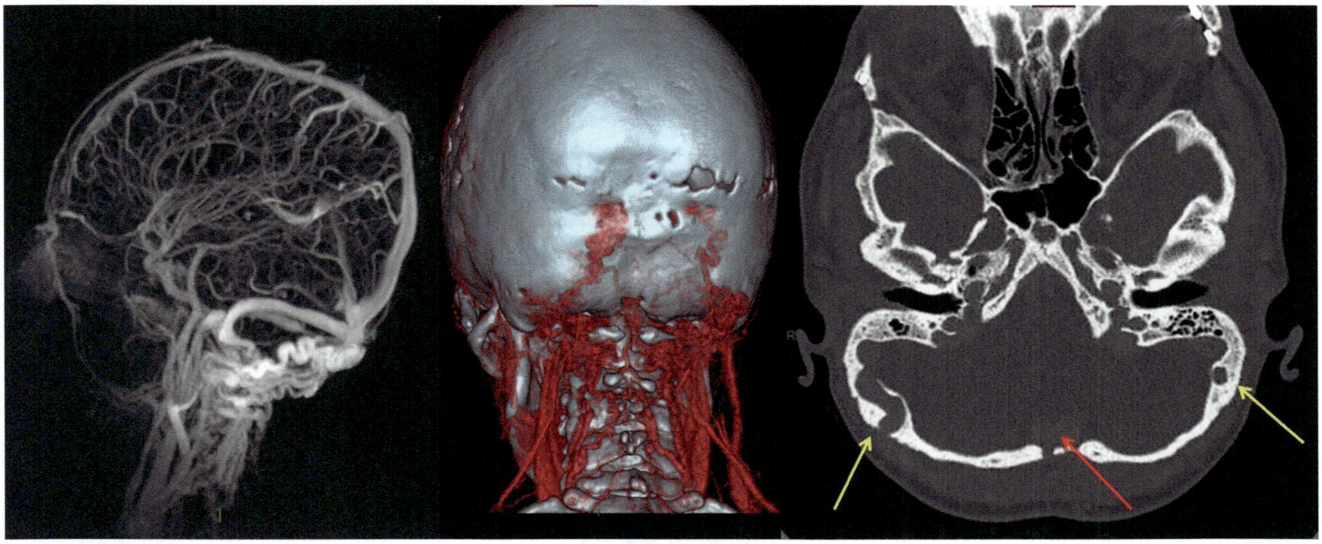

Fig. 2.4 Magnetic Resonance Venogram is fundamental preoperatively to evaluate venous drainage

2.2 Technical Tips for PVE with Distraction

For best results, the osteotomy around the posterior pole is carried out as inferiorly as possible. The occipital insertions of the posterior neck muscles can be partially detached or carefully interrupted at the desired location of the lower horizontal osteotomy line. Abnormally large collateral veins are frequently encountered at this location—a stigma of abnormal intracranial venous outflow (Fig. 2.4). These veins are preferably preserved if possible. The lower horizontal osteotomy carries the most risk during the procedure as the sigmoid sinuses are usually detected underneath.

This lower osteotomy line is preferably performed centripetally using a 3 to 4-mm Kerrison rongeur or a Boehler rongeur. The internal occipital crest is then exposed, intercalated through the dura mater between the cerebellar hemispheres. It is crucial to completely interrupt this crest while avoiding any dural lacerations. An incomplete osteotomy at this location impedes the posterior translocation of the bony flap and hampers intracranial expansion.

Three expansion approaches in PVE may be undertaken.

1. Spring-assisted expansion (Fig. 2.5).
2. Internal distractors (Fig. 2.6).
3. Brain-mediated expansion (without or with low-flow shunt) (Fig. 2.7).

In severe cases where brain constriction causes extremely thin and perforated bone that precludes the use of internal distractors, PVE craniotomies are performed to release the constriction and the intracranial pressure is harnessed to drive cranial expansion posteriorly.

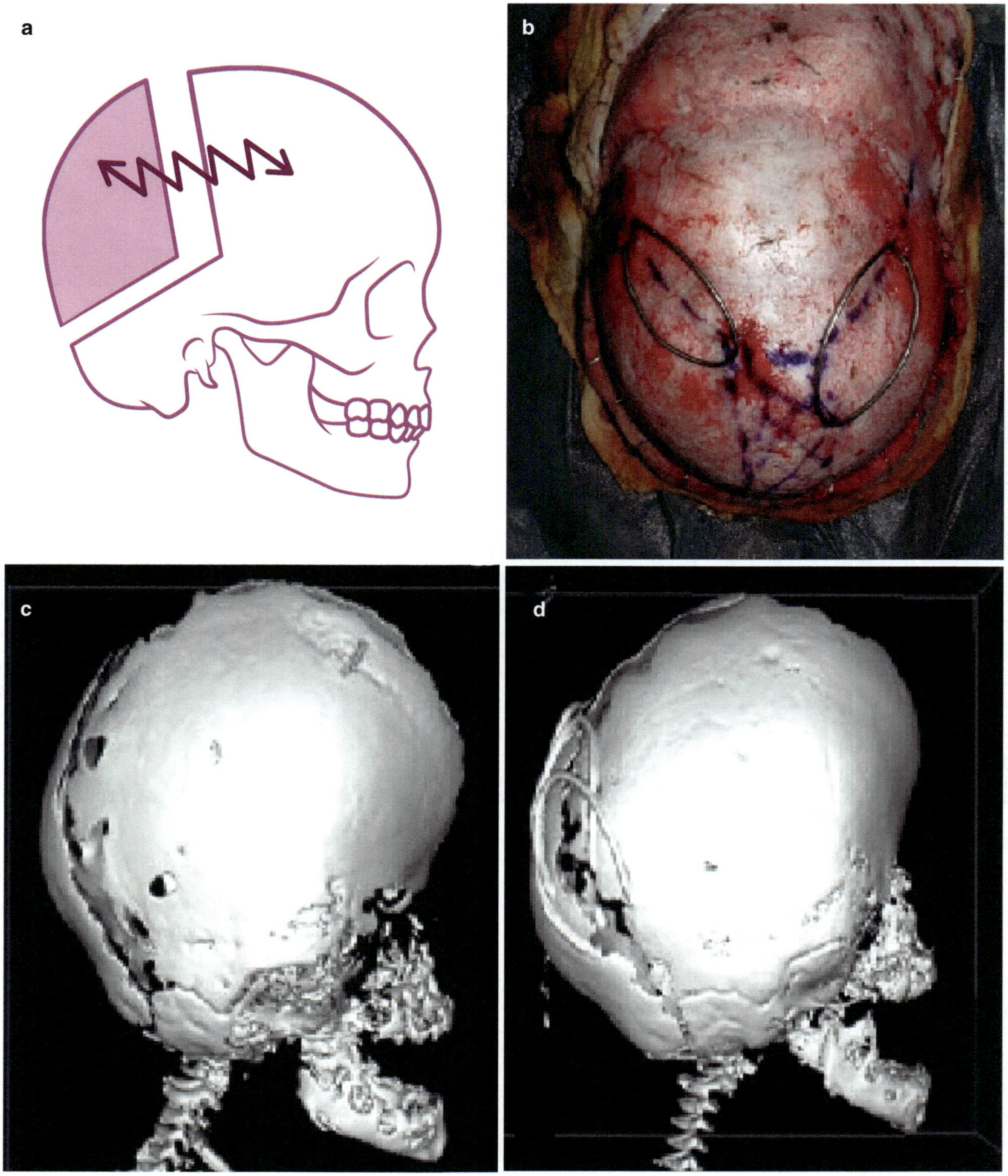

Fig. 2.5 Spring-assisted posterior vault expansion. (**a**) Diagram representing spring-assisted trans-lambdoid expansion. (**b**) Intraoperative view with two springs inserted across lambdoid sutures. (**c**) Preoperative CTscan. (**d**) Postoperative CT scan. © Cassandra Vion

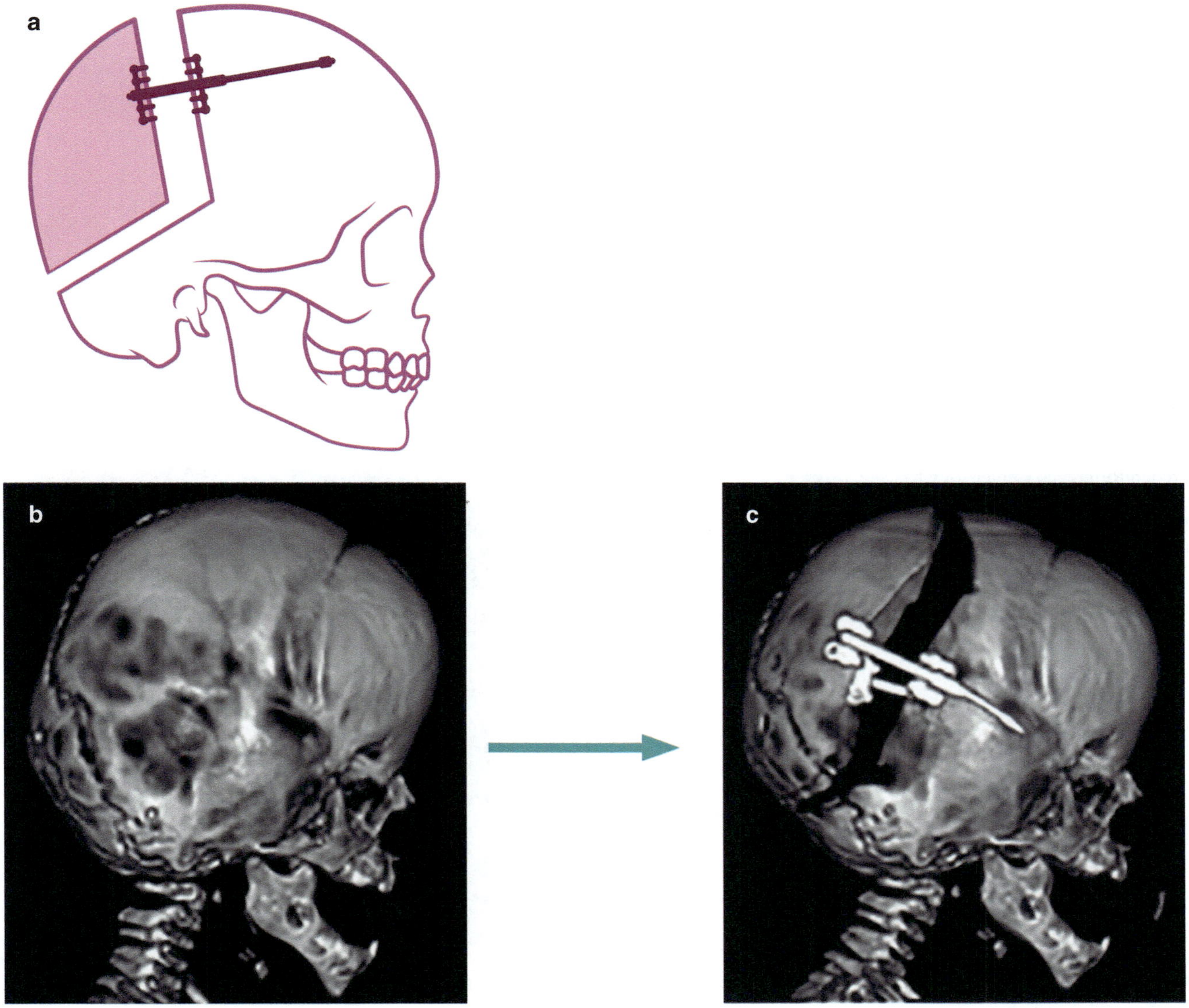

Fig. 2.6 Posterior vault distraction using internal distractors. This technique is currently the standard of care at our institution. (**a**) Diagram representing PVE with internal distractors. (**b**) Before PVE with distractors. (**c**) After PVE with distractors. © Cassandra Vion

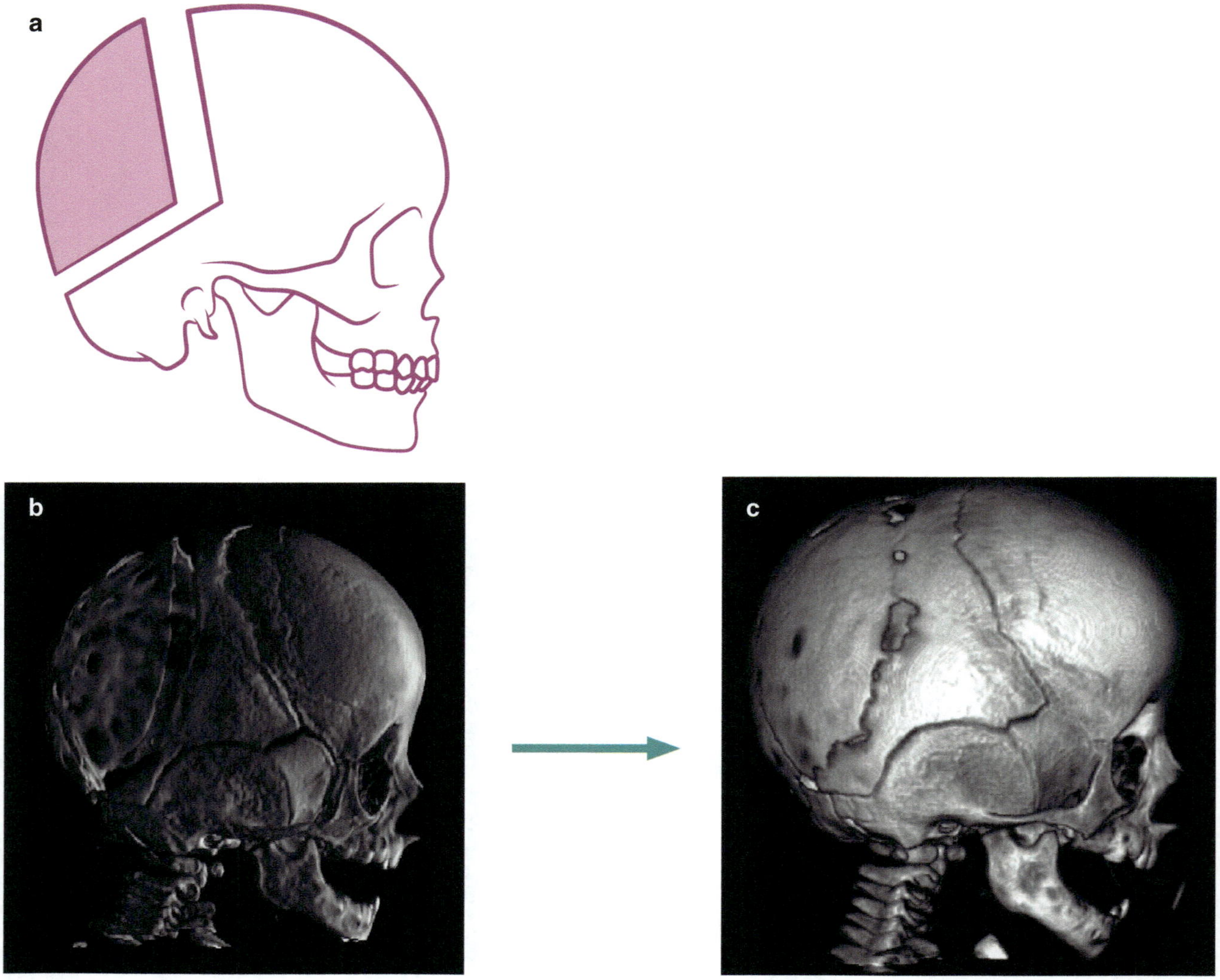

Fig. 2.7 Brain mediated posterior vault expansion. (**a**) Diagram representing brain mediated expansion. (**b**) Right after occipital craniotomy. (**c**) After occipital craniotomy. © Cassandra Vion

2.3 Spring-Assisted Expansion (Figs. 2.5, 2.8, 2.9, 2.10, 2.11, and 2.12)

This technique is less used at our institution for PVE. The main limitation of springs is that they deliver their maximum power at the beginning of the expansion when little force is needed to separate the bone segments. Their power inevitably wears out as the bone segments move away from each other and the elastic soft tissue forces grow stronger [1–4] (Fig. 2.8). Spring-assisted expansion initially stemmed from an orthodontic principle of applying forces across an open suture. Morbidity is minimal but the effect is limited. When applied across the lambdoid sutures, the FM diameter does not seem to improve. We have only exceptionally applied springs to distract a craniotomy site, when a preexisting nearby shunt contraindicated the use of distractors because of the risk of bacterial contamination through the percutaneous activation arms.

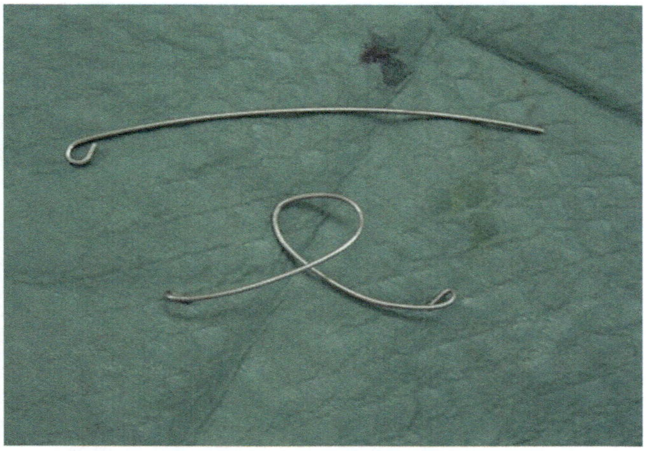

Fig. 2.8 The first springs proposed by the Göteborg team were simply made with a roll of high-quality stainless steel wire. Adding a loop reduced the strength between arms

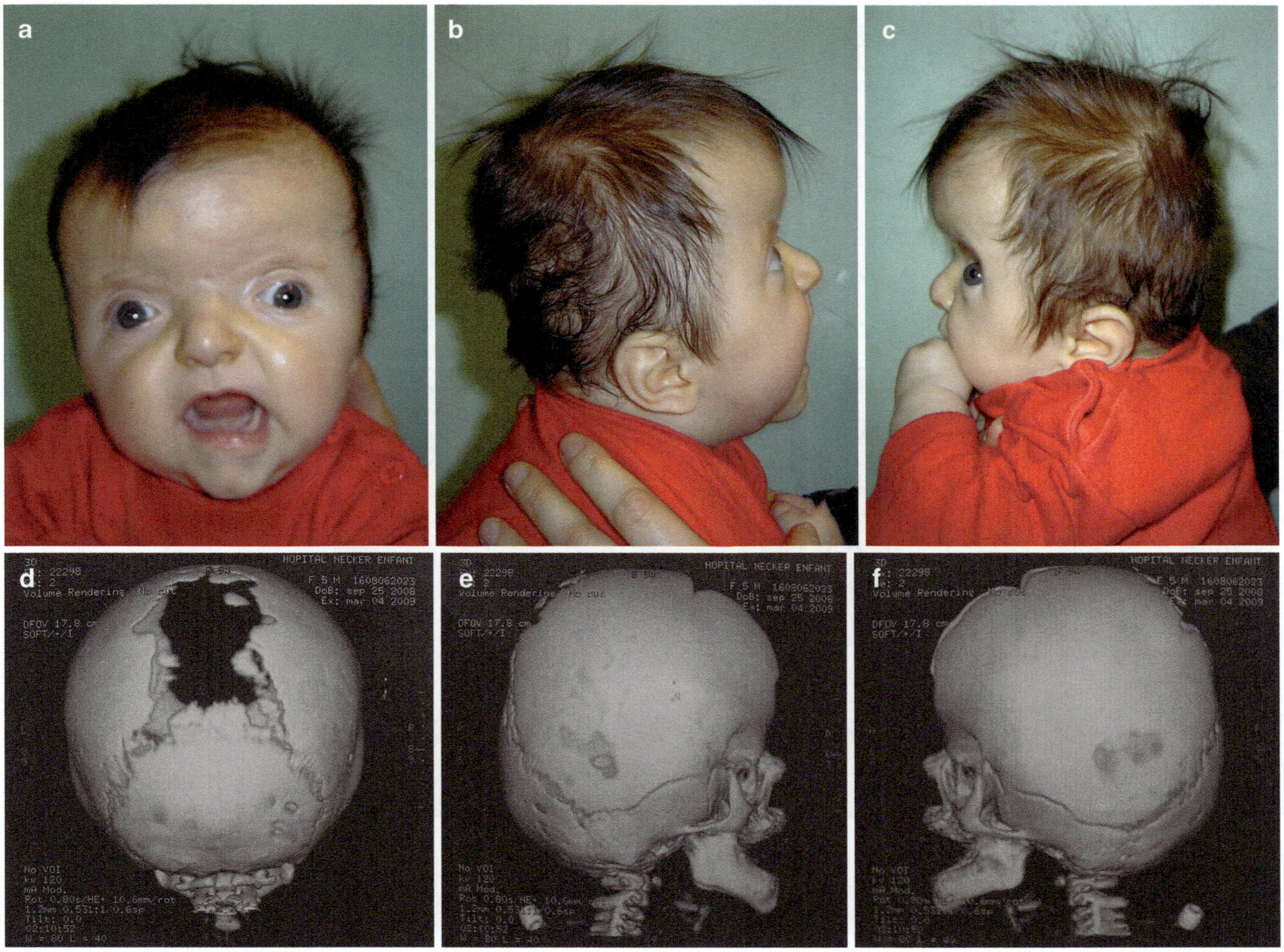

Fig. 2.9 (**a**, **b**, **c**) A young patient with Apert syndrome at 4 months of age (**d**, **e**, **f**). Intraoperative CT scans of a 4-month-old patient with Apert syndrome. Insertion of 2 springs across lambdoid sutures at 6 months of age in a patient with Apert syndrome. (**h**, **i**) Postoperative profile views 2 months after spring insertion. Lateral positioning was necessary. (**j**, **k**, **l**). Postoperative views at 18 months of age, 12 months after spring insertion. (**m**, **n**). Postoperative CT scans 7 months after spring removal at 18 months of age

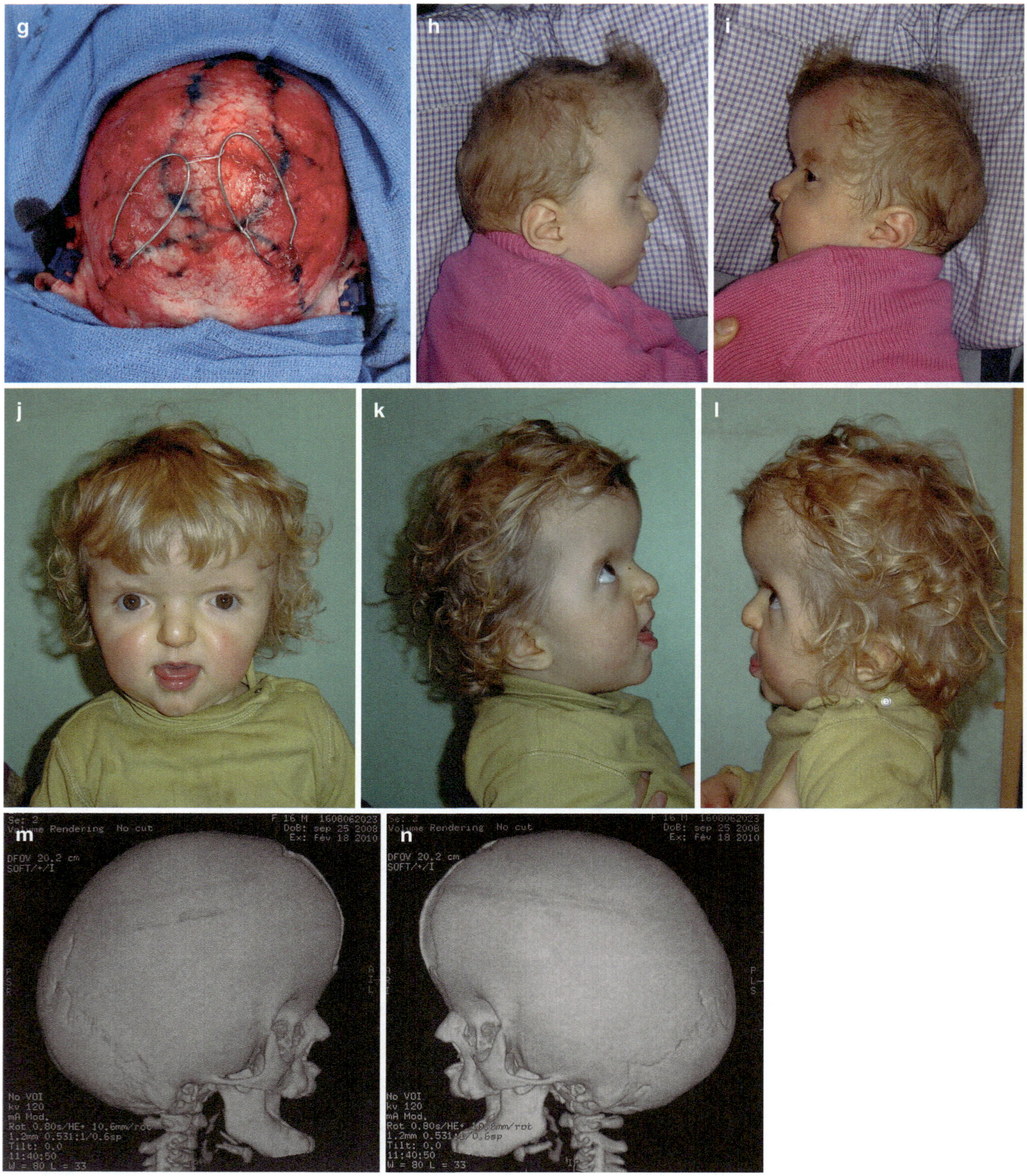

Fig. 2.9 (continued)

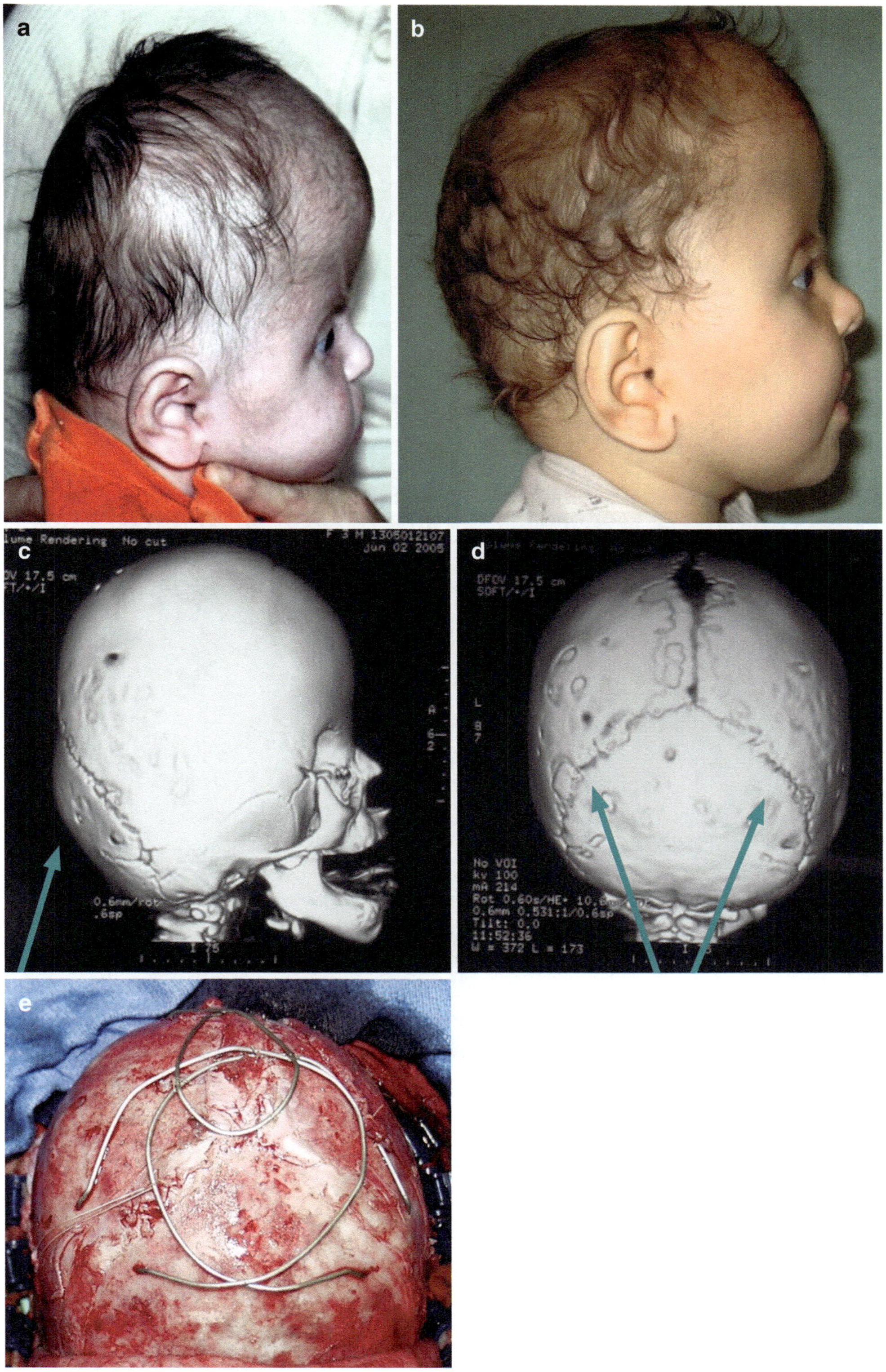

Fig. 2.10 (**a**, **b**) Clinical results of spring-mediated expansion at the lambdoid suture level in a child with Apert syndrome: (**a**) preoperative picture at 5 months of age showing turribrachycephaly, (**b**) one-year postoperative picture at 18 months of age demonstrating moderate improvement of posterior flattening. (**c**, **d**) Preoperative CT scans at 5 months of age showing bicoronal craniosynostosis and posterior skull flattening. The lambdoid sutures are normal. (**e**) Intraoperative picture at age 7 months. Two springs were used for expansion at the level of the lambdoid sutures, and one spring was used for transversal contraction at the level of the sagittal suture. (**f**, **g**) CT scans before and 12 months after initial distraction, lateral views, showing the correction of the posterior flatness. (**h**, **i**) CT scans before and 12 months after initial distraction, posterior views

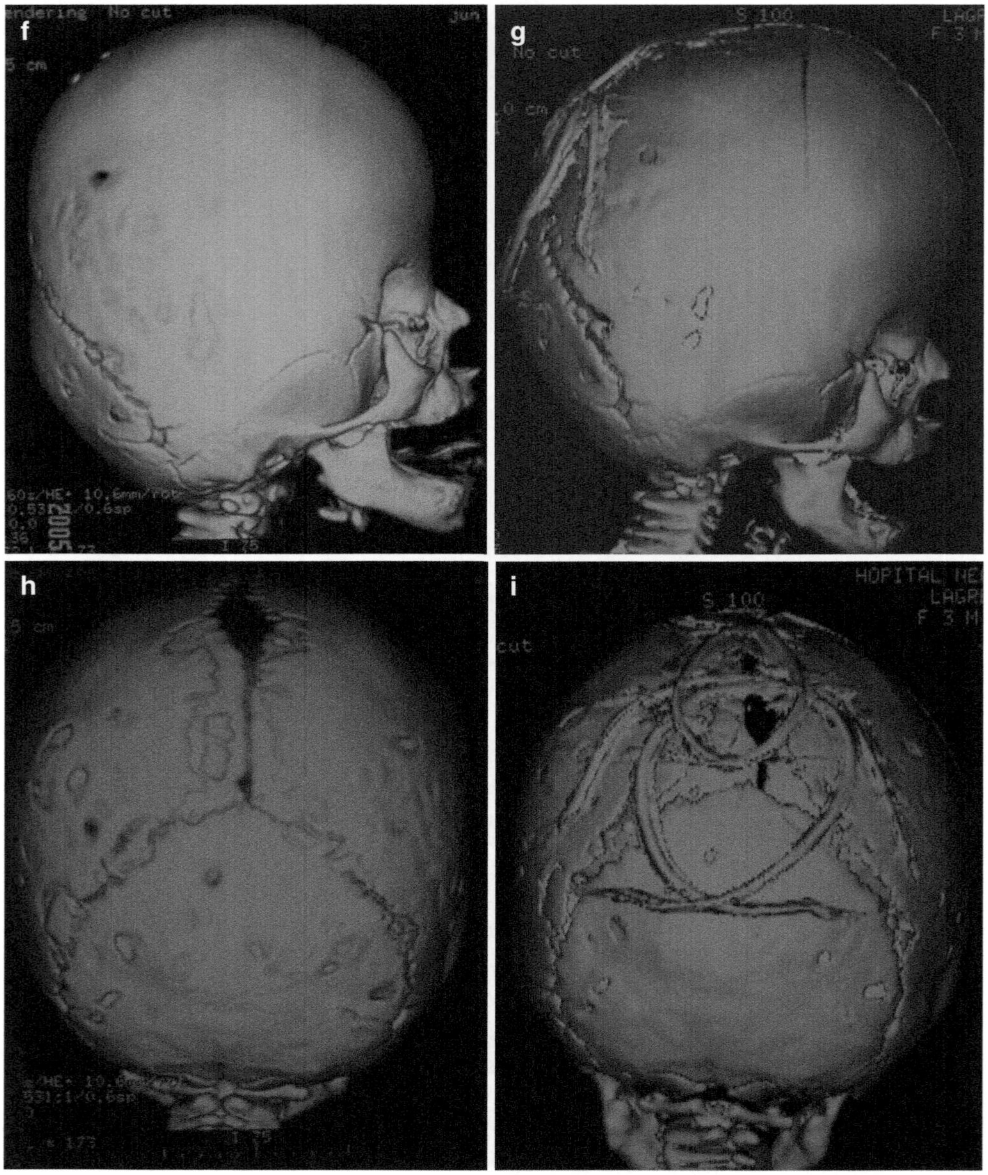

Fig. 2.10 (continued)

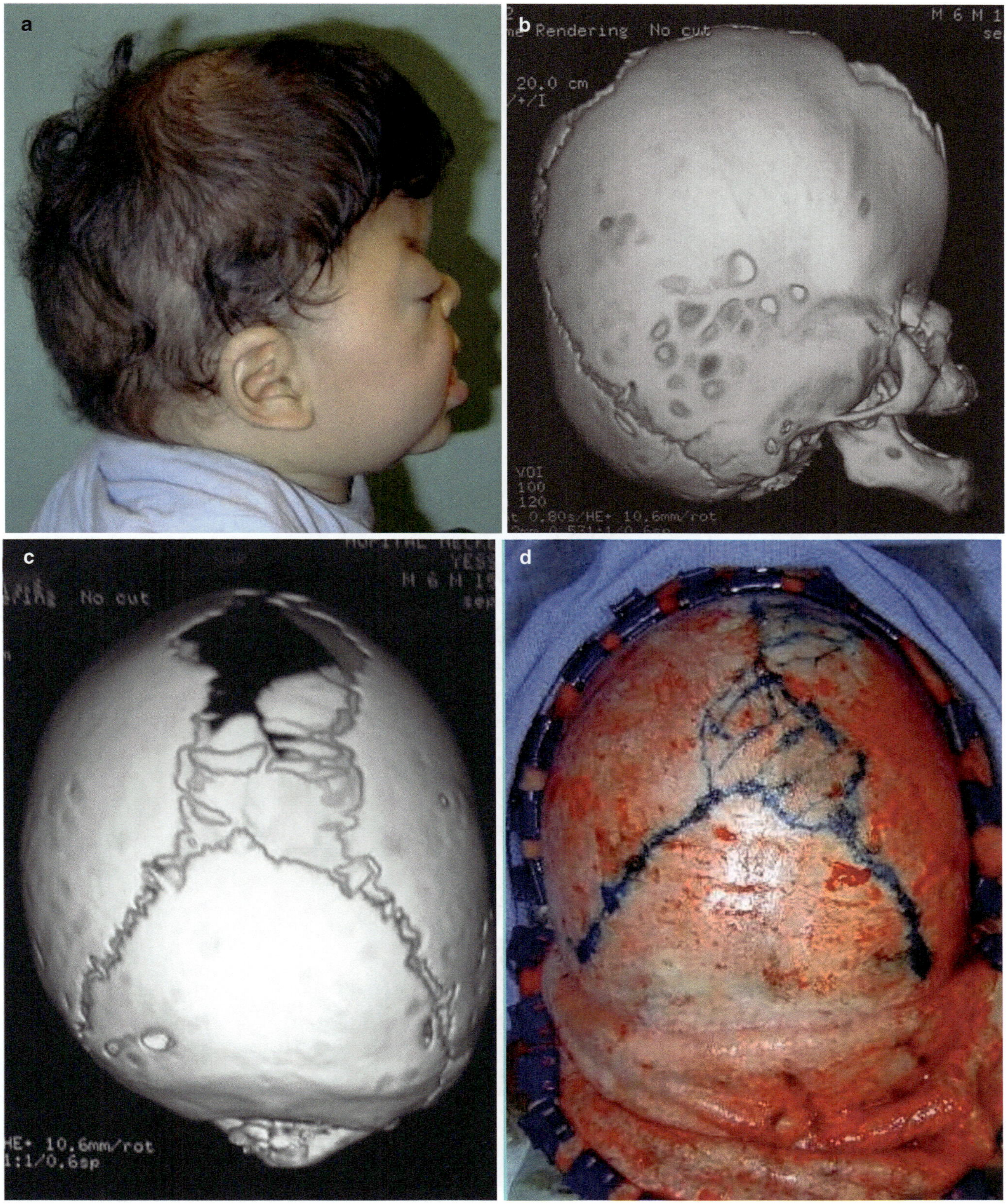

Fig. 2.11 (**a**, **b**) Severe turribrachycephaly in a 7-month patient with Apert syndrome and bicoronal craniosynostosis, with widely open sagittal and lambdoid sutures and posterior flattening. Posterior skull expansion with springs. (**c**, **d**) CT scan and intraoperative picture demonstrating a wide posterior fontanelle. (**e**) Insertion of 2 springs across lambdoid sutures at 8 months of age. (**f**, **g**) Effective posterior vault expansion was obtained in 10 weeks. (**h**, **i**) CT scan at age 18 months demonstrating adequate ossification. Despite satisfactory posterior vault expansion with springs, no improvement of the forehead shape was achieved between 7 and 18 months of age

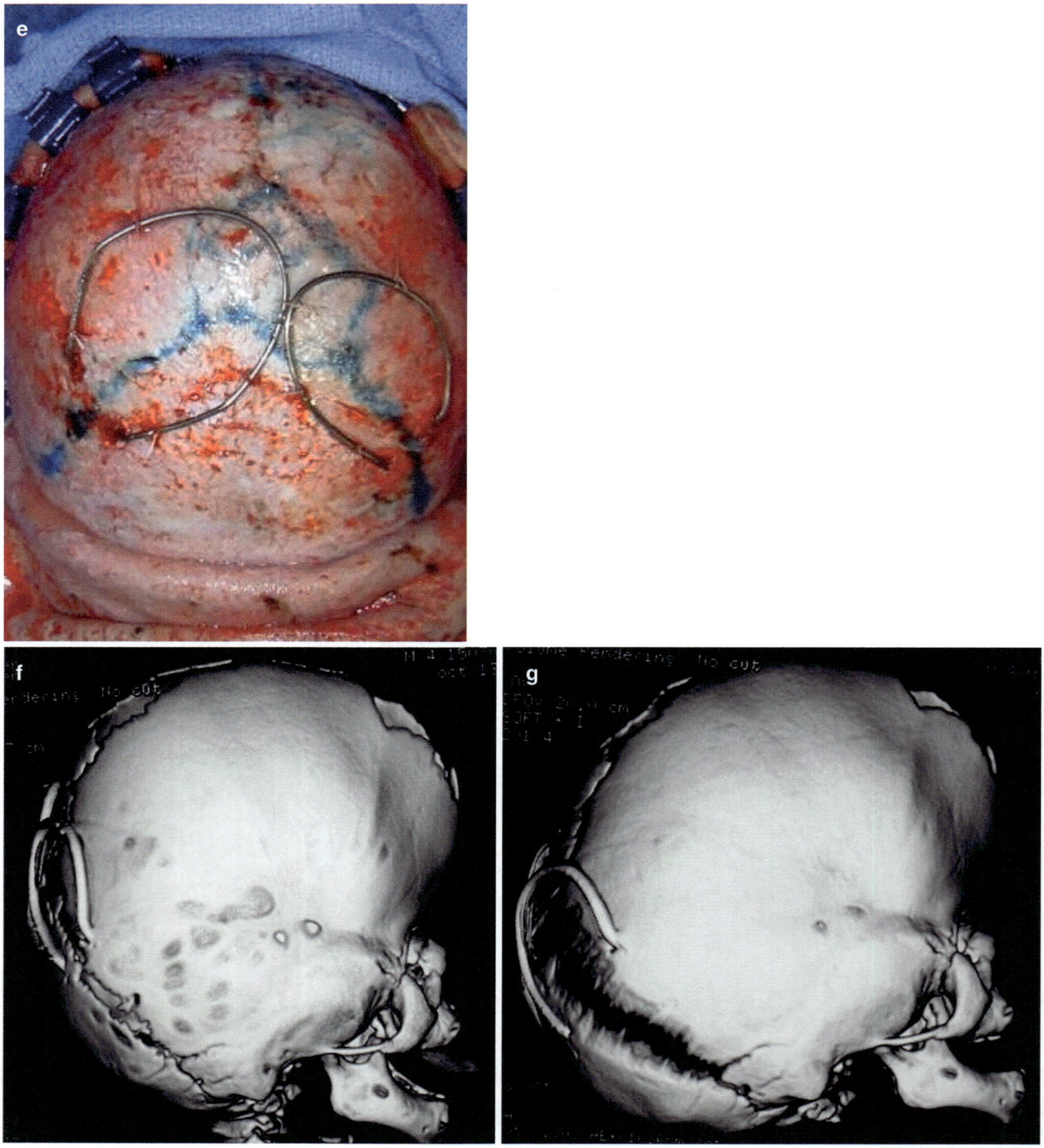

Fig. 2.11 (continued)

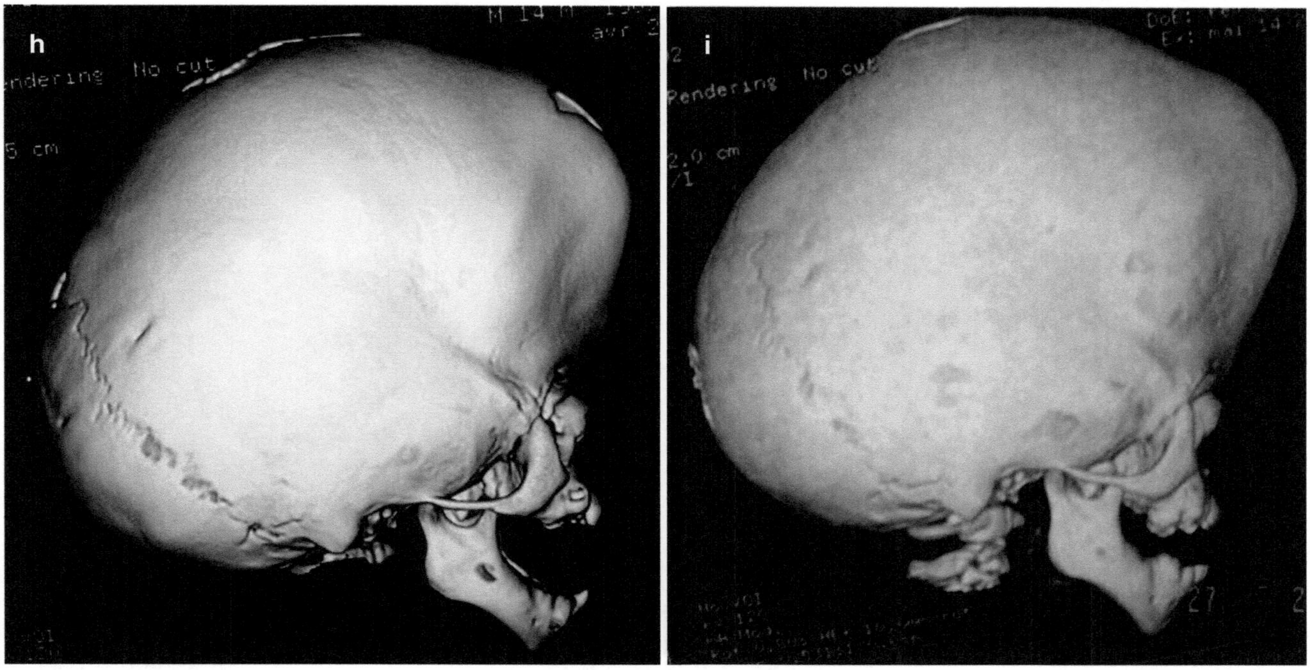

Fig. 2.11 (continued)

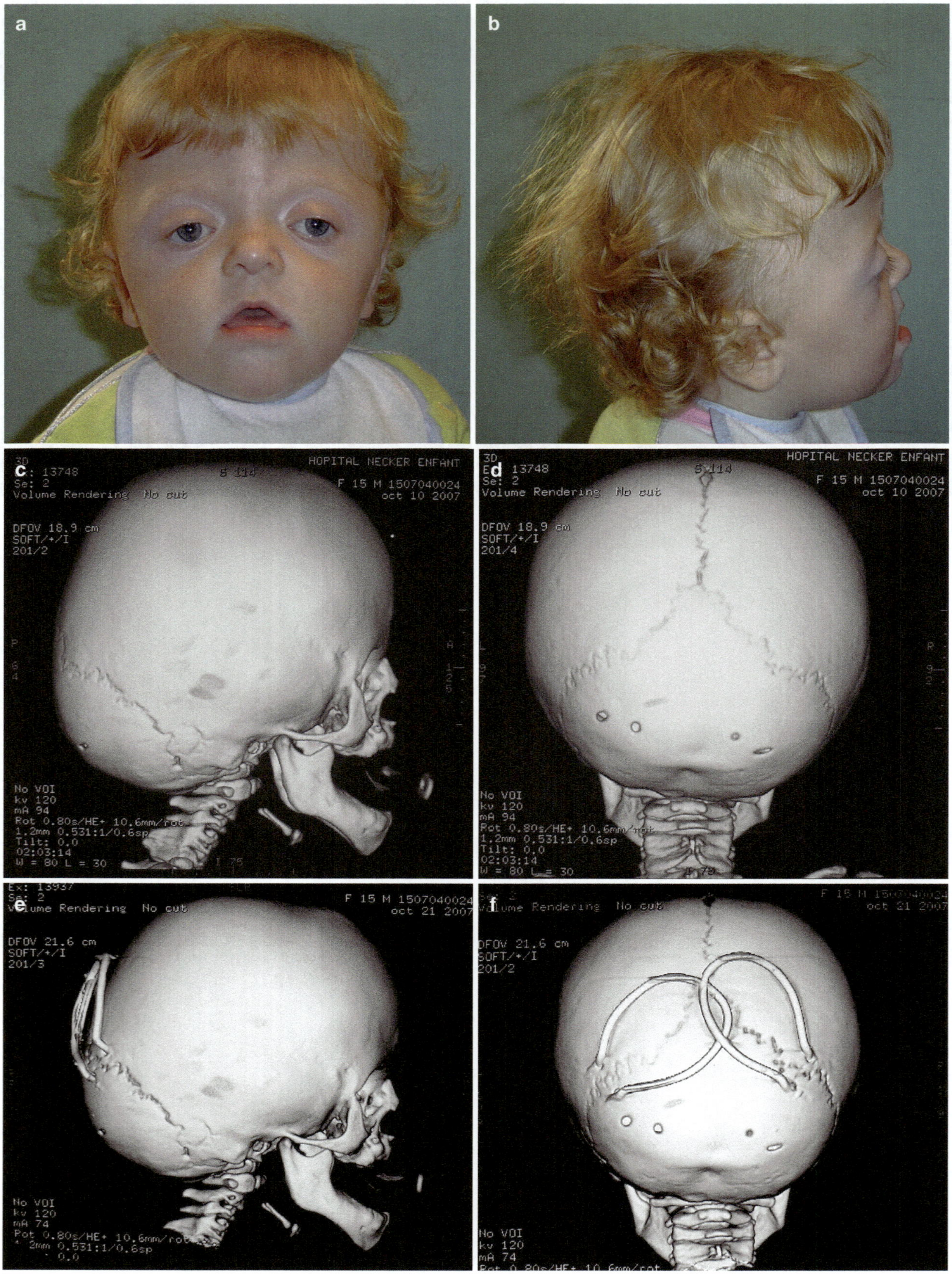

Fig. 2.12 (**a**, **b**) Patient with Apert syndrome at 7 months of age. (**c**, **d**) CT-scan of patient with Apert syndrome at 7 months of age. CT scans showing posterior flattening and open sagittal and lambdoid sutures. (**e**, **f**) Patient with Apert syndrome at 7 months of age immediately after spring insertion. (**g**) Patient with Apert syndrome at 10 months of age, 3 months after spring insertion—lateral clinical view. (**h**, **i**) Patient with Apert syndrome at 10 months of age, 3 months after spring insertion—CT scan controls. (**j**, **k**) Patient with Apert syndrome at 12 months of age, 5 months after trans-lambdoid spring insertion—CT scan controls

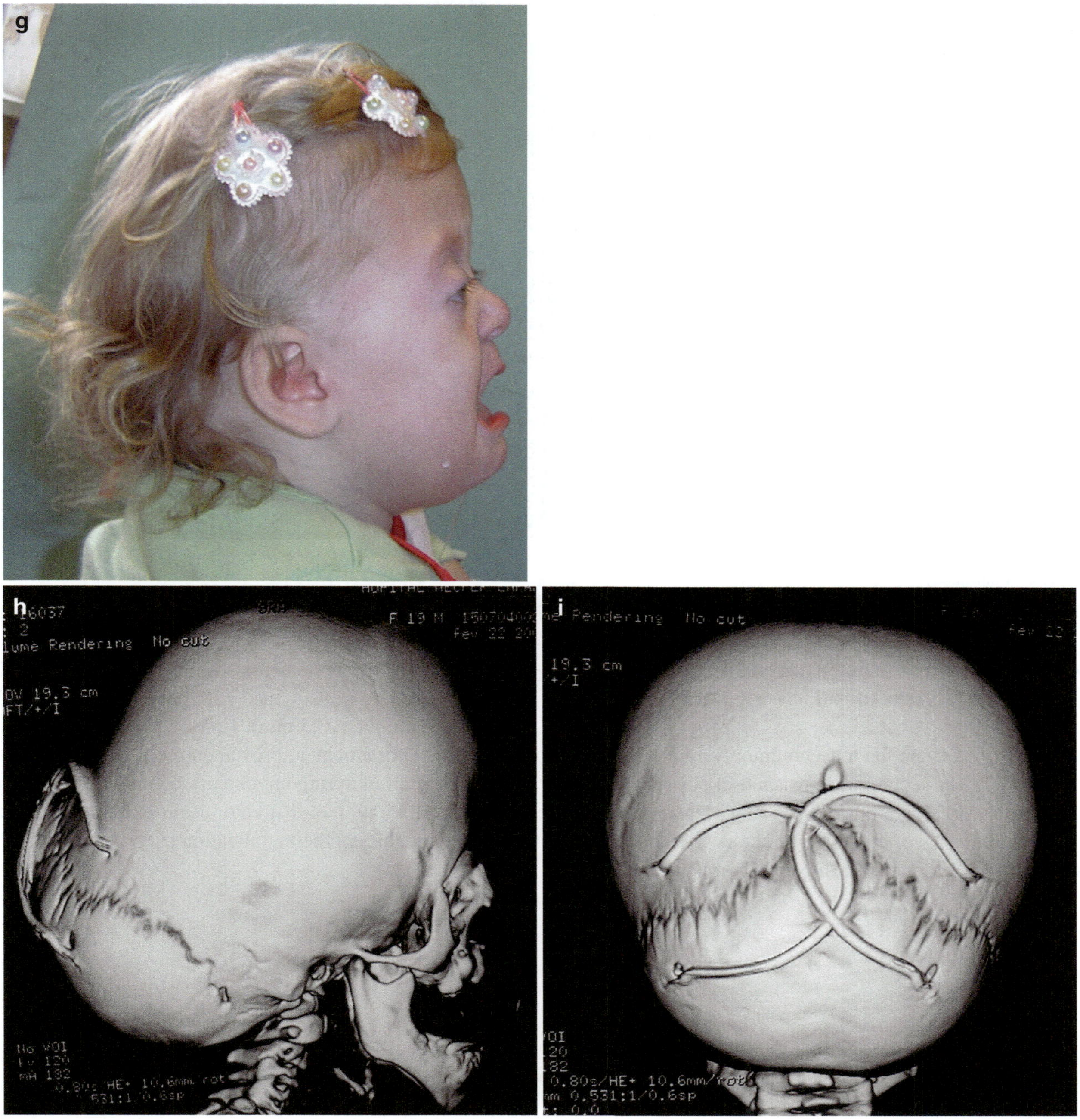

Fig. 2.12 (continued)

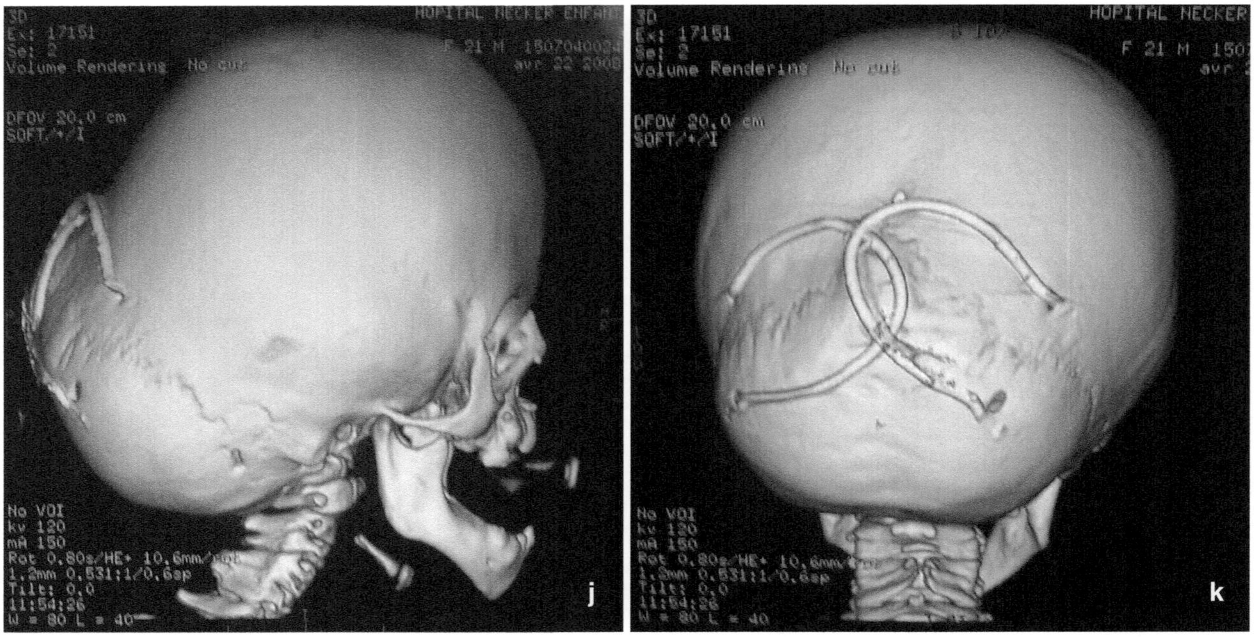

Fig. 2.12 (continued)

2.4 Posterior Vault Expansion with Distractors (Figs. 2.13 and 2.14)

Internal distractors are the most commonly applied hardware to drive PVE. The technique consists of a posterior craniotomy around an occipital bony flap, going as low as the torcular if possible. Two cranial distractors (Arnaud cranial distractors, KLS Martin, Tuttlingen, Germany) are screwed or welded into the bone across the craniotomy (Fig. 2.13). The distraction is carried out 1 mm per day until the end of the distractor course (25 mm). Consolidation time is around 3 months. Subsequent improvement of tonsillar herniation and prevention of syringomyelia are common MRI findings [5–8]. The limitation of distractor use is extremely thin parietal bone precluding their application (Fig. 2.14).

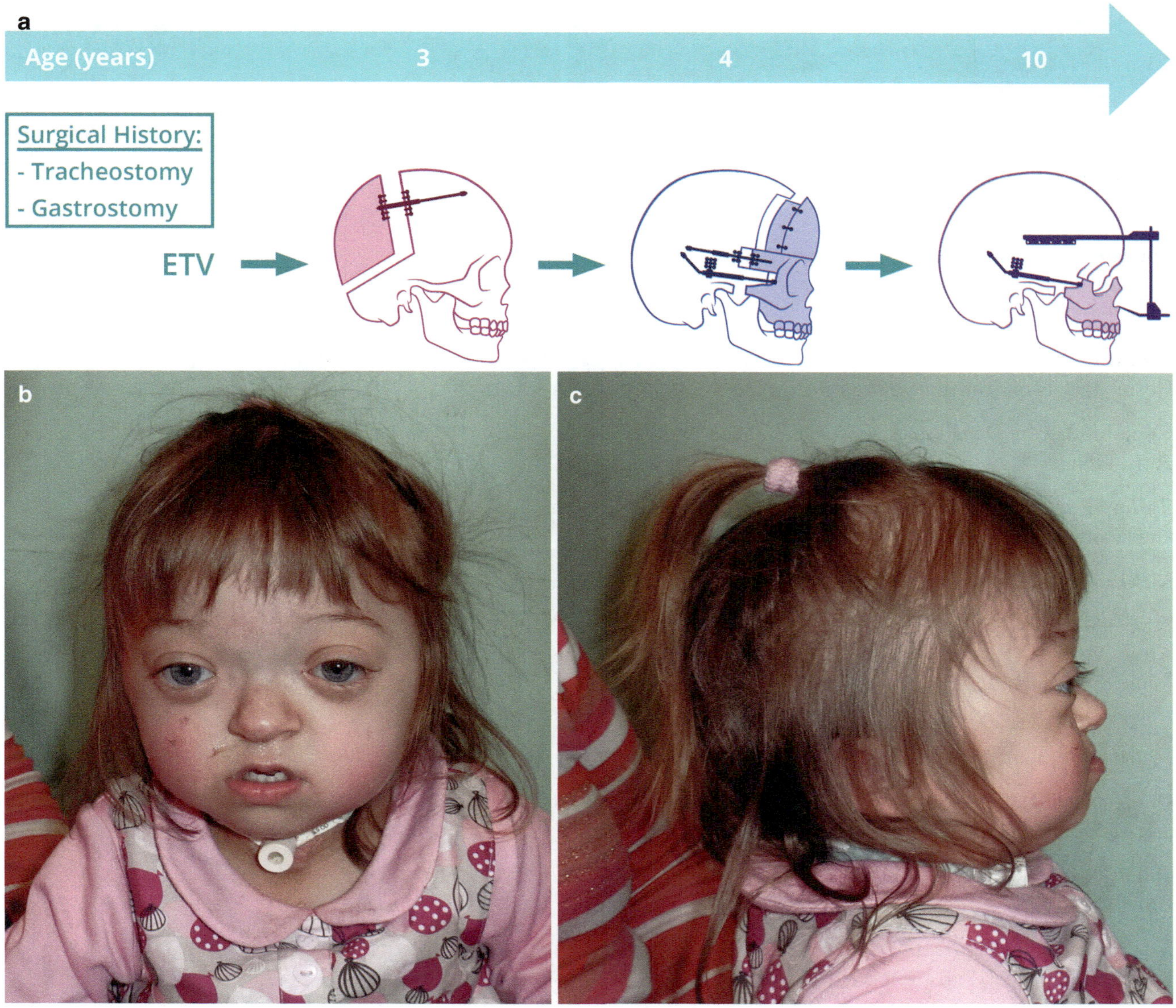

Fig. 2.13 (**a**, **b**, **c**) Two-year-old patient with Crouzon and Acanthosis Nigricans syndrome (FGFR3 mutation) presenting with tracheostomy and gastrostomy. Obstructive hydrocephalus and tonsillar herniation were detected on MRI along with cervical syringomyelia. ETV was performed at age 27 months with successful resumption of CSF circulation through the floor of the third ventricle. However, tonsillar herniation remained unresolved and was due to crowding of the posterior fossa. PVE was performed at age 32 months using internal distractors. The consolidation period lasted 4 months. © Cassandra Vion. (**d**, **e**) T2-weighted MRI at age 27 months showing cerebellar tonsillar herniation with hydrocephalus and cervical syringomyelia. (**f**) After ETV: presence of CSF flow at the floor of the third ventricle. Tonsillar herniation remains unchanged. (**g**) After PVE with distraction: resolution of cerebellar tonsillar hernia. (**h**, **i**). CT scans at age 36 months before and after distractor removal. Resolution of posterior fossa crowding. (**j**, **k**) Clinical photographs at age 42 months showing midface hypoplasia, class III malocclusion, and exorbitism. Polysomnography with a capped tracheostomy cannula showed OSA (AHI = 13 per hour). Tonsillectomy and adenoidectomy followed by FFMBA were indicated to attempt decannulation. (**l**) FFMBA performed at 45 months of age, 9 months after distractor removal for PVE, and 4 months after tonsillectomy and adenoidectomy. Distractors were removed after 3 months of consolidation. Polysomnography demonstrated the resolution of sleep apnea (AHI = 0 per hour). The patient was decannulated. She subsequently required a secondary Le Fort III facial advancement at age 10 years which successfully treated relapsing OSA

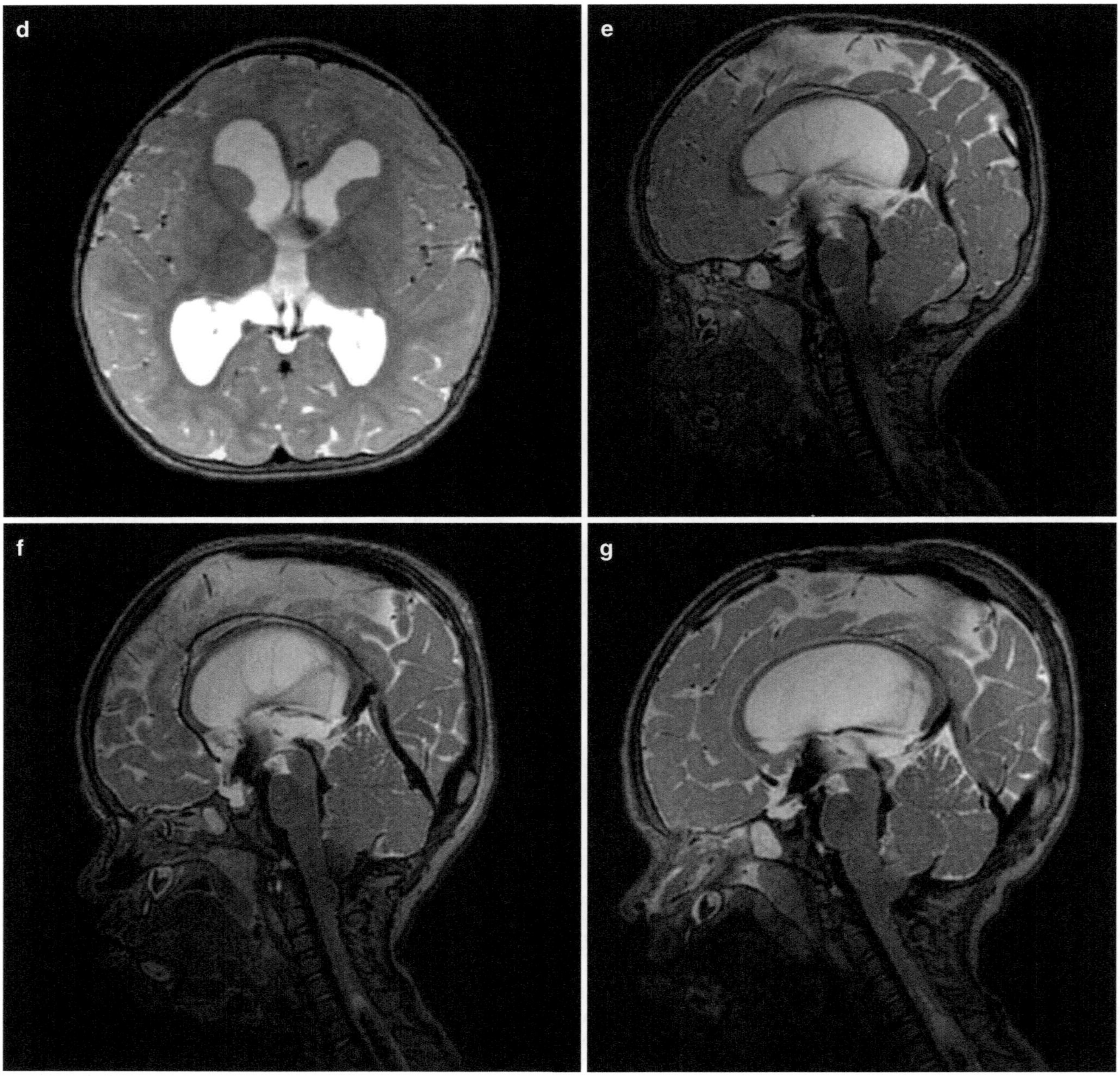

Fig. 2.13 (continued)

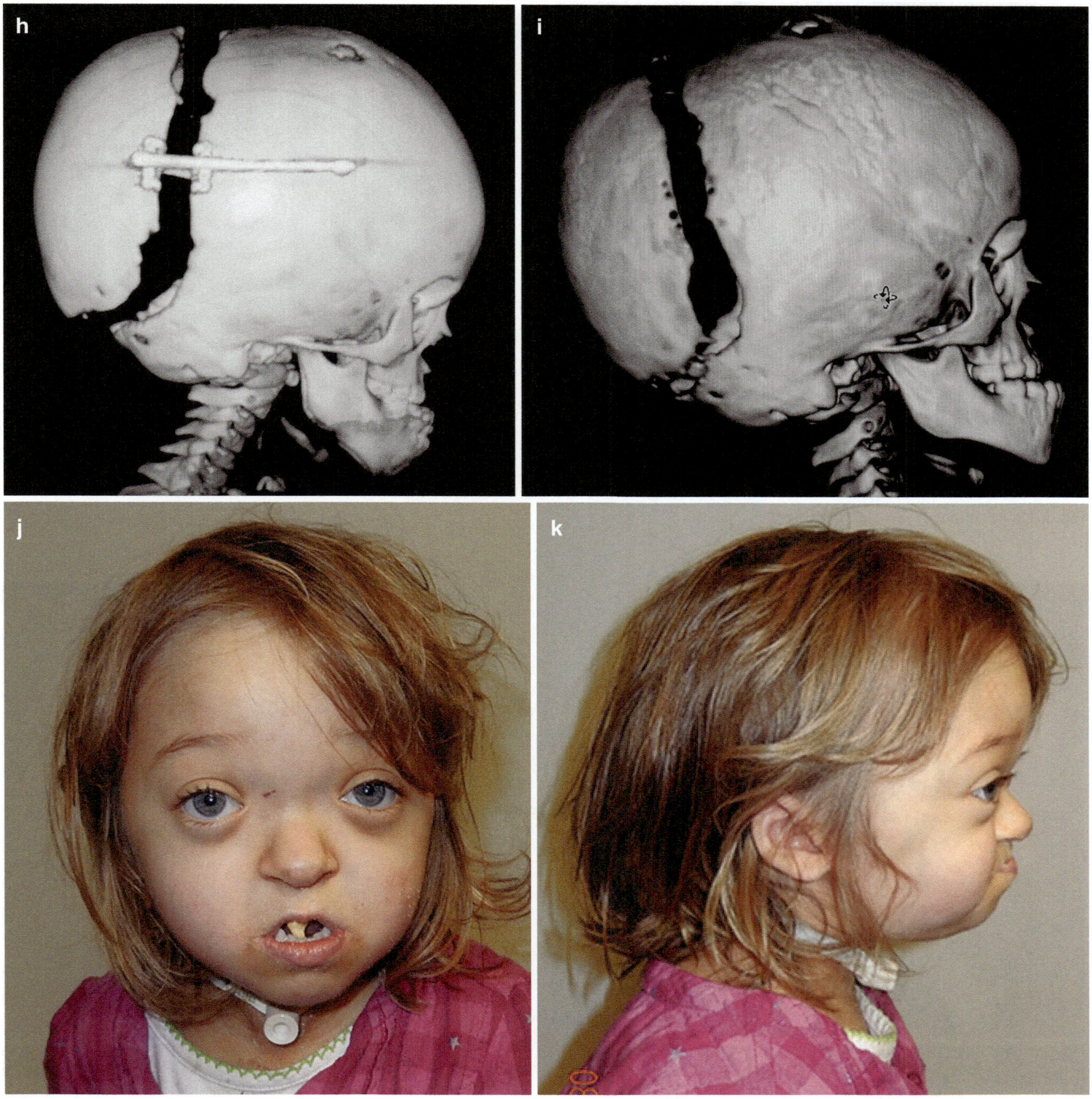

Fig. 2.13 (continued)

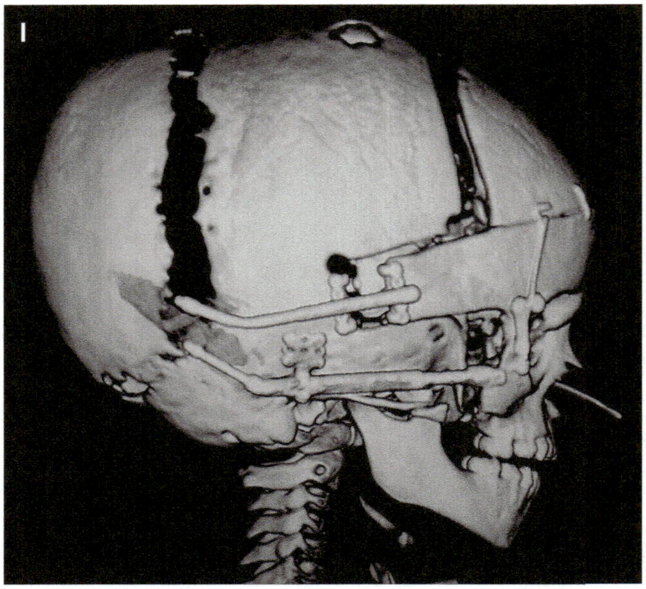

Fig. 2.13 (continued)

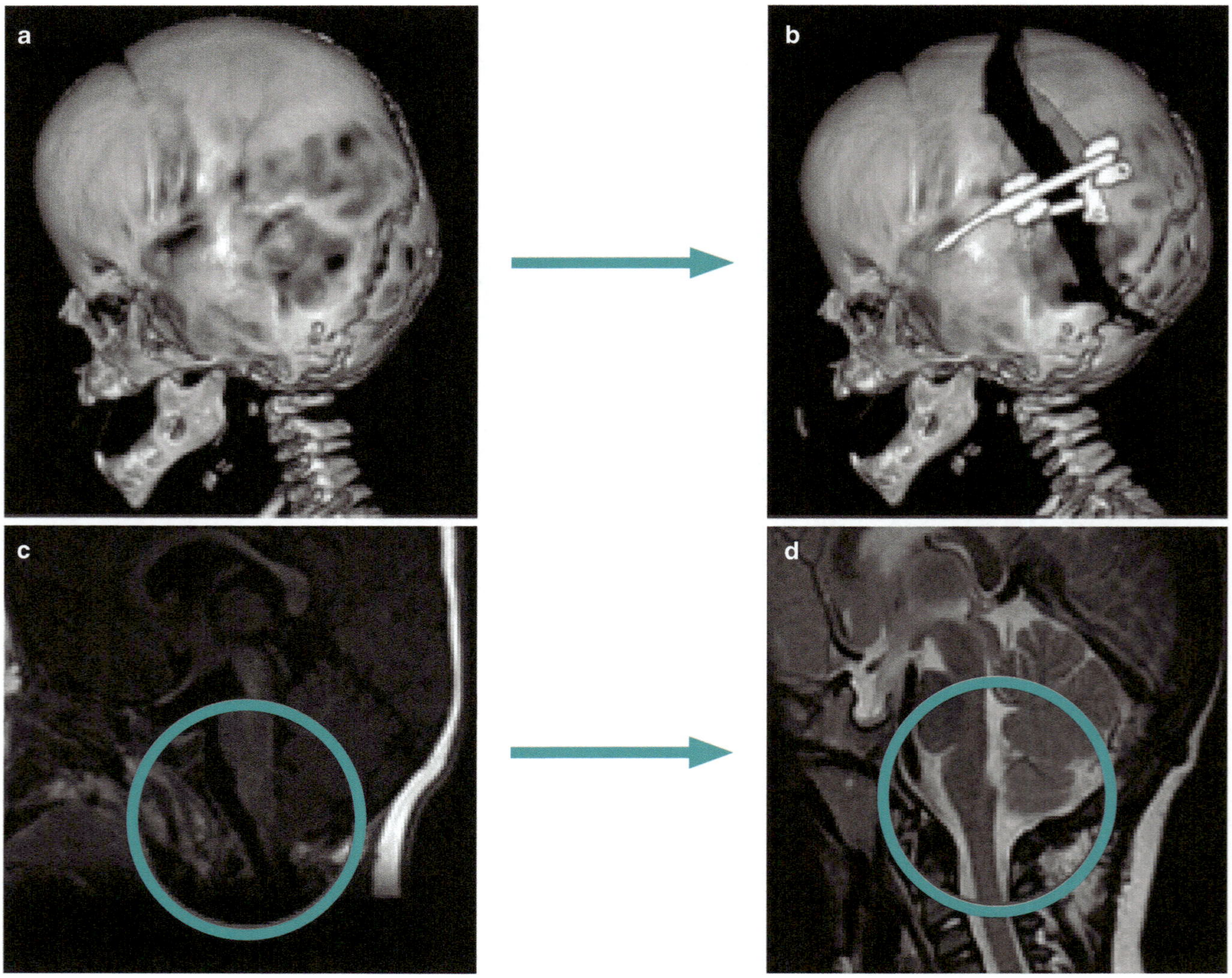

Fig. 2.14 (**a-d**) Improvement of tonsillar herniation after 6 months following a PVE with distraction performed at 8 months of age in a patient with Crouzon syndrome

2.5 PVE without Springs or Distractors (Figs. 2.15, 2.16, and 2.17)

When the calvarial bone is so thin (copper-beaten skull) that no device is applicable, posterior cranial expansion may be driven by brain growth, especially when intracranial pressure is raised [7] (Figs. 2.15, 2.16, and 2.17).

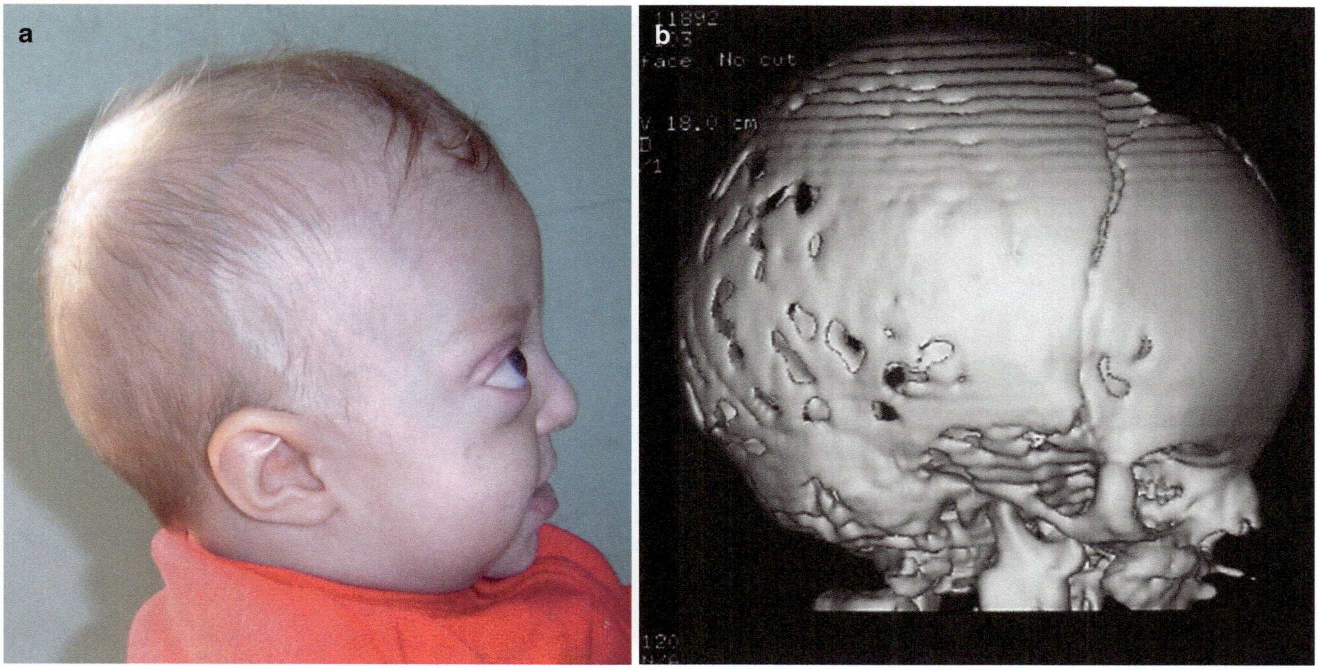

Fig. 2.15 (**a**, **b**) Patient with Pfeiffer syndrome aged 5 months with bilateral lambdoid craniosynostosis. Despite the round head shape, PVE was indicated to increase intracranial volume and prepare for the upcoming FFMBA. (**c**, **d**) Clinical and CT scan aspect at 8 months of age, 1 month after brain-driven PVE. (**e**) CT scan aspect 3 months after surgery, at 10 months of age: beginning of ossification with bony bridges across the osteotomy line and decreased copper-beaten appearance. This patient later underwent FFMBA

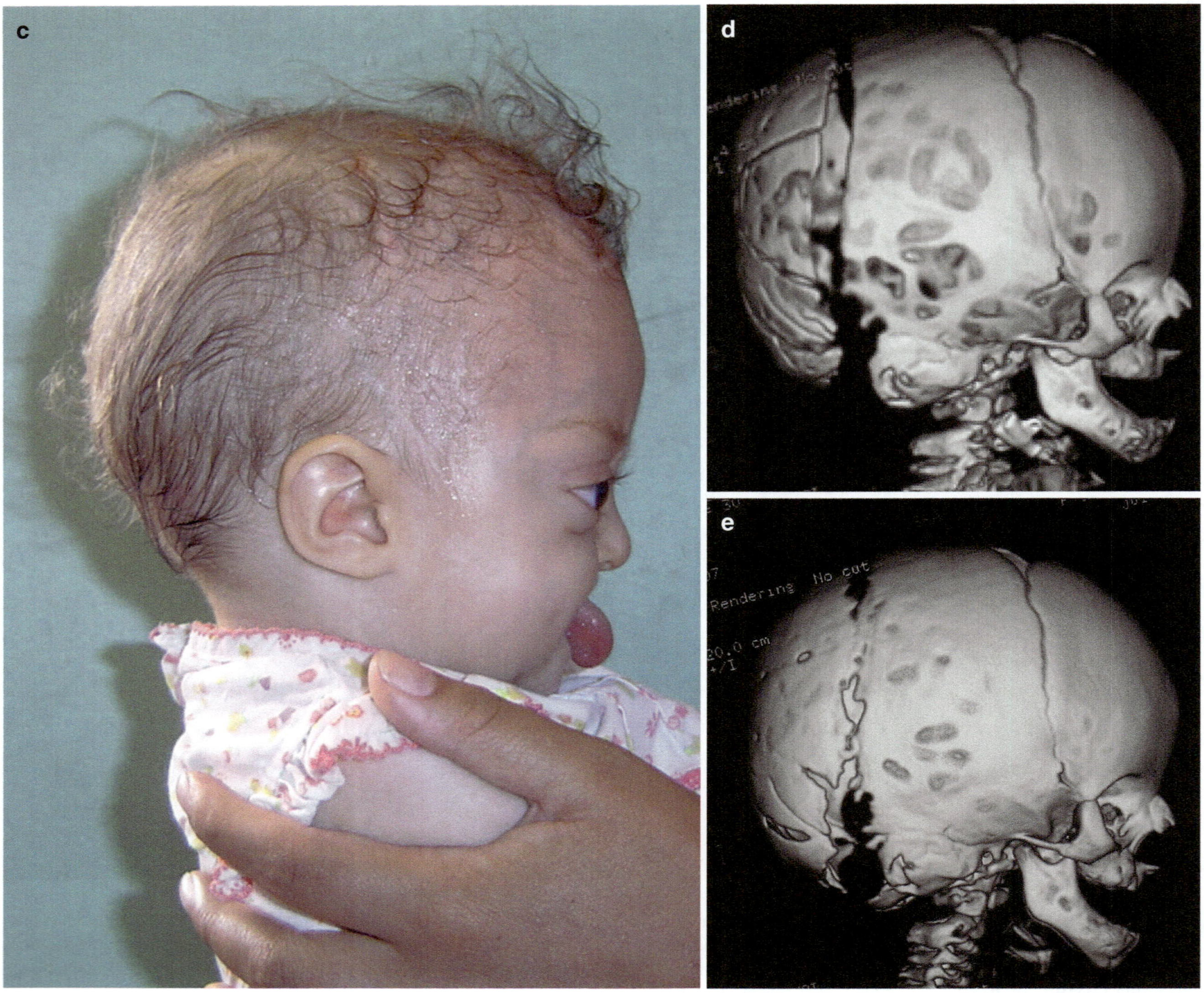

Fig. 2.15 (continued)

Fig. 2.16 (**a**) Five-month-old boy with Pfeiffer syndrome (p. Cys342Ser mutation) presenting with severe maxillary hypoplasia, exorbitism, and severe OSAS (AHI = 25 per hour). Turbinectomy and adenoidectomy were performed and nocturnal positive airway pressure was initiated. © Cassandra Vion. (**b, c**) CT scan showing extremely thin parietal bone and crowding of the posterior fossa with tonsillar herniation obstructing CSF flow. PVE was indicated. (**d**) Two-day-postoperative CT scan at age 6 months showing the osteotomies of brain-mediated PVE. The thin parietal bone precluded the use of internal distractors. (**e**) Three-month postoperative CT scan demonstrating improved skull roundness and rapid re-ossification of the osteotomy lines despite the posterior compression related to prolonged CPAP use. (**f**) Three-month postoperative MRI demonstrating the resolution of cerebellar tonsillar herniation and the normalization of CSF flow at age 8 months. (**g, h**) The systematic ophthalmologic follow-up detected Frisén stage 3 papilledema at age 11 months. Urgent secondary PVE was indicated and bone thickness allowed internal distractor use this time. The two-day postoperative CT scan demonstrates the position of the new osteotomy lines anterior to the old osteotomy lines to reduce the risk of dural laceration. The squamous part of the temporal bone was spared for the upcoming FFMBA. (**i, j**) CT scan during the activation phase of distraction demonstrating the improvement in skull roundness and the enlargement of the posterior fossa with improvement of the inclination of the tentorium cerebelli (This case is further detailed in Fig. 10.11)

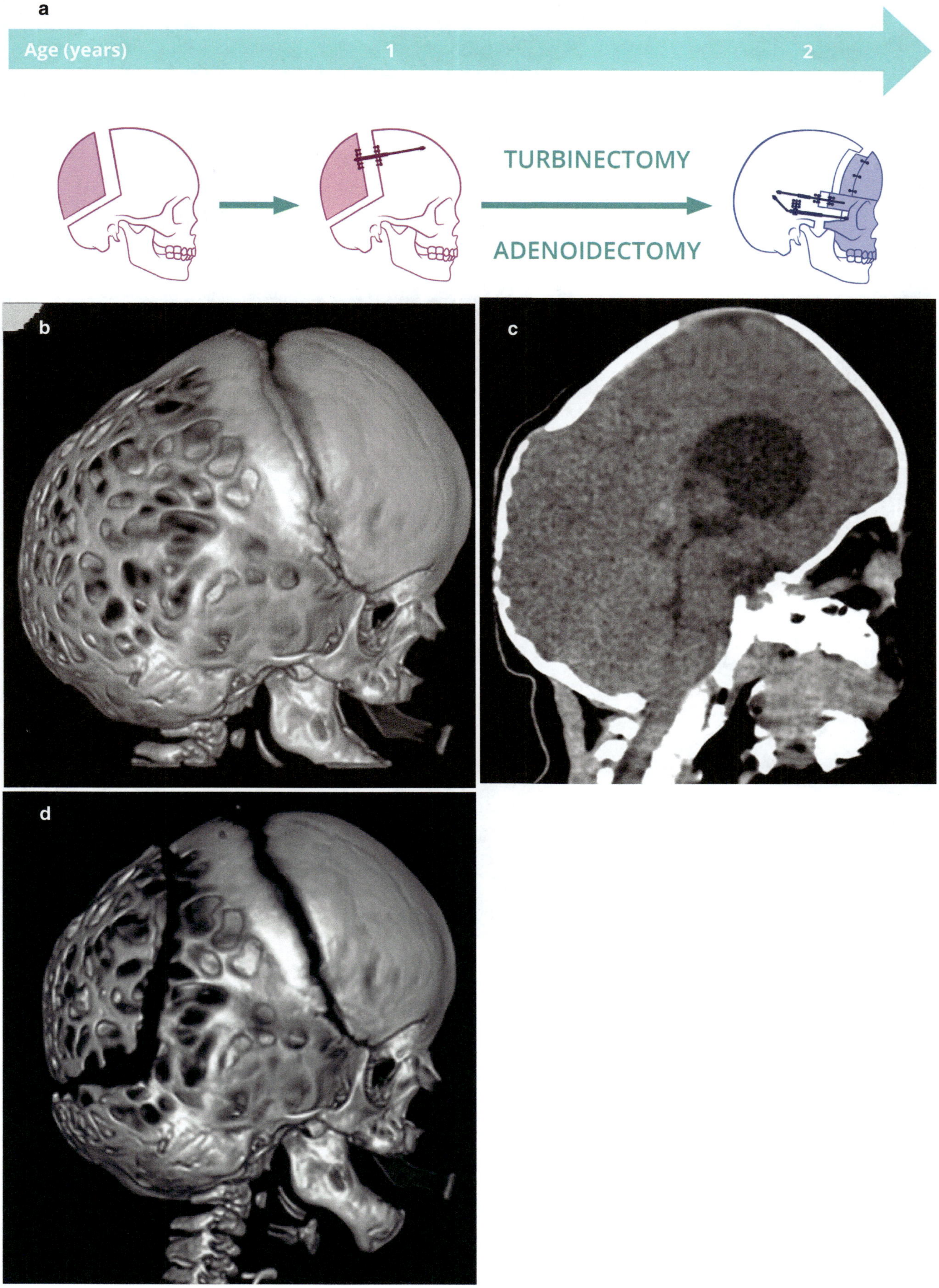
a
Age (years)
1
2
TURBINECTOMY
ADENOIDECTOMY
b
c
d

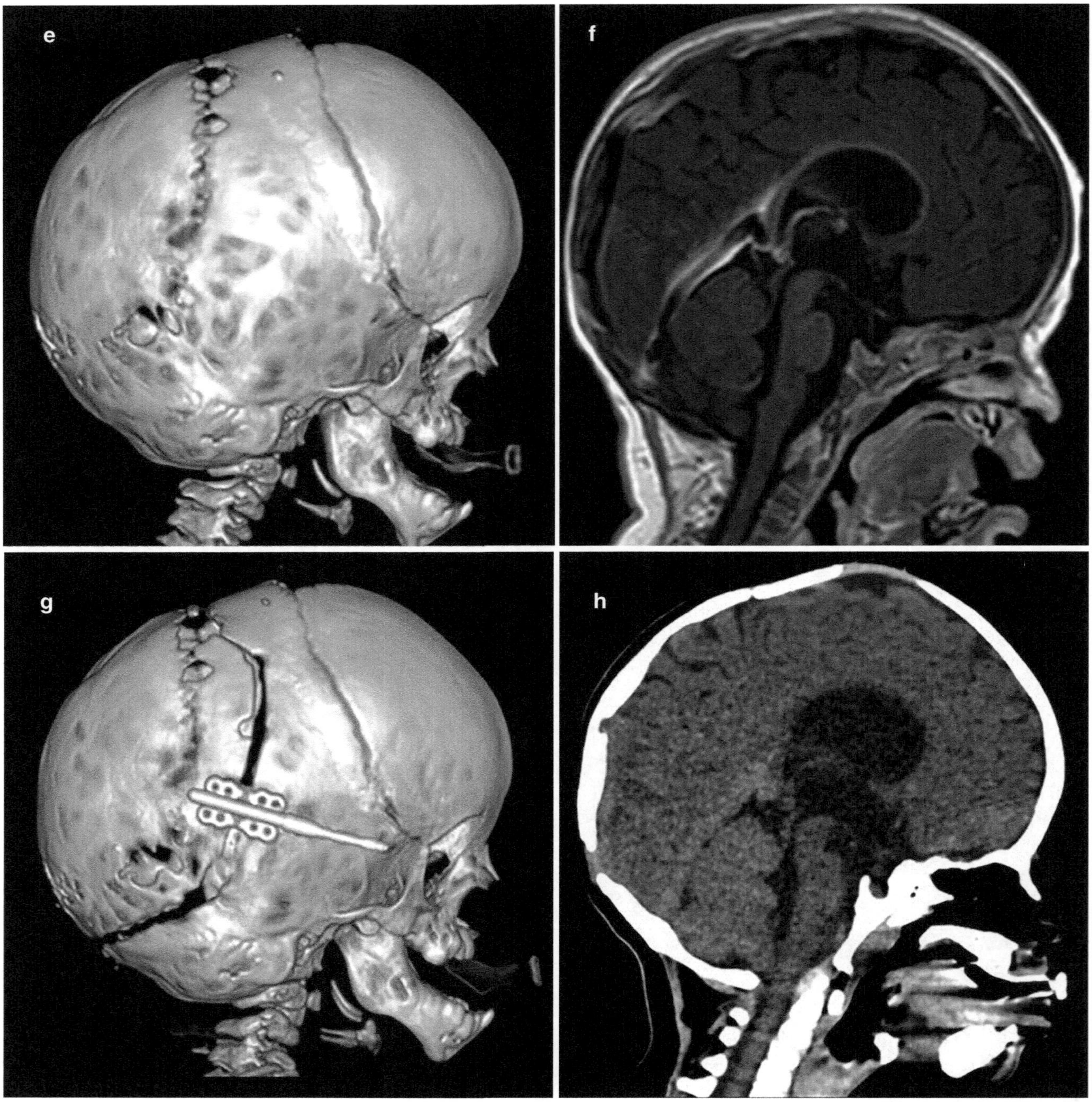

Fig. 2.16 (continued)

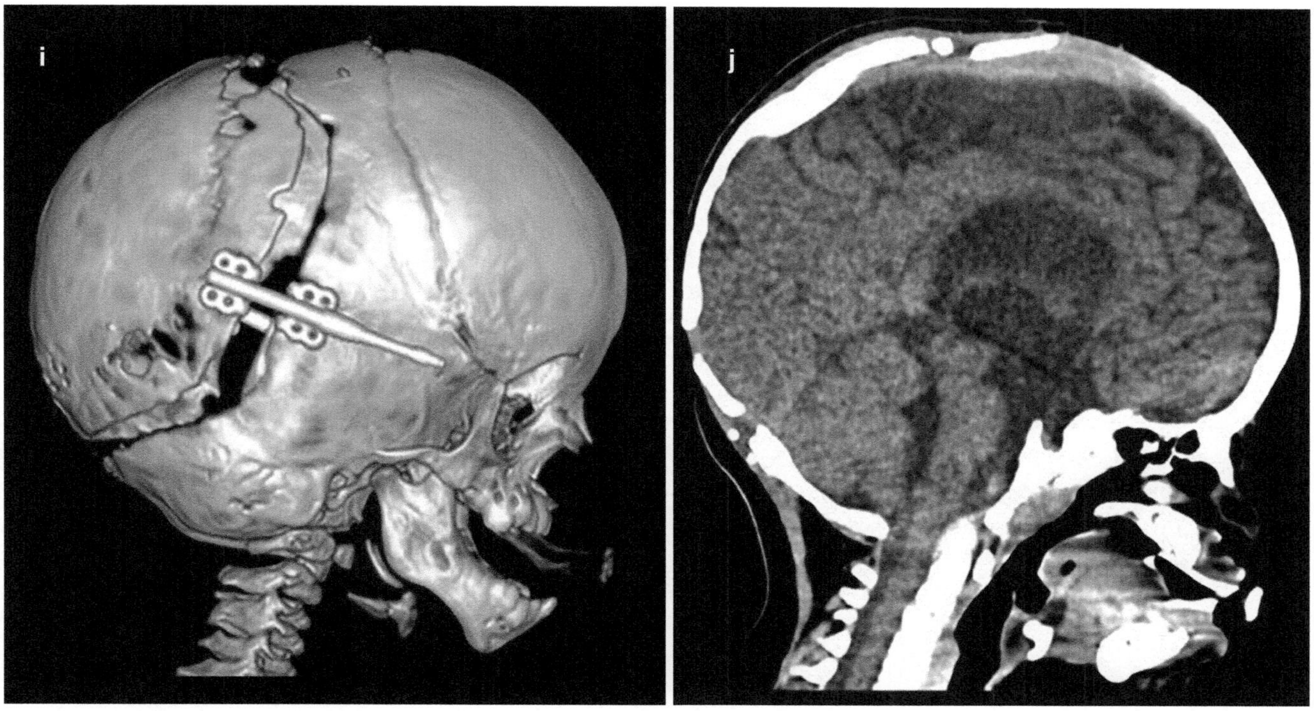

Fig. 2.16 (continued)

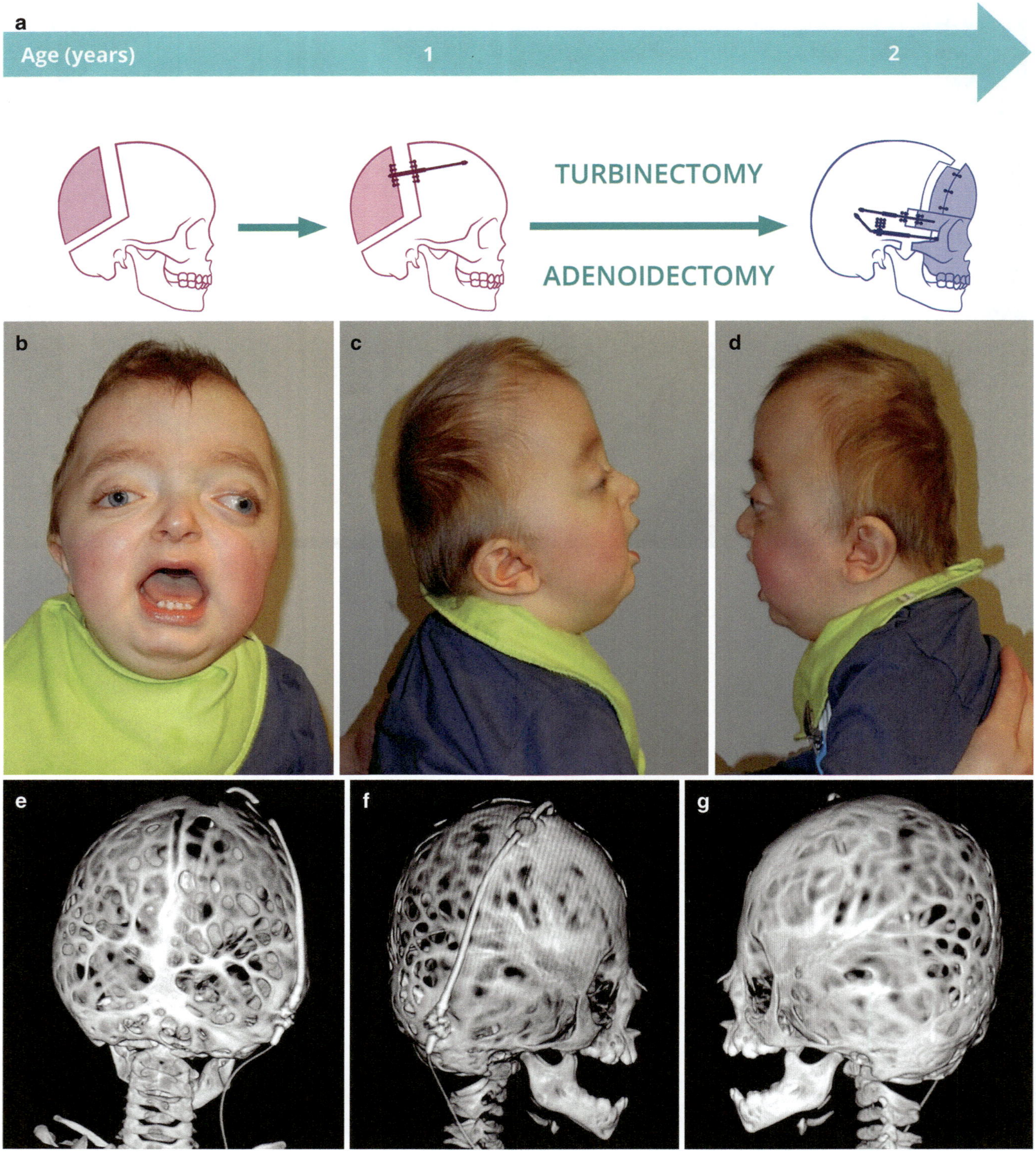

Fig. 2.17 (**a**, **b**, **c**, **d**) Patient with Pfeiffer syndrome aged 8 months with turricephaly. © Cassandra Vion. (**e**, **f**, **g**) CT scan demonstrating severe copper-beaten appearance of the skull at 8 months of age, a stigma of increased intracranial pressure—a pressure-regulated shunt had been inserted in another hospital. (**h**, **i**, **j**, **k**) Intraoperative view before craniotomy—the markings are asymmetrical: posterior to the shunt on the right side. (**i**, **j**) Asymmetric osteotomies with replacement of the valve by a flow-regulated device. (**l**, **m**, **n**) At 12 months of age, decreased flattening of the posterior aspect of the skull. (**o**, **p**, **q**) CT scan at 13 months of age demonstrating decreased copper-beaten appearance and thicker bone

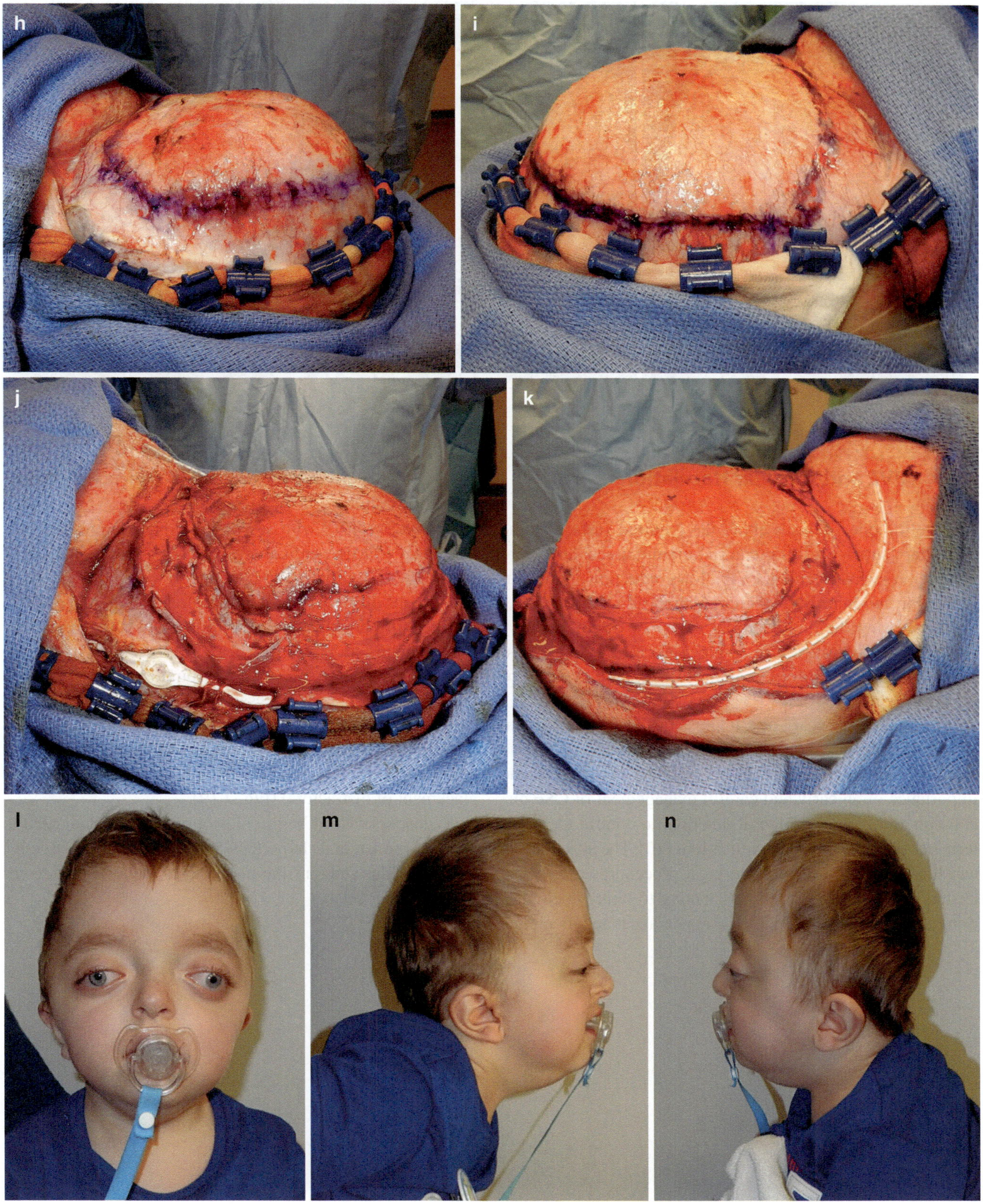

Fig. 2.17 (continued)

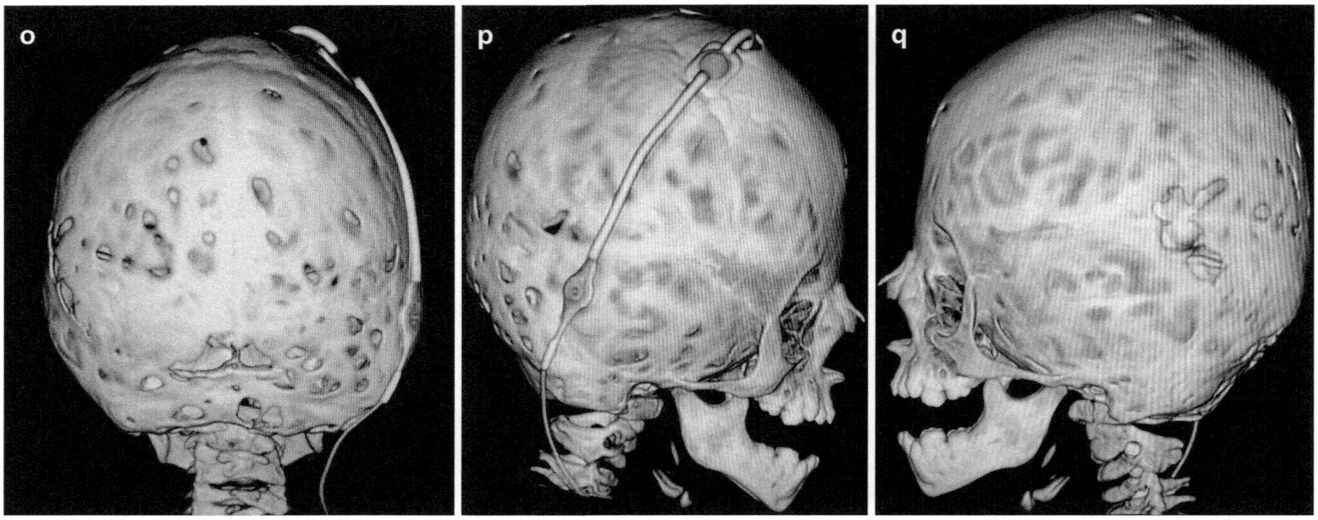

Fig. 2.17 (continued)

2.6 PVE and Tonsillar Herniation

Despite the open debates about the required surface of the bony flap, supra- or infra-tentorial craniotomies, and dural opening, it seems clear that PVE allows reduction of tonsillar herniation and improved CSF circulation [9].

Considering the multifactorial nature of Chiari anomaly in faciocraniosynostoses, in some cases, a FM decompression needs to be performed, combined with PVE or as a separate procedure [4, 10].

In the last few years, the interest in the craniovertebral junction anomalies and the discovery of large syringomyelia cases at late follow-up of FCST patients highlighted the importance of an early and careful management of CSF circulation at the craniovertebral junction, to control the long-term risk of neurological complications [10]. The introduction and the application of other surgical procedures need to be evaluated such as IVth ventricle stenting to improve circulation and reduce syringomyelia appearance and occipito-cervical fusion or C1-C2 fusion in very particular conditions of clear instability.

In any case, PVE with or without FM decompression may help delay FFMBA until after 2 years of age (Fig. 2.18).

After an initial PVE, usually performed around 5–6 months of age, a relapse in intracranial hypertension was reported in some patients, usually manifesting as papilledema. In this circumstance, the indication of FFMBA has to be considered based on age and respiratory status: if airway obstruction has been successfully tackled by ENT procedures and/or CPAP, we prefer to postpone FFMBA and perform in the meantime another PVE with distraction (by the second operation, bone thickness most generally allows the placement of distractors) (Fig. 2.19).

Endoscopic Third Ventriculostomy (ETV) is indicated to control intracranial hypertension in case of obstructive hydrocephalus and tonsillar herniation to delay skull decompression (Fig. 2.19).

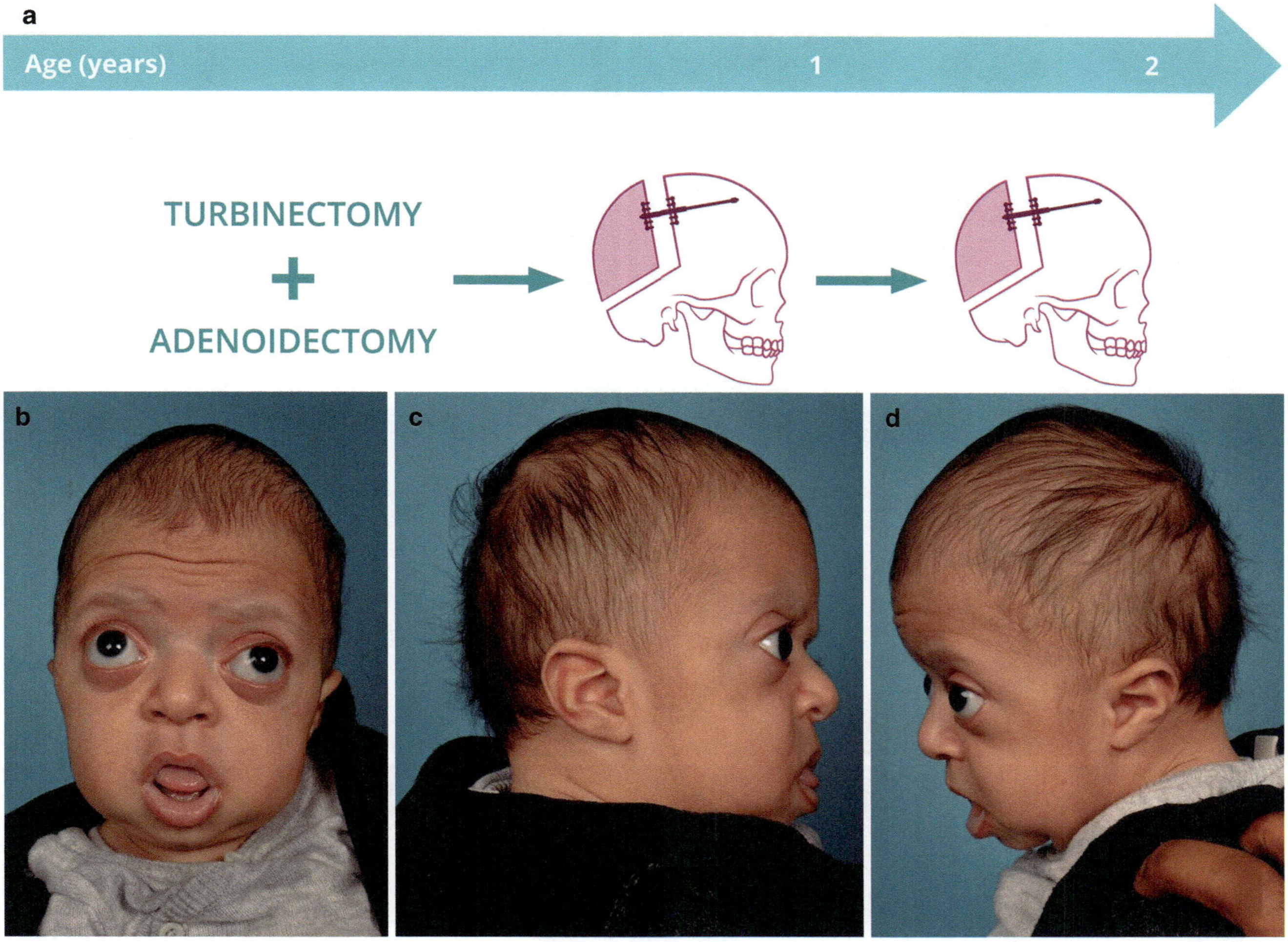

Fig. 2.18 (**a**) Patient with Pfeiffer syndrome presenting at age 2 months with a history of respiratory distress at birth, nasal airway obstruction, and feeding problems. Polysomnography revealed severe OSAS (AHI = 28 per hour). © Cassandra Vion. Turbinoplasty and adenoidectomy were performed by the pediatric ENT team and noninvasive ventilation was started. (**b**, **c**, **d**) Clinical photographs at age 2 months demonstrating exorbitism and maxillary hypoplasia. (**e**, **f**, **g**, **h**) CT scan at age 2 months demonstrating a very partial fusion of the coronal sutures. (**i**, **j**) Cerebral MRI at age 2 months demonstrated the absence of both tonsillar herniation and ventriculomegaly. (**k**, **l**, **m**) Ophthalmologic follow-up detected Frisén Stage 2 papilledema at age 7 months. PVE was indicated. Preoperative CT scan demonstrated complete fusion of both coronal sutures and fingerprinting of the skull bone. Bone thickness allowed the use of internal distractors. (**n**, **o**, **p**) Two-day postoperative CT scan at age 7 months demonstrating the PVE osteotomy and the hardware. Intraoperative 8 millimeter distraction is shown to immediately relieve intracranial pressure. (**q**, **r**, **s**) Fifteen-day postoperative CT scan demonstrating the increase in intracranial volume. (**t**-**w**) Brain MRI at age 14 months demonstrating the absence of cerebellar tonsillar herniation and hydrocephalus on T1- and T2-weighted sequences (**t** and **w**, respectively). Black Bone sequence demonstrated partial re-ossification (**u**). Inhance 3D velocity MRI sequence showed improved intracranial venous circulation. (**x**, **y**, **z**) Clinical photographs at age 15 months showing aggravation of maxillary hypoplasia and exorbitism, partly due to nocturnal noninvasive ventilation. Notice the external tarsorrhaphy that was performed as an ancillary procedure during the previous PVE. The head shape is round and satisfactory. (**a'**-**f'**) The ophthalmologic follow-up detected a relapse of papillary edema at age 16 months (Frisén stage 3). Urgent secondary PVE with distraction was indicated to protect the visual function and release brain compression. (**a'**, **b'**, **c'**) Preoperative CT scan demonstrating partial re-ossification of the previous osteotomies. (**d'**, **e'**, **f'**) CT scan at postoperative day 22 after the end of distraction demonstrating the new osteotomy line. The temporal region was spared for the upcoming FFMBA. (**g'**, **h'**) Postoperative brain MRI showing the absence of cerebellar tonsillar herniation and adequate CSF spaces

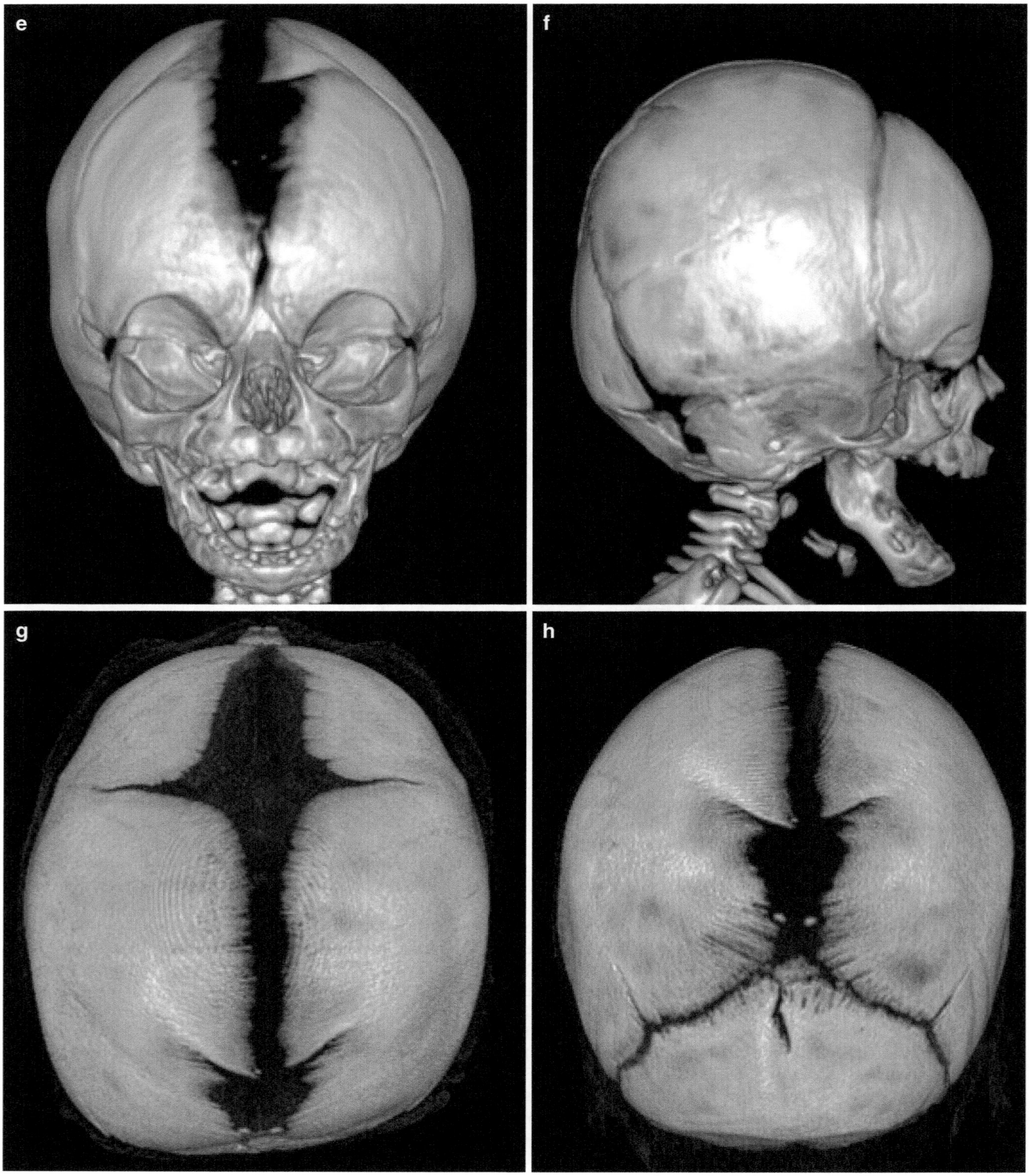

Fig. 2.18 (continued)

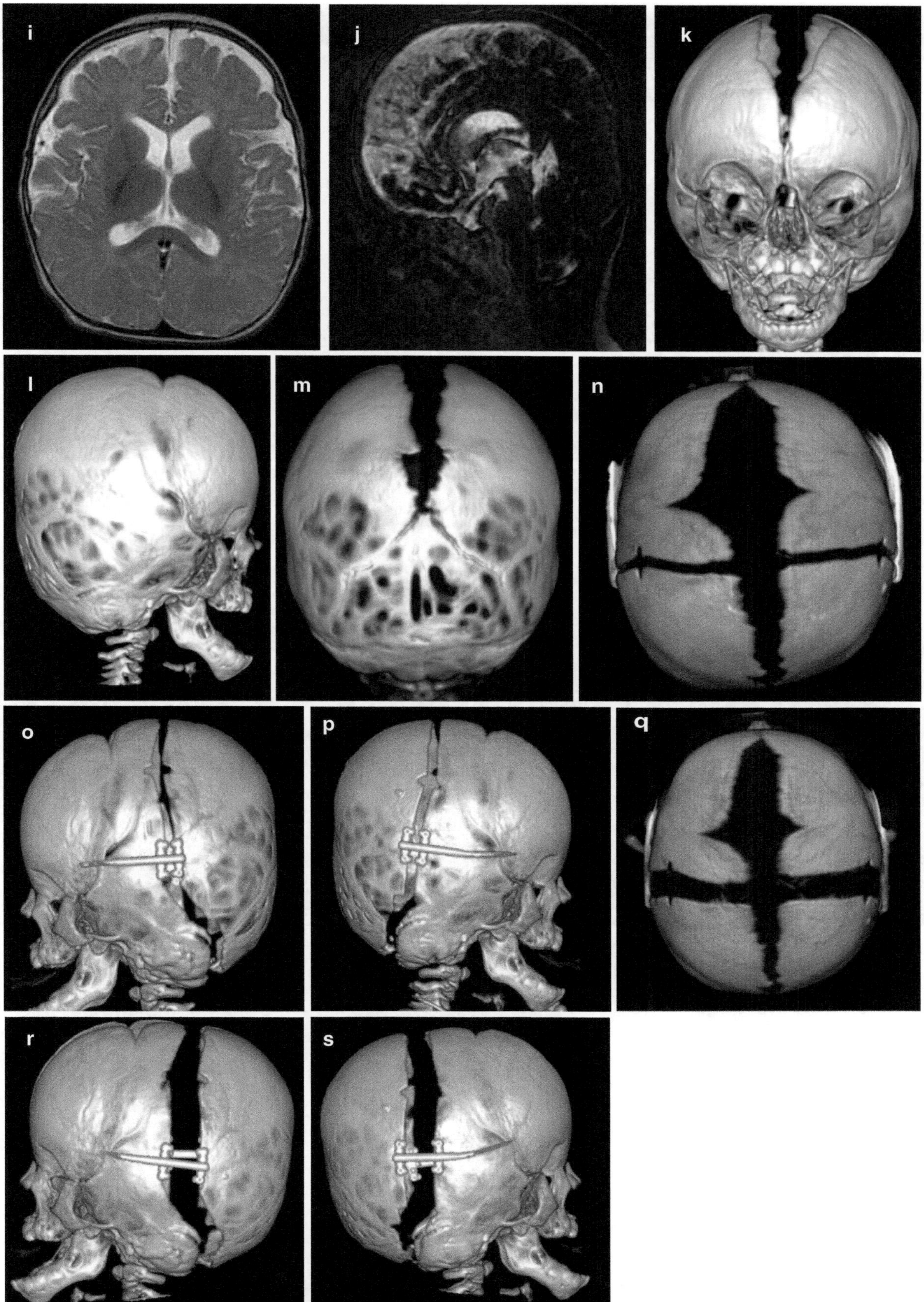

Fig. 2.18 (continued)

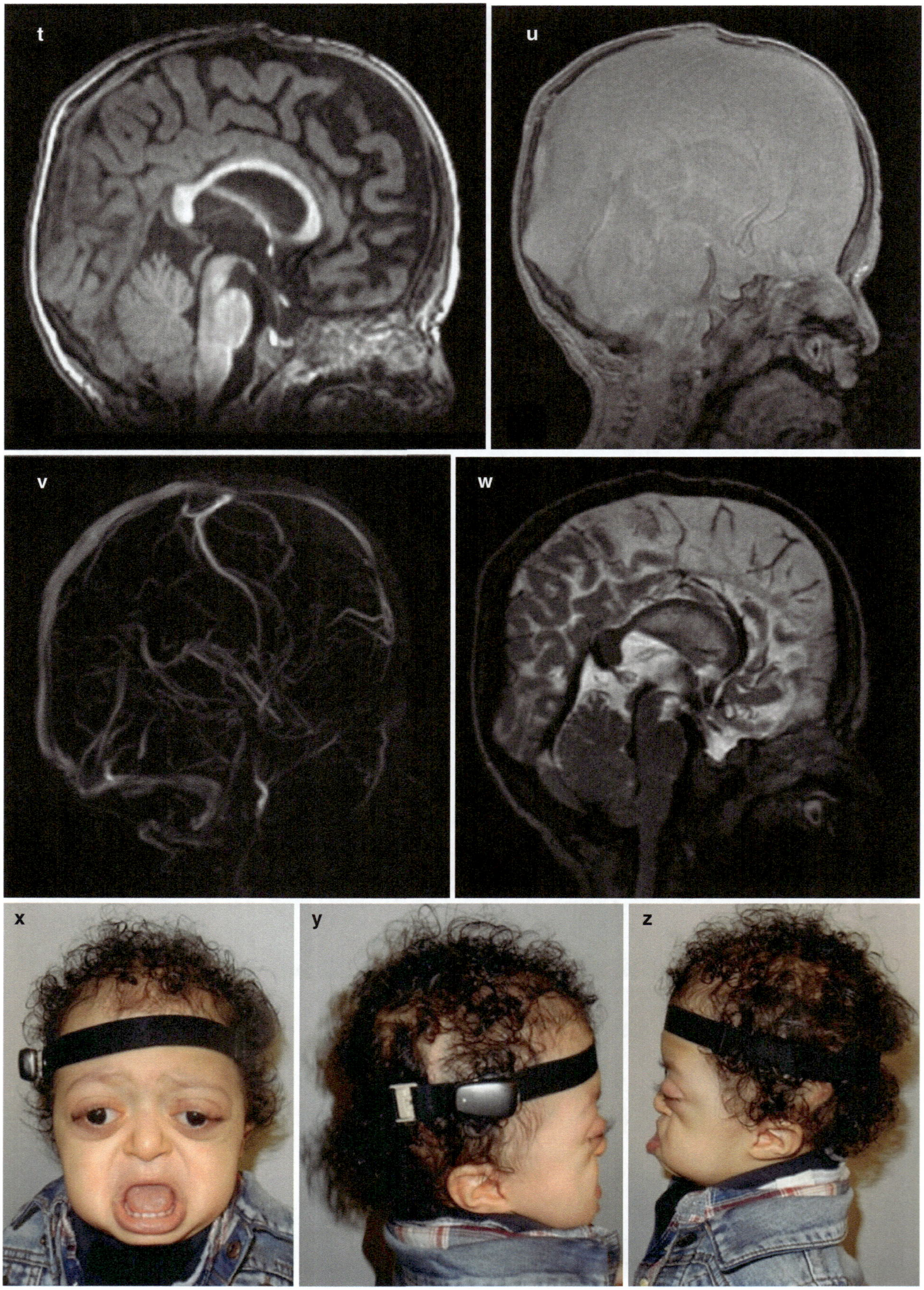

Fig. 2.18 (continued)

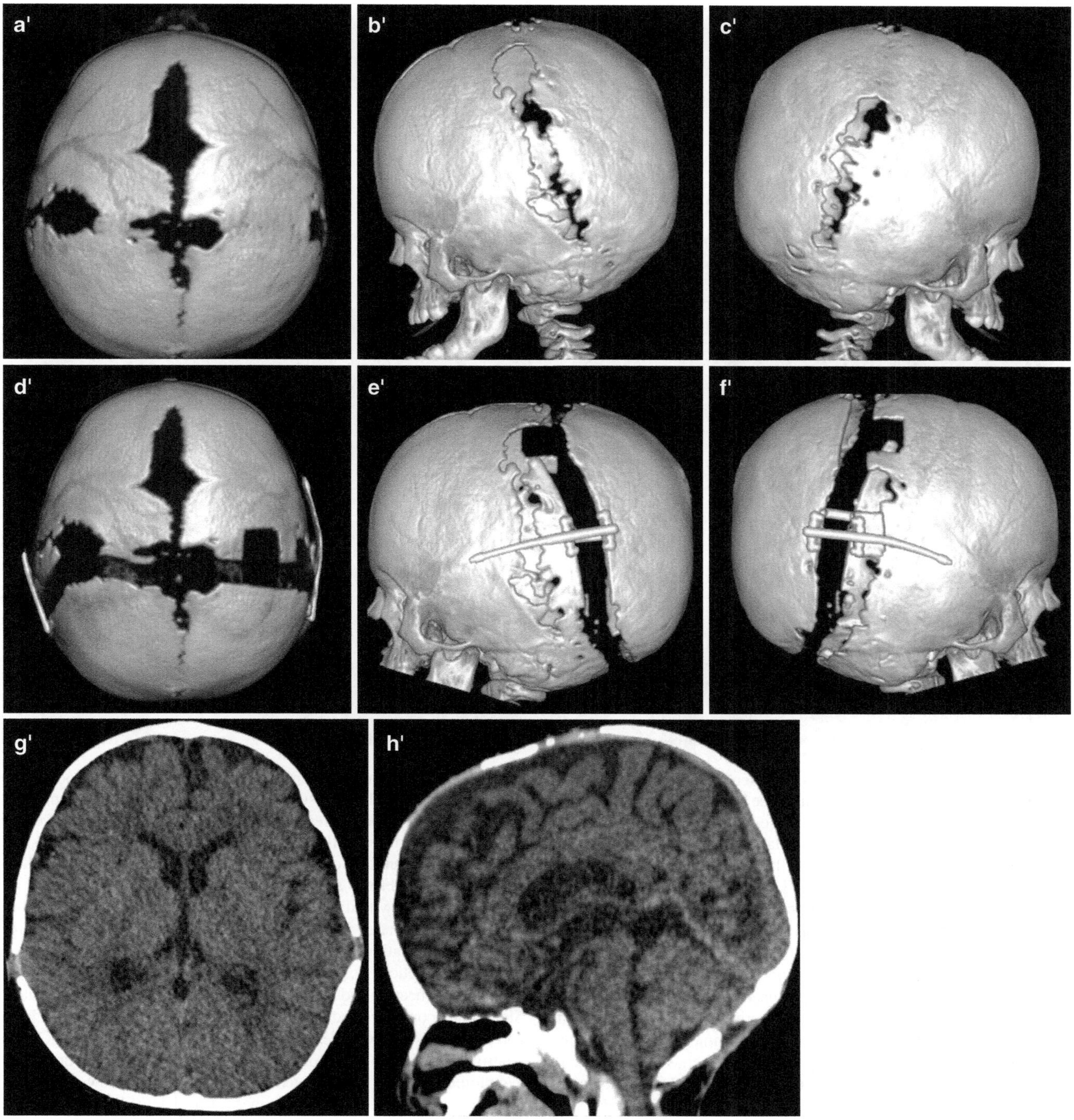

Fig. 2.18 (continued)

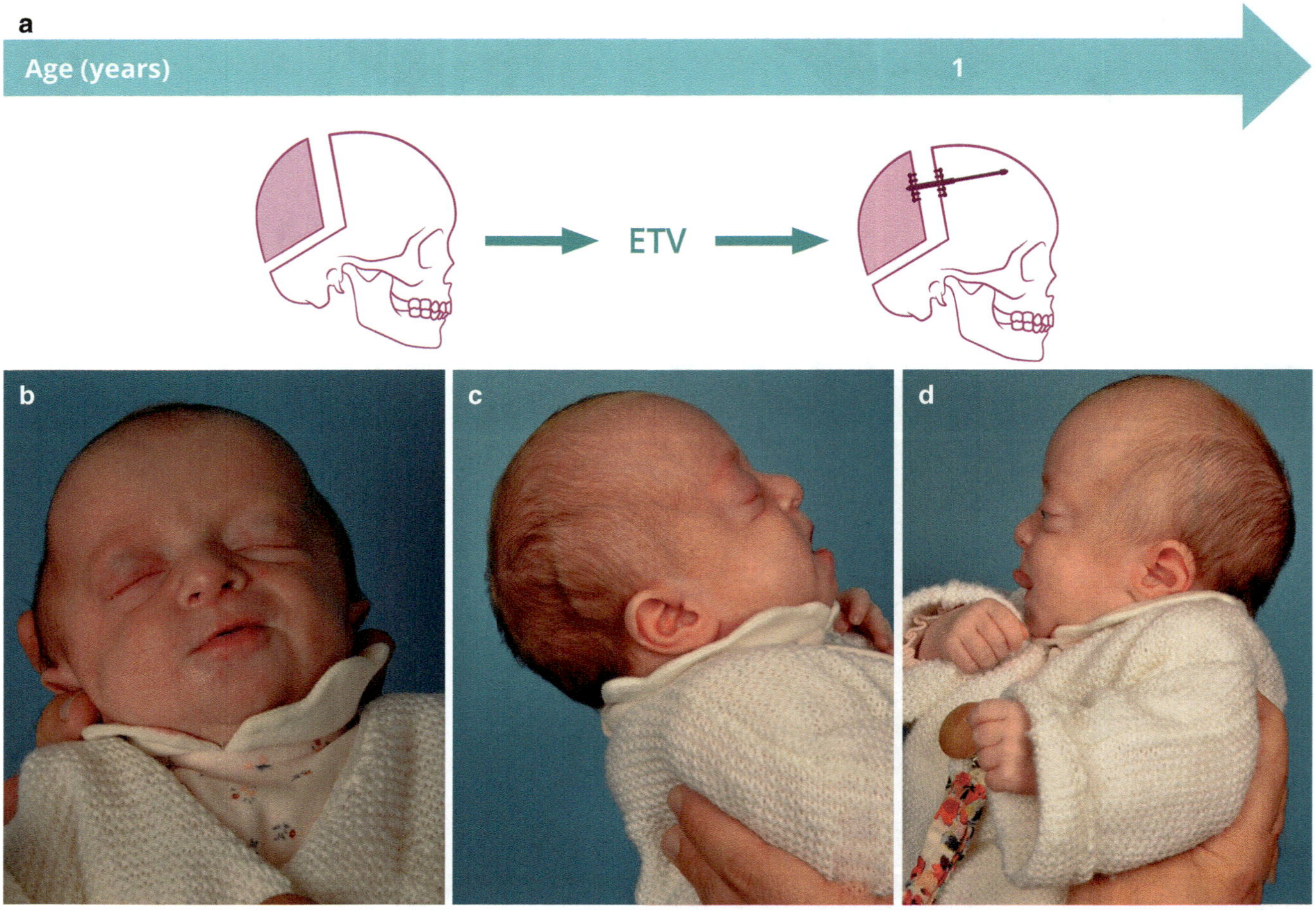

Fig. 2.19 (**a**, **b**, **c**, **d**) Three-week-old patient with Pfeiffer syndrome presenting with turribrachycephaly, midface hypoplasia, exorbitism, and bilateral deafness. © Cassandra Vion. (**e**, **f**, **g**, **h**, **i**) CT scan at age 3 months demonstrating sagittal and bi-lambdoid craniosynostosis with hydrocephalus without cerebellar tonsillar herniation. Nasal endoscopy was impossible due to the small nares. (**j**, **k**, **l**) Brain MRI at age 3 months demonstrating hydrocephalus with transependymal CSF resorption. Stenosis of the right sigmoid sinus and the left transverse sinus and collateral venous veins were evident on Inhance 3D velocity MRI. Despite the absence of papilledema on fundoscopy, PVE was indicated to relieve brain compression and treat hydrocephalus. Bone thinness precluded the use of internal distractors. (**m**, **n**) Postoperative CT scan demonstrating the osteotomies of brain-mediated PVE and immediate brain decompression. (**o**, **p**) Three-month-postoperative T2-weighted MRI showed a slightly increased ventricular size with transependymal resorption and a bulging floor of the third ventricle. The patient also developed papilledema. ETV was indicated to treat hydrocephalus. (**q**) T2-weighted MRI after ETV at age 7 months demonstrating CSF flow at the floor of the third ventricle. Papilledema subsided. (**r**, **s**) CT scan at age 13 months. The patient developed severe OSA which was aggravated by upper respiratory infections (AHI = 48.4 per hour). Medical treatment was initiated including antibiotics and topical nasal corticosteroids as well as nocturnal CPAP. Frisen stage 2 papillary edema was also detected on fundoscopy. PVE with distractors was indicated. (**t**, **u**) Two-day postoperative CT scan after PVE with distractors. (**v**, **w**) CT scan at age 15 months illustrating the volumetric gain after the end of the activation phase of distraction. (**x**, **y**) Clinical photographs at age 19 months with the patient's hearing aid in place. CPAP ceased to be well tolerated. Sleep fibroscopy revealed airway obstruction due to inferior turbinate and adenoid hypertrophy despite adequate medical treatment and GERD control. Turbinectomy and adenoidectomy were performed followed by symptomatic relief 1 month later. This case illustrates how ENT management and PVE/ETV can be harnessed to delay FFMBA until age 2 years at the least, without shunting

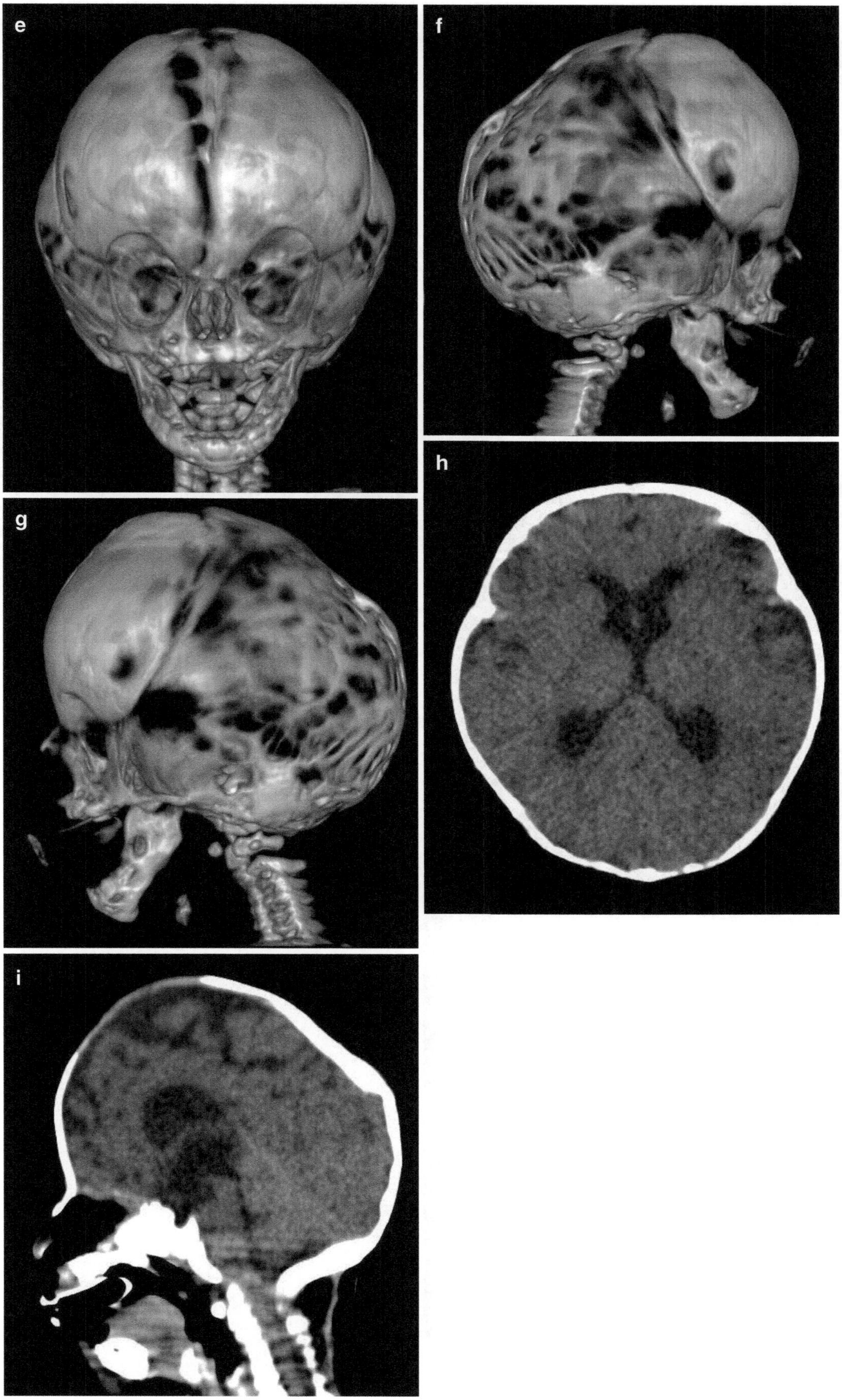

Fig. 2.19 (continued)

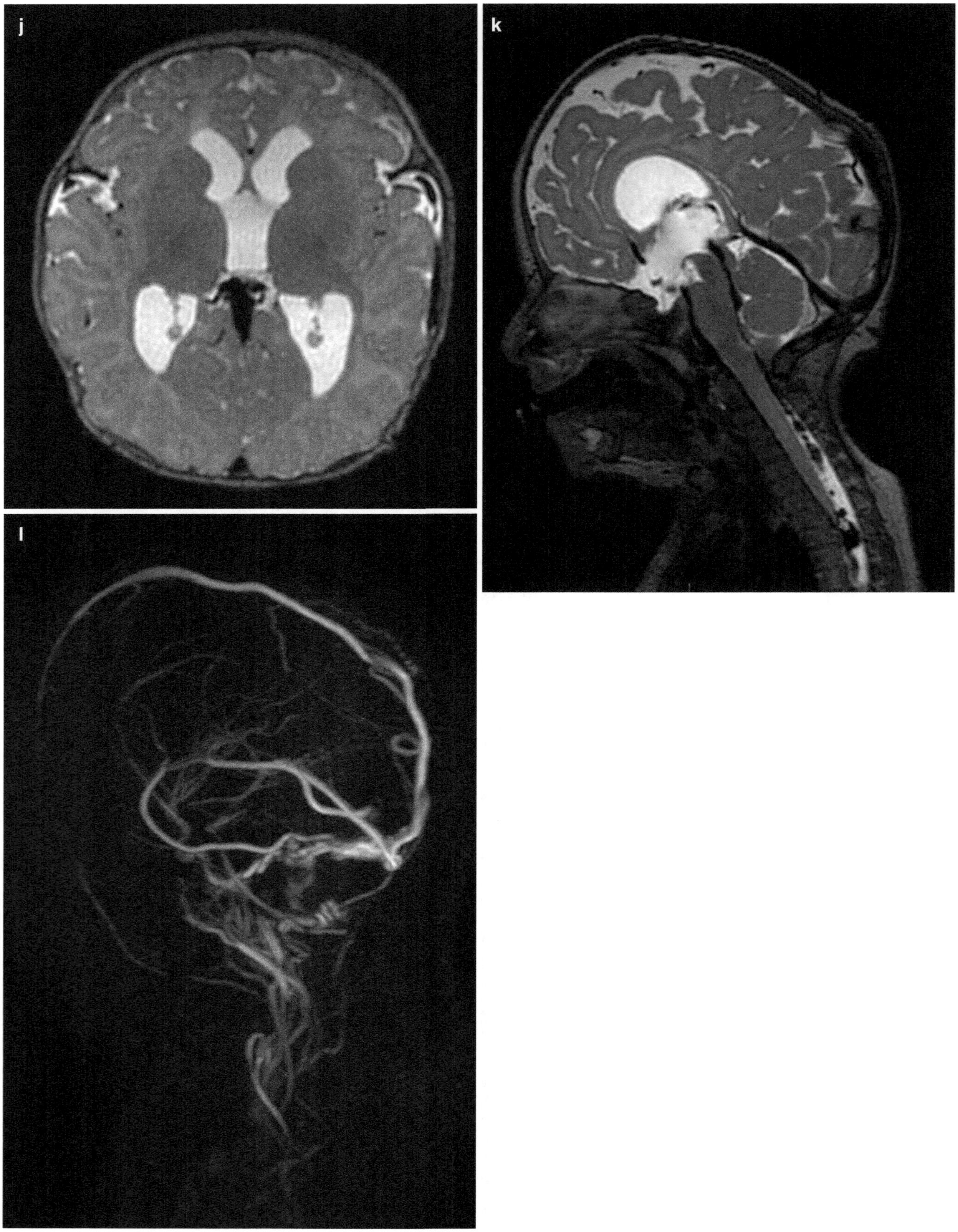

Fig. 2.19 (continued)

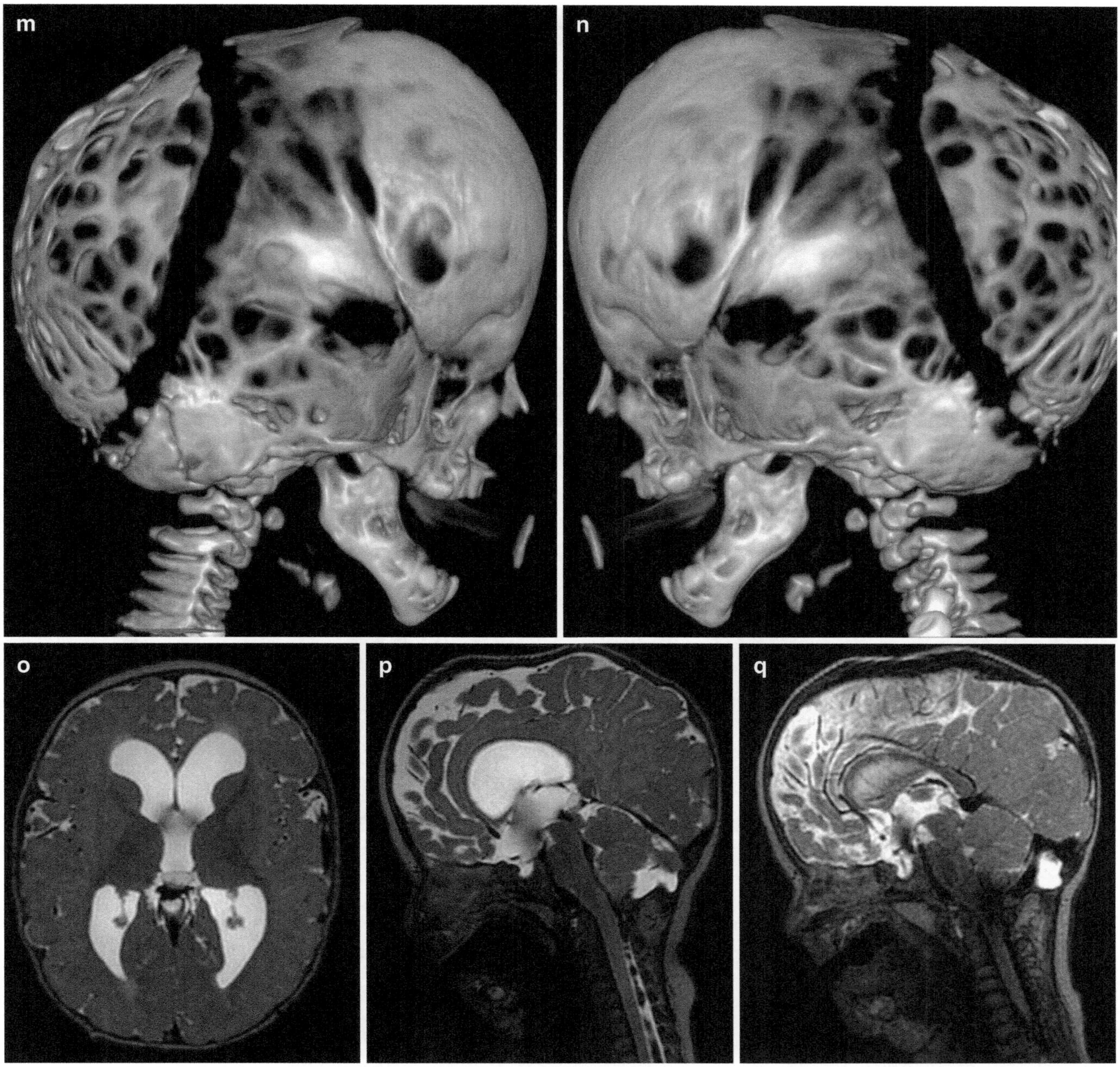

Fig. 2.19 (continued)

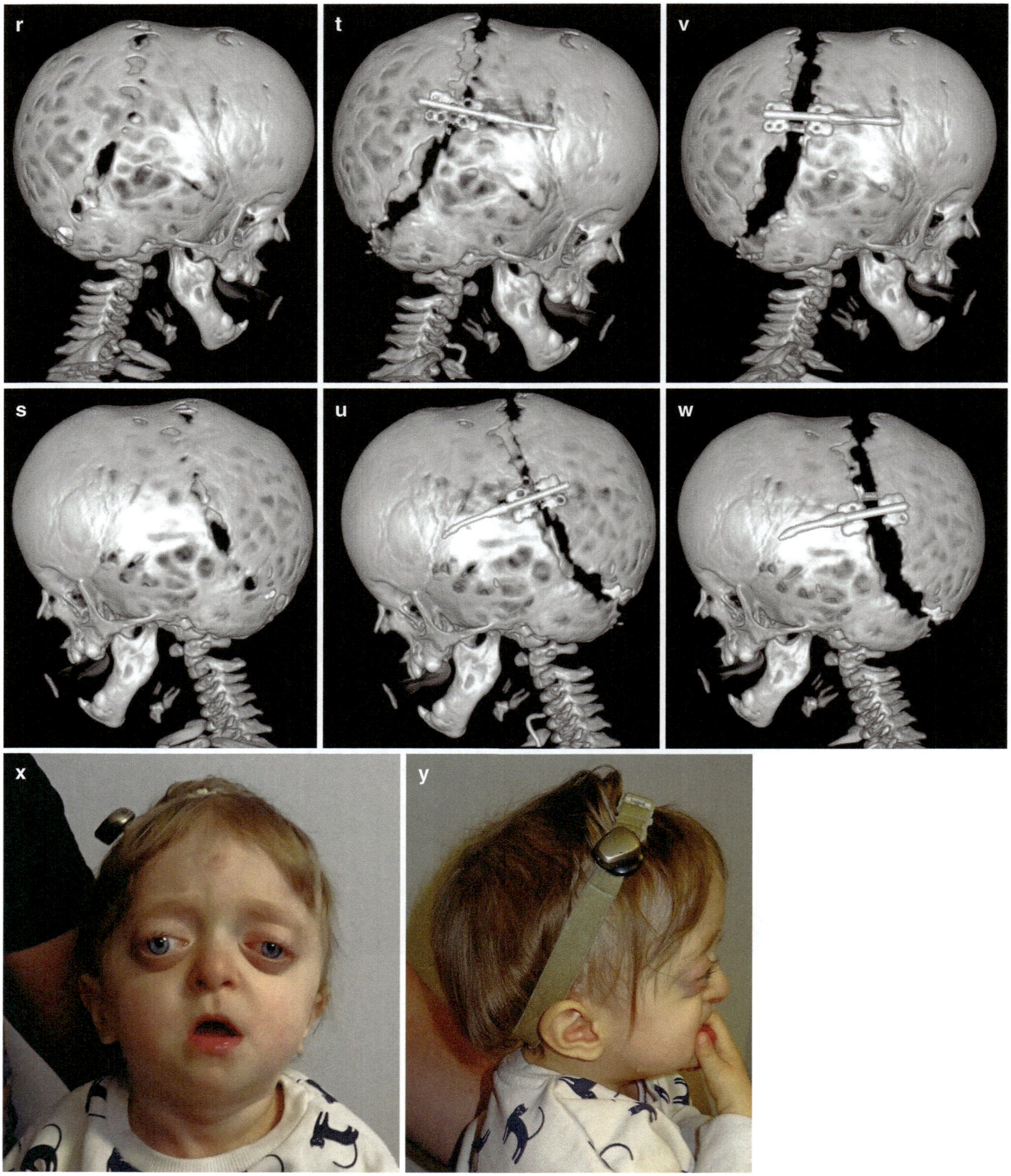

Fig. 2.19 (continued)

2.7 Biparietal Decompression

More generally, even in the presence of hydrocephalus, increased ICP has to be considered as the consequence of multiple factors: craniocerebral disproportion, venous outflow obstruction, and obstruction to CSF flow [11–14].

In this context, cranial vault procedures and decompression surgeries are preferred and performed before considering the insertion of a VP shunt. Biparietal decompression can be indicated for the management of secondarily increased ICP, when the anteroposterior skull diameter is maximal after the first PVE (Figs. 2.20 and 2.21).

In older patients presenting late and with intracranial hypertension, the initial step is usually PVE with distraction. The second step may include biparietal remodeling simultaneously to the FFMBA (Fig. 2.22).

In case of a normal posterior fossa and a rather dolichocephalic head shape, biparietal decompression is considered first line before FFMBA.

Shunt insertion is considered a last resort. When a shunt has to be placed, a flow-regulated valve is preferred at our institution [15, 16].

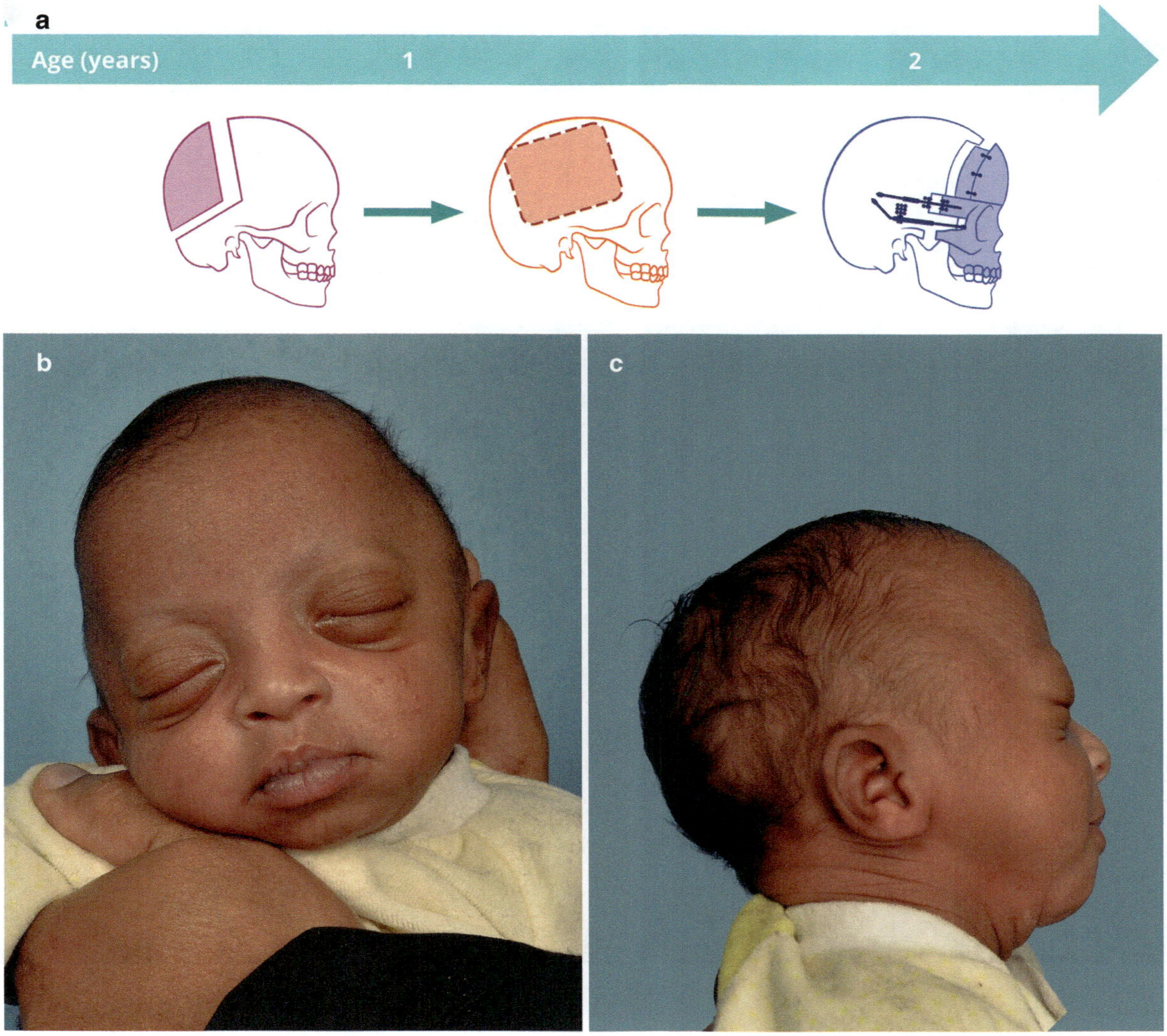

Fig. 2.20 (**a**, **b**, **c**) Three-week-old patient with Pfeiffer syndrome presenting with turribrachycephaly and exorbitism with wide toes and thumbs. Polysomnography revealed OSAS (AHI = 12 per hour). Noninvasive ventilation was started. Ophthalmology follow-up detected papilledema on fundoscopy at age 5 months prompting PVE. © Cassandra Vion. (**d**) Preoperative CT scan demonstrating very thin lateral skull bone precluding the possibility of hardware used for distraction. Urgent brain-mediated PVE was indicated at age 5 months. (**e**) Preoperative cerebral MRI revealed cerebellar tonsillar herniation causing obstructive hydrocephalus. (**f**, **g**) Two-day-postoperative CT scan demonstrating the osteotomy lines. The inferior horizontal component of the osteotomy is inferior to the occipital tuberosity. (**h**, **i**) Six-week-postoperative CT scan demonstrating a two-centimeter expansion with increased intracranial volume and decompression of the posterior cranial fossa. (**j**, **k**) Papillary edema relapsed at age 18 months while cerebellar tonsillar herniation did not obstruct the foramen magnum. Urgent cranial decompression was indicated again. As the posterior pole already had adequate projection, biparietal expansion was indicated rather than a repeat PVE with distraction to avoid ending up with a scaphocephalic head shape after the FFMBA to come. (**l**, **m**) CT scan 3 months after biparietal expansion: the osteotomy lines spare the temporal region for the upcoming FFMBA internal distractors. (**n**, **o**) Clinical pictures at age 2 years demonstrating severe maxillary retrusion aggravated by nocturnal noninvasive ventilation. FFMBA was performed at age 25 months

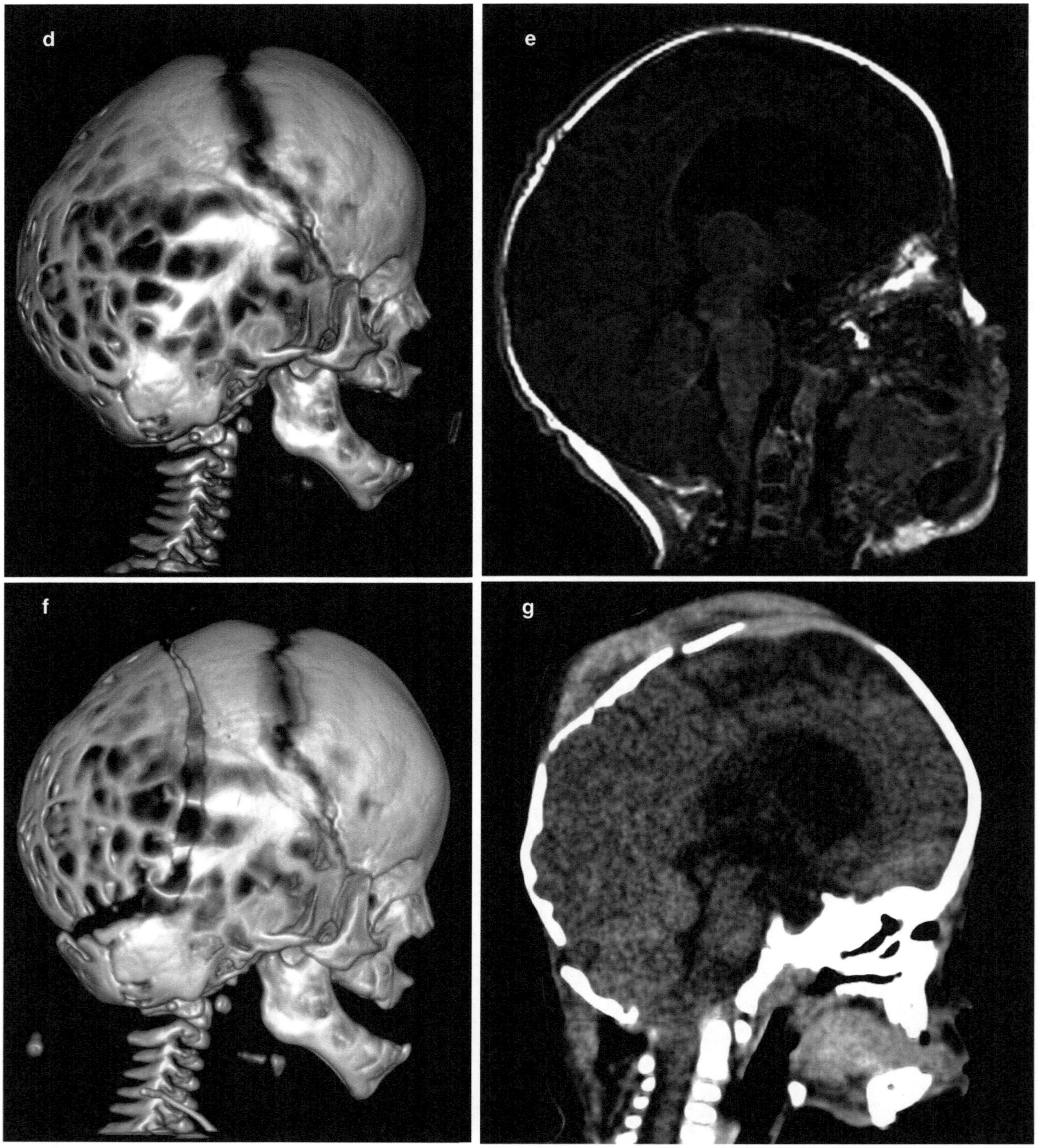

Fig. 2.20 (continued)

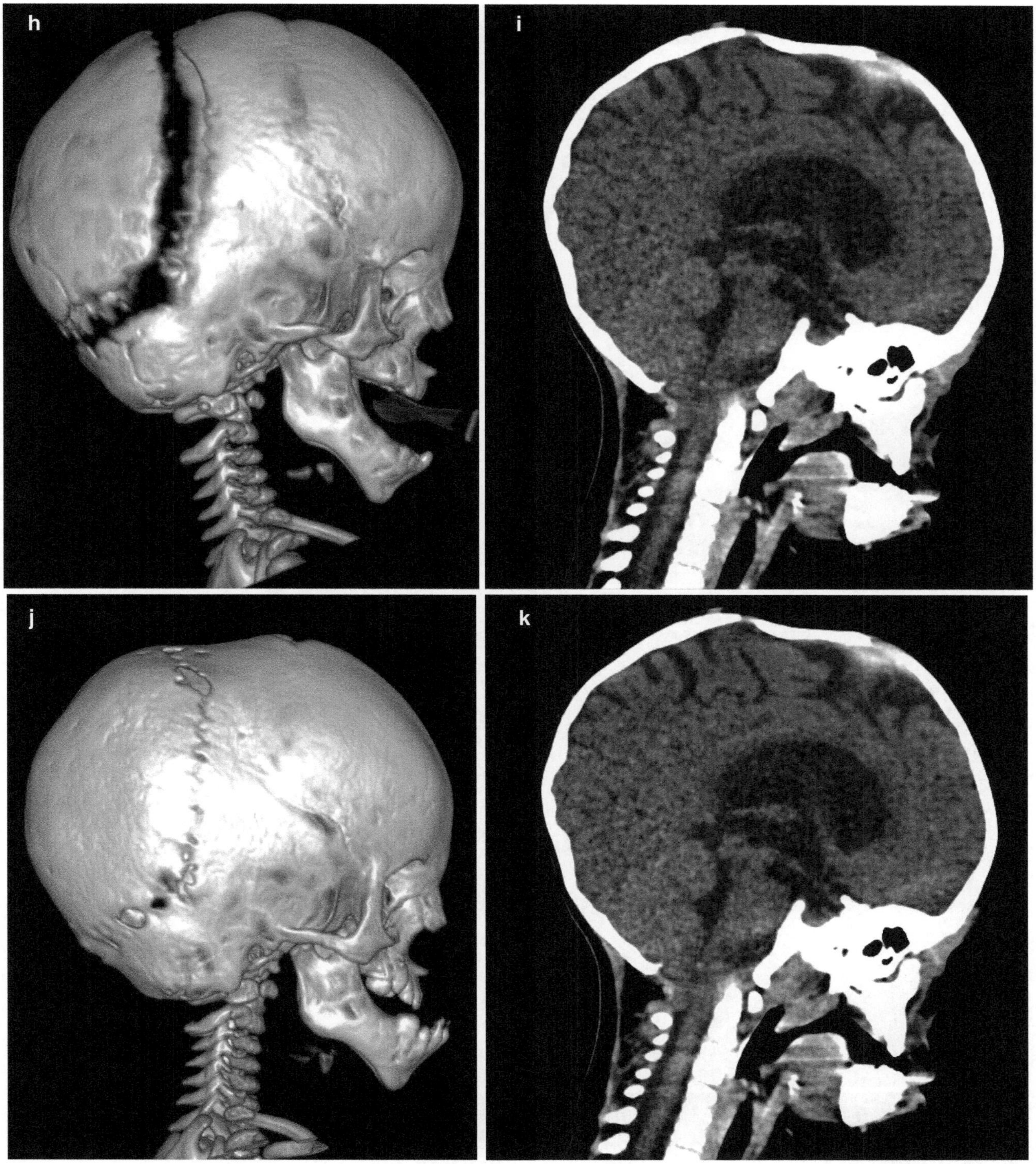

Fig. 2.20 (continued)

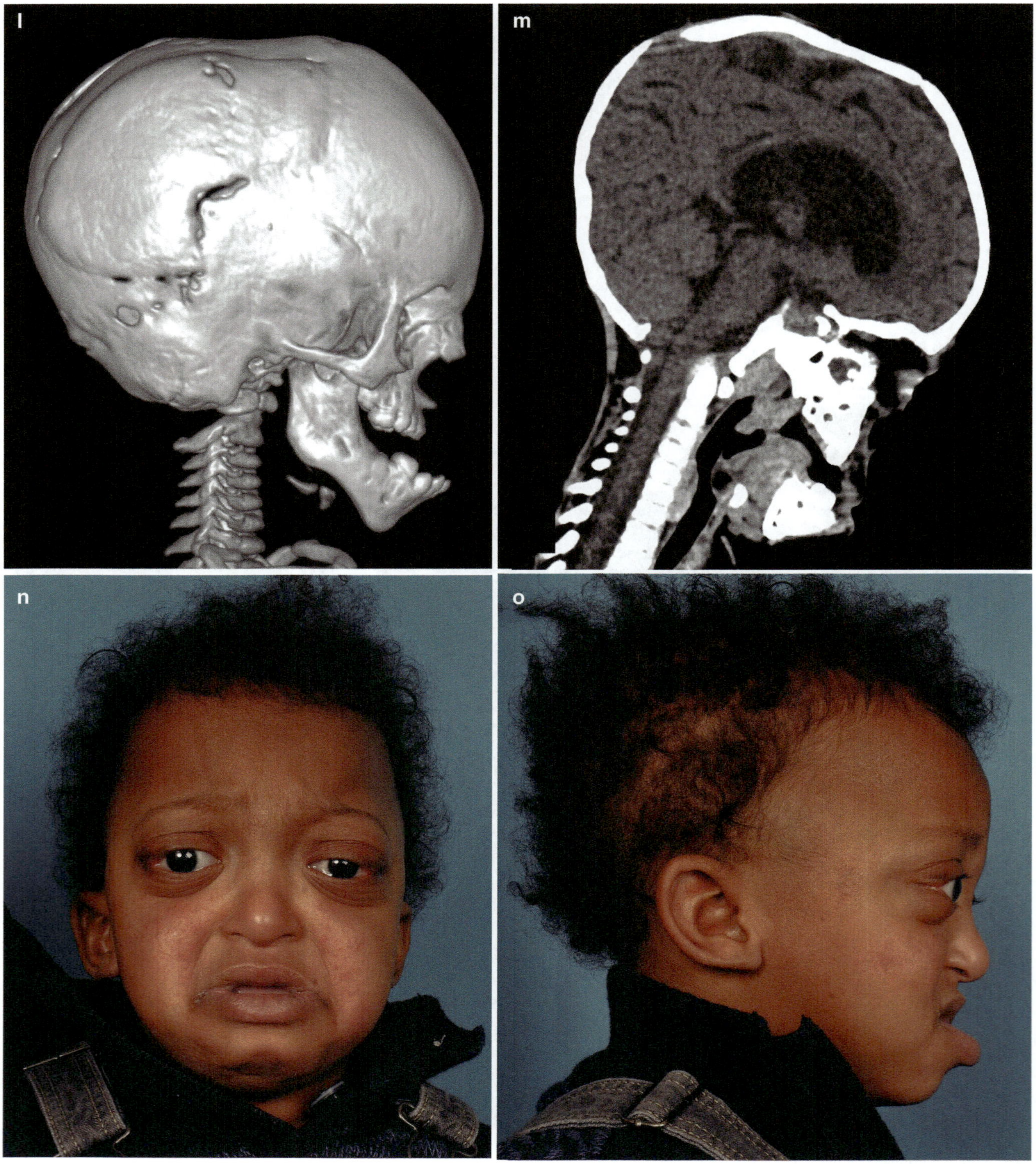

Fig. 2.20 (continued)

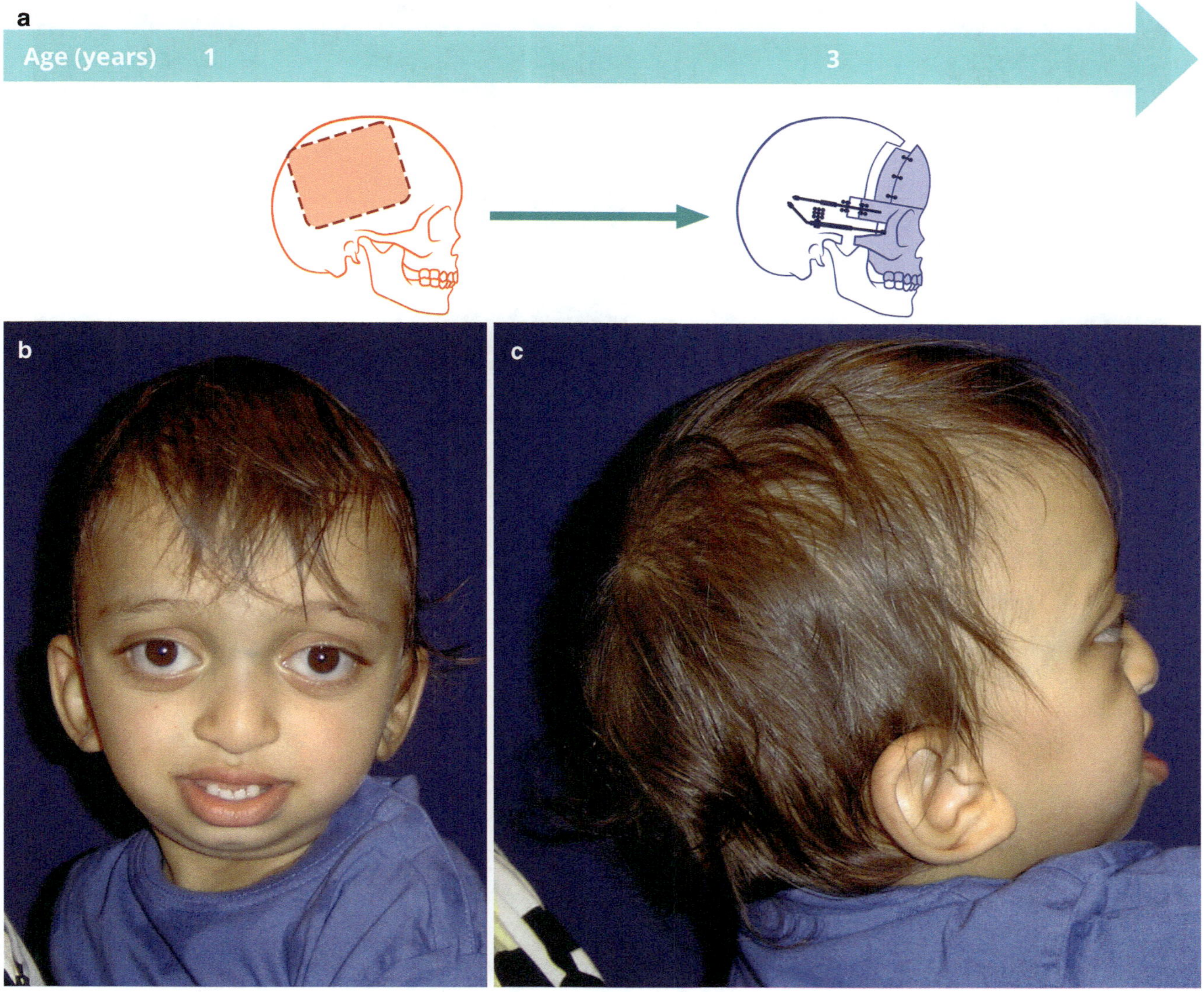

Fig. 2.21 (**a**, **b**, **c**) Eighteen-month-old patient with Crouzon syndrome presenting with maxillary hypoplasia and exorbitism. Head shape is normocephalic with reduced biparietal width. The posterior skull has a full round shape. Fundoscopic examination reveals papillary edema. Emergent skull decompression is indicated. CT scan shows pansynostosis. Given the head shape, biparietal decompression was decided rather than PVE to increase biparietal width. © Cassandra Vion. (**d**, **e**) Immediate postoperative CT scan aspect after biparietal decompression was performed at 18 months of age. (**f**, **g**) Clinical results at 23 months of age, 5 months after biparietal decompression. Papilledema was resolved. (**h**, **i**, **j**) CT scan at 23 months of age, 5 months after biparietal decompression, demonstrating biparietal expansion. Biparietal decompression allowed to delay FFMBA 1 year, when this patient developed severe OSA requiring FFMBA at age 33 months (AHI = 21 per hour)

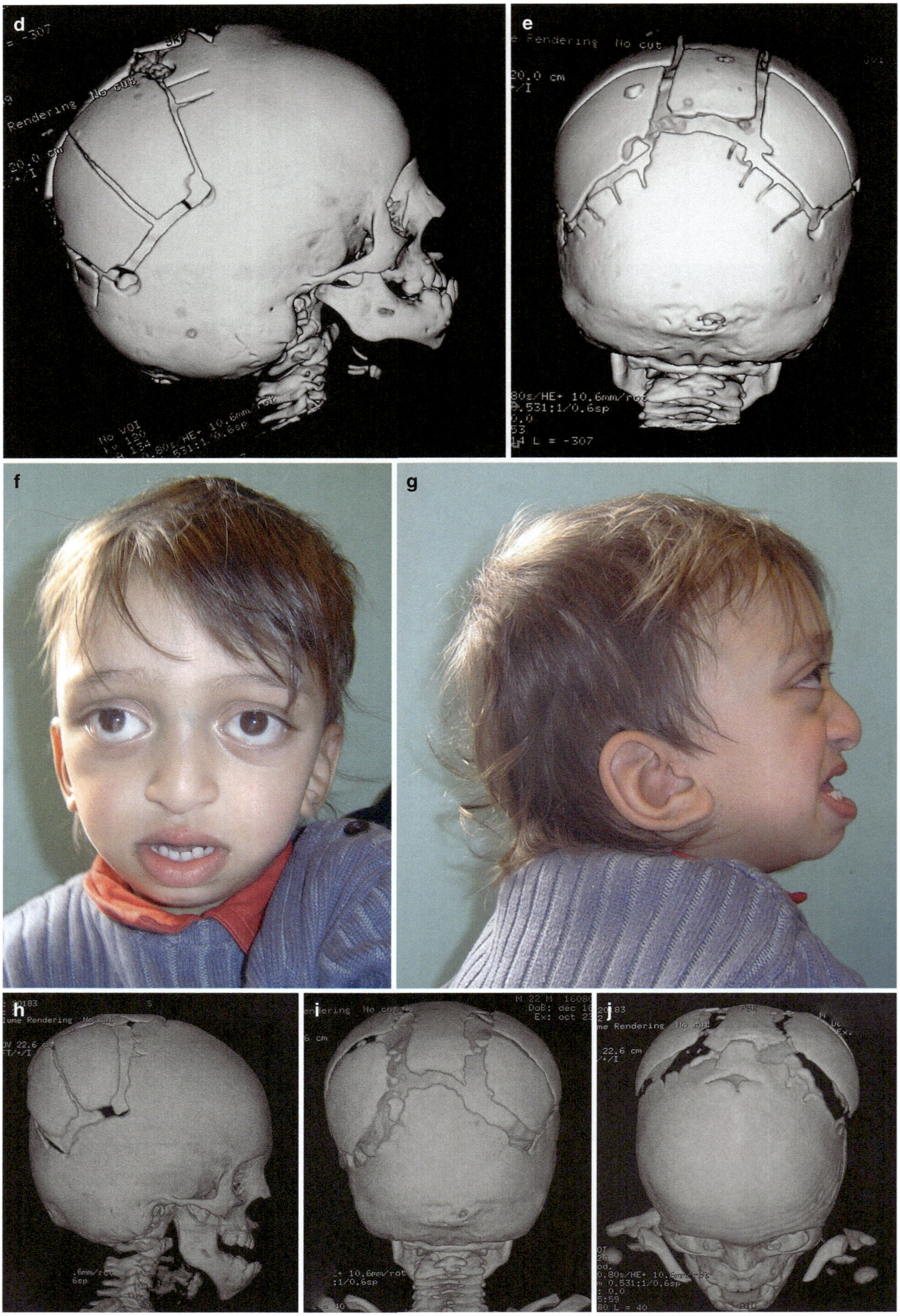

Fig. 2.21 (continued)

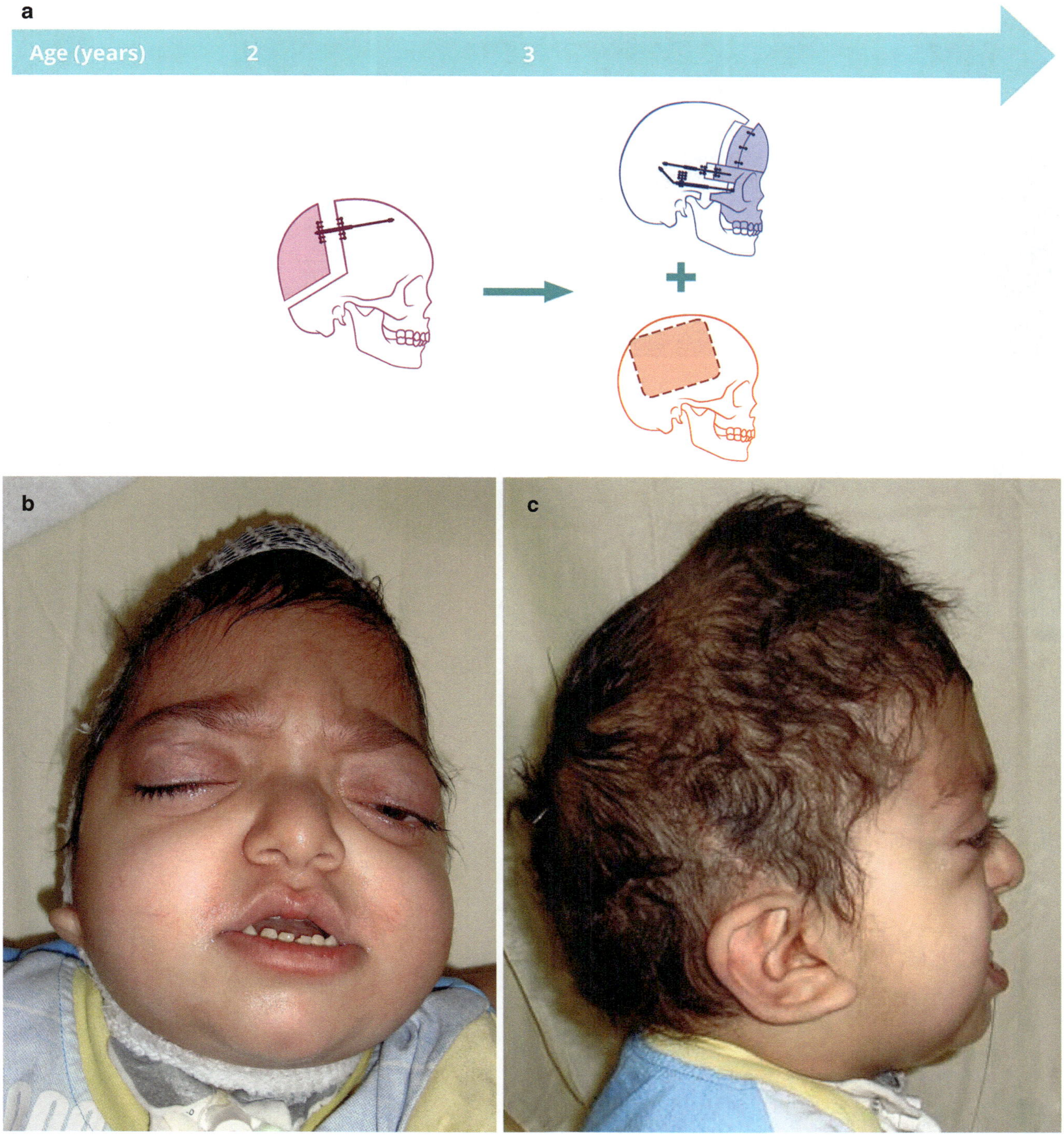

Fig. 2.22 (**a**, **b**, **c**) Thirty-month-old Crouzon patient with turricephaly and severe OSA (Apnea-Hypopnea Index was 41 per hour) presenting with tracheostomy. © Cassandra Vion. (**d**, **e**, **f**) PVE performed at 30 months of age with progressive distraction at 1 week, 3 weeks, and 6 weeks. (**g**, **h**, **i**) Clinical photographs 3 months after PVE. (j-m) Intraoperative photographs and postoperative CT scan of FFMBA associated with parietal enlargement and bregmatic hump removal were performed at 36 months of age. (**n**, **o**, **p**) Clinical results 3 months after FFMBA demonstrating overcorrection at the orbital level with enophthalmos and an edge-to-edge occlusion. (**q**, **r**, **s**) Clinical results 6 months after FFMBA demonstrating partial relapse and correction of enophthalmos. Internal distractors were removed and decannulation was performed. (**t**, **u**, **v**) Clinical results 12 months after FFMBA: exorbitism was properly corrected while occlusion was only partially improved. Polysomnography revealed the resolution of OSAS (AHI = 4 per hour)

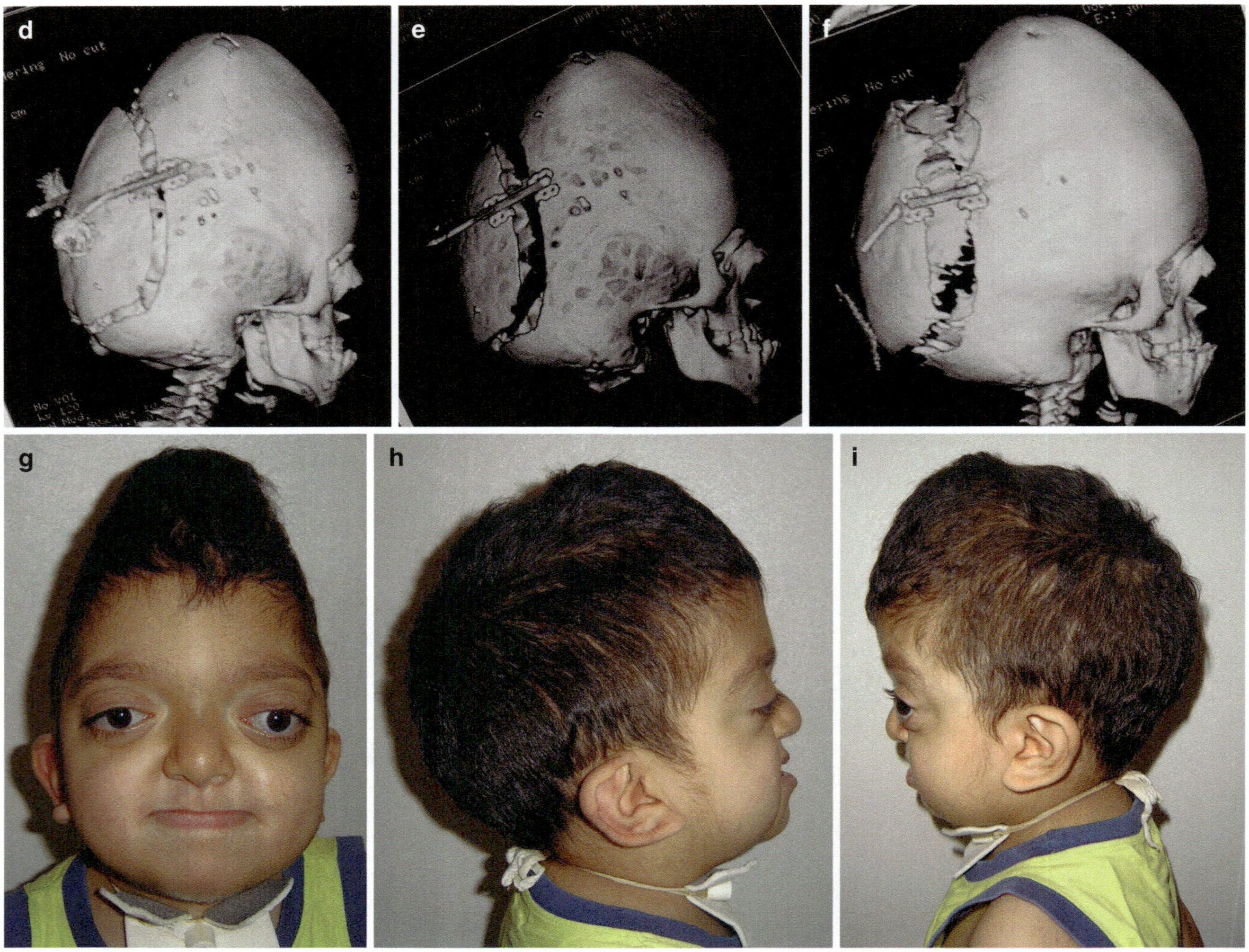

Fig. 2.22 (continued)

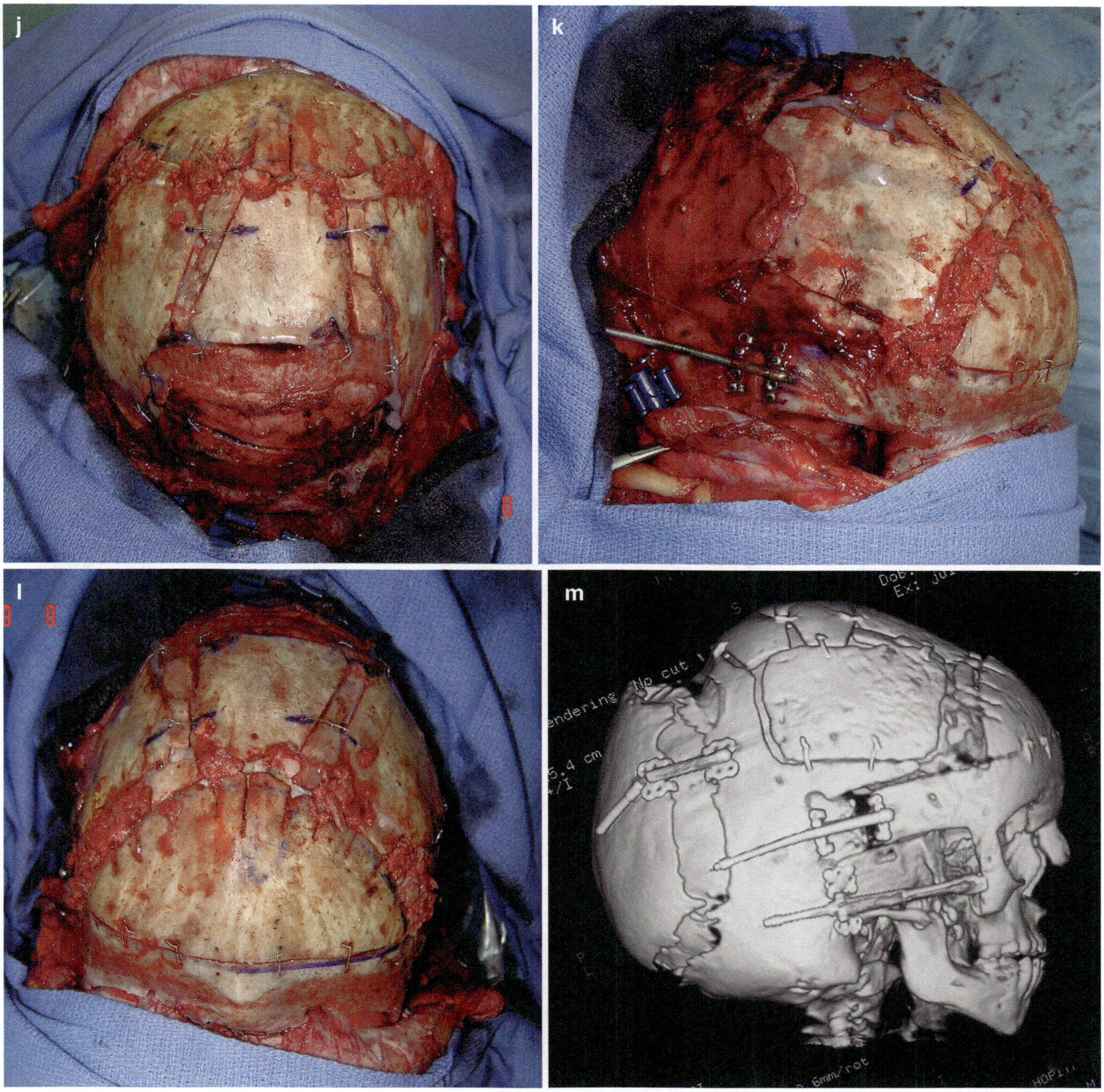

Fig. 2.22 (continued)

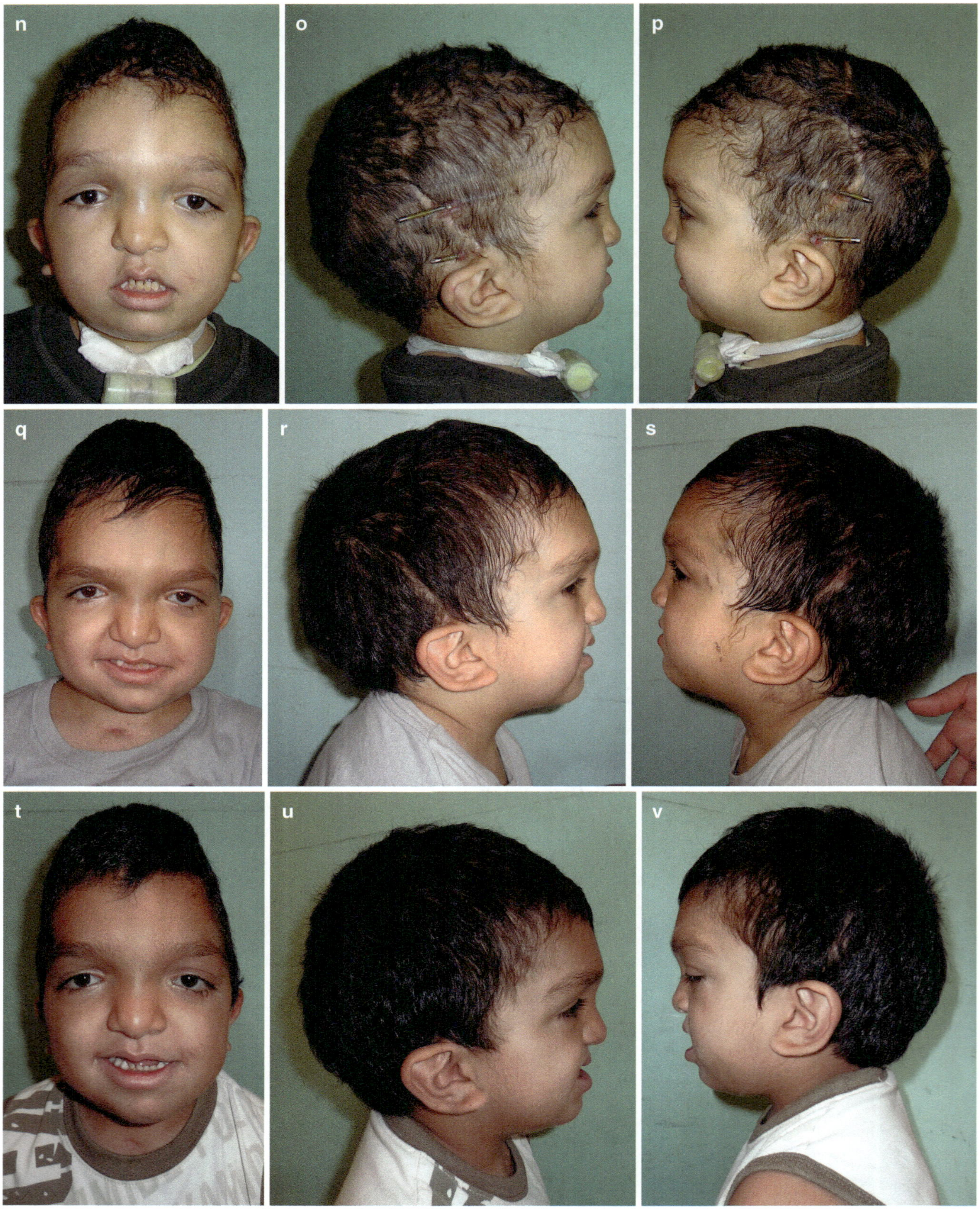

Fig. 2.22 (continued)

2.8 Posterior Expansion as an Essential Tool to Correct Turricephalic Head (Fig. 2.22)

In case of a patient presenting late (more than 2 years) with untreated Crouzon resulting in turricephalic appearance, PVE with distractors was successfully used to expand primarily the skull, and then at the time of FFMBA, biparietal expansion flaps were associated.

References

1. Arnaud E, Marchac A, Jeblaoui Y, et al. Spring-assisted posterior skull expansion without osteotomies. Childs Nerv Syst. 2012 Sep;28(9):1545–9.
2. Bozkurt S, Borghi A, van de Lande LS, et al. Computational modelling of patient specific spring assisted lambdoid craniosynostosis correction. Sci Rep. 2020 Oct 29;10(1):18693.
3. Rodgers W, Glass GE, Schievano S, et al. Spring-assisted Cranioplasty for the correction of nonsyndromic Scaphocephaly: a quantitative analysis of 100 consecutive cases. Plast Reconstr Surg. 2017 Jul;140(1):125–34.
4. Mathijssen IMJ, Driessen C, Versnel SL, et al. Posterior distraction using springs in syndromic and multisuture Craniosynostosis: improving the technique. J Craniofac Surg. 2020 Oct;31(7):2095–6.
5. Derderian CA, Wink JD, McGrath JL, et al. Volumetric changes in cranial vault expansion: comparison of fronto-orbital advancement and posterior cranial vault distraction osteogenesis. Plast Reconstr Surg. 2015 Jun;135(6):1665–72.
6. Sgouros S, Goldin JH, Hockley AD, et al. Posterior skull surgery in craniosynostosis. Childs Nerv Syst. 1996 Nov;12(11):727–33.
7. Nowinski D, Di Rocco F, Renier D, et al. Posterior cranial vault expansion in the treatment of craniosynostosis. Comparison of current techniques. Childs Nerv Syst. 2012 Sep;28(9):1537–44.
8. Swanson JW, Samra F, Bauder A, et al. An algorithm for managing syndromic Craniosynostosis using posterior vault distraction Osteogenesis. Plast Reconstr Surg. 2016 May;137(5):829e–41e.
9. Heller JB, Lazareff J, Gabbay JS, et al. Posterior cranial fossa box expansion leads to resolution of symptomatic cerebellar ptosis following Chiari I malformation repair. J Craniofac Surg. 2007 Mar;18(2):274–80.
10. Coll G, Lemaire J-J, Di Rocco F, et al. Human foramen magnum area and posterior cranial fossa volume growth in relation to Cranial Base Synchondrosis closure in the course of child development. Neurosurgery. 2016 Nov;79(5):722–35.
11. Hayward R. Venous hypertension and craniosynostosis. Childs Nerv Syst. 2005 Oct;21(10):880–8.
12. Florisson JMG, Barmpalios G, Lequin M, et al. Venous hypertension in syndromic and complex craniosynostosis: the abnormal anatomy of the jugular foramen and collaterals. J Craniomaxillofac Surg. 2015 Apr;43(3):312–8.
13. Ghali GZ, Zaki Ghali MG, Ghali EZ, et al. Intracranial venous hypertension in craniosynostosis: mechanistic underpinnings and therapeutic implications. World Neurosurg. 2018 Aug;6
14. Cornelissen MJ, de Goederen R, Doerga P, et al. Pilot study of intracranial venous physiology in craniosynostosis. J Neurosurg Pediatr. 2018 Jun;21(6):626–31.
15. Beuriat P-A, Puget S, Cinalli G, et al. Hydrocephalus treatment in children: long-term outcome in 975 consecutive patients. J Neurosurg Pediatr. 2017 Jul;20(1):10–8.
16. Hirsch JF, Hoppe-Hirsch E, Sainte-Rose C. Overdrainage in the treatment of hydrocephalus. Pediatrie. 1991;46(8–9):617–23.

3 Standardization of the Fronto-facial Monobloc Advancement Technique Developed at Necker-Enfants Malades Hospital

Between 2000 and 2020, 175 FFMBA have been performed. Although slight modifications were introduced along the way, the technique was rather well standardized and could be summarized as follows.

FFMBA is performed in a supine position with oral intubation (Figs. 3.1 and 3.2). The tube is sutured to the lower jaw using nonabsorbable braided sutures (Fig. 3.3). Bilateral tarsorrhaphies are placed using nonabsorbable monofilament sutures (Fig. 3.4). The child is positioned on a headrest and two chest rolls—one under the thighs and one under the shoulders—are taped to the operating table to prevent him from sliding down during the procedure (Fig. 3.2). An instrument table is fixed to the operating table at approximately 20–25 centimeters from the chin of the patient (Fig. 3.1).

Skin markings are made for a zigzag or undulated bicoronal incision (Fig. 3.5). Usually, the scar from a previous posterior vault expansion is used. The hair is shaved over a 3-cm wide band around the incision line. Infiltration in subgaleal and subdermal planes using 1 mg/l adrenaline solution is performed along the incision line.

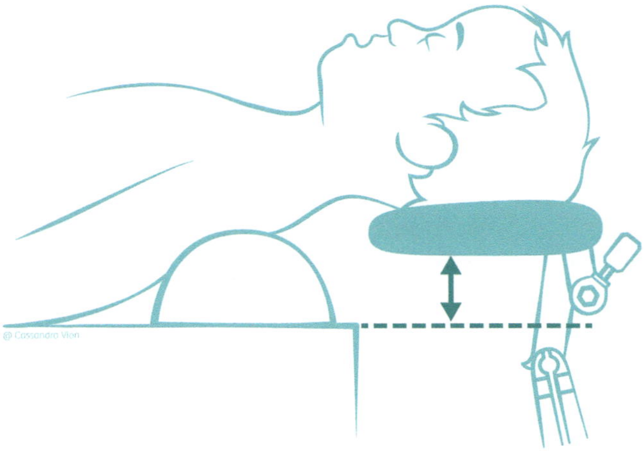

Fig. 3.2 Position of the headrest relative to the operating table © Cassandra Vion

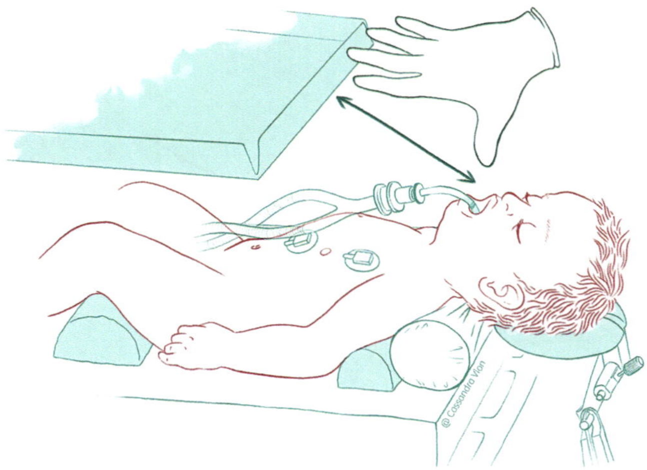

Fig. 3.1 Operating room set up and patient positioning © Cassandra Vion

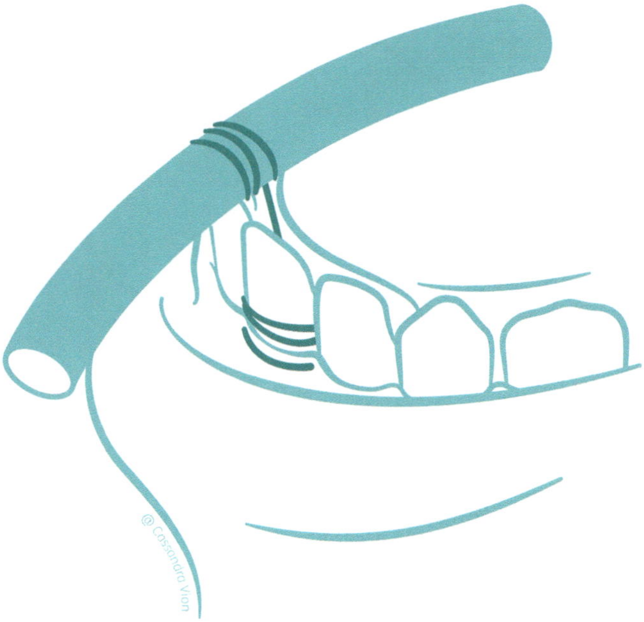

Fig. 3.3 Fixation of the tube to the lower jaw © Cassandra Vion

E. Arnaud et al., *Frontofacial Monobloc Advancement with Internal Distraction*, https://doi.org/10.1007/978-3-031-07574-2_3

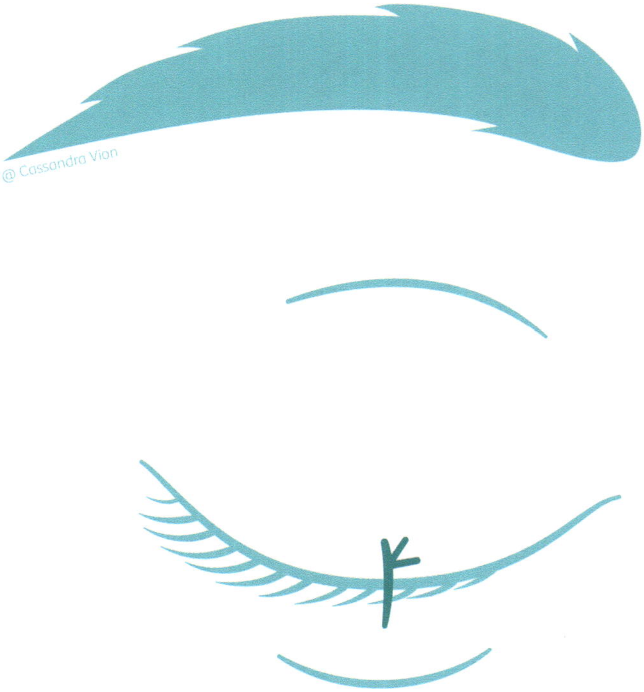

Fig. 3.4 Tarsorrhaphy © Cassandra Vion

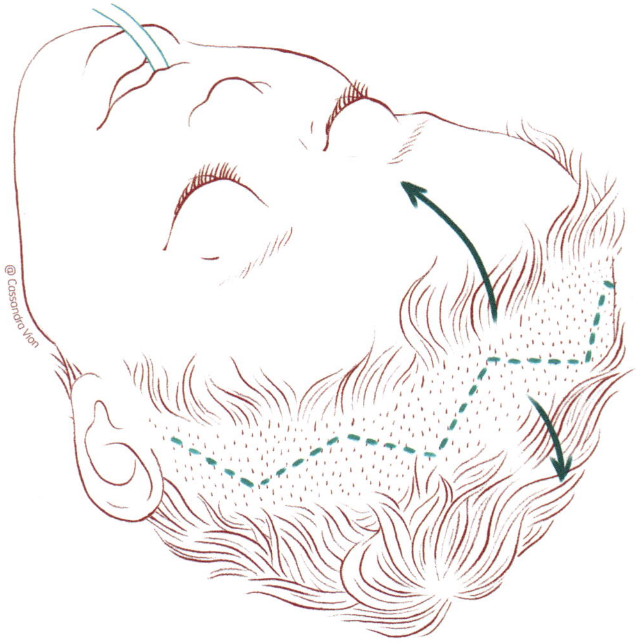

Fig. 3.5 Skin incision © Cassandra Vion

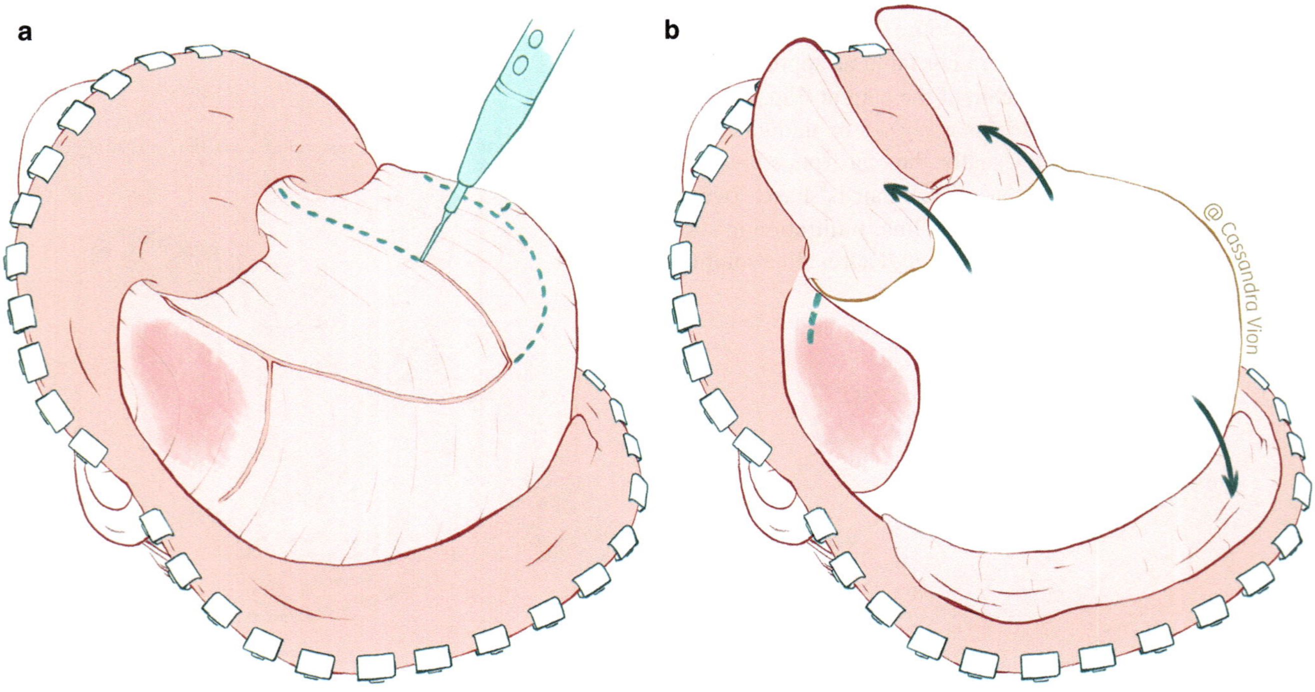

Fig. 3.6 (**a**, **b**) Elevation of the periosteal flaps and exposure of the skull vault © Cassandra Vion

The subgaleal plane is undermined down to the superior orbital ridge and on the surface of the superficial layer of the deep temporal fascia, in order to avoid facial nerve branch injuries. Two periosteal flaps are elevated and irrigated by the supraorbital and supratrochlear pedicles (Figs. 3.6, and 3.7). A small horizontal incision of the superficial layer of the deep temporal fascia is performed in order to prepare for the Tessier maneuver (Fig. 3.8a). The orbital roofs and the

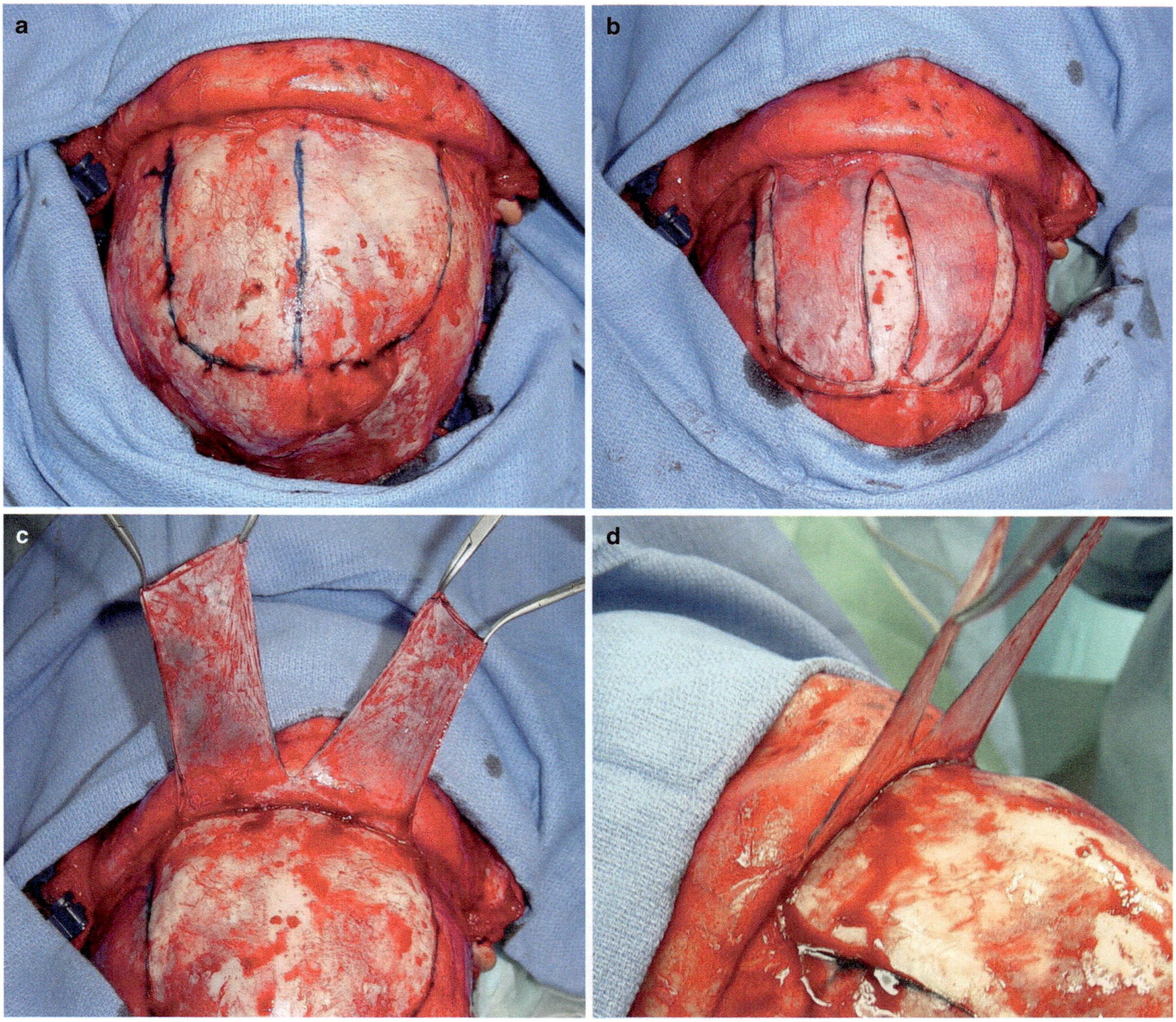

Fig. 3.7 (**a**, **b**, **c**, **d**) Elevation of the periosteal flaps, intraoperative view

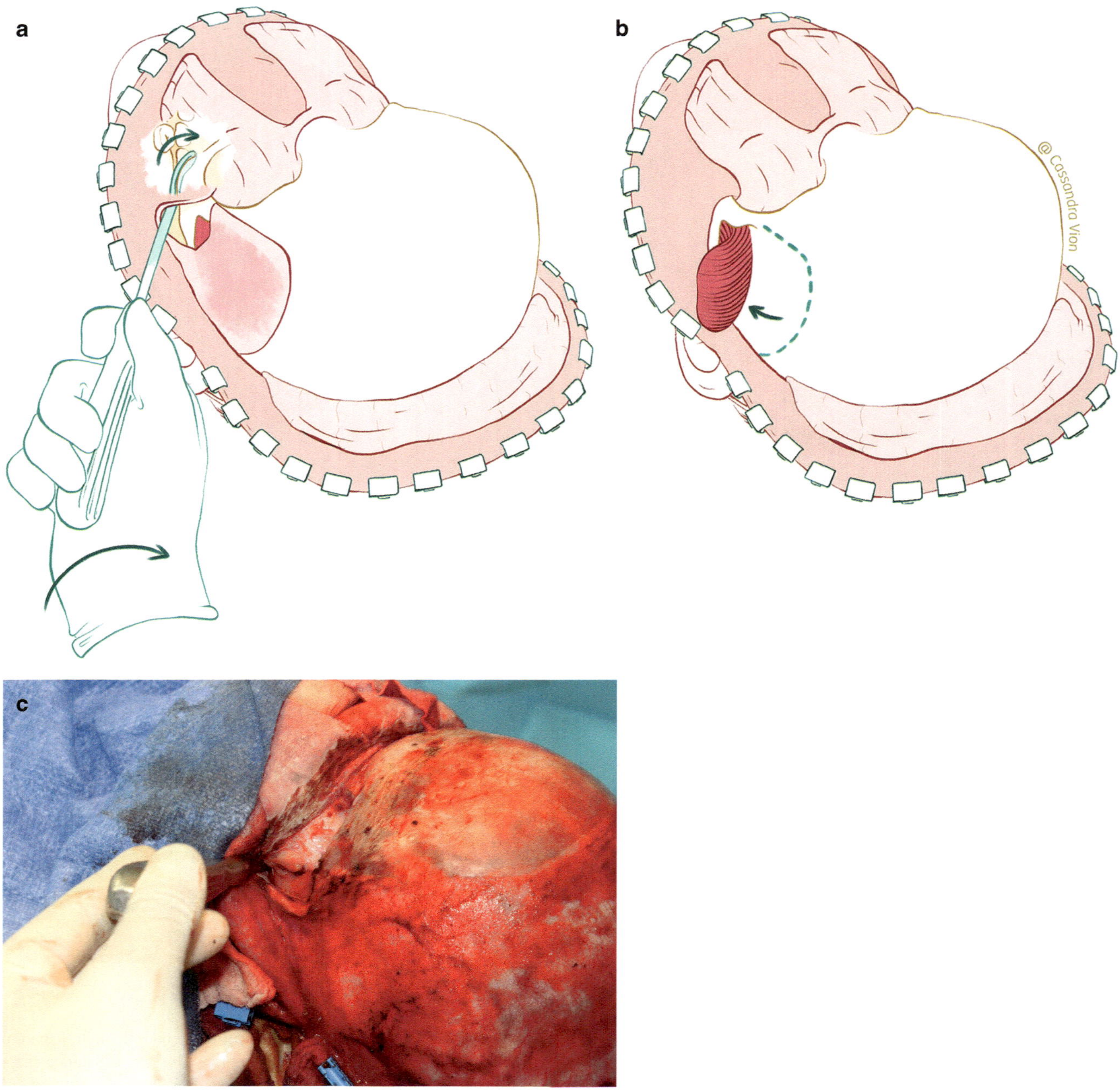

Fig. 3.8 (**a**) Tessier maneuver exposing the zygomatic surface and the zygomatic arch, performed before raising the temporal muscle but after dissecting the lateral orbital wall from the orbital contents. © Cassandra Vion (**b**) Raising of the temporal muscle and exposure of the lateral orbital wall. © Cassandra Vion (**c**) Intraoperative photograph demonstrating the Tessier maneuver

lateral orbital walls are dissected using a periosteal elevator. The bony vertex is exposed.

The surface of the zygoma and the zygomatic arch are exposed using the Tessier maneuver before raising the temporal muscles (Fig. 3.8a, c). The temporal muscles are then raised, providing exposure to the lateral orbital wall (Fig. 3.8b).

Burr holes are performed lateral to the forehead, in sufficient numbers to safely raise the forehead bone as a unit (Figs. 3.9, 3.10, and 3.11). The lower limit of the forehead is located 1 cm above the upper orbital rim. The forehead and two laterally adjacent coronal bony segments (Paternoster side-wings) are raised using a craniotome and/or piezosurgery. The tongue and groove designs of the temporal osteotomies are illustrated in Fig. 3.13.

Deep tongue and groove designs are performed in the temporal regions with an anteroposterior length of 5 cm. An oscillating saw can be used for a cleaner cut of the vertical osteotomy at the edge of the tongue and groove (Figs. 3.11 and 3.12). Piezoelectric surgery can alternatively be used to

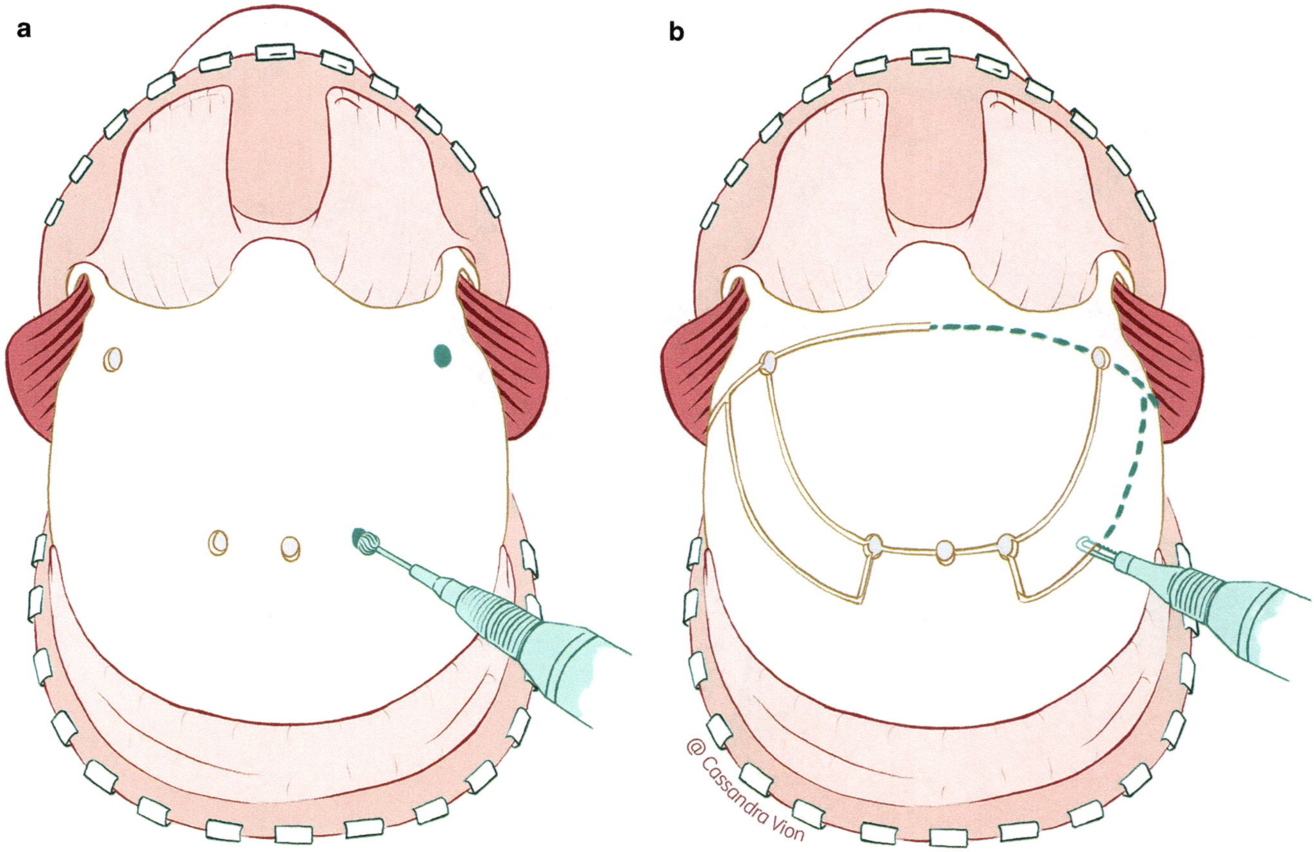

Fig. 3.9 (**a**) Burr holes lateral to the forehead, which is sectioned 1 cm above the upper orbital rim. (**b**) Two lateral coronal side-wings are raised on both sides of the forehead © Cassandra Vion

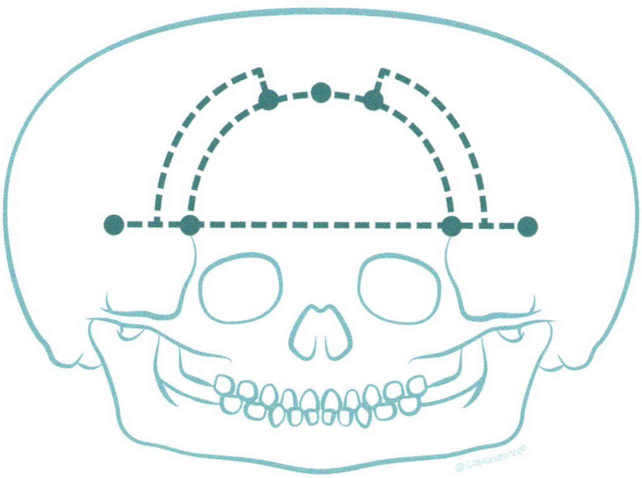

Fig. 3.10 Frontal osteotomy design © Cassandra Vion

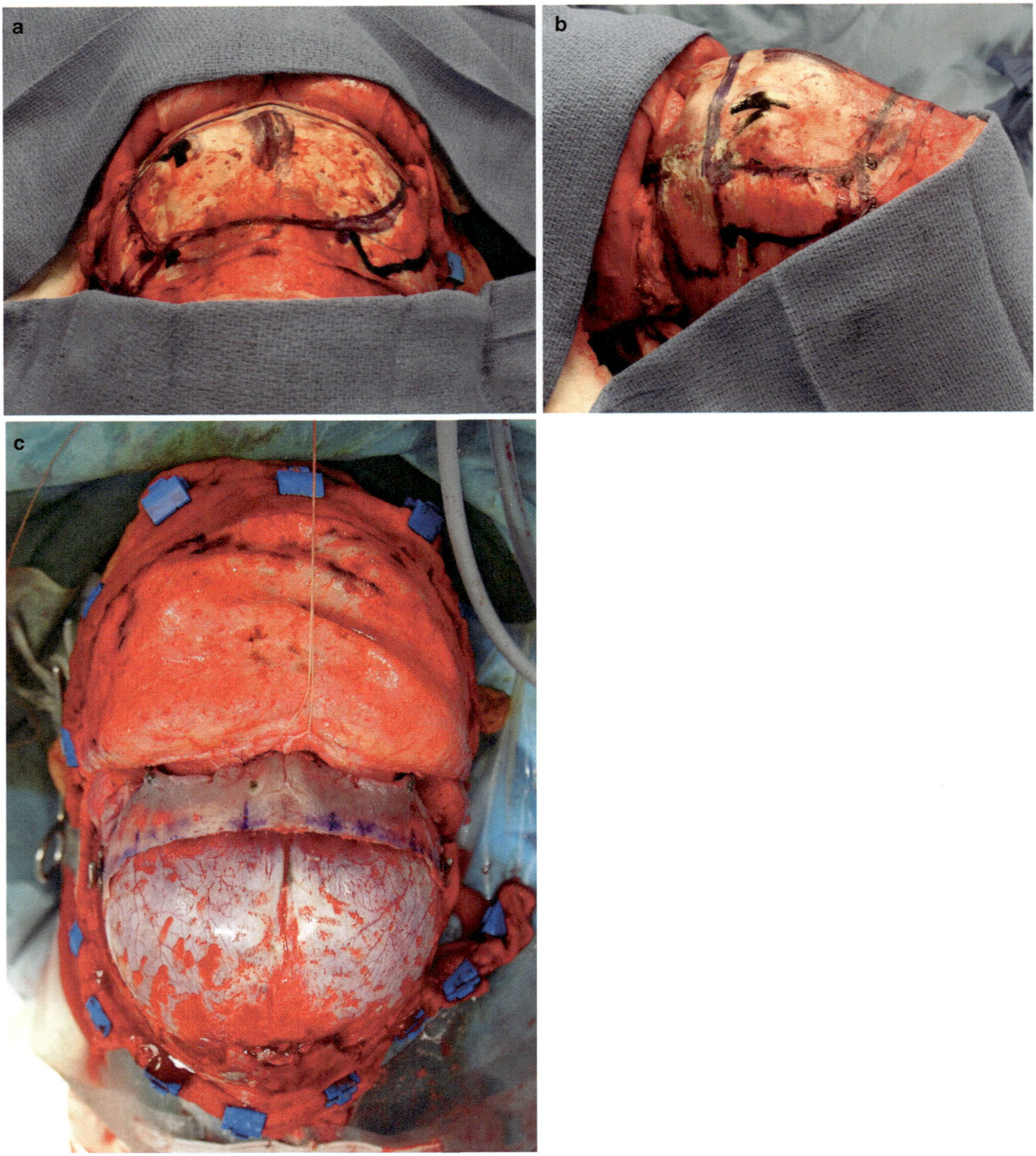

Fig. 3.11 (**a, b**) Lateral coronal bony side-wings. (**c**) Forehead raised 1 cm above the upper orbital rim

perform all the previous steps. The zygomatic arches are sectioned using a reciprocating saw (Fig. 3.13).

The lateral orbital wall is sectioned with the reciprocating saw directed upward, until the osteotomy line meets the previous osteotomy at the lower border of the temporal tongue and groove design (Fig. 3.14). The reciprocating saw is then oriented downward inside that same lateral orbital osteotomy line, to cut the body of the zygoma and the lateral part of the orbital floor.

The osteotomy of the orbital floor is performed using the reciprocating saw 2 mm anterior to the inferior orbital fissure. The osteotomy is extended toward the medial orbital

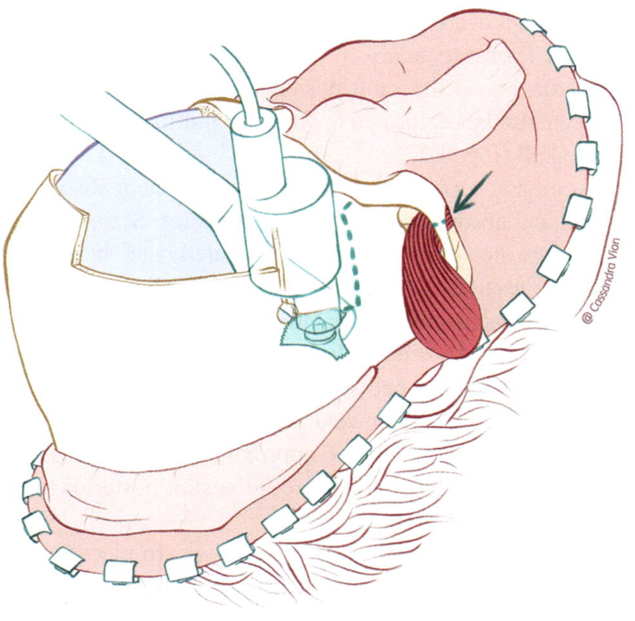

Fig. 3.12 Tongue and groove temporal osteotomies and section of the zygomatic arches © Cassandra Vion

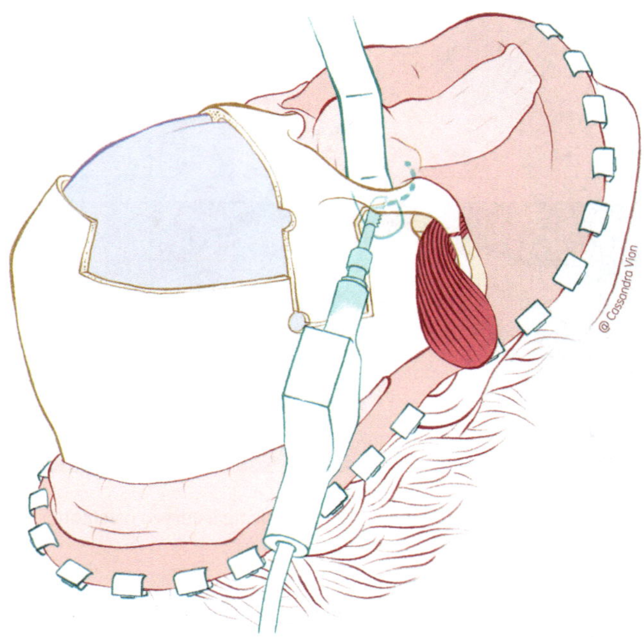

Fig. 3.14 Osteotomy of the lateral orbital wall © Cassandra Vion

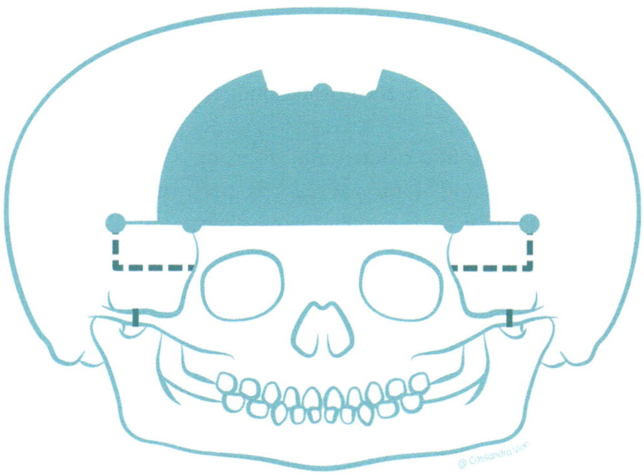

Fig. 3.13 Tongue and groove design after forehead elevation © Cassandra Vion

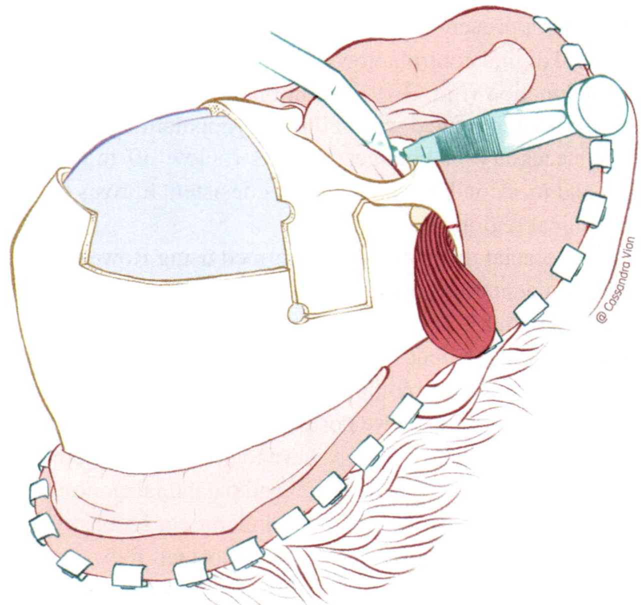

Fig. 3.15 Osteotomies of the orbital floor and medial orbital wall using a curved osteotome © Cassandra Vion

wall using a curved osteotome oriented posteriorly, while applying extreme caution not to section the inferior orbital rim (Figs. 3.15 and 3.16). In fact, the orbits are very shallow in FCST and the osteotomy line has to be posterior enough to avoid sectioning the inferior orbital rim anteriorly. A critical instrument in this step of the procedure is a curved lighted retractor with built-in suction. It allows visualizing the orbital floor and protecting the orbital content while performing the osteotomy.

Three malleable retractor blades are then used to protect the temporal lobe under the lesser wing of the sphenoid bone, the eyeball, and the frontal lobe dura mater. The orbital roof osteotomy is then performed using a reciprocating saw starting at the posterior border of the lesser wing toward the midline (Fig. 3.17a). Piezoelectric surgery can also be used for this step of the procedure.

On the midline, a small dural extension is a constant anatomic finding within the foramen caecum (Fig. 3.17b). It is dissected using bipolar electrocautery (Fig. 3.17c, d). The midline osteotomy of the ethmoid and the septum/vomer is performed using the reciprocating saw (and/or with the sup-

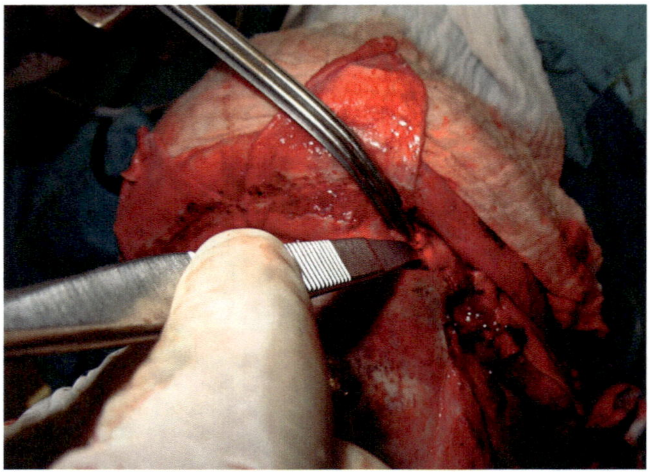

Fig. 3.16 Osteotomy of the orbital floor using a curved osteotome and an illuminated retractor with built-in suction

port of piezosurgery) (Fig. 3.17f). It is then completed with a curved osteotome all the way down to the vomer (Figs. 3.17e and 3.18).

Pterygomaxillary disjunction is performed using an infratemporal approach with an elevator or a curved osteotome. Intraoral digital control allows assessing the completeness of the disjunction (Fig. 3.19). Additional disjunction using an elevator that is rotated within the pterygopalatine junction is often necessary in younger patients (below 30 months of age) and in secondary cases, due to consistent fibrosis of this anatomical region.

Craniofacial disjunction is performed using Rowe forceps without indentations protected intra-orally by silicon sleeves (Figs. 3.20 and 3.21). A counterclockwise movement (when the head of the patient is directed toward the right side) produces the disjunction, completed by careful lateral and clockwise movements to achieve posterior disjunctions in the nasal and oral areas. The two forceps have to be handled together in order to avoid midline disjunction and palatal lacerations.

The anterior midline gap of the skull base is reconstructed using the two initially designed periosteal flaps, pulled through the orbital roof osteotomies (Figs. 3.22 and 3.23). One flap is used to cover the midline gap and is sutured to the bandeau using two trans-osseous 5.0 nonabsorbable nylon sutures and then glued. The other flap is used as a secondary cover, sutured to the bandeau, and also glued. No sutures are performed on the dura in order to avoid tears during distraction.

The forehead is remodeled using barrel-stave osteotomies (Figs. 3.24, 3.25, and 3.26). Its inferior border is trimmed laterally to allow a posterior tilt after fixation. Forehead barrel-staving is performed to control curvature and triangular lateral trimming allows inducing a posterior tilt after fixation. This tilt decreases the volume of the frontal dead space that will form secondary to the fronto-facial advancement. Barrel-staving of the vault posterior to the forehead osteotomy can also be performed in order to optimize the curvature of the skull (Fig. 3.27).

Fixation is performed using 4.0 monofilament absorbable sutures and absorbable osteosynthesis plates. Stainless steel sutures are not used anymore. The Paternoster bony side-wings are used to cover the lateral defects and fixed laterally to the forehead using absorbable sutures.

Internal cranio-orbital distractors are placed and fixed using 4 mm blunt-tipped screws with potentially additional absorbable rivets (Sonicweld Rx®, KLS Martin Group). Intraoperative distraction of approximately 5 mm is performed. The activation arm pierces the skin posterior to the coronal incision line (Fig. 3.28a).

Internal temporo-zygomatic distractors are placed under the temporal muscle and fixed using the superior fixation zone only—the inferior fixation zone has to be sectioned. The anterior arm of the temporo-zygomatic distractor is positioned low on the zygoma, close to the zygomatic arch osteotomy line. A small notch to secure the position of the anterior arm can be performed on the posterior aspect of the external orbital wall using gouge forceps. The activation arm is extruded posterior to the coronal incision line (Figs. 3.28b, 3.29, and 3.30).

Fronto-zygomatic osteosynthesis using a curved 1.5 mm titanium plate and 4 mm screws is performed to prevent fronto-zygomatic disjunction during distraction (Fig. 3.31).

When present, a vertex bulge can be remodeled using a sand dollar design and repositioned using fibrin glue (Fig. 3.32).

In younger patients (before 30 months of age), transfacial pinning using a 2.1 Kirschner wire can be discussed, through the bodies of the zygoma, in order to avoid maxilla-zygomatic disjunction during distraction (Figs. 3.33 and 3.34). Transfacial pins are also used for external traction in very early FFMBA. Due to frequent severe facial retrusion in younger cases with small zygoma, the pinning can be difficult and lead to considerable damage to the tooth germs.

The temporal muscle is repositioned over the distractors and fixed using 4.0 monofilament absorbable sutures, in order to prevent temporal hollowing (Fig. 3.35). A lower back-cut of the muscle can be required to allow adequate transposition anteriorly.

Residual bone gaps are filled using bone powder collected during the procedure. The powder is secured using fibrin glue (Fig. 3.36).

External canthopexies are performed using surgical stainless steel sutures and fixed to the fronto-zygomatic plates with moderate over-correction (Figs. 3.37, 3.38, and 3.39).

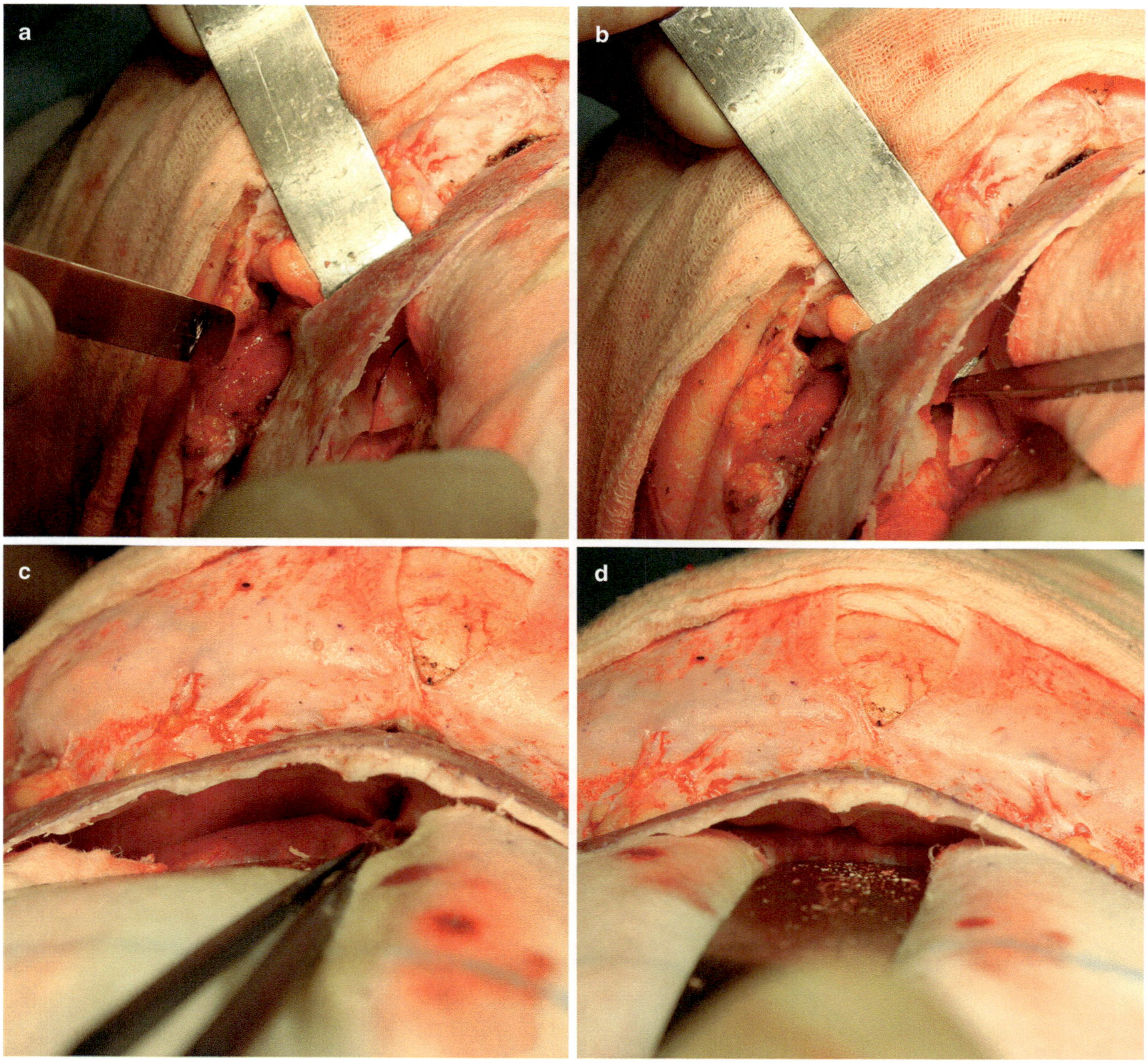

Fig. 3.17 (**a**) Osteotomy of the orbital roof starting at the lesser sphenoid wing. Malleable retractor blades protect the eyeball and the temporal lobe beneath the lesser sphenoid wing. (**b**) Complete release is verified at the convergence point of three osteotomies: lateral orbital, lesser wing, and inferior tenon. (**c**) Midline dural extension penetrating the foramen cecum. (**d**) Dissection of the foramen caecum using gentle bipolar electrocautery to retract the dura. (**e**) Skull base osteotomy using the reciprocating saw. Malleable blades are used to protect the dura mater and the orbital content © Cassandra Vion. (**f**) The skull base osteotomy is extended inferiorly at the medial wall of the orbit using a curved osteotome oriented posteriorly to the posterior lacrimal crest © Cassandra Vion

The posterior periosteum is redraped anteriorly to cover the bone fragments and glued (Fig. 3.40a). Suspension using absorbable 4.0 monofilament sutures can be used to drape the periosteum over the vault surface. Bilateral external drainage is used without aspiration, in case of unnoticed cerebrospinal fluid leak (Fig. 3.40b). The skin is closed using 3.0 and 4.0 braided absorbable sutures with minimal subcutaneous points. Nasopharyngeal tubes with transseptal fixation are used to maintain airway patency. The tips of the transfacial pin are protected using silicon tubes (Fig. 3.40c). A non-compressive dressing is made. All patients are managed in the pediatric intensive care unit after surgery. Extubation occurs on days 3–5, and nasopharyngeal tubes and tarsorrhaphies are removed at the same time. The activation phase of distraction generally starts on day 2 after a control CT scan.

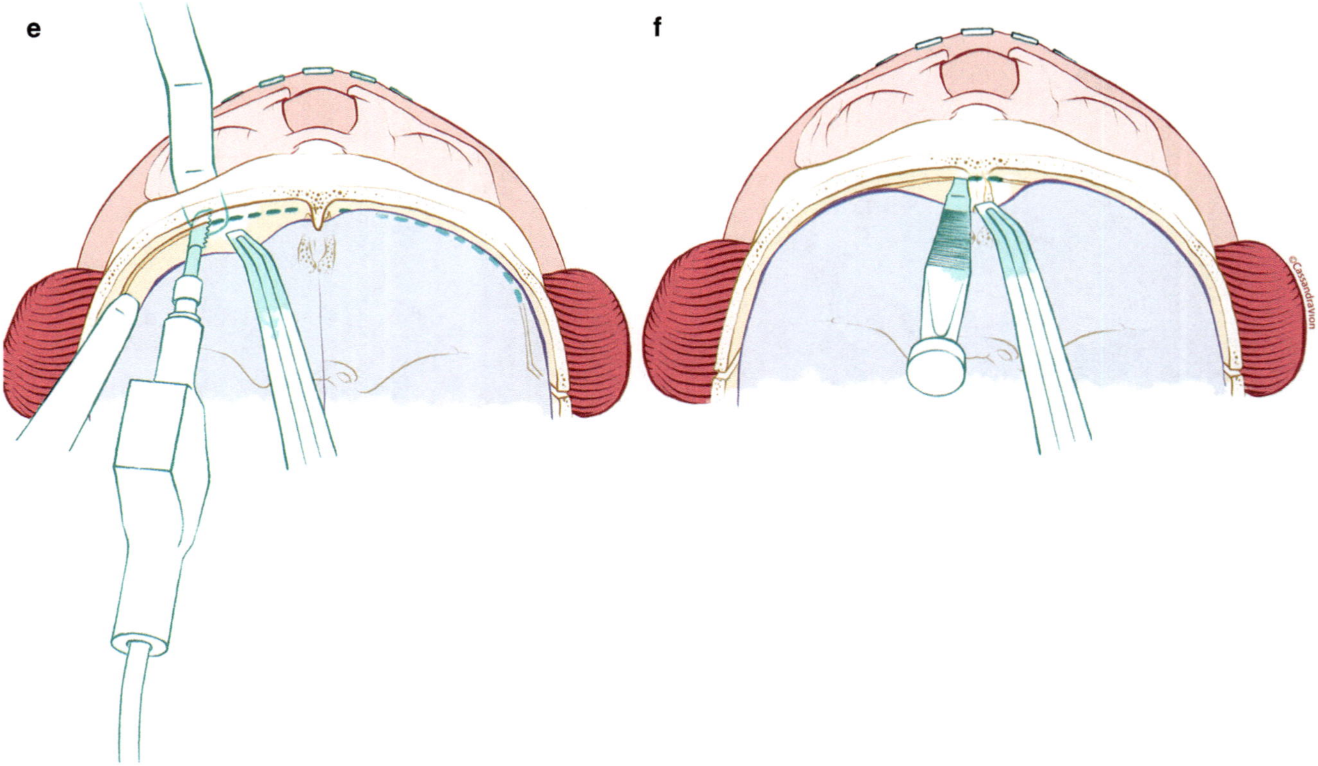

Fig. 3.17 (continued)

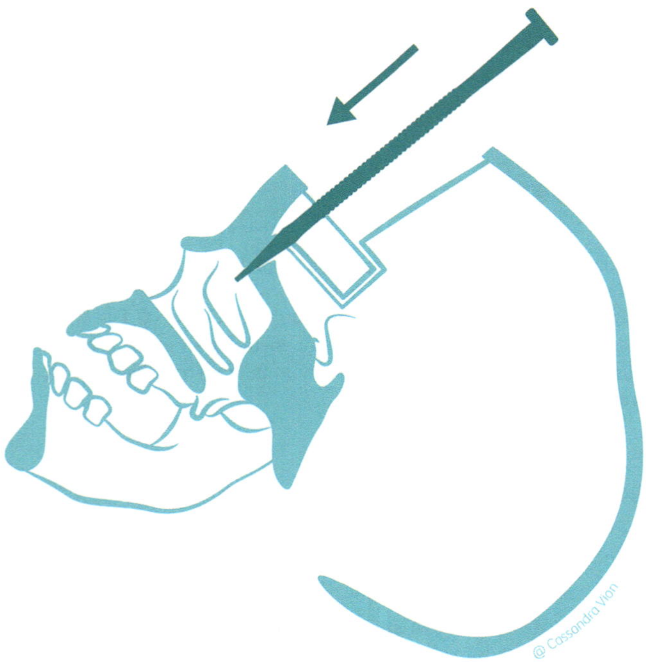

Fig. 3.18 Position of the osteotome when performing the midline osteotomy of the ethmoid and the vomer on a sagittal view © Cassandra Vion

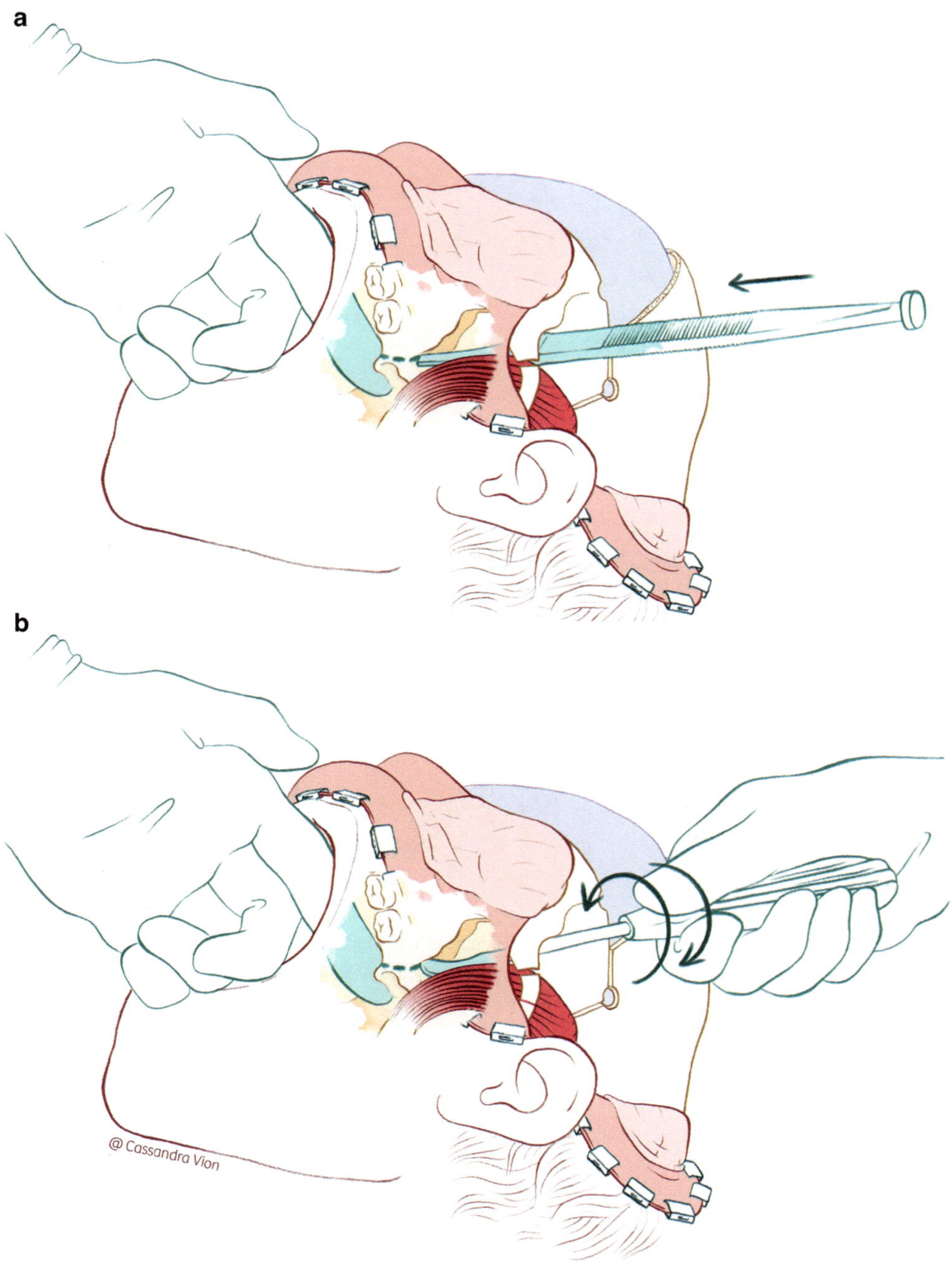

Fig. 3.19 (**a**) Pterygomaxillary disjunction using a curved osteotome. (**b**) Additional disjunction using an elevator © Cassandra Vion

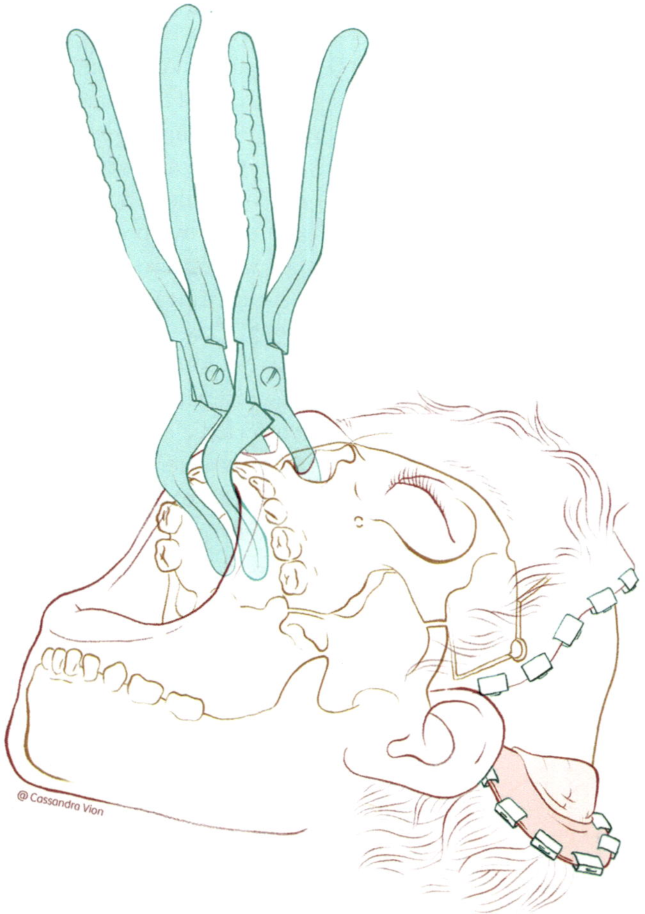

Fig. 3.20 Craniofacial disjunction using Rowe forceps © Cassandra Vion

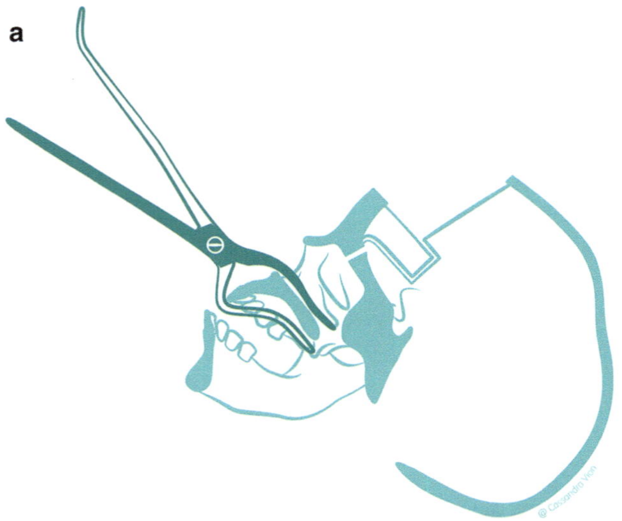

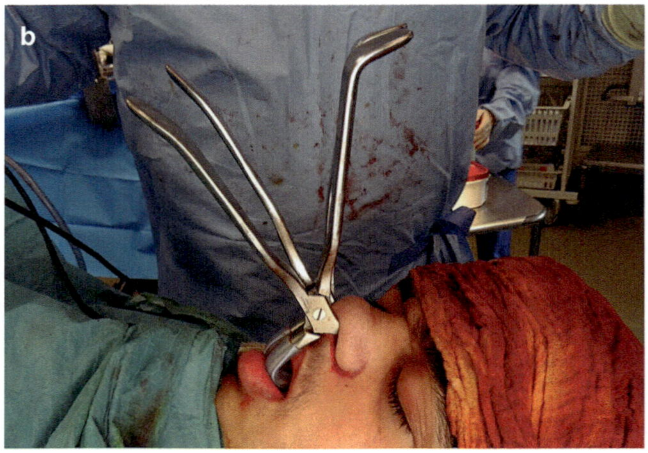

Fig. 3.21 (**a**) Position of the Rowe forceps on a sagittal section before performing craniofacial disjunction. (**b**) Intraoperative view of the position of the Rowe forceps before craniofacial disjunction

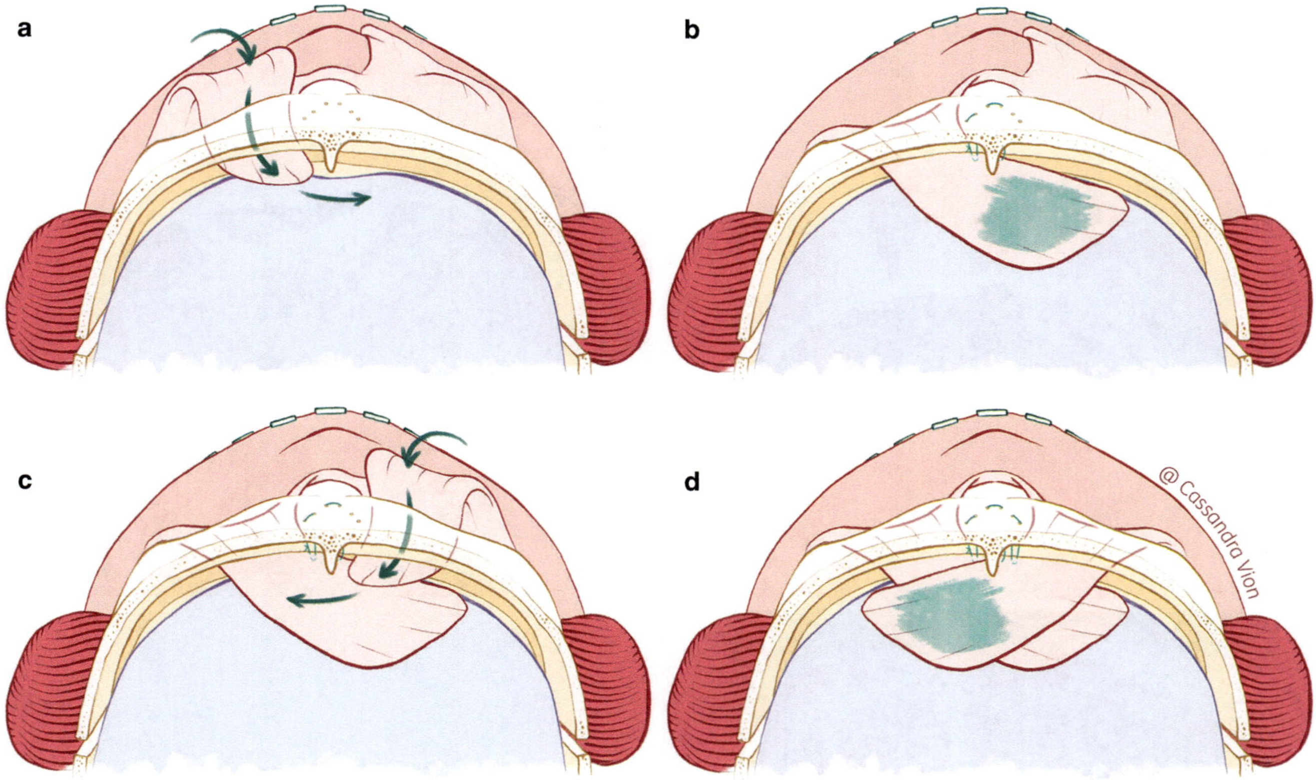

Fig. 3.22 (**a**) Anterior skull base transposition of transorbital periosteal flaps. (**b**) The left flap is sutured to the bandeau toward the right side and glued. (**c**) The same procedure is performed with the right flap toward the left side © Cassandra Vion

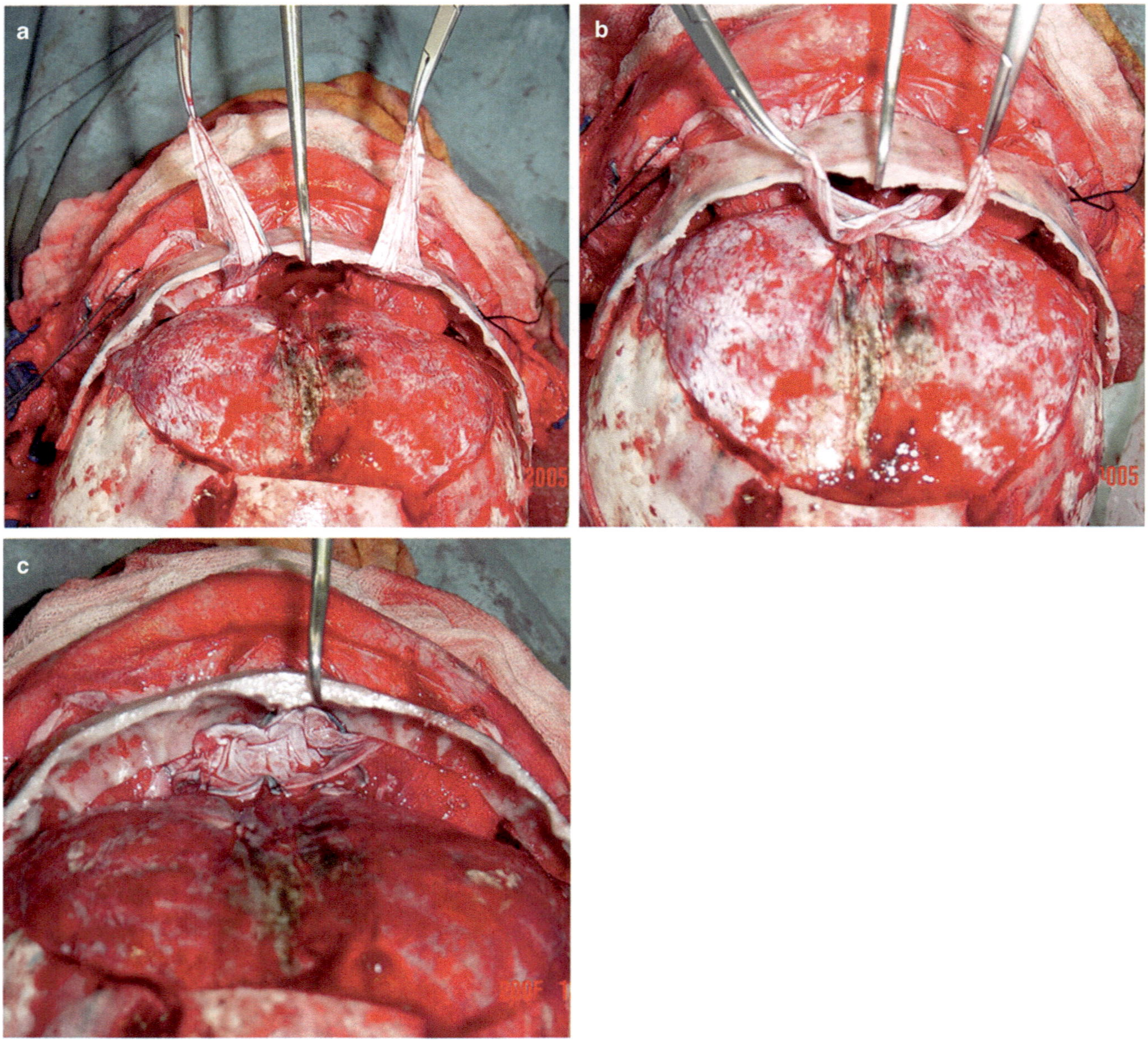

Fig. 3.23 Intraoperative views of anterior skull base reconstruction. (**a**) Transorbital periosteal flaps. (**b**) Crossing of the flaps and coverage of the anterior midline. (**c**) Final sealing using trans-osseous sutures and glue

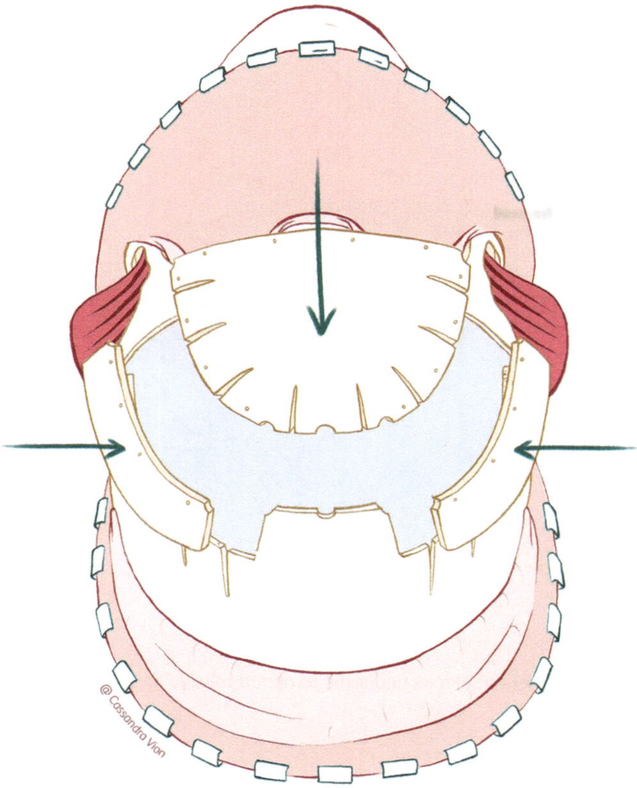

Fig. 3.24 Forehead reconstruction after lateral trimming and barrel-stave osteotomies. Positioning of the two lateral bony side-wings © Cassandra Vion

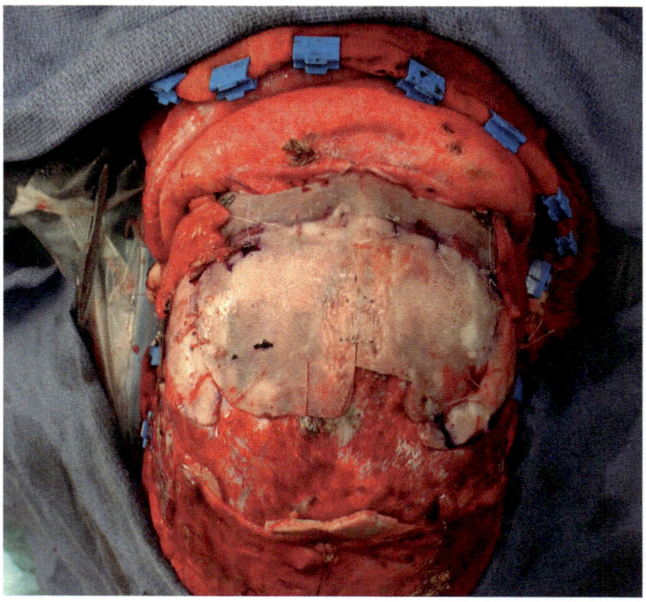

Fig. 3.25 Intraoperative view of a reconstructed forehead after lateral trimming, barrel-stave osteotomies, and fixation of the lateral bony side-wings. Fixation is performed using a combination of monofilament absorbable sutures and absorbable osteosynthesis plates

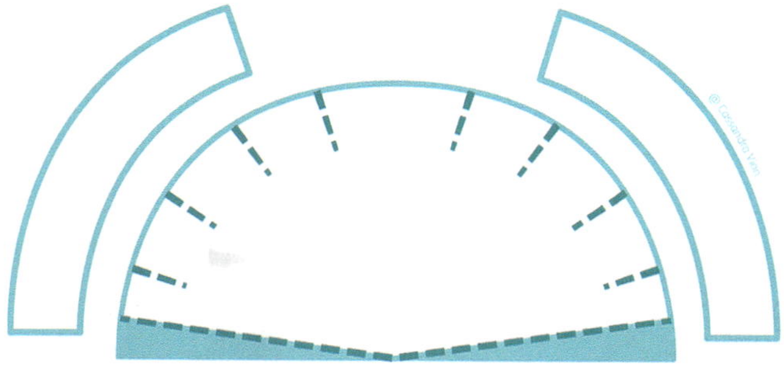

Fig. 3.26 Lateral triangular trimming of the inferior border of the forehead in order to induce a posterior tilt after firm fixation to the bandeau © Cassandra Vion

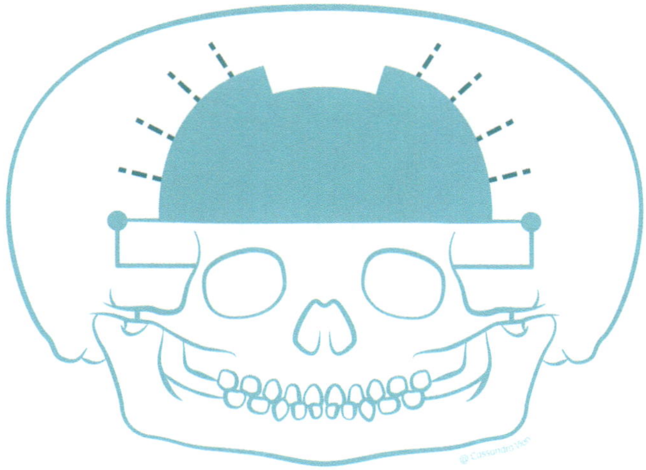

Fig. 3.27 Barrel-stave osteotomies of the skull vault posterior of the forehead osteotomy line © Cassandra Vion

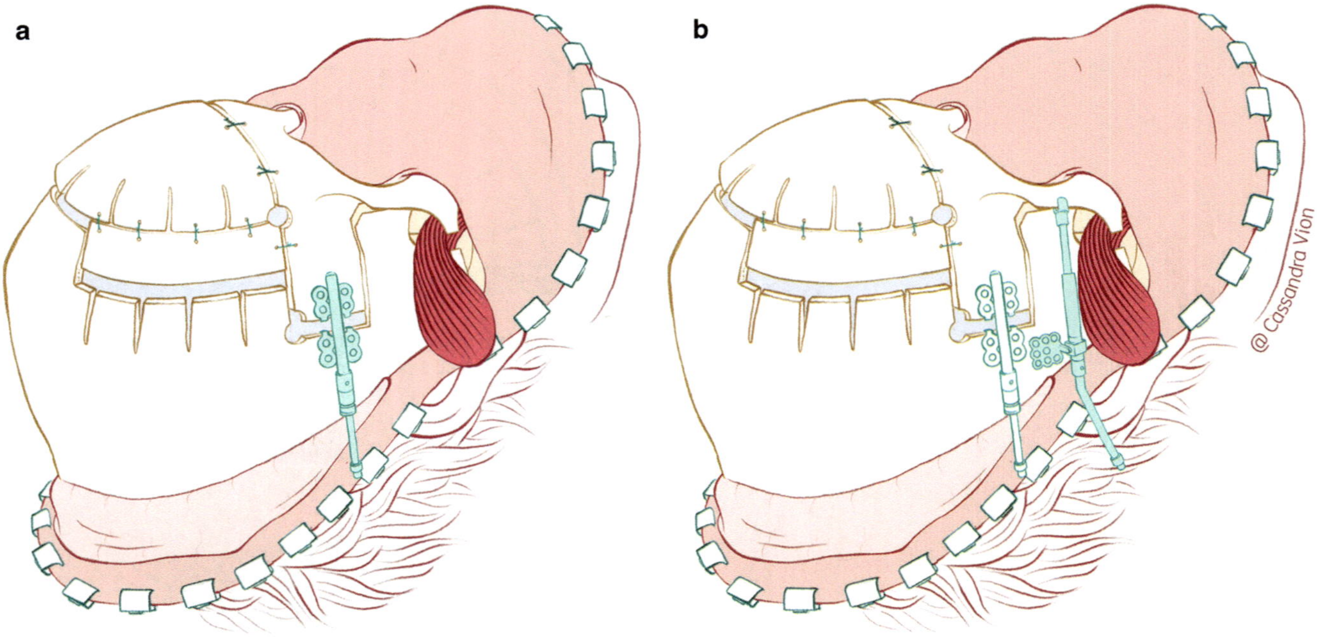

Fig. 3.28 (**a**) Internal cranio-orbital distraction. (**b**) Internal temporo-zygomatic distraction, placed under the temporal muscle © Cassandra Vion

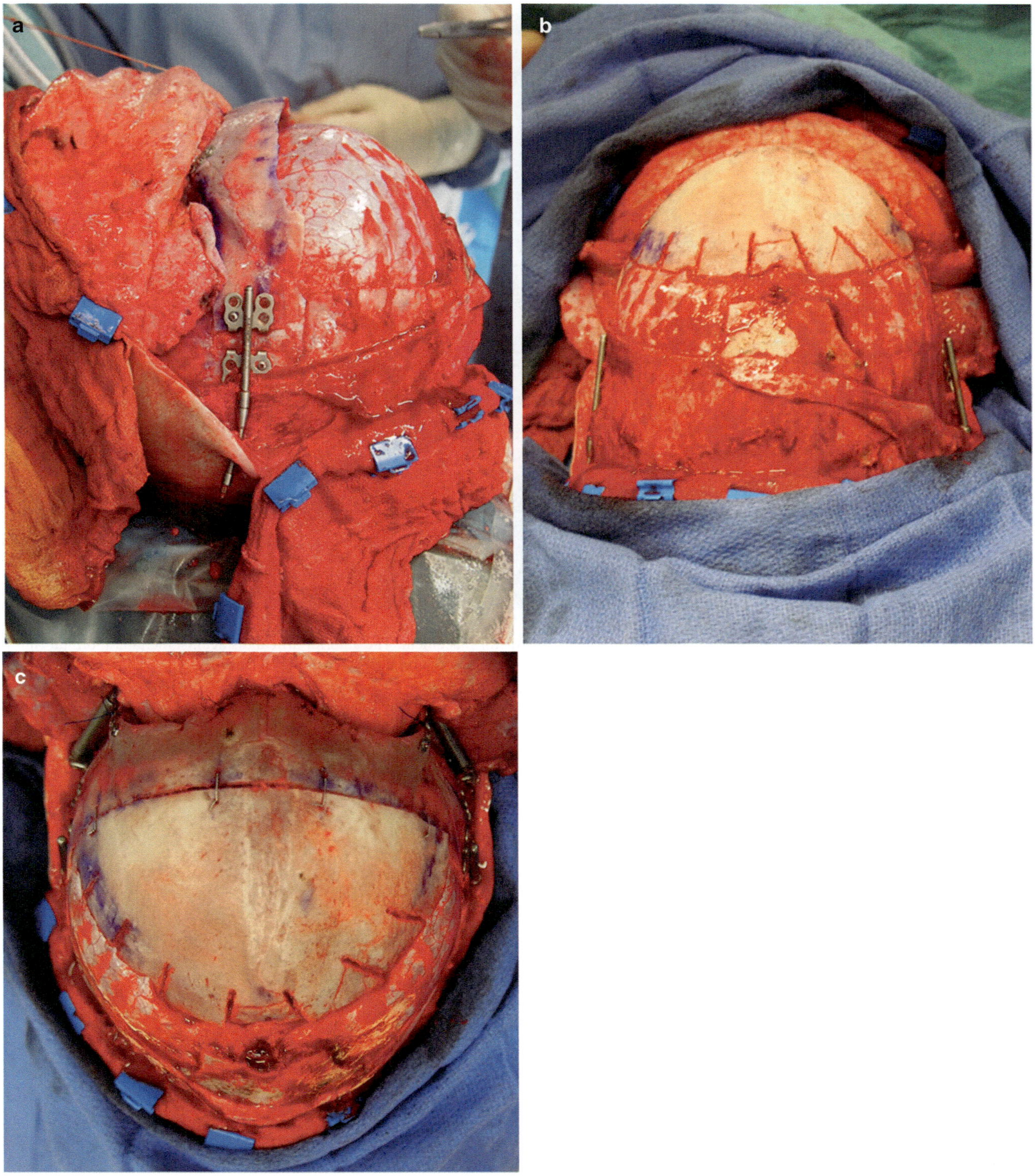

Fig. 3.29 (**a, b, c**) Intraoperative view of internal cranio-orbital distractor placement

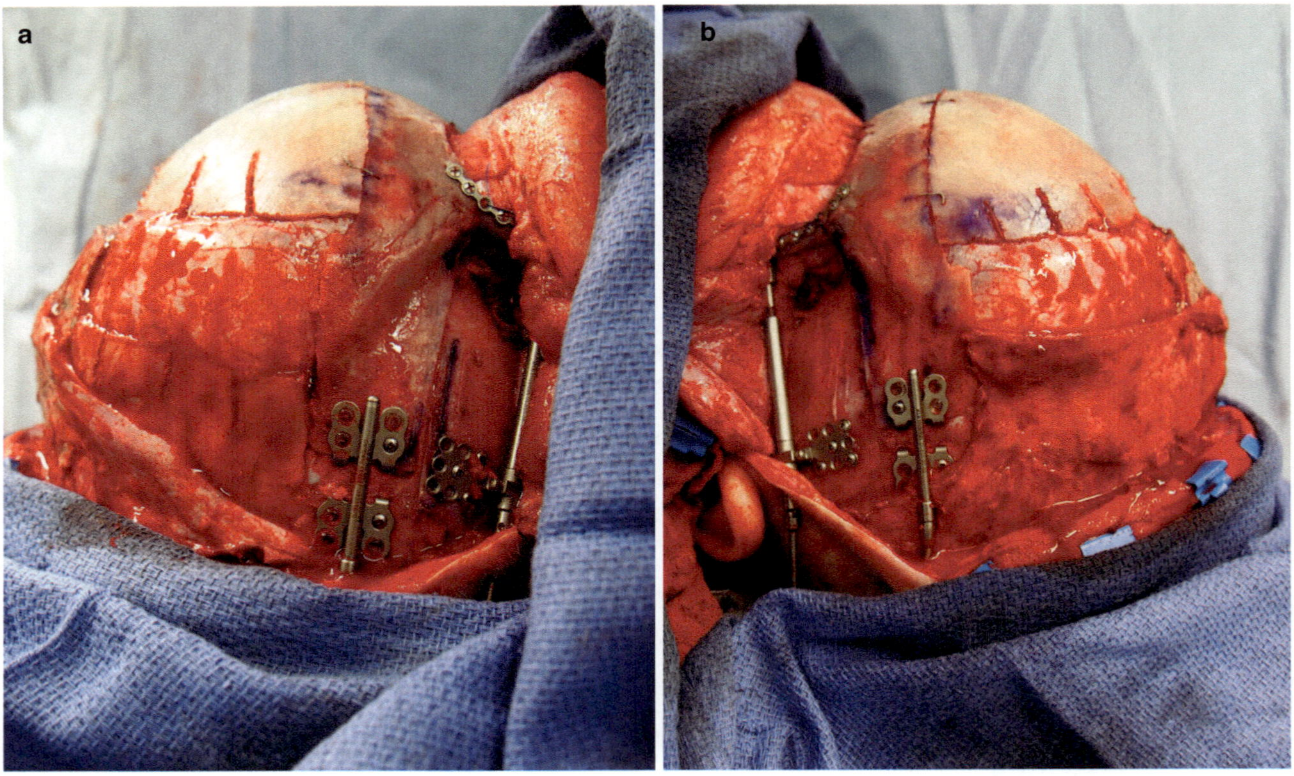

Fig. 3.30 (**a, b**) Intraoperative view of internal temporo-zygomatic distractor placement. The anterior arm abuts against the lateral orbital rim. It is positioned low, at the level of the zygoma, and secured by performing a small notch on the external orbital rim

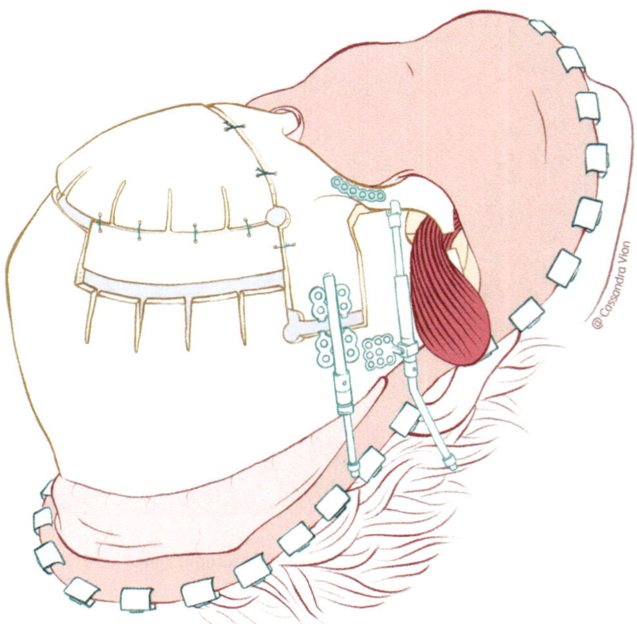

Fig. 3.31 Fronto-zygomatic osteosynthesis using a curved 1.5 mm titanium plate © Cassandra Vion

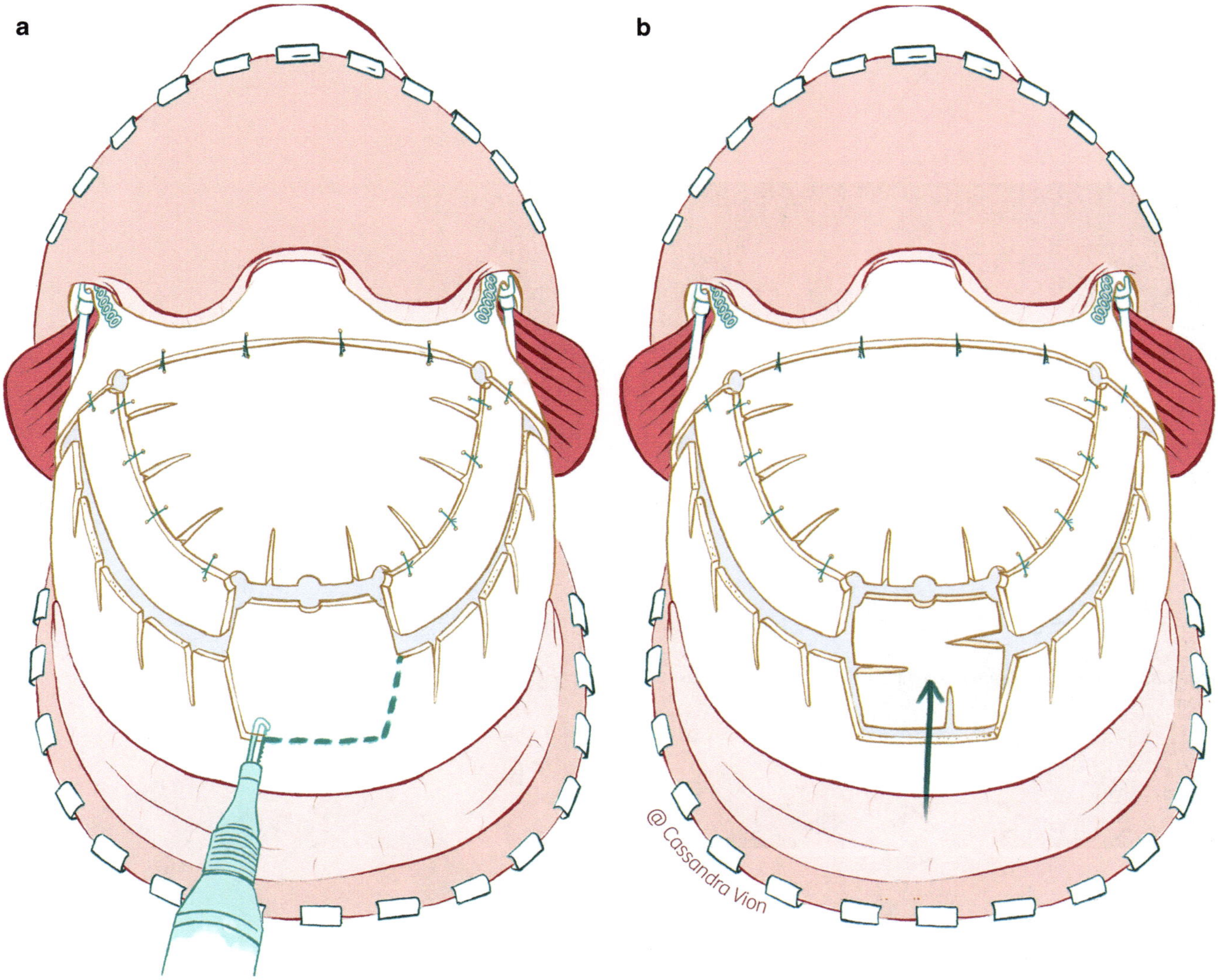

Fig. 3.32 (**a**) Vertex bulge osteotomy. (**b**) Vertex remodeling using a sand dollar design and repositioning using glue © Cassandra Vion

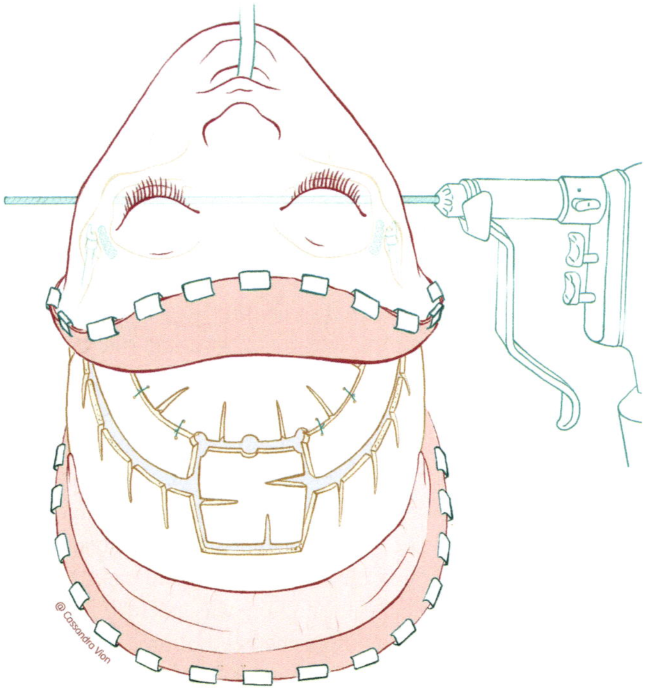

Fig. 3.33 Transfacial pinning using a 2.1 Kirschner wire © Cassandra Vion

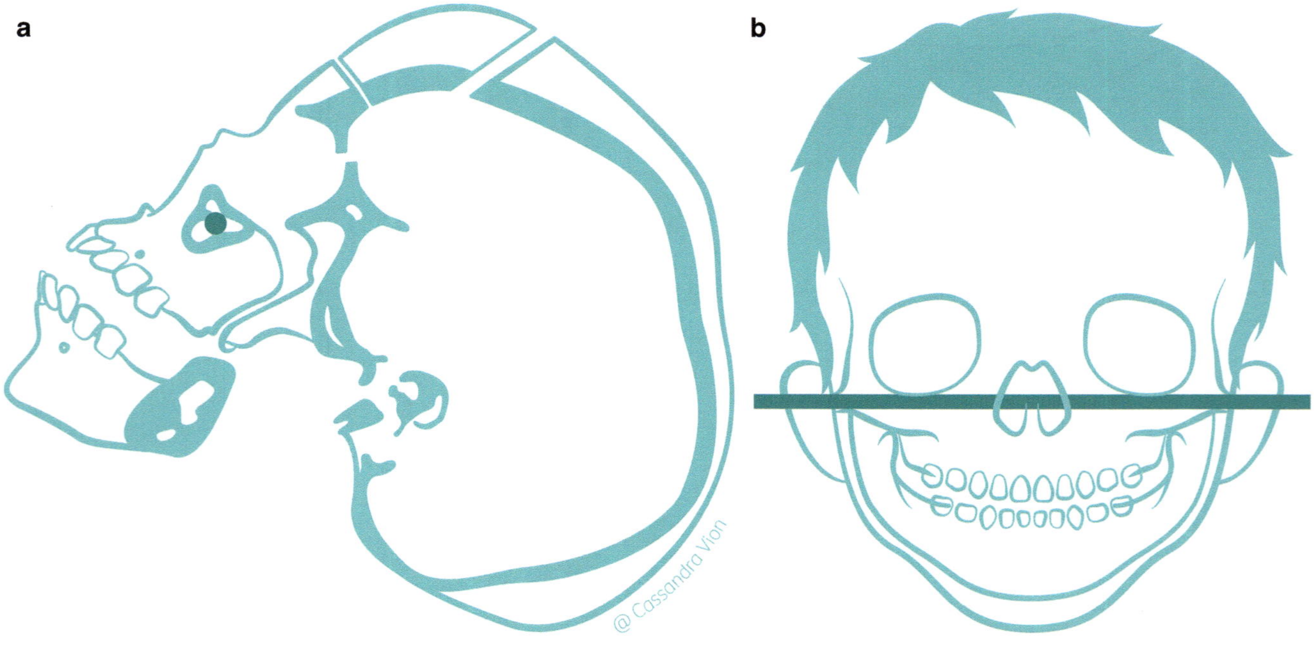

Fig. 3.34 (**a**) Sagittal section showing the trans-zygomatic position of the wire. (**b**) Frontal view showing the proximity of the pin with the orbital cavity © Cassandra Vion

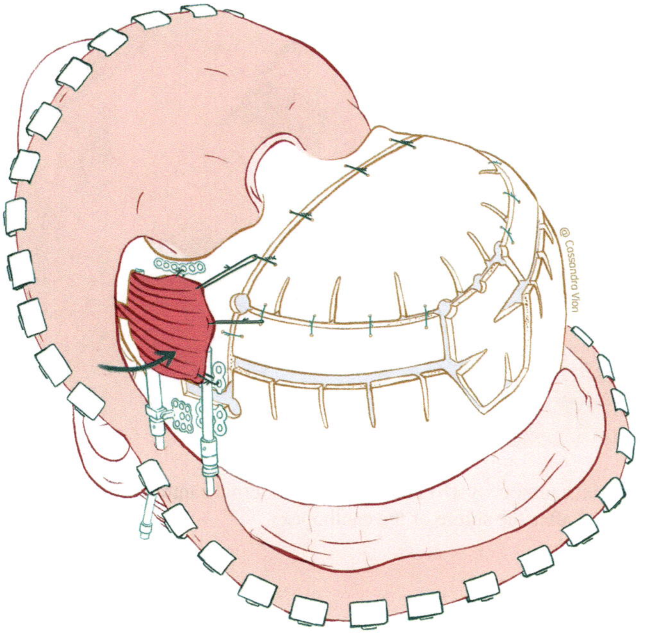

Fig. 3.35 Temporal muscle repositioning after anterior rotation assisted by a low back-cut © Cassandra Vion

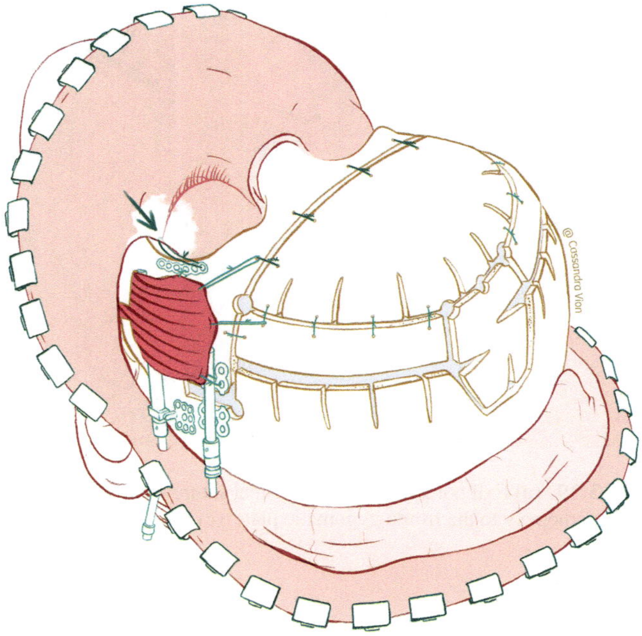

Fig. 3.37 External canthopexy using stainless steel sutures © Cassandra Vion

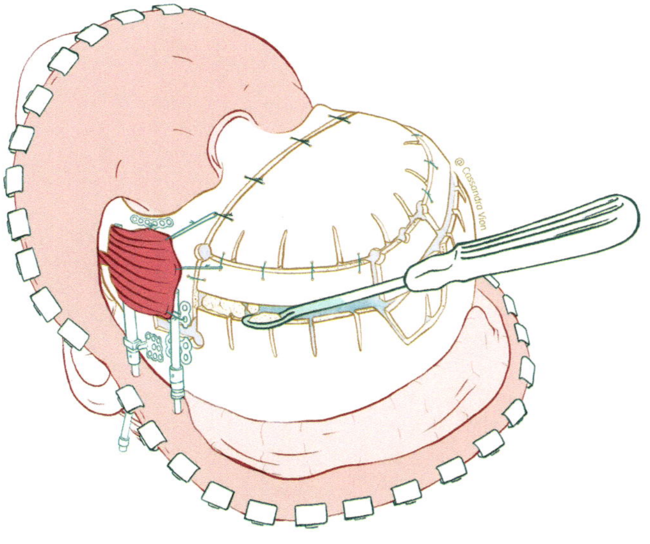

Fig. 3.36 Filling the bony gaps using glued bone powder © Cassandra Vion

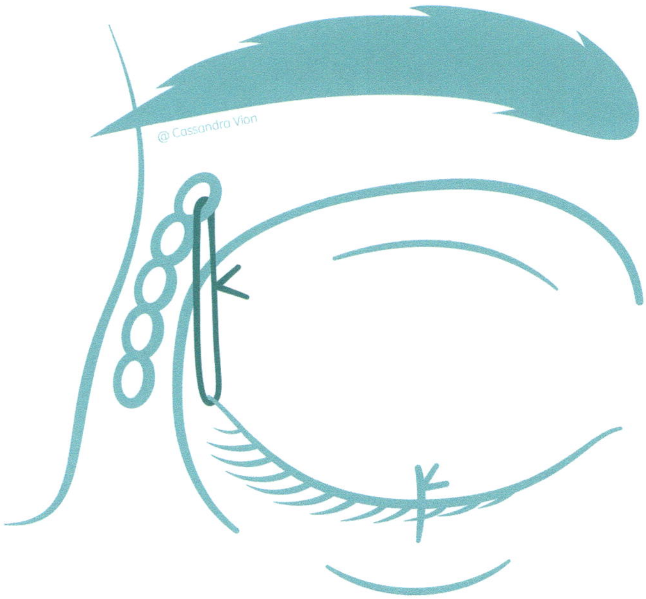

Fig. 3.38 Direction of the suture in external canthopexies © Cassandra Vion

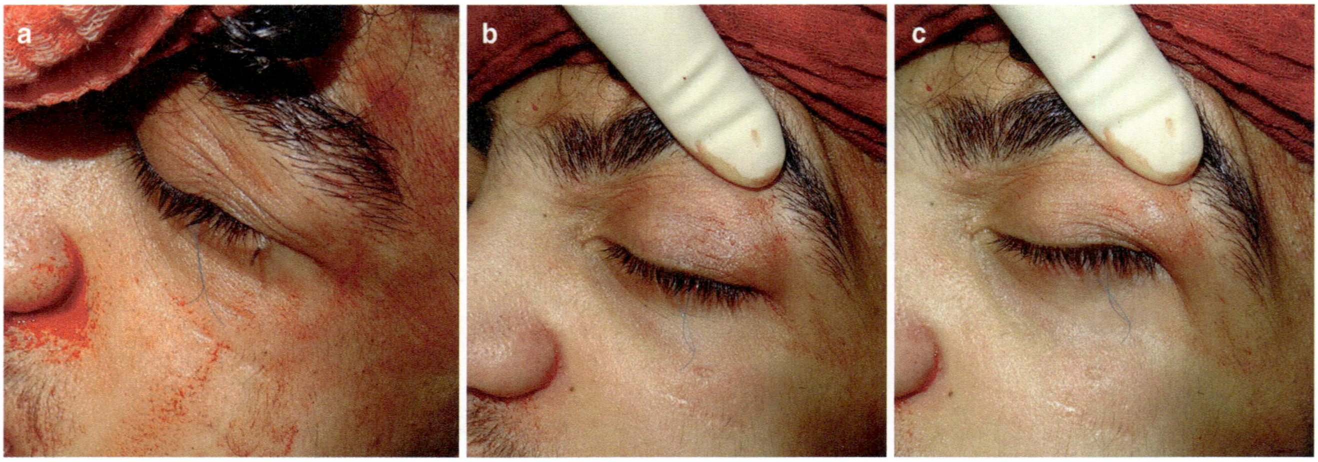

Fig. 3.39 (**a**) Exit point of the stainless steel suture when performing an external canthopexy. (**b**) Position of the external canthus before suturing the canthopexy to the fronto-zygomatic plate. (**c**) Position of the external canthus after the suture of the canthopexy

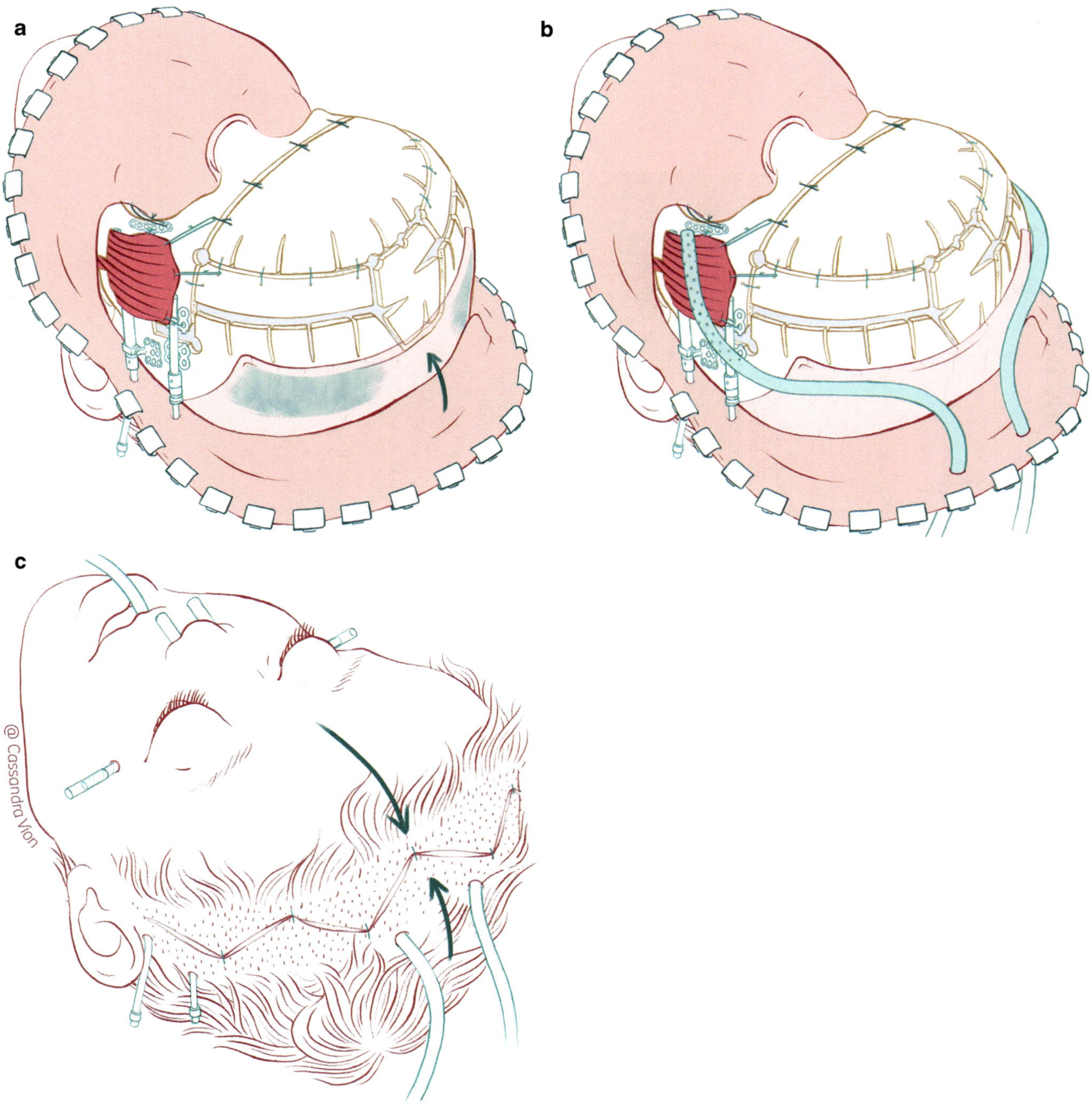

Fig. 3.40 (**a**) Periosteal draping over the skull vault surface. (**b**) External drainage without aspiration. (**c**) Skin closure using 4–0 running Vicryl Rapide (Ethicon) with eversion of the wound edges. Inverted sutures are avoided and reduced to a minimum to avoid suture extrusion. Nasopharyngeal tubes are inserted and the tips of an eventual transfacial pin are covered using silicon sleeves © Cassandra Vion

4 Postoperative Analysis after Fronto-facial Monobloc Advancement

4.1 Anterior Skull Analysis After FFMBA

1. Re-ossification in the coronal region after FFMBA is partial.
2. Re-ossification of the zygomatic arch after FFMBA is partial.
3. Re-ossification at the anterior skull base after FFMBA is associated with a pericranial flap transposition through the orbits bilaterally.
4. Despite early bone mineralization on CT scan, partial relapse may still occur.
5. Postoperative re-ossification is reduced in Pfeiffer syndrome compared to Apert and Crouzon syndromes.
6. Supraorbital ridge protrusion after FFMBA is correlated with later age at surgery and specific mutations in both Crouzon and Apert syndromes.
7. Supraorbital ridge thickening may warrant secondary aesthetic refinement, especially in female adults.

FFMBA osteotomies leave large coronal and skull base bony gaps behind the advanced forehead, raising the question of re-ossification in several critical craniofacial areas. We evaluated re-ossification after FFBMA in the frontal, coronal, and skull base regions [1–4] (Fig. 4.1).

4.1.1 Frontal and Zygomatic Arch Re-ossification after FFMBA

We assessed the re-ossification of the cranium and zygomatic bone after FFMBA in 40 patients (22 Crouzon, 11 Apert, and 7 Pfeiffer syndrome patients), with a mean of 2.1 years of follow-up [1]. Bone regeneration was evaluated at the coronal and zygomatic osteotomy gaps on CT scans postoperatively using a dedicated scoring scale.

The association was studied between re-ossification and other clinical parameters (type of syndrome, existence of previous anterior craniofacial procedure, use of bone paste, and the age at operation) to determine influencing factors.

The possibility of increased ICP, hydrocephalus, or CSF obstruction as the cause of this persistent gap has been excluded in all cases.

Good or Fair re-ossification of the coronal gap was found in 68.2% of patients with Crouzon and 54.5% of patients with Apert syndrome. In contrast, 85.7% of patients with Pfeiffer syndrome had Poor or Absent re-ossification. Re-bridging of the zygomatic arch osteotomy gap in Pfeiffer was also the poorest among three syndromes. The history of previous operations performed before FFMBA was associated with decreased re-ossification. In the group of patients with autologous bone paste application on the coronal osteotomy gap, bone formation was significantly improved.

In brief, our results suggest that the re-ossification of the coronal osteotomy gap in Pfeiffer syndrome was poorer than that in Crouzon and Apert syndromes. Bone paste seemed effective in increasing osteogenesis even in patients with Pfeiffer syndrome or patients with previous surgeries.

4.1.2 Anterior Skull Base Re-ossification after FFMBA

FFMBA includes an osteotomy of the skull base that causes communication of the anterior cranial fossa with the nasal cavities. Pericranial flaps (PF) are systematically transposed through the orbits in our center to seal off the anterior cranial fossa from the ethmoid air cells and nasal cavities. This maneuver was found technically challenging in secondary FFMBA cases because of fibrous adhesions and insufficient pericranial tissue (Figs. 3.22, and 3.23 and Fig. 4.2). The postoperative

E. Arnaud et al., *Frontofacial Monobloc Advancement with Internal Distraction*, https://doi.org/10.1007/978-3-031-07574-2_4

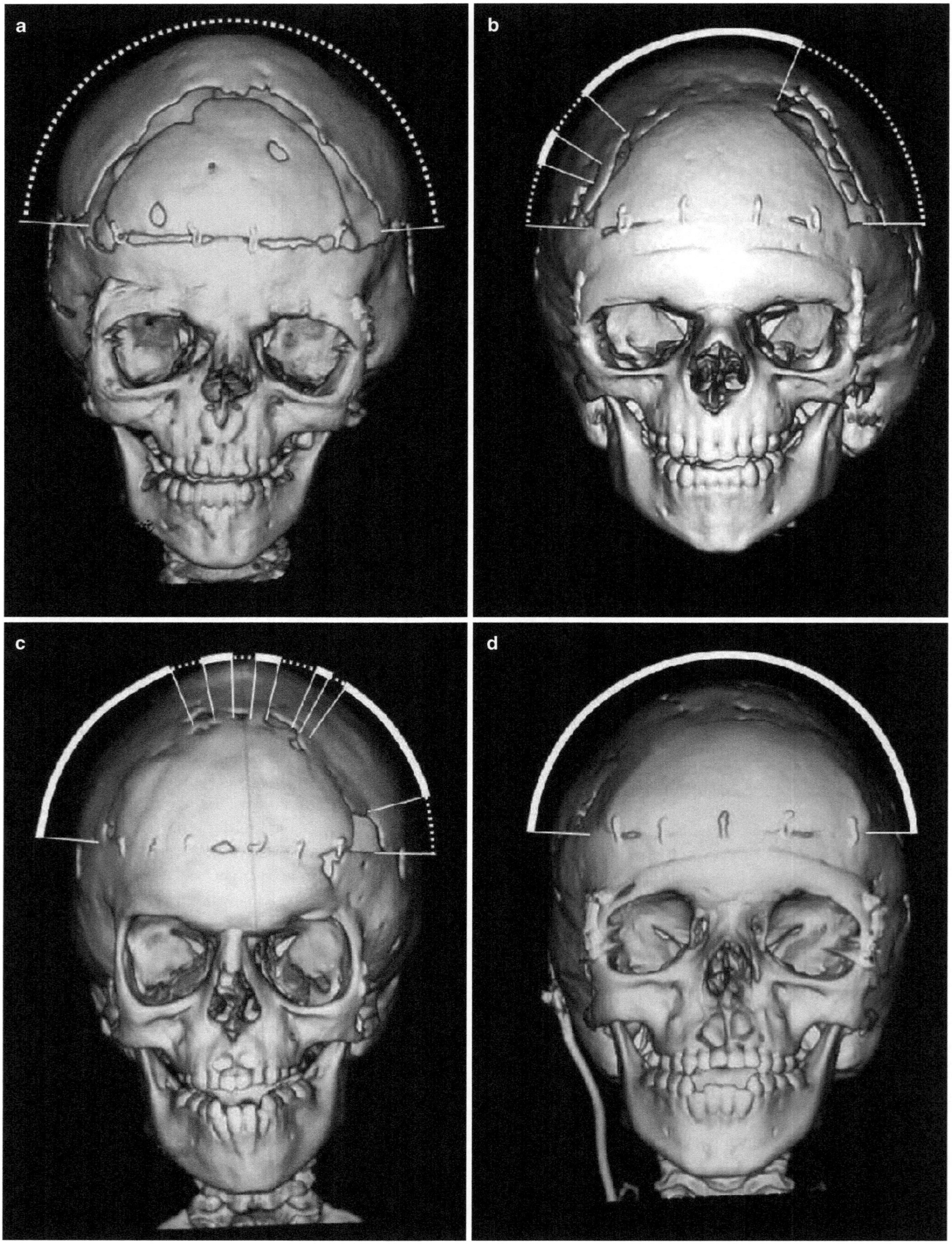

Fig. 4.1 Grading of re-ossification on the coronal distraction gap. The solid lines indicated the area of bone linkage, and the broken lines indicate the lack of bone linkage. *A*, Bone linkage = 0% (0–24%), graded "absent." *B*, Bone linkage = 46% (25–50%), graded "poor." *C*, Bone linkage = 70% (51–74%), graded "fair." *D*, Bone linkage = 100% (75–100%), graded "good"

ossification of the anterior skull base was assessed and we attempted to identify factors influencing this ossification [2].

The measurements of ossification were performed on CT scans at the nasofrontal (NF) and the naso-ethmoïdo-frontal (NEF) junctions in operated patients and healthy controls (Fig. 4.3). The total bone thickness of the skull vault was measured and a qualitative defect score for the anterior skull base was computed (Fig. 4.4). We included 22 patients who underwent FFMBA at a median age of 3.1 years (range 1.9–3.6): 14 patients with Crouzon syndrome, 5 patients with Pfeiffer syndrome, and 3 patients with Apert syndrome.

One year and 5 years postoperatively, the anterior skull base distraction gap was completely ossified at midline in all patients. The ossification of PF significantly increased bone thickness compared to unoperated healthy controls at these two time points. At one year postoperatively, patients with Pfeiffer

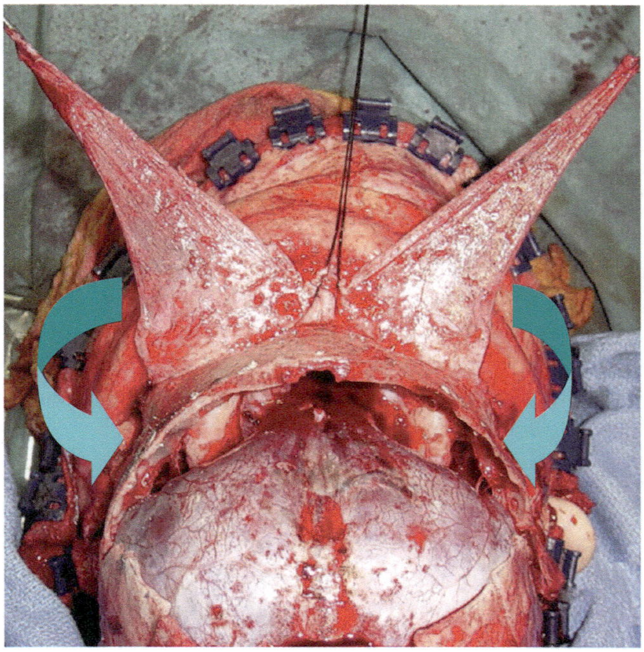

Fig. 4.2 Operative view of the double pericranial pedicled flaps

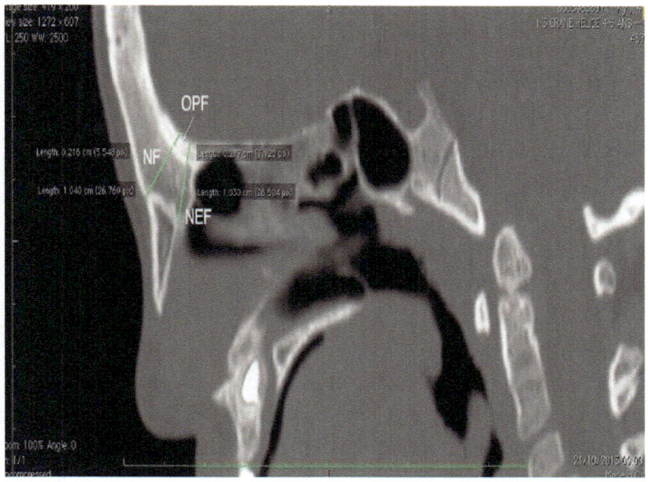

Fig. 4.3 Thickness measurements on the anterior skull base and ossified pericranial flaps thickness on midline sagittal CT scan sections. *NF* nasofrontal landmark, *NEF* naso-ethmoido-frontal landmark, *OPF* ossified pericranial flap. Measurements were performed perpendicular to the inner table of the skull [2]

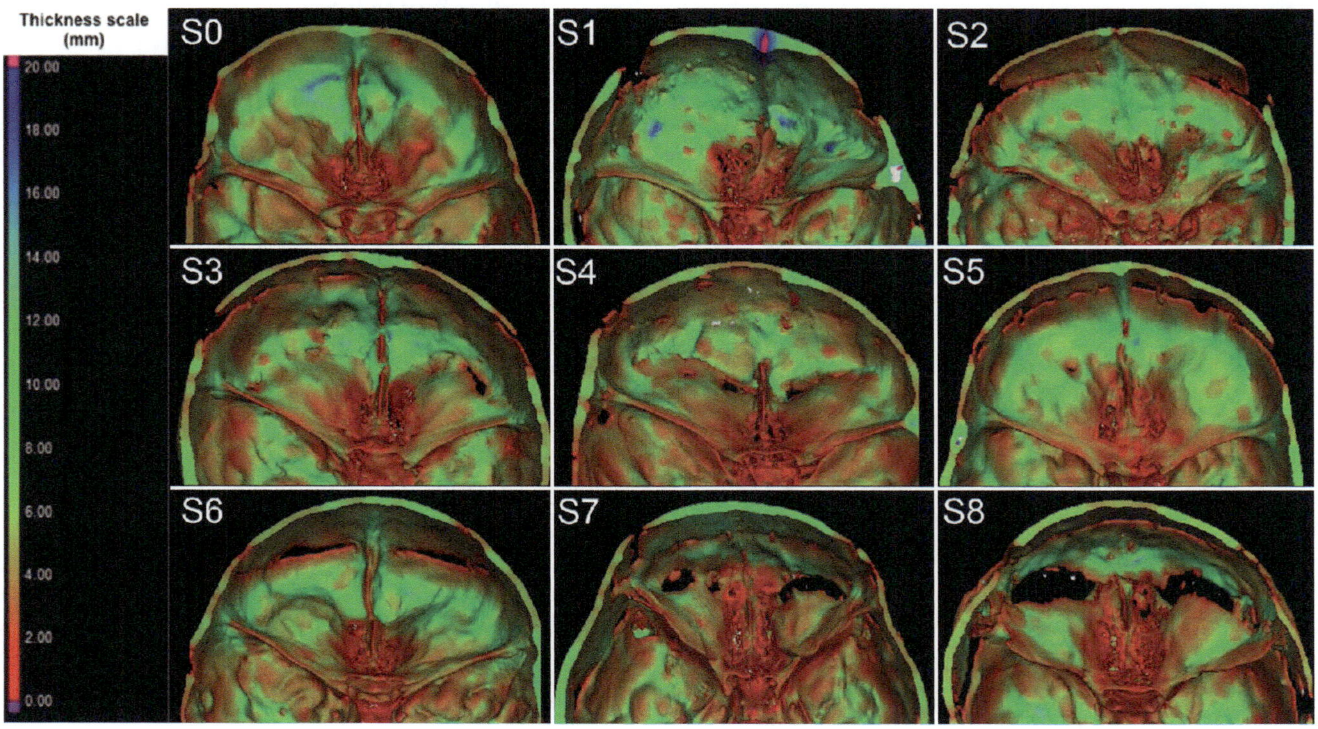

Fig. 4.4 One year postoperative 3D CT scan (superior view of the anterior skull base) showing defect scores (S). The defect score was computed as follows: S = 8: presence of two defects, affecting each orbital roof = 4 (score of the right defect) + 4 (score of the left defect) = 8

syndrome had significantly thicker bone at midline and lower defect scores than patients with Crouzon or Apert syndromes.

Performing PF in FFMBA seems to promote anterior skull base re-ossification. Surprisingly, in contrast with our previous results concerning coronal re-ossification, Pfeiffer syndrome was associated with better anterior skull base ossification than Crouzon and Apert syndromes, potentially indicating differential effects of activating *FGFR2* mutations in specific craniofacial territories.

4.1.3 Supraorbital Ridge Bone Thickness

Supraorbital bar protrusion is a common clinical observation after FFMBA. We conducted a morphometric study to assess this issue. Before FFMBA, children with Crouzon syndrome had significantly thicker frontal bones, unlike children with Apert syndrome. Age and sex were not statistically correlated to frontal bone thickness. A significant increase in frontal bone thickness was reported after FFMBA in both Crouzon and Apert syndromes. The postoperative increase in frontal bone thickness was independent of age, gender, and *FGFR2* mutations. Nevertheless, in Crouzon syndrome, two *FGFR2* mutations (Phe276Val and Ser347Cys) seemed to be related to thicker frontal bones after FFMBA but larger numbers are required to confirm these trends. Similar findings were reported in Apert syndrome with the Ser252Trp mutation. Regarding age at FFMBA: the older the patients, the thicker the frontal bone postoperatively (Fig. 4.5).

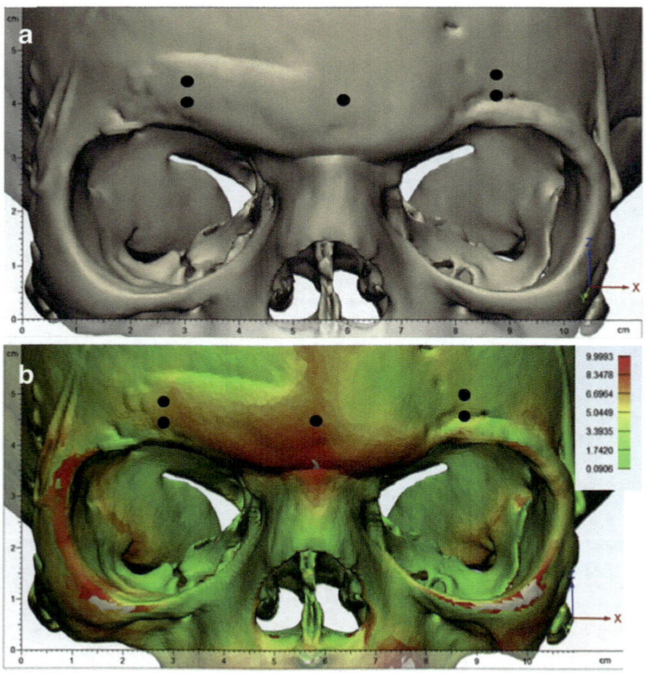

Fig. 4.5 Bone thickness measurements were performed on the frontal bone. Green-yellow-red (respectively, 0-5-10 mm) continuous color map for thickness values plotted over the 3D rendering of the supraorbital rim and frontal bone, showing bandeau thickening in a postoperative case of Crouzon syndrome [5]

4.2 Orbital Shape and Optic Nerve Modifications after FFMBA in Crouzon Syndrome

1. Exorbitism due to smaller and shallower orbits is a constant phenotypic trait of FCST.
2. FFMBA is a powerful tool to enlarge the orbit.
3. Orbital shape and volume overcorrection were obtained immediately after FFMBA and remained stable 2 years postoperatively.
4. The best orbital volume enlargement and shape modification were obtained when FFMBA was performed between 1.5 and 5 years of age.
5. Orbital shape asymmetry was better corrected when FFMBA was performed before 2 years of age.
6. Despite lateral canthopexy during FFMBA, downslanting of the palpebral fissures may occur as a result of distraction.
7. In Apert syndrome, LF3 with bipartition is a common secondary procedure to correct residual orbital dysmorphology.

The correction of orbital dysmorphology is a key point in faciocraniosynostosis care. Malformations of both the bony structure and the soft tissues interact to produce the pathologic phenotype.

4.2.1 Eyelids and FFMBA

Soft tissue anomalies of the orbits in Crouzon and Apert syndrome mostly consist of downslanting palpebral fissures, more specifically in Apert syndrome [6, 7]. FFMBA by itself does not correct this morphological characteristic [6]. In fact, FFMBA can even aggravate lateral canthal descent because of sub-periorbital circumferential dissection and separation of the external canthus from the lateral orbital rim [8]. To avoid this risk, we systematically perform external canthopexy during FFMBA to pull the external canthus upwards [8]. We evaluated this technique in Apert syndrome following LF3 with facial bipartition [7] but formal assessment is lacking following FFMBA.

4.2.2 FFMBA Is a Powerful Tool to Enlarge the Orbit and Reduce Exorbitism

Exorbitism, a central sign in FCST and a major functional concern, is mainly the consequence of bony orbital malformations. In fact, morphometric assessment of the orbit in

28 Crouzon and 14 Apert syndrome cases has shown that the orbital cavity in both syndromes is shallow with increased vertical height and hypertelorism [9], confirming previous reports [10–12]. Interestingly, larger ocular globe volumes have been reported in both Crouzon and Apert syndromes [11], potentially contributing to ocular proptosis, although this contribution is most probably clinically irrelevant.

To assess the effects of FFMBA on intrinsic orbital anomalies in Crouzon syndrome, the volume and shape of the orbits have been assessed before and after FFMBA. Quantitative time-related postoperative orbital shape modifications were studied. Twenty-four patients with Crouzon syndrome and 48 control patients were included. CT scans at four time points—preoperative, early postoperative, 6 months postoperative, and 12 months postoperative—were used to compute orbital volume and orbital shape parameters based on a semiautomatic orbital segmentation method. These parameters included Maximum Absolute Distance (MAD), Hausdorff Distance (HD), and Dice Similarity Coefficient (DSC). Symmetry was evaluated by computing DSC after superimposing each orbit with the mirror image of its contralateral orbit (Figs. 4.6, 4.7, and 4.8) [9].

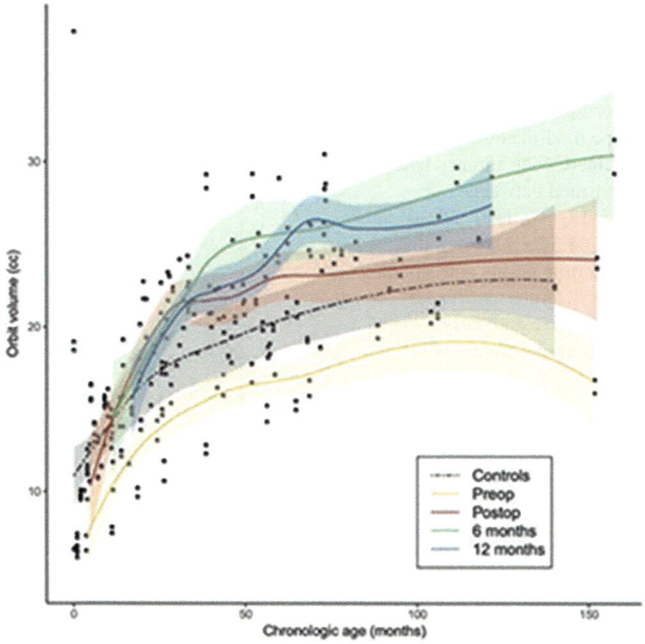

Fig. 4.6 Model curves of orbital growth in control, preoperative, and postoperative groups. Fronto-facial monobloc advancement induces a stable overcorrection of the orbital volume [13]

Orbital volumes were smaller in Crouzon syndrome and surgery allowed a stable overcorrection of this parameter. Crouzon orbits were significantly more asymmetrical than controls and surgery did not correct this parameter. Nevertheless, surgery performed before 20.65 [16.30–25.36] months improved symmetry. Orbital morphology quantified by MAD, HD, and DSC was improved by fronto-facial advancement, and the improvement was stable in the long term. Maximal shape modification was obtained when surgery was performed between 13.73 [+/− 1.40] and 64.57 [+/− 1.89] months. Over 80% of orbital growth was achieved in all groups at the age of 64.57 [+/− 1.89] months [13].

Orbital morphology was thus deeply modified by FFMBA. We defined a critical period between 1 and 5.5 years of age during which the effects of fronto-facial advancement are maximal on the orbital shape. This period corresponds to a peak in orbital growth, accounting for the major influence of surgery on shape parameters.

Interestingly, we showed that during the distraction phase of FFMBA in Crouzon syndrome, the optic nerve is significantly elongated (Fig. 4.9): on the same cohort of patients, the mean left optic nerve length was 19.4 mm before FFMBA and 23.0 mm after FFMBA ($p = 0.001$), and the mean right optic nerve length was 19.6 mm before FFMBA and 22.8 mm after FFMBA ($p = 0.001$). We could not find specific elongation patterns in the subgroup of patients who had vision issues during the activation phase after FFMBA but these findings may explain the rare cases of vision loss during fronto-facial advancement.

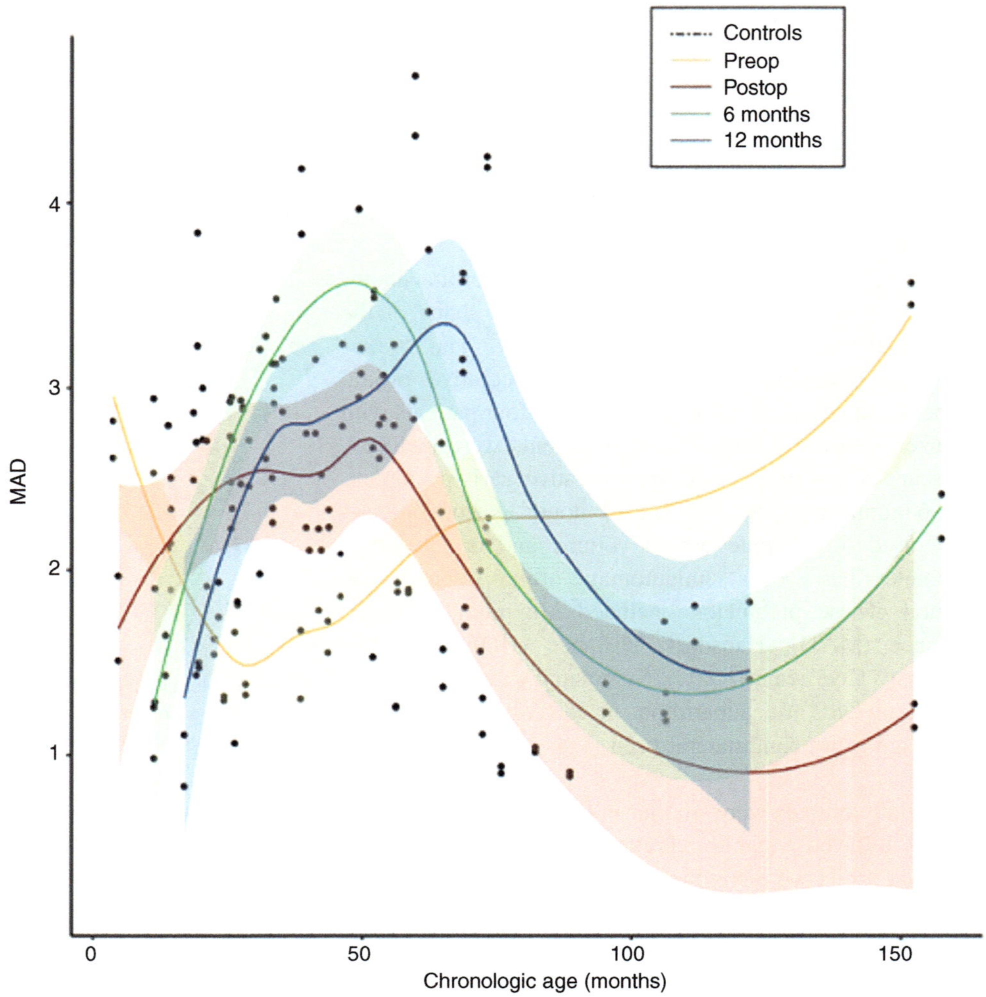

Fig. 4.7 Evolution of the mean absolute distance between Crouzon orbits and age-matched control according to age. Maximal shape modification was obtained when surgery was performed between m1 = 13.73 ± 1.40 and m2 = 64.57 ± 1.89 months. These time points correspond to the two intersections of preoperative and early postoperative curves

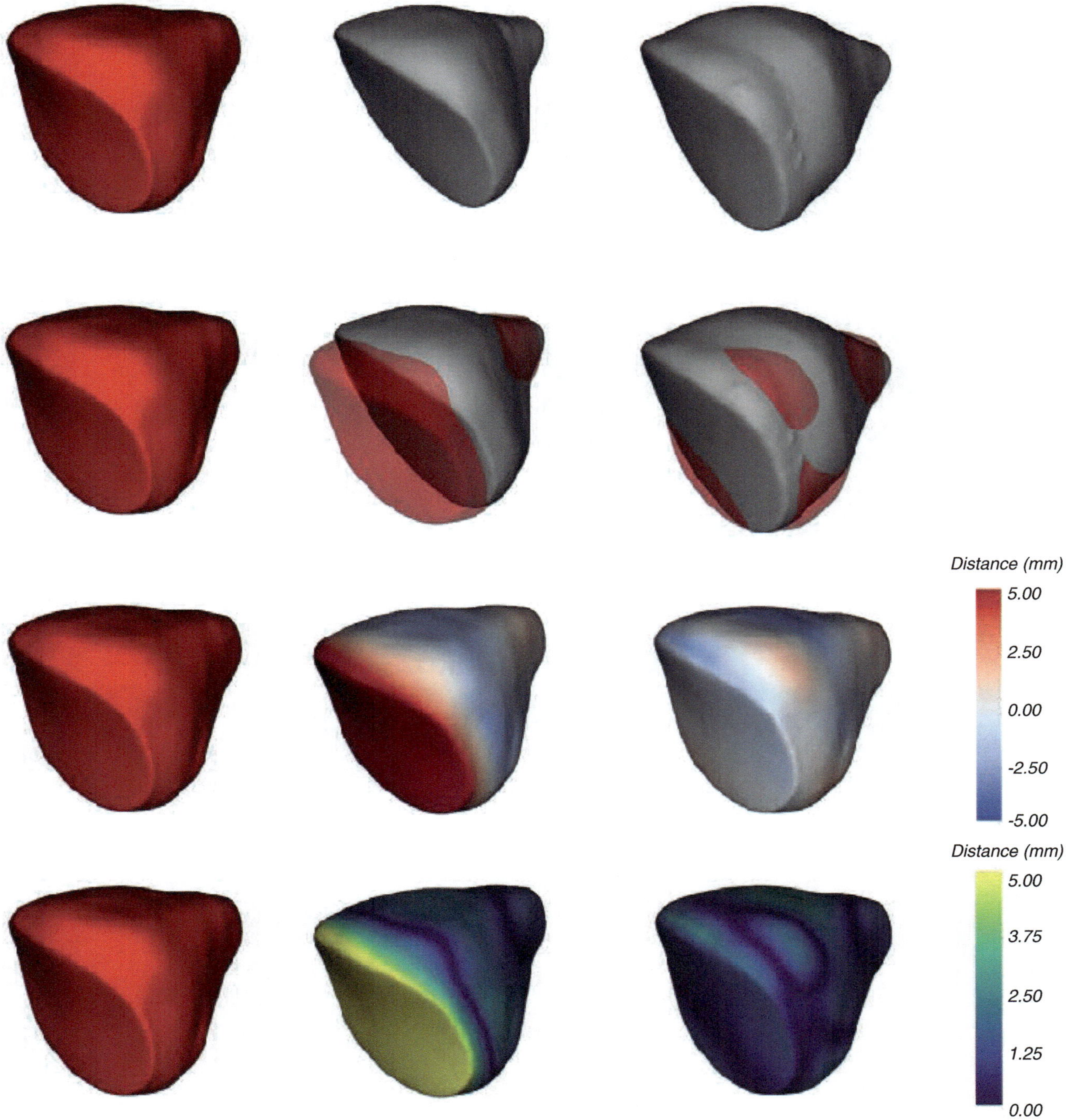

Fig. 4.8 Three-dimensional shape model of the orbit in Crouzon syndrome before and after fronto-facial monobloc advancement osteotomy. Age group: 0–5 years. Columns: (Left) Control age-matched orbit; (Center) Before surgery; (Right) 12 months after surgery. Lines: (First) Mean model of the orbital shape; (Second) Superimposition of the mean model with the age-matched control (rendered in transparent red); (Third) Signed distance map; (Fourth) Unsigned distance map. The global shape of the orbit is qualitatively closer to normal after surgery

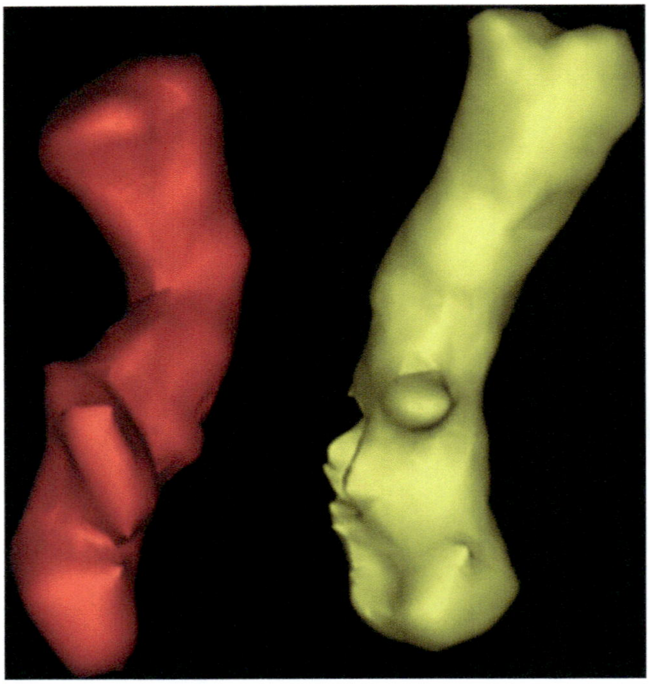

Fig. 4.9 FFMBA induces significant optic nerve elongation: left = before distraction, right = at the end of distraction

4.3 FFMBA Improves OSAS in Faciocraniosynostosis

1. FFMBA normalizes sleep apnea in almost half of FCST cases treated in our center. The other half shows significant improvement.
2. Tracheostomy is usually avoided or removed by applying a protocol including FFMBA.
3. ENT procedures (tonsillectomy/adenoidectomy/turbinectomy), as well as PVE should be performed whenever possible before FFMBA for best respiratory results.
4. Delaying FFMBA improves its respiratory effects.

OSAS is specifically prevalent in children with FCST and is associated with poor cognitive outcomes and added risk of intracranial hypertension [14, 15] (Fig. 4.10). FFMBA advances the midface and is often performed for OSAS management [16, 17] (Figs. 4.11 and 4.12). The aim here was to provide a definitive quantitative and prospective assessment

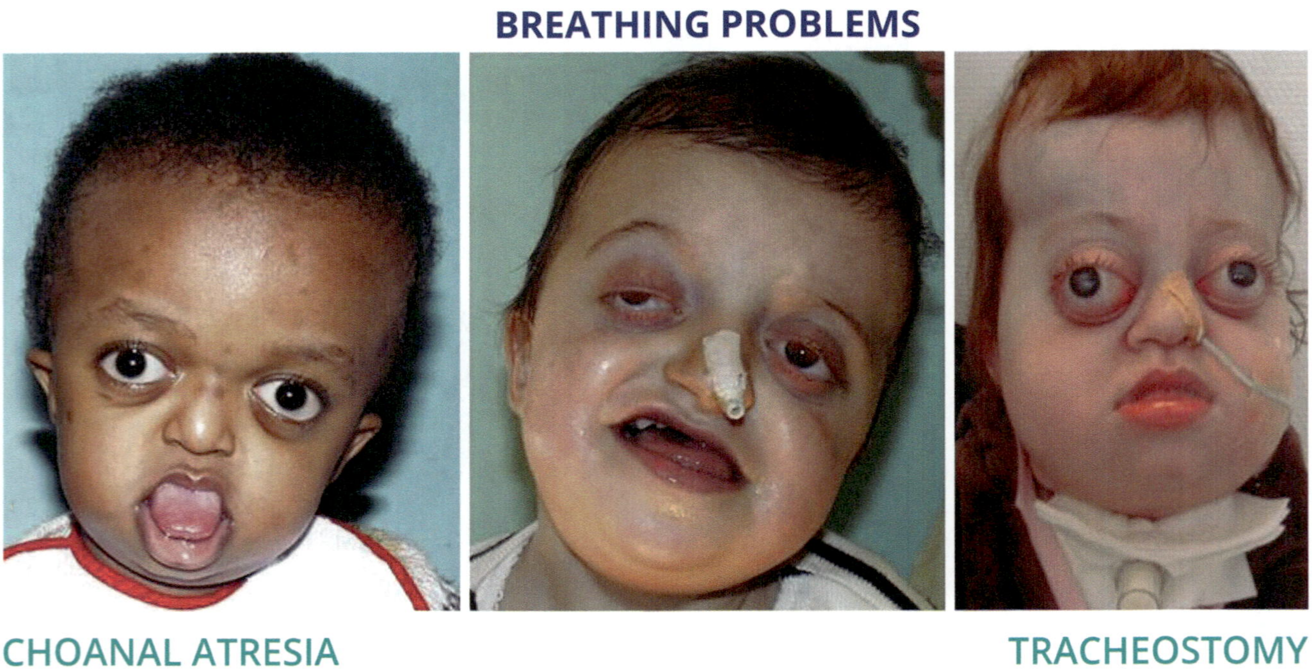

Fig. 4.10 Most patients with faciocraniosynostosis present with some degree of choanal atresia. Nasopharyngeal tubes may improve the situation but tracheostomy is sometimes required

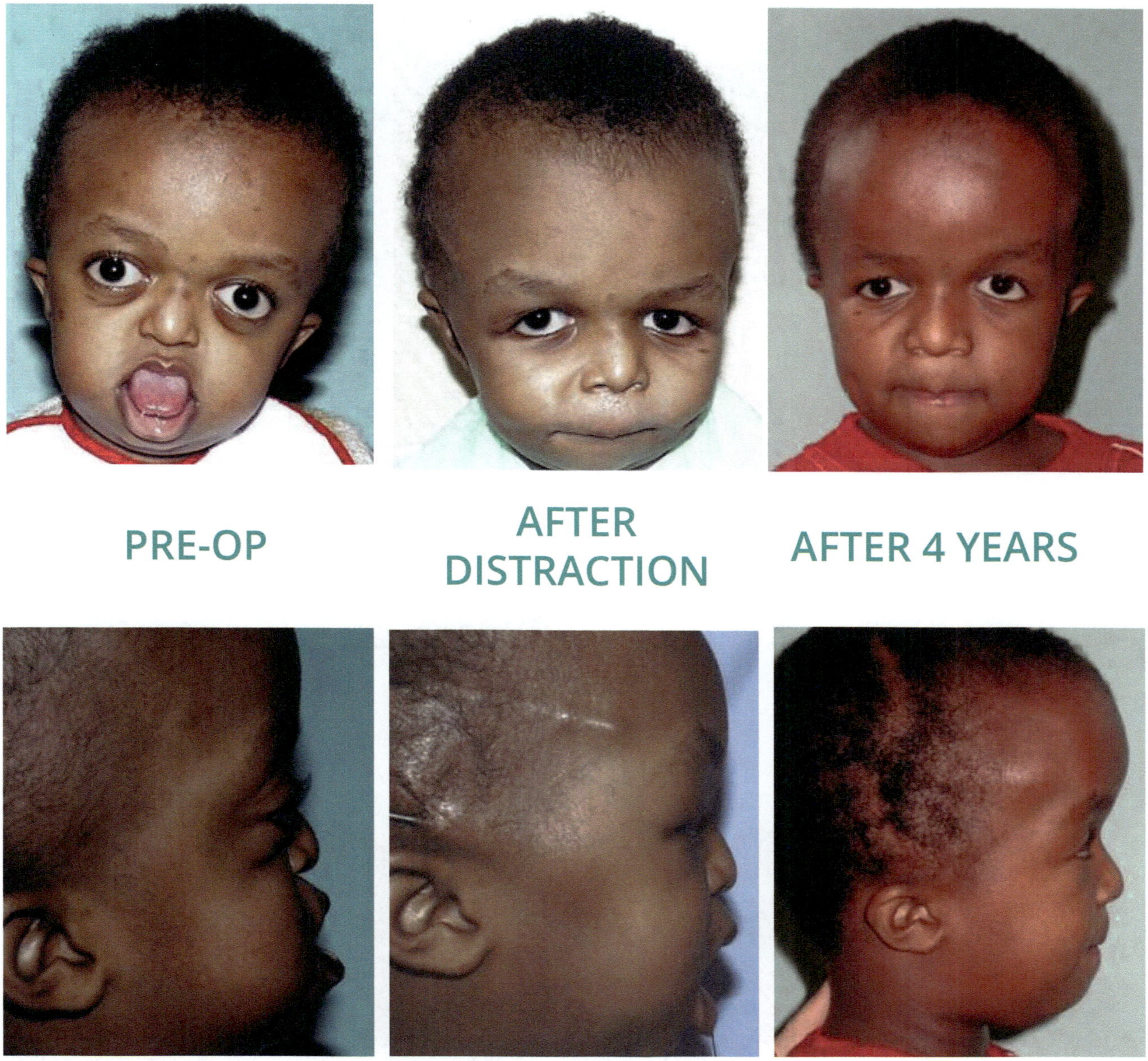

Fig. 4.11 (left) A 30-month-old patient with Crouzon syndrome presenting with complete choanal atresia and maxillary hypoplasia causing severe obstructive sleep apnea. (middle) He underwent FFMBA with choanal permeation and subsequent complete resolution of sleep apnea. (right) Stability of facial advancement 4 years postoperatively

of the effects of FFMBA on OSAS in children with faciocraniosynostosis. At the beginning of our experience patients were only monitored by oxymetries. For more than 20 years now, all patients have been screened using polysomnography. Of 149 patients who underwent FFMBA, 108 presented with OSAS.

Most breathing problems in faciocraniosynostosis are obstructive [18]. Exceptionally, when a cerebellar tonsillar herniation has been neglected, central apneas may occur requiring PVE or FM decompression. Modern evaluation includes a systematic PSG at all stages of the follow-up. PSG may quantify the severity of the obstructive apnea syndrome, and quantify evolution before and after each treatment step.

Among the surgical tools to treat OSAS, tonsillectomy, and adenoidectomy are systematic when the structures are present even of a normal size. Choanal repermeation at an early stage is more and more emphasized nowadays, as it may correct a mild to moderate OSAS and differ the osteotomy [19–21]. Osteotomies and facial distraction (early FFMBA or LF3) remain the workhorse of OSAS management in faciocraniosynostosis [16, 22, 23].

In order to assess the effects of FFMBA on OSAS, faciocraniosynostosis patients with OSAS managed in our unit

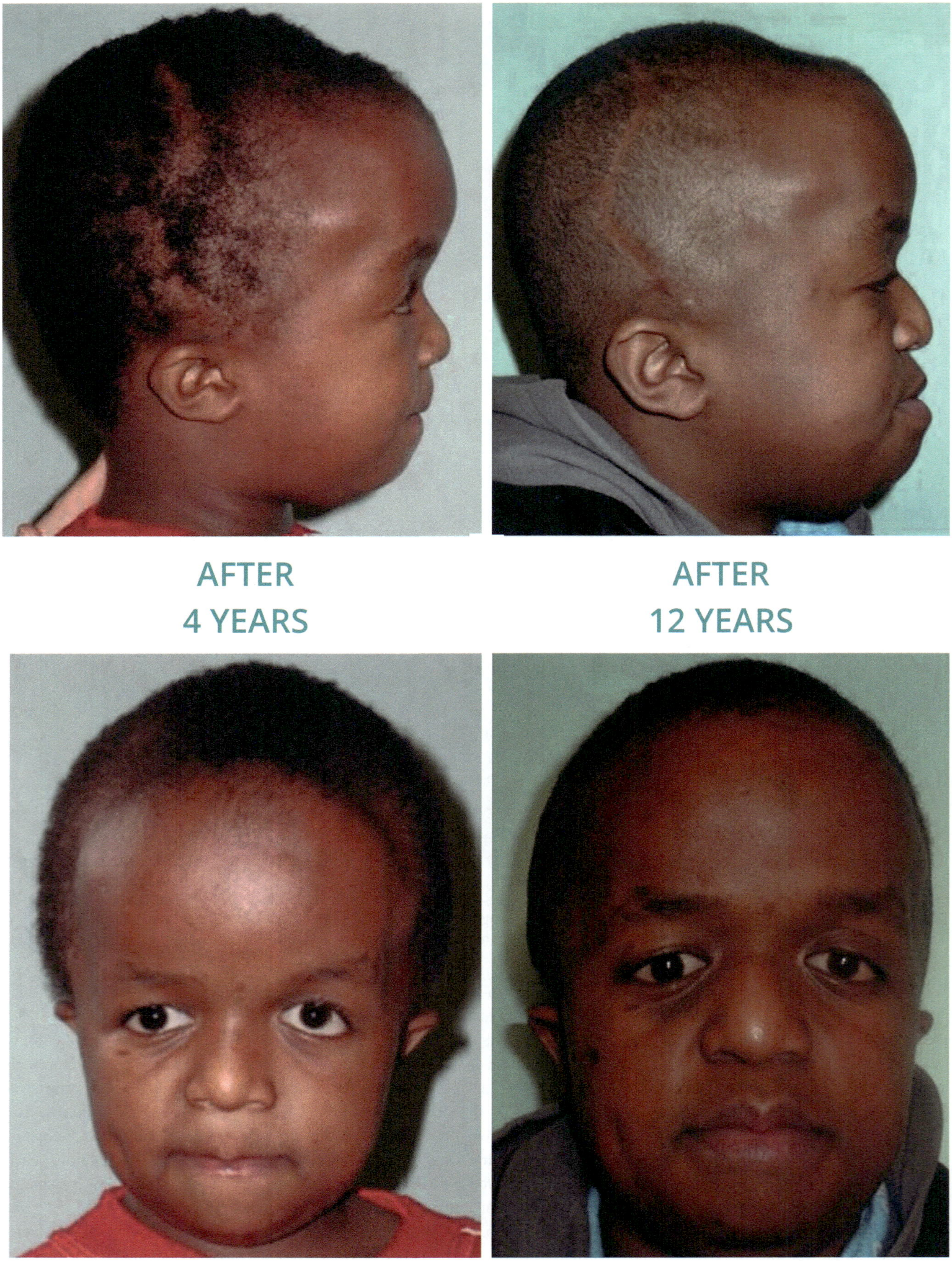

Fig. 4.12 Long-term follow-up of the same patient as in 4.11. (left) Four year postoperative pictures. (right) Clinical presentation at 15 years of age, 12 years after FFMBA. The patient still has a normal AHI but he has developed Angle class III malocclusion. The patient declined to undergo orthognathic surgery and lateral canthopexy, which would have been aesthetically beneficial

Table 4.1 Average AHI values before and after FFMBA in a series of 108 patients with faciocraniosynostosis and OSAS

Preoperative	Six-month postoperative distractor removal	One-year postoperative
22.5 /h	12.5 /h	8.4 /h

Table 4.2 Average postoperative AHI after FFMBA in patients who have or have not previously undergone airway optimization (tonsillectomy, turbinectomy, and/or adenoidectomy)

Preoperative AHI		Previous ENT airway optimization	No previous ENT airway optimization
<10 /h	Preoperative AHI	5	6
	Postoperative AHI	5	8
10 /h to 20 /h	Preoperative AHI	16	17
	Postoperative AHI	11	18
>20 /h	Preoperative AHI	43	43
	Postoperative AHI	15	12

Table 4.3 Endoscopy under sedation before and after FFMBA in 20 patients with Crouzon syndrome

Standardized airway endoscopy under sedation		
Dysfunction		
Before FFMBA		After FFMBA
Ventilation	57%	28%
Tongue tonus	65%	29%
Pharyngeal tonus	65%	36%
Larynx tonus	28%	14%

were prospectively included over a period of 14 years and followed up for their AHI based on PSG studies, before and after FFMBA.

AHI values were assessed using several linear and logistic multivariate models, in order to quantify (1) the preoperative AHI values, (2) the absolute decrease in AHI values after FFBMA, (3) AHI normalization (AHI < 5) after FFMBA, (4) the need for a secondary facial advancement, and (5) genotype–phenotype correlations [17].

Preoperatively, AHI values were similar in Crouzon, Apert, and Pfeiffer syndromes. Preoperative lateral and/or posterior skull vault expansion was associated with more AHI decrease. Preoperative tonsillectomy and/or adenoidectomy, older age at FFMBA surgery, and Pfeiffer syndrome were associated with more AHI normalization.

In brief, our results suggest that FFMBA is efficient in treating OSAS in FCST (Tables 4.1 and 4.2). Preoperative tonsillectomy and lateral and/or posterior skull decompression are recommended before FFMBA in order to improve the respiratory results of the fronto-facial advancement. Delaying surgery when allowed by the neurosurgical and respiratory medicine teams is also a parameter favoring better respiratory outcomes. Of note, neglected tonsils or adenoids before FFMBA undergo transient enlargement by inflammation immediately after procedure, which accounts for several of the cases that showed transient respiratory worsening.

Sleep endoscopy has emerged as a useful tool to localize airway obstruction and optimize FFMBA [24]. At our institution, the evolution of OSAS was analyzed with a preliminary dynamic assessment of airways with endoscopy through a standardized protocol under sedation (unpublished data). Our results suggest an improvement of 4 dynamic functional parameters. Dysfunctions of ventilation, tongue tonus, and pharyngeal tonus—evaluated based on a 1–4 score—were reported in about 60% of cases before FFMBA and were reduced by half after surgery (Table 4.3).

References

1. Oyama A, Arnaud E, Marchac D, et al. Reossification of cranium and zygomatic arch after monobloc frontofacial distraction advancement for syndromic craniosynostosis. J Craniofac Surg. 2009 Sep;20(Suppl 2):1905–9.
2. Morice A, Paternoster G, Ostertag A, et al. Anterior Skull Base and Pericranial flap ossification after Frontofacial Monobloc advancement. Plast Reconstr Surg. 2018;141(2):437–45.
3. Noordzij N, Brouwer R, van der Horst C. Incomplete Reossification after Craniosynostosis surgery. J Craniofac Surg. 2016 Jan;27(1):e105–8.
4. Thenier-Villa JL, Sanromán-Álvarez P, Miranda-Lloret P, et al. Incomplete reossification after craniosynostosis surgery-incidence and analysis of risk factors: a clinical-radiological assessment study. J Neurosurg Pediatr. 2018;22(2):120–7.
5. Bouaoud J, Hennocq Q, Paternoster G, et al. Excessive ossification of the bandeau in Crouzon and Apert syndromes. J Craniomaxillofac Surg. 2020 Apr;48(4):376–82.
6. Taylor JA, Bartlett SP. What's new in syndromic Craniosynostosis surgery? Plast Reconstr Surg. 2017 Jul;140(1):82e–93e.
7. Chetty V, Haber SE, Khonsari RH, et al. Improvement of periorbital appearance in Apert syndrome after subcranial Le fort III with bipartition and distraction. J Craniofac Surg. 2020 May;31(3):711–5.
8. Arnaud E, Paternoster G, James S, et al. Craniofacial strategy for syndromic craniosynostosis. Ann Chir Plast Esthet. 2016 Oct;61(5):408–19.
9. Khonsari RH, Way B, Nysjö J, et al. Fronto-facial advancement and bipartition in Crouzon–Pfeiffer and Apert syndromes: impact of fronto-facial surgery upon orbital and airway parameters in FGFR2 syndromes. J Cranio-Maxillofac Surg. 2016 Oct 1;44(10):1567–75.
10. Kreiborg S, Cohen MM. Ocular manifestations of Apert and Crouzon syndromes: qualitative and quantitative findings. J Craniofac Surg. 2010 Sep;21(5):1354–7.
11. Forte AJ, Steinbacher DM, Persing JA, et al. Orbital Dysmorphology in untreated children with Crouzon and Apert syndromes. Plast Reconstr Surg. 2015 Nov;136(5):1054–62.

12. Lu X, Forte AJ, Sawh-Martinez R, et al. Anterior convex lateral orbital wall: distinctive morphology in Apert syndrome. Br J Oral Maxillofac Surg. 2018 Nov;56(9):864–9.
13. Khonsari RH, Hennocq Q, Nysjö J, et al. Defining critical ages for orbital shape changes after Frontofacial advancement in Crouzon syndrome. Plast Reconstr Surg. 2019;144(5):841e–52e.
14. Gozal D. Morbidity of obstructive sleep apnea in children: facts and theory. Sleep Breath. 2001;5(1):35–42.
15. Guilleminault C, Korobkin R, Winkle R. A review of 50 children with obstructive sleep apnea syndrome. Lung. 1981;159(5):275–87.
16. Bannink N, Nout E, Wolvius EB, et al. Obstructive sleep apnea in children with syndromic craniosynostosis: long-term respiratory outcome of midface advancement. Int J Oral Maxillofac Surg. 2010 Feb;39(2):115–21.
17. Khonsari RH, Haber S, Paternoster G, et al. The influence of fronto-facial monobloc advancement on obstructive sleep apnea: an assessment of 109 syndromic craniosynostoses cases. J Cranio-Maxillofac Surg. 2020 Jun 1;48(6):536–47.
18. Driessen C, Mathijssen IMJ, De Groot MR, et al. Does central sleep apnea occur in children with syndromic craniosynostosis? Respir Physiol Neurobiol. 2012 May 31;181(3):321–5.
19. Amonoo-Kuofi K, Phillips SP, Randhawa PS, et al. Adenotonsillectomy for sleep-disordered breathing in children with syndromic craniosynostosis. J Craniofac Surg. 2009 Nov;20(6):1978–80.
20. Willington AJ, Ramsden JD. Adenotonsillectomy for the management of obstructive sleep apnea in children with congenital craniosynostosis syndromes. J Craniofac Surg. 2012 Jul;23(4):1020–2.
21. Zandieh SO, Padwa BL, Katz ES. Adenotonsillectomy for obstructive sleep apnea in children with syndromic craniosynostosis. Plast Reconstr Surg. 2013 Apr;131(4):847–52.
22. Uemura T, Hayashi T, Satoh K, et al. A case of improved obstructive sleep apnea by distraction osteogenesis for midface hypoplasia of an infantile Crouzon's syndrome. J Craniofac Surg. 2001 Jan;12(1):73–7.
23. Tsui WK, Yang Y, Cheung LK, et al. Distraction osteogenesis as a treatment of obstructive sleep apnea syndrome: a systematic review. Medicine (Baltimore). 2016 Sep;95(36):e4674.
24. Doerga PN, Spruijt B, Mathijssen IMJ, et al. Upper airway endoscopy to optimize obstructive sleep apnea treatment in Apert and Crouzon syndromes. J Craniomaxillofac Surg. 2016 Feb;44(2):191–6.

5 Secondary Le Fort III Facial Advancement after Primary Fronto-facial Monobloc Advancement: Effects on Sleep Apnea Syndrome

1. Secondary LF3 with distraction efficiently corrects sleep apnea and exorbitism after FFMBA.
2. LF3 is most often performed around mixed dentition age using the same bicoronal incision that was used for PVE and FFMBA as well as an additional intra-oral upper vestibular incision.
3. Both internal and external distractors can be used to optimize vector control and facilitate a long consolidation phase with early removal of the rigid external device.
4. Overcorrection is key in non-adult patients.
5. External canthopexy prevents downslanting of the palpebral fissures due to soft tissue sagging.
6. Bipartition of the LF3 segment is particularly useful in Apert syndrome to simultaneously correct hypertelorbitism and the narrow arched palate along with the maxillary retrusion.

Le Fort III facial advancement treats maxillary and malar retrusion. This procedure aims to improve exorbitism and OSAS, but cannot expand intracranial volume. Unlike traditional orthognathic surgery, LF3 does not intend to obtain Angle class I occlusion.

LF3 can be safely performed at any age above 4 years. Nevertheless, its most appropriate timing is usually during or right after mixed dentition. On the one hand, this period corresponds to the stabilization of brain growth and the relief from the risk of intracranial hypertension. On the other hand, it provides the growing child/teenager attending school a chance to breathe normally and avoid nocturnal C-PAP, with potential severe worsening to the preexisting maxillary retrusion. In addition to those direct advantages, LF3 during/after mixed dentition greatly facilitates orthognathic surgery procedures proposed at the end of growth.

The LF3 procedure usefully completes a FOA when a staged strategy has been chosen instead of a FFMBA. However, as mentioned before, the staged strategy does not address OSAS until the LF3 is performed and therefore should be reserved to mild cases.

Unfortunately, all FFMBA do not improve sufficiently the OSAS. In order to assess the functional effects of LF3 performed after FFMBA, we focused on FFMBA patients in whom normalization of AHI was not obtained [1, 2].

We considered a population of 17 patients (16%) who benefited from secondary LF3 after FFMBA, within a population of 108 patients with faciocraniosynostosis with OSAS who underwent FFMBA (Fig. 5.1). The mean age at FFMBA in this cohort was 2.6 ± 1.7 years, and the mean age at secondary LF3 was 9.6 ± 3.9 years, which corresponds to a 7-year gap between FFMBA and LF3. The mean follow-up after this secondary LF3 was 4.0 ± 3.1 years.

Most patients normalized their AHI after LF3 (15 patients, 88%). One-half of those with preoperative tracheostomy were decannulated postoperatively (two of four patients). The AHI

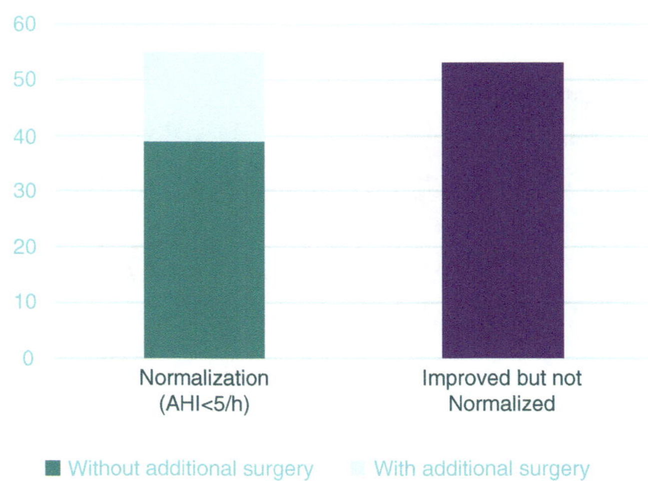

Fig. 5.1 LF3 after FFMBA may contribute to normalization in patients with persistent OSAS

E. Arnaud et al., *Frontofacial Monobloc Advancement with Internal Distraction*, https://doi.org/10.1007/978-3-031-07574-2_5

significantly decreased: from an average of 21.5 per hour before LF3 to 3.9 per hour postoperatively ($p = 0.003$). This normalization was progressive postoperatively: it required 27 months on average and the improvement was long-lasting. Higher preoperative AHI was predictive of higher AHI postoperatively.

Bipartition and medial rotation of the LF3 segment were associated with more AHI improvement. The main indication of this technical variation was Apert syndrome, to treat mild hypertelorbitism, to correct downslanting of eyelids fissures, and to widen the narrow V-shaped palate. This marked improvement in AHI might be explained a posteriori by the ensuing expansion of the hard palate and the nasal fossae, and the subsequent decrease in nasal airway resistance.

In conclusion, secondary LF3 improves residual or relapsing sleep apnea in faciocraniosynostoses patients who have previously had FFMBA.

5.1 Operative Technique: Secondary Le Fort III Facial Advancement with External and Internal Distraction (Fig. 5.2)

Surgery was performed through a bicoronal approach with sub-galeal undermining until the supraorbital rims. Care was taken to separate the deep temporal fascia from the skin-

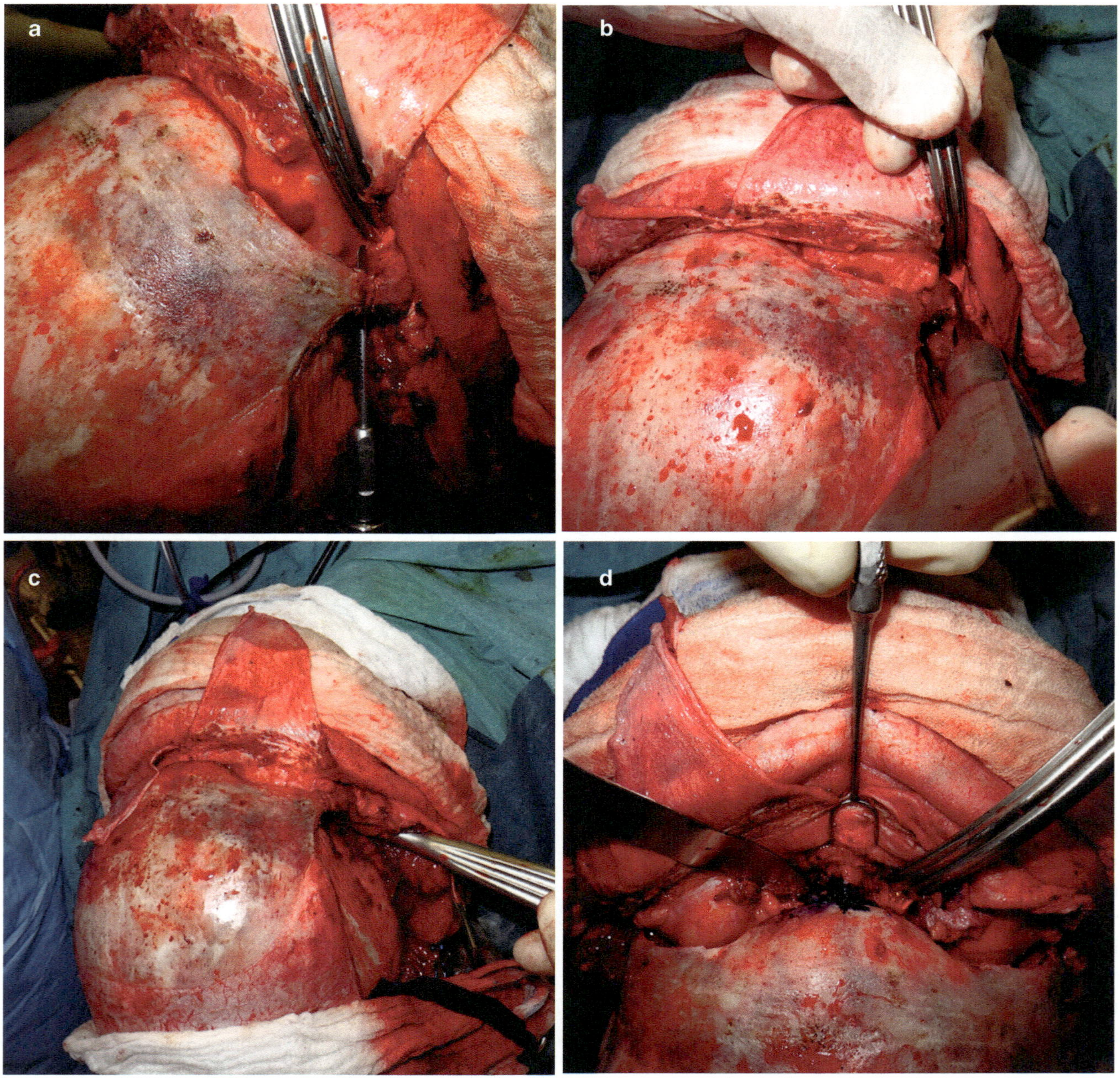

Fig. 5.2 (**a**) Lateral orbital wall osteotomy using a reciprocating saw. (**b**) Osteotomy of the zygomatic arch. (**c**) Pterygo-zygomatic disjunction: direction of insertion of the osteotome and elevator. (**d**) osteotomy of the nasal bones and the medial orbital walls behind the posterior lacrimal crest

galea flap before the temporal muscle flaps were detached from bone. The zygomatic arch was denuded through the superficial temporal fat pad to avoid exposing the frontal branch of the facial nerve. Sub-periorbital dissection extended to the orbital floor and the medial wall of the orbit behind the posterior lacrymal crest until the inferior-medial angle. Le Fort III osteotomies were carried out, followed by pterygopalatine disjunction. The facial segment was mobilized with Rowe forceps. Orbital advancement was usually simple to obtain and at the estimated ideal position, the lateral wall of the orbit was osteosynthetized with a microplate and one micro-screw at each extremity (1.5 mm in diameter, 4–6 mm in length).

Internal distractors were posteriorly anchored to the temporal bones using metallic screws with blunt tips (neuro-screws, KLS Martin, Tuttlingen, Germany) to avoid trauma to the underlying dura mater. Anteriorly, the distractors had a grooved cylindrical tip intended to clutch the lateral orbital rim and push forward. They were positioned as low as possible, just above the zygomatic arch (Fig. 5.3). The activation arms exited the skin through a stab wound behind the incision line.

The temporal muscle flap was transposed anteriorly to fill the temporal defect and cover the hardware to protect the thin overlying skin. Through an upper vestibular incision, a linear titanium microplate bridged the anterior maxilla from side to side. Two 3–0 surgical steel wires were passed through the plate bilaterally. They exited through the nasolabial folds, 5–10 mm lateral to the alar creases. Lateral canthopexy was performed with overcorrection of upward pull while avoiding pupillary obstruction (Fig. 5.4).

Two drainage tubes were inserted. The skin-galea flap was redraped. Closure was performed using 4–0 Vicryl Rapide running suture. Buccal mucosa was closed after a V-Y plasty with a running 4–0 Vicryl suture. A Rigid External Distraction (RED) device was installed, and the fixation pins were gently turned manually while avoiding palpable bone defects from previous surgeries. Nasopharyngeal tubes were inserted bilaterally. They were removed along with tarsorrhaphy sutures 2–3 days later. A loose headwrap with a moist dressing was made and the patient was transferred to the ICU with a wire cutter at bedside as a security measure in case of emergency intubation.

A latency phase of 2–3 days was allowed before the activation phase of the distraction. The distraction rate was one millimeter per day until an overcorrected class II malocclusion was achieved. Both internal and external distractors were activated during the same sedation session. At the end of the distraction period, the activation arms of the internal distractors were detached, and the RED device was removed (Fig. 5.5). Consolidation lasted 3–4 months with internal devices only.

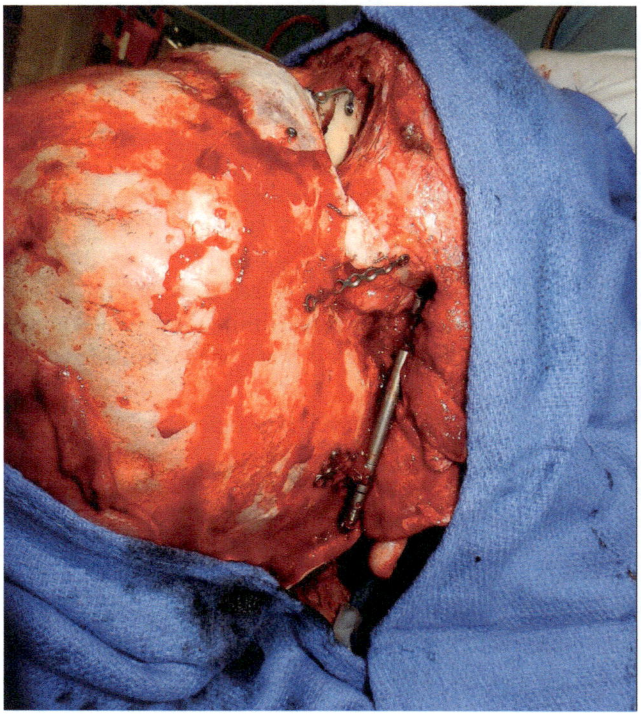

Fig. 5.3 Position of the temporo-zygomatic internal distractors

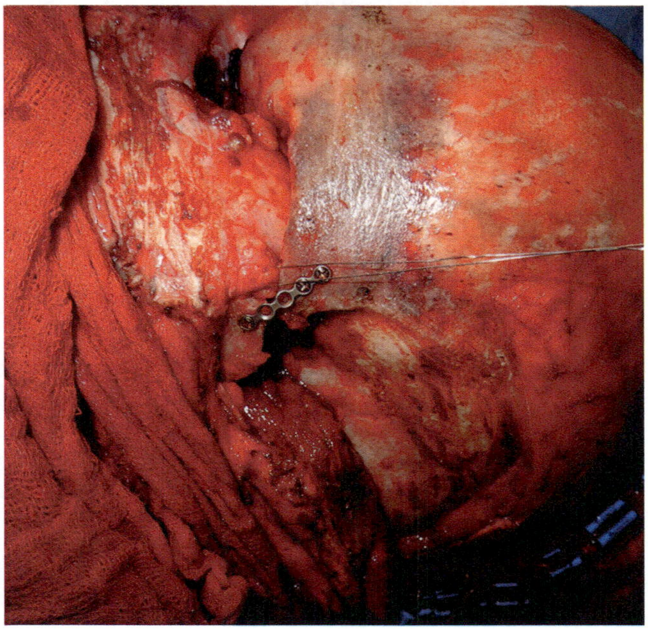

Fig. 5.4 Suspension of the lateral canthopexy wires to the fronto-zygomatic plates were used to determine facial advancement

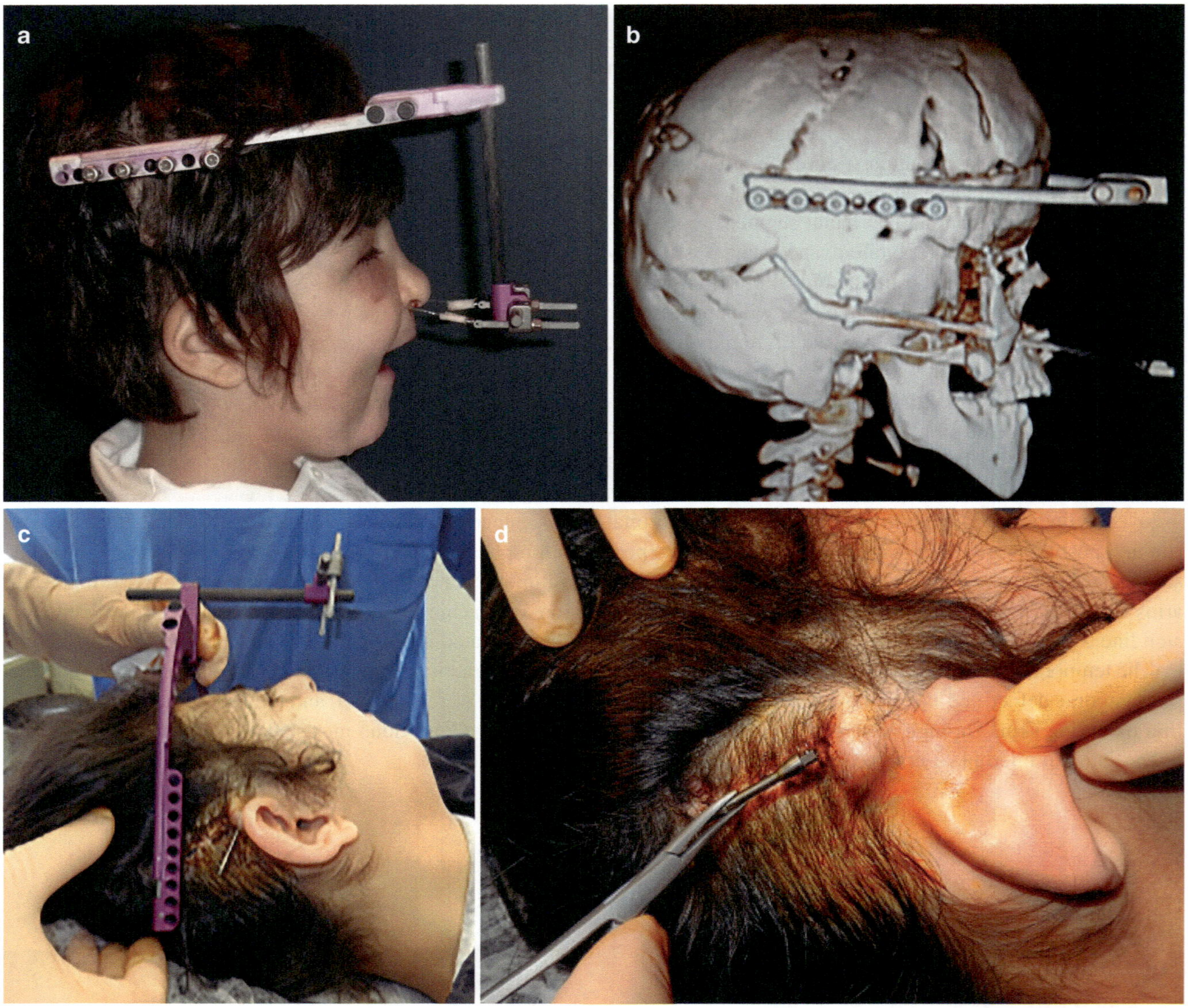

Fig. 5.5 (**a, b**) Rigid external device and internal distractors. (**c**) Removal of the rigid external device at the end of the distraction period. (**d**) Detachment of the activation arms of the internal distractors at the end of the distraction period (KLS Martin, Tuttlinger, Germany)

5.2 Technical Adaptations

The efficacy of primary LF3 on OSAS is established in faciocraniosynostoses. However, in secondary LF3, the main concern is the extent of scarring of the deep tissues from the previous FFMBA. Theoretically, this scarring could limit the amount of advancement that can be achieved, as well as potentially increase the relapse risk of the maxillary retrusion. The bipartition of the LF3 segment increases the airways as it has been proved before (Fig. 5.6).

Technical adaptations have been introduced to the secondary LF3 to optimize the amount and durability of the advancement.

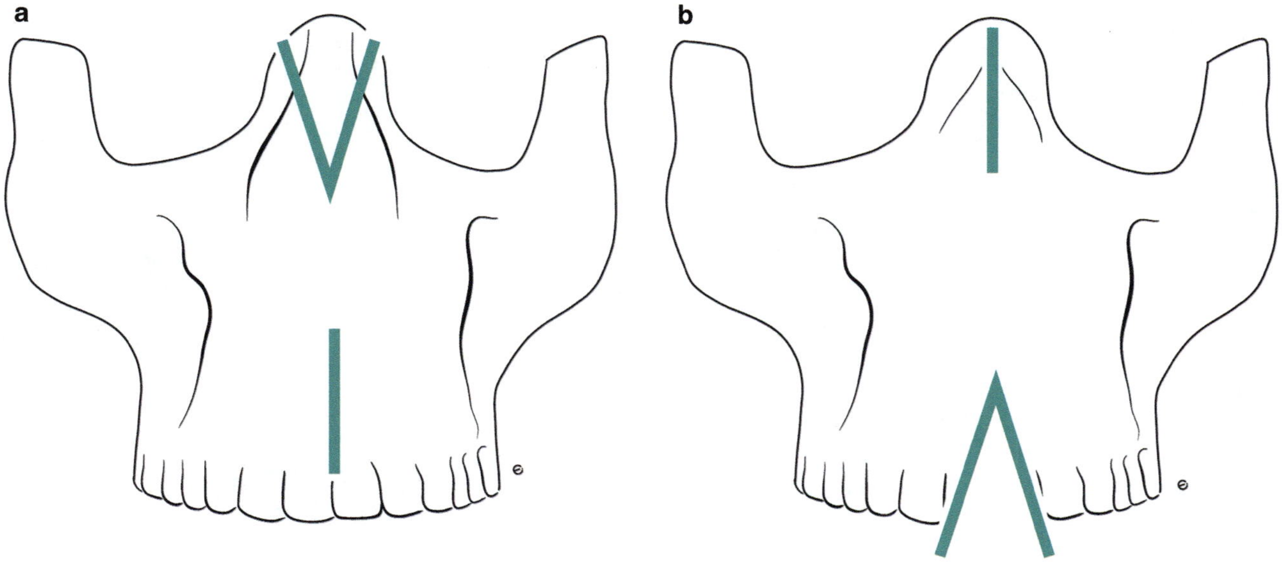

Fig. 5.6 (**a**) Variation: LF3 with bipartition, involving a V-shaped resection at the root of the nose and a medial split of the palate. (**b**) After rotation of both hemifaces, narrowing at the interorbital level and enlargement at the palatal level are obtained. ©Cassandra Vion

5.3 Amount of Advancement

Overcorrection is the hallmark of this stage of the strategy of care. Distraction osteogenesis potentiates the amount of advancement that can be achieved. Distraction progressively distends the soft tissues and induces simultaneous bone formation, bridging the distraction gap with bony osteoid that mineralizes secondarily.

The distraction devices employed in the secondary LF3 have a relatively important range of motion to allow such massive advancement. The Rigid External Distraction (RED) Device and the Marchac-Arnaud temporo-zygomatic internal distractors both offer important distraction amplitudes.

A differential maxillary advancement is usually required in the secondary LF3. Advancement is usually more important inferiorly than superiorly. Inferiorly, at the level of the maxillary arch, the anterior movement must achieve Angle class II malocclusion with substantial overcorrection of the maxillary retrusion. Superiorly, at the level of the inferior orbital rims, the amount of advancement is less important. It aims to correct the negative vector, scleral show, and malar retrusion without causing enophthalmos. This difference in endpoints is justified by the (unpublished) observation of more important retrusion forces inferiorly than superiorly, and by the unaesthetic aspect of enophthalmos that, if attained, tends to persist and is difficult to correct surgically. Conversely, at the occlusal level, any persisting overcorrection or anterior open bite can subsequently be addressed by orthognathic surgery at dental maturity.

The disposition of the internal and external distraction devices has been optimized to allow such a differential distraction. In short, a rotational component to the advancement is introduced by using a microplate bilaterally at the level of the fronto-zygomatic osteotomy. Only one 5-mm screw is used at each side of the plate to allow counterclockwise rotation and forward translation of the maxilla. The fronto-zygomatic osteotomy line is designed oblique forward and downward, and the frontal process of the zygomatic bone is positioned anterior to the zygomatic process of the frontal bone. This allows both a translational (forward) and a rotational hinge movement of the maxilla (mobile segment) around the zygomatic process of the frontal bone (fixed segment).

5.4 Durability of the Advancement

At the end of the activation phase, the external device is removed under sedation while the internal devices are kept in place for 3 to 4 months for consolidation.

Two examples of secondary LF3 after FFMBA are given in Figs. 5.7 and 5.8.

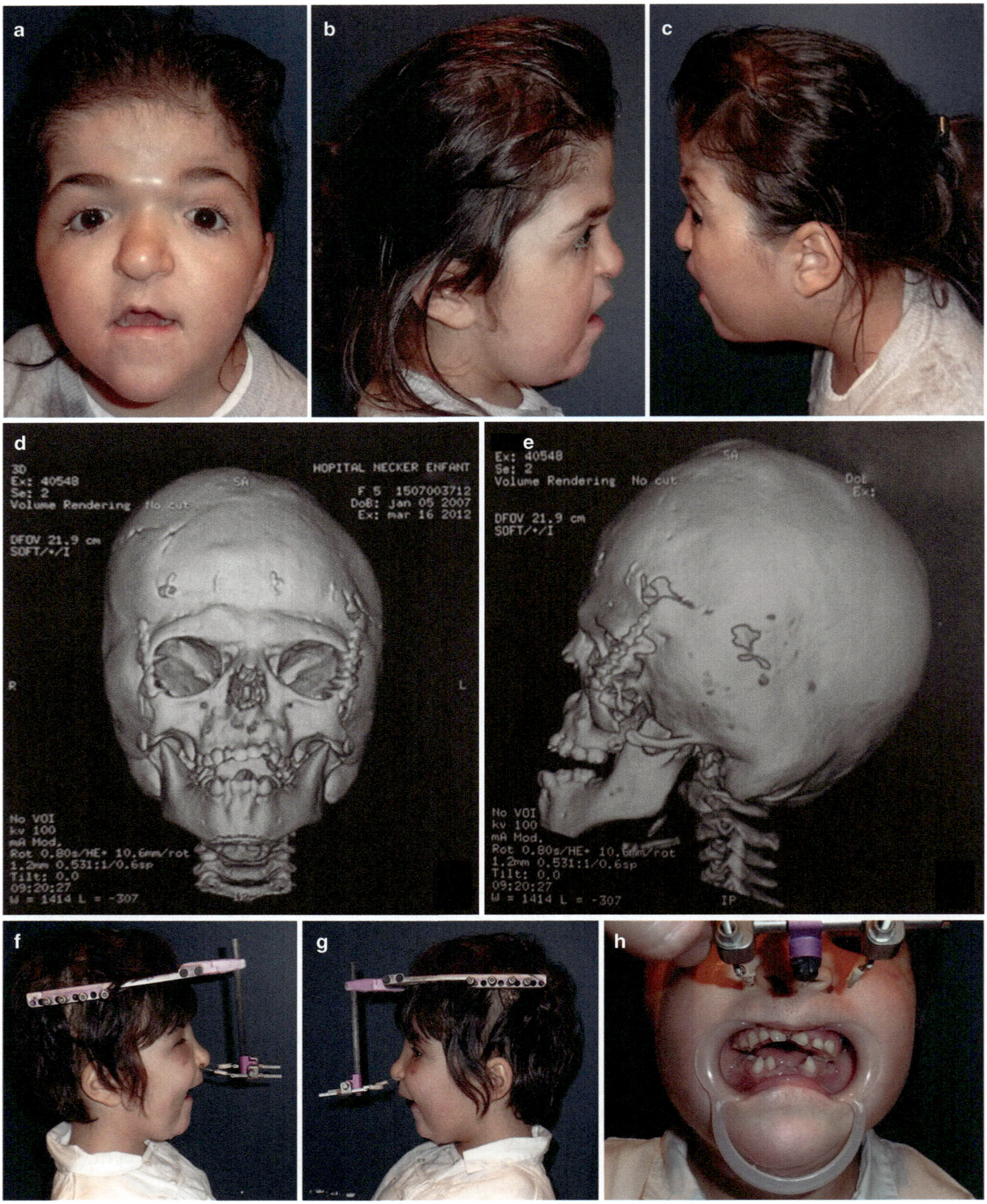

Fig. 5.7 (**a**, **b**, **c**) Patient with Apert syndrome at 6 years of age, 4 years after FFMBA presenting with midface hypoplasia and obstructive sleep apnea (AHI = 8 per hour). (**d**, **e**) CT scan at 6 years of age before secondary LF3. (**f**, **g**, **h**) Rigid external distraction device in place and distraction in progress. No internal distractors were used. (**i**, **j**) CT scan with the RED in place demonstrates the advancement. (**k**, **l**, **m**) Clinical results at 7 years of age, 12 months after LF3, with clear overcorrection. Normalization of AHI: 0.5 per hour. (**n**, **o**, **p**) Progressive relapse and loss of the overcorrection at 10 years of age, 4 years after the LF3. No relapse of sleep apnea (AHI = 0 per hour)

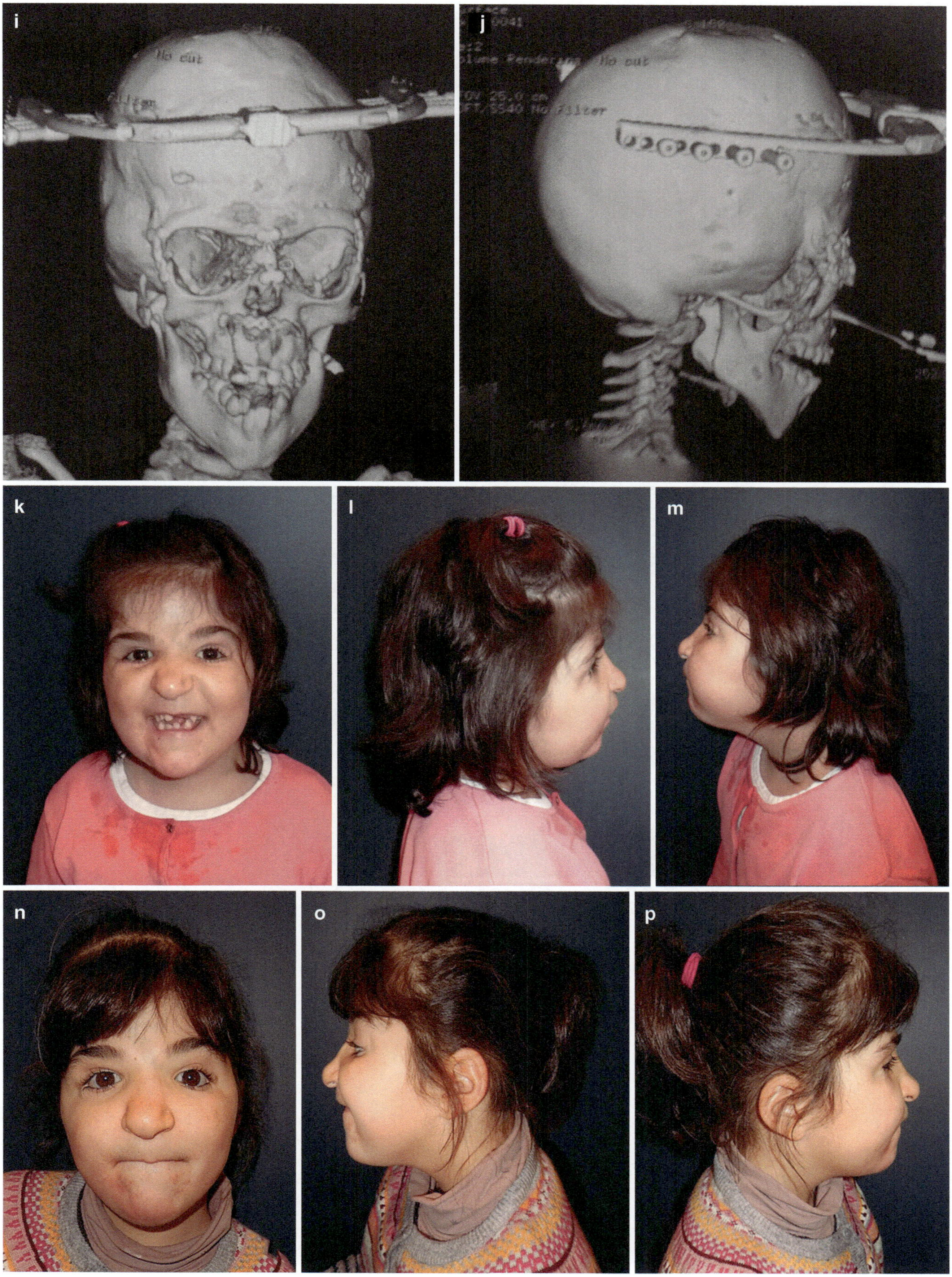

Fig. 5.7 (continued)

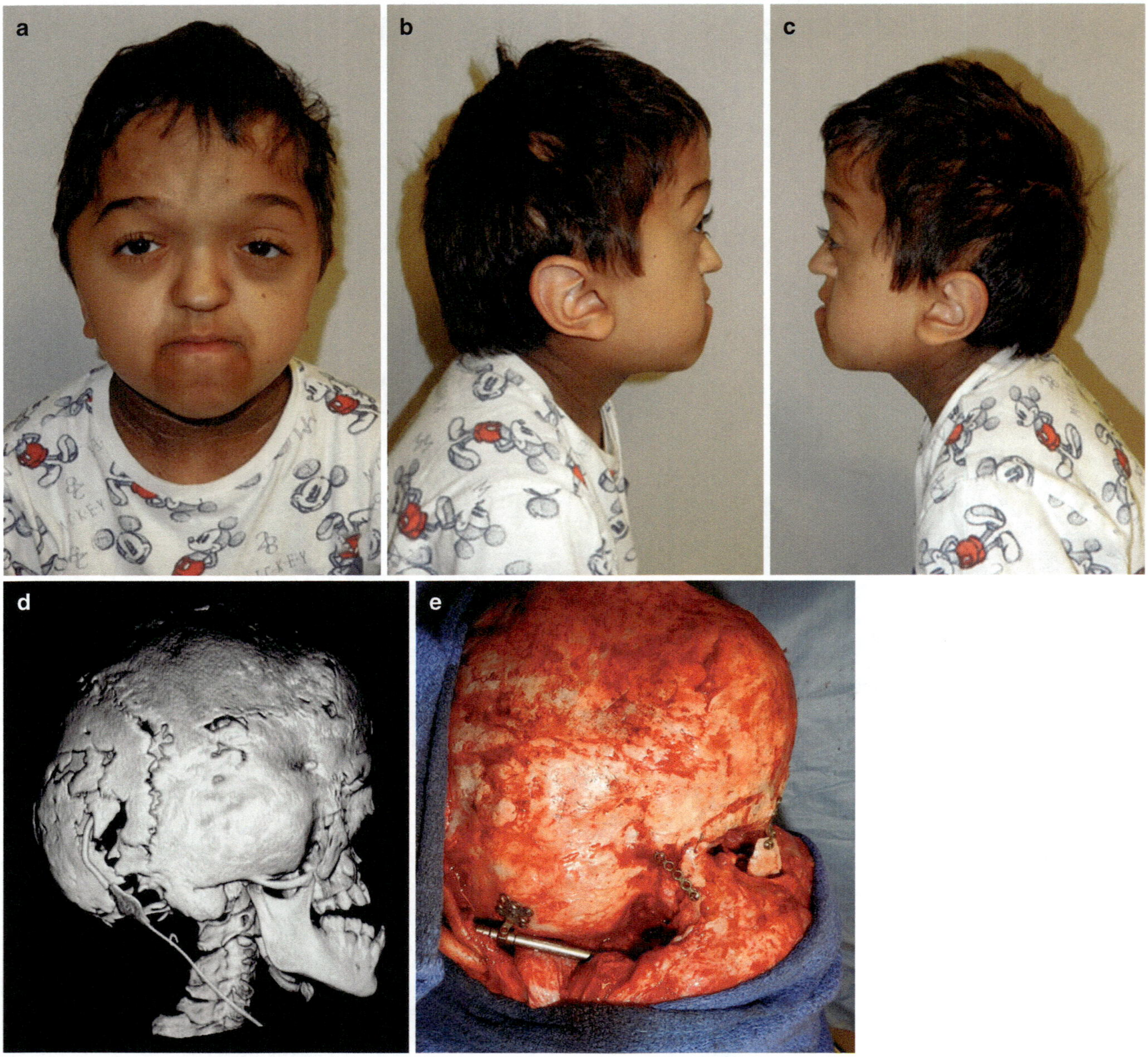

Fig. 5.8 (**a**, **b**, **c**) Patient with Crouzon with acanthosis nigricans at 8 years of age, 6,5 years after PVE, shunt, and FFMBA. Observe the moderate exorbitism, but OSAS was severe. (**d**) CT scan at 8 years of age, before secondary LF3. (**e**) Per-operative view showing the facial advancement, the fronto-zygomatic plate, and the internal temporo-zygomatic distractors. (**f**, **g**, **h**) Result at 10 years of age 2 years after the LF3 showing insufficient correction of the midface hypoplasia. (**i**) CT scan at 10 years, 2 years after secondary LF3, showing a relapse of the midface hypoplasia

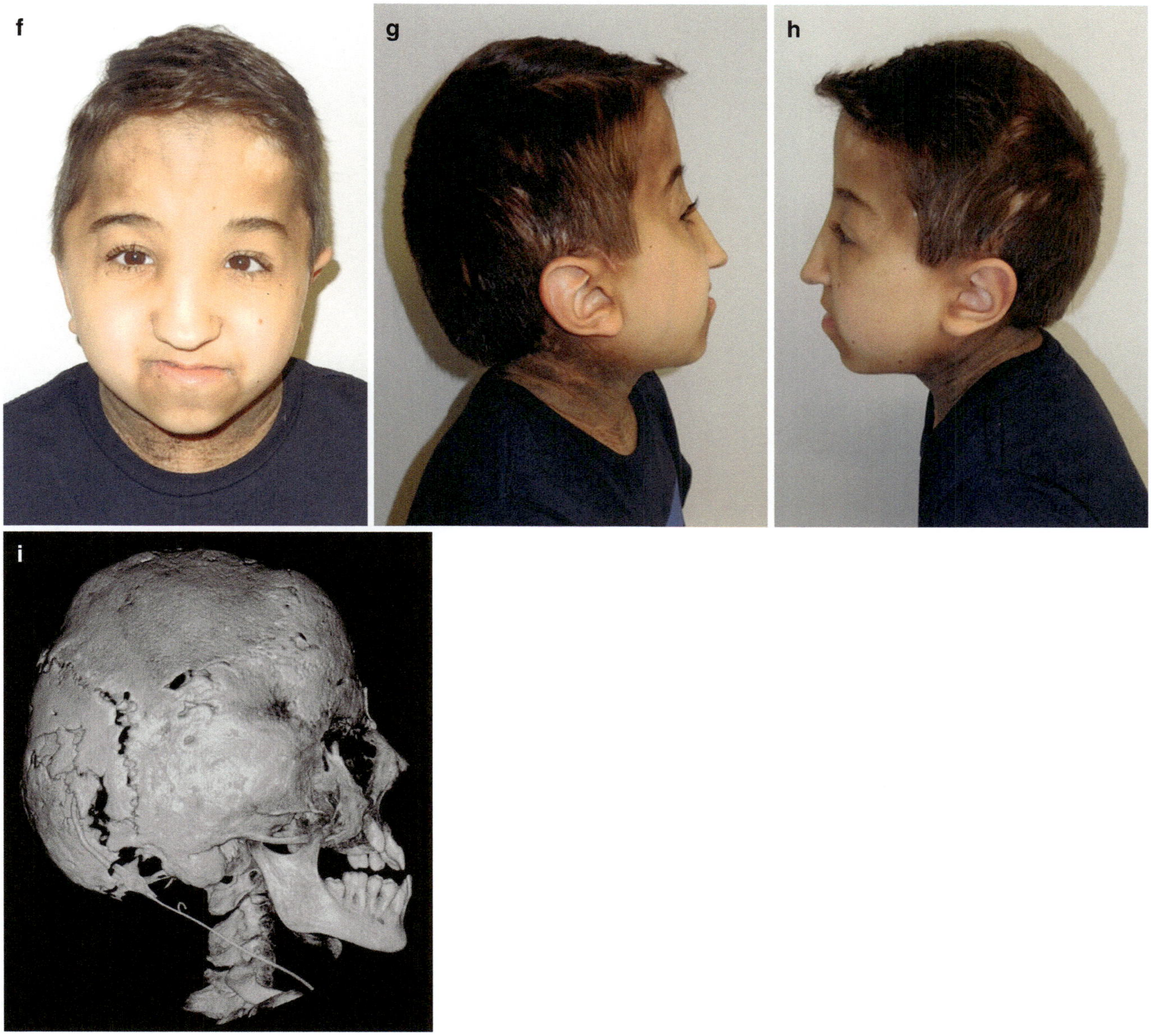

Fig. 5.8 (continued)

References

1. Haber SE, Khonsari RH, Leikola J, et al. S3–18 Session 3: Faciocraniosynostosis–PART I secondary facial advancement in syndromic craniosynostoses: a prospective assessment of 109 cases. Plast Reconstr Surg–Global Open. 2019 Aug;7(8S-2):40–1.
2. Haber SE, Leikola J, Nowinski D, et al. Secondary Le fort III after early Fronto-facial Monobloc normalizes sleep Apnea in Faciocraniosynostosis: a cohort study. J Plast Reconstr Aesthet Surg. 2022 Aug;75(8):2706–18.

Very Early Monobloc: A Procedure for Extreme Conditions with Transfacial External Traction and Internal Distraction

6

1. Before 18 months of age, FFMBA is only indicated in rare extreme conditions: life-threatening situations, in case of risk for blindness and/or to avoid tracheostomy.
2. Very early FFMBA (VEM) requires technical adaptations consisting of external traction associated with internal distractors.
3. Overcorrection is key but limited by optic nerve elongation.
4. VEM almost invariably leads to the relapse of mid-face retrusion, requiring secondary LF3 at later ages.
5. An experienced pediatric anesthesia team is crucial in the management of very early FFMBA.

Performing FFMBA in the first year of life presents specific difficulties that require technical adaptations. We associate internal distraction and an external traction system using a transfacial Kirschner wire [1, 2]. Between March 2008 and July 2016, seven patients (5 with Pfeiffer syndrome, 2 with Crouzon syndrome including 1 CAN) benefited from very early fronto-facial advancement (7 procedures) with the placement of a trans-zygomatic K-wire (Kirshner 2-2,2 mm) after the osteotomies. External traction was applied to the Kirschner wire using pulleys and strings (between 2–3 kg). Continuous postoperative sedation was maintained during the first 7 days postoperatively. The traction system was then released and the patient extubated. The activation phase of internal distraction was then engaged, followed by 3–6 months of consolidation (Fig. 6.1). The median follow-up was 5,2 ± 2,1 years.

Exorbitism improved in all patients. All patients were weaned off noninvasive ventilation postoperatively. Fifty percent of tracheotomized patients were decannulated. One year postoperatively, all patients had a better occlusion. At 5 years of follow-up, 57% were still in class II occlusion. Two complications occurred: one pin-tract infection was solved after removal of the Kirschner wire and one transient brachial plexus palsy due to overextension of the neck during traction.

The traction/distraction system is a reliable ancillary procedure for very young patients with FCST in whom an early progressive facial advancement is mandatory. A longer follow-up and a greater series of patients is advisable before applying this technique in less complex/urgent cases. In five other cases, a very early monobloc was performed and a Kirschner wire inserted without the need of an external traction: In those latter cases, the trans-zygomatic K-wire was used as a stabilizer of the young skeleton.

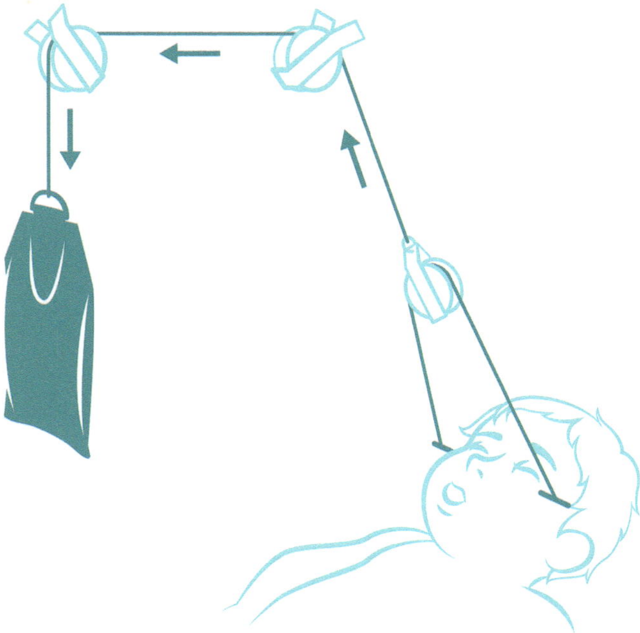

Fig. 6.1 Diagram illustrating the components of the external traction system in the very early FFMBA. ©Cassandra Vion

E. Arnaud et al., *Frontofacial Monobloc Advancement with Internal Distraction*, https://doi.org/10.1007/978-3-031-07574-2_6

The importance of a dedicated pediatric anesthesia team cannot be stressed enough. All the anesthesia physicians, nurses, and staff members as well as the pediatric ICU team have to be experienced in the peculiarities of craniofacial surgery procedures and the postoperative pediatric intensive care unit management of these patients. Decision-making is closely coordinated with the surgical team and strategies are evaluated daily to ensure the highest safety standards are constantly met. This coordination between surgeons and anesthesiologists is specifically crucial for very early FFMBA.

Several examples of this rare procedure including external traction applied to the transfacial pin are given (Figs. 6.2, 6.3, 6.4, 6.5, and 6.6).

Fig. 6.2 (**a**, **b**, **c**) Patient with Pfeiffer syndrome who benefited from initial posterior expansion. ©Cassandra Vion. (**d**, **e**, **f**) Very early FFMBA was performed at the age of 12 months. Intraoperative views of the osteotomies. (**g**) During the distraction phase with external traction. (**h**) At the removal of the transfacial pin after 14 days of external traction. (**i**, **j**) Clinical and CT scan lateral views after the completion of the distraction, at 16 months of age. (**k**) Clinical outcome 10 months after very early FFMBA, at the age of 22 months. (**l–o**) CT scan aspect outcome 10 months after very early FFMBA, at the age of 22 months

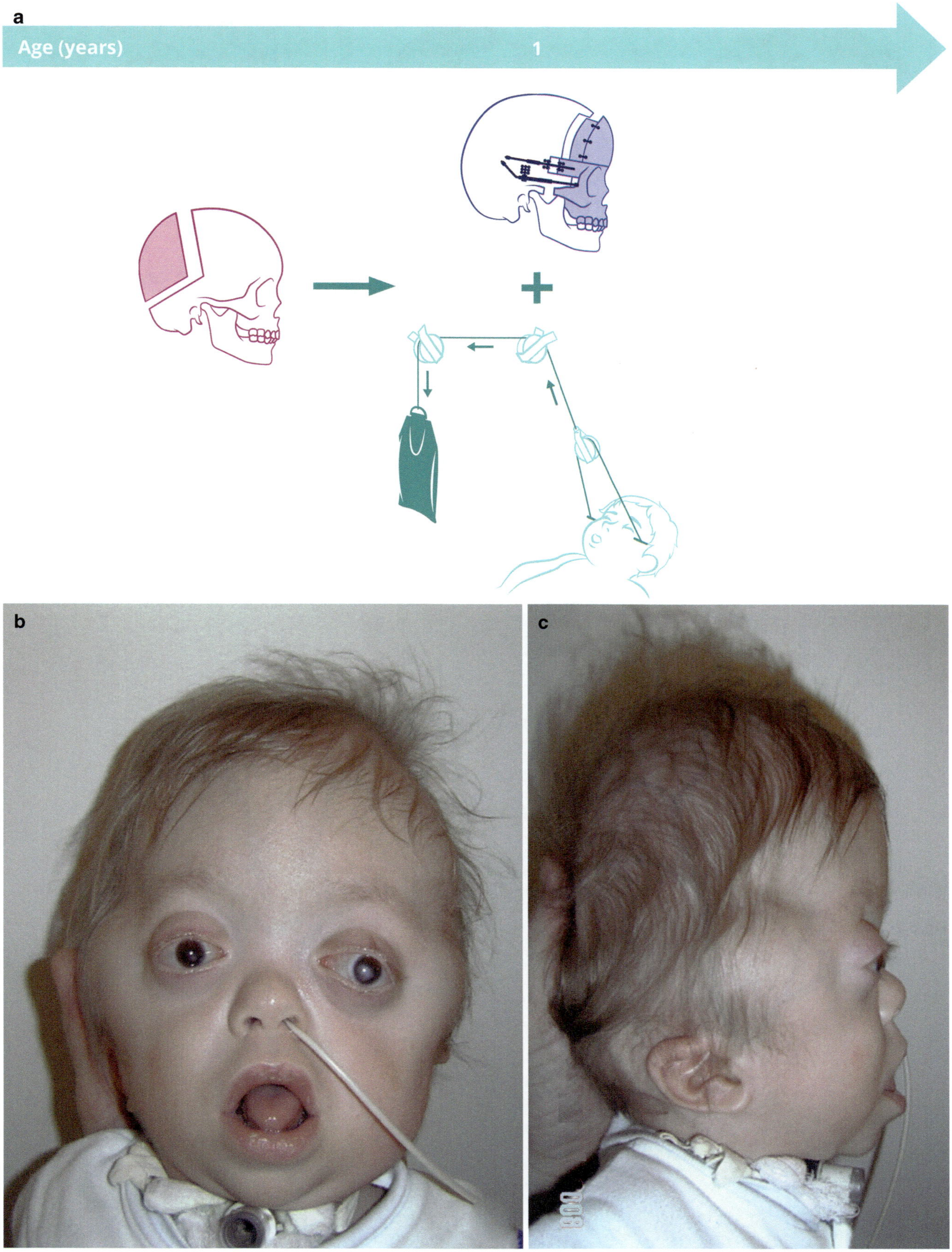
a
Age (years)
1
b
c

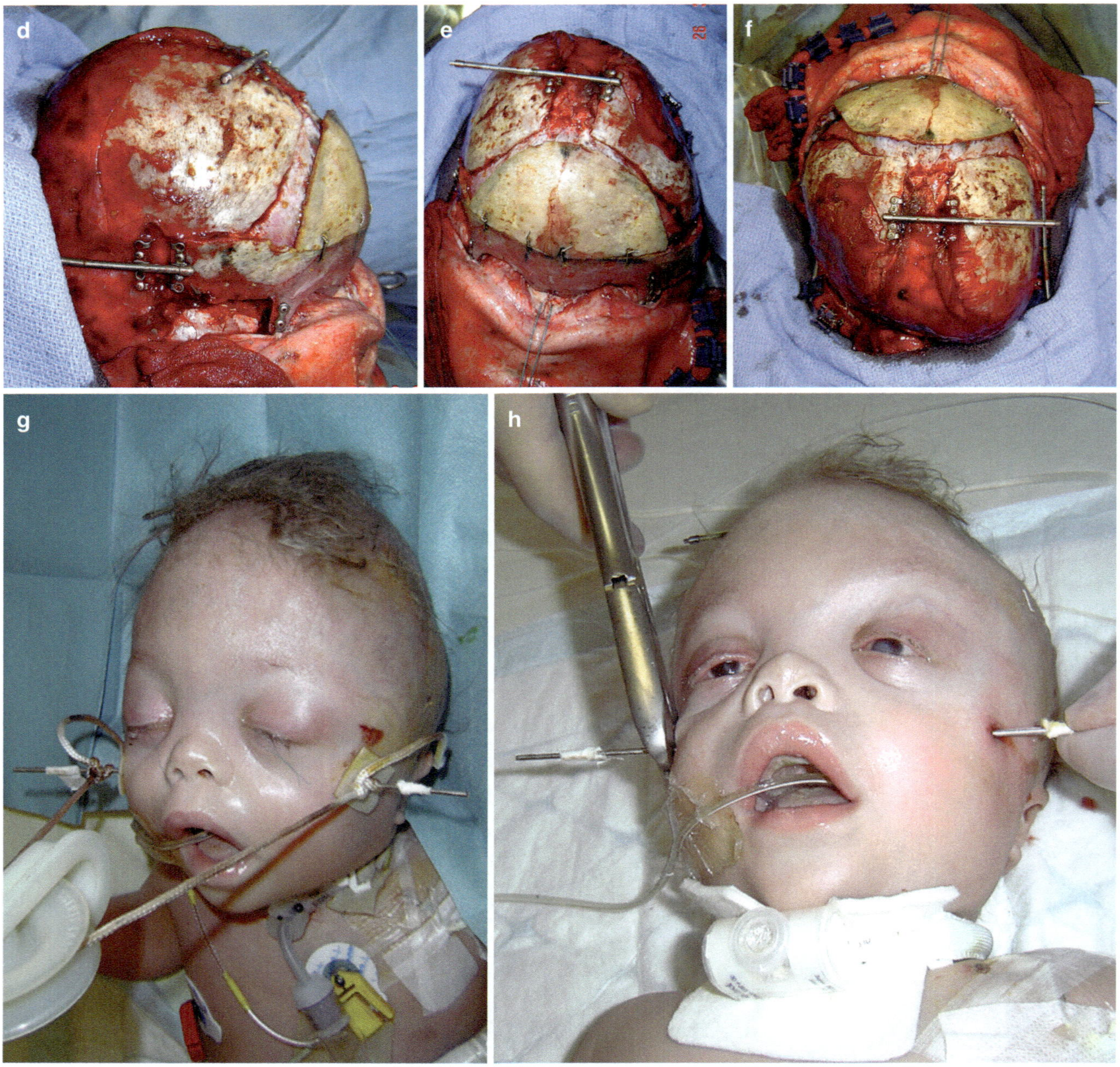

Fig. 6.2 (continued)

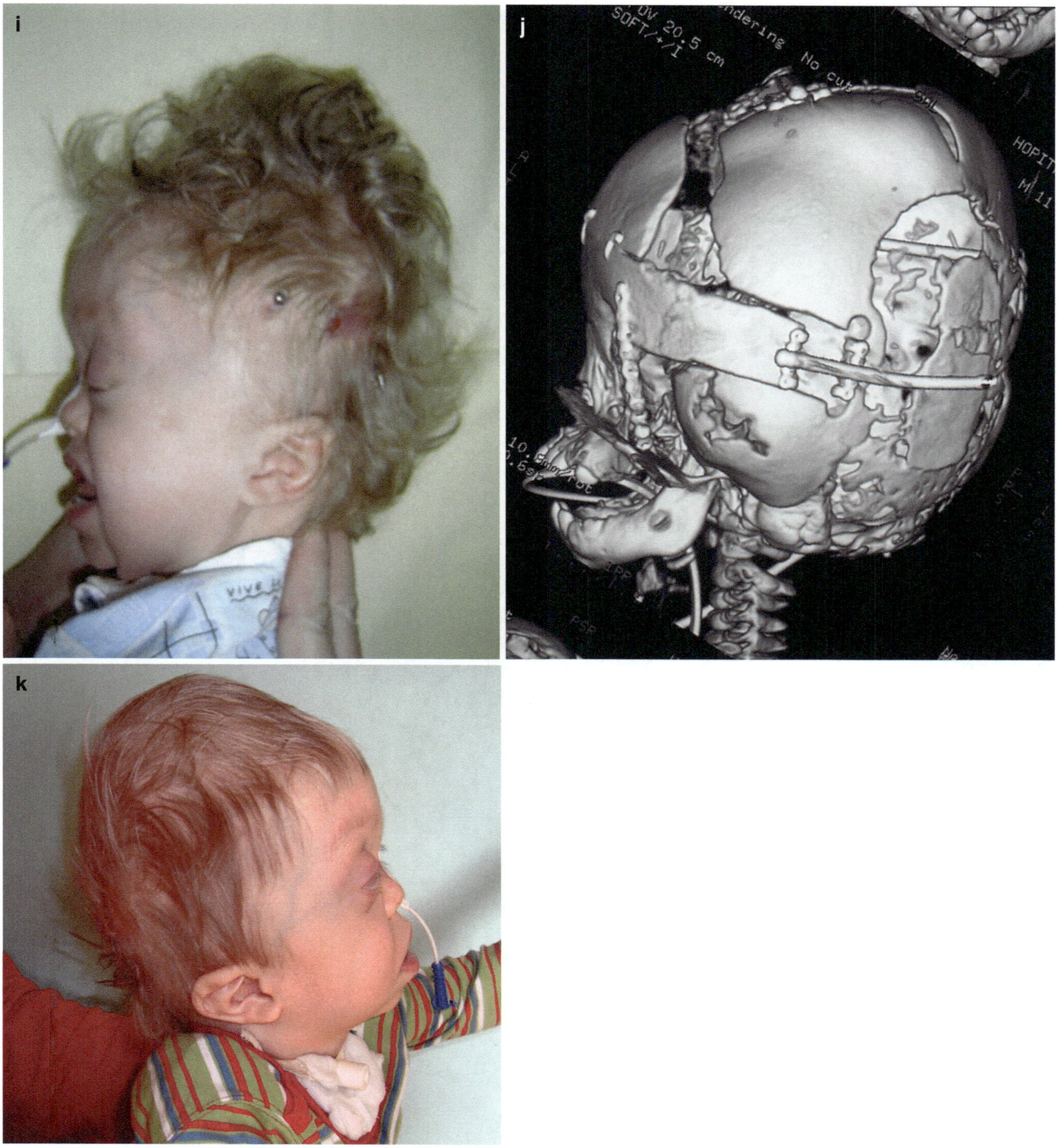

Fig. 6.2 (continued)

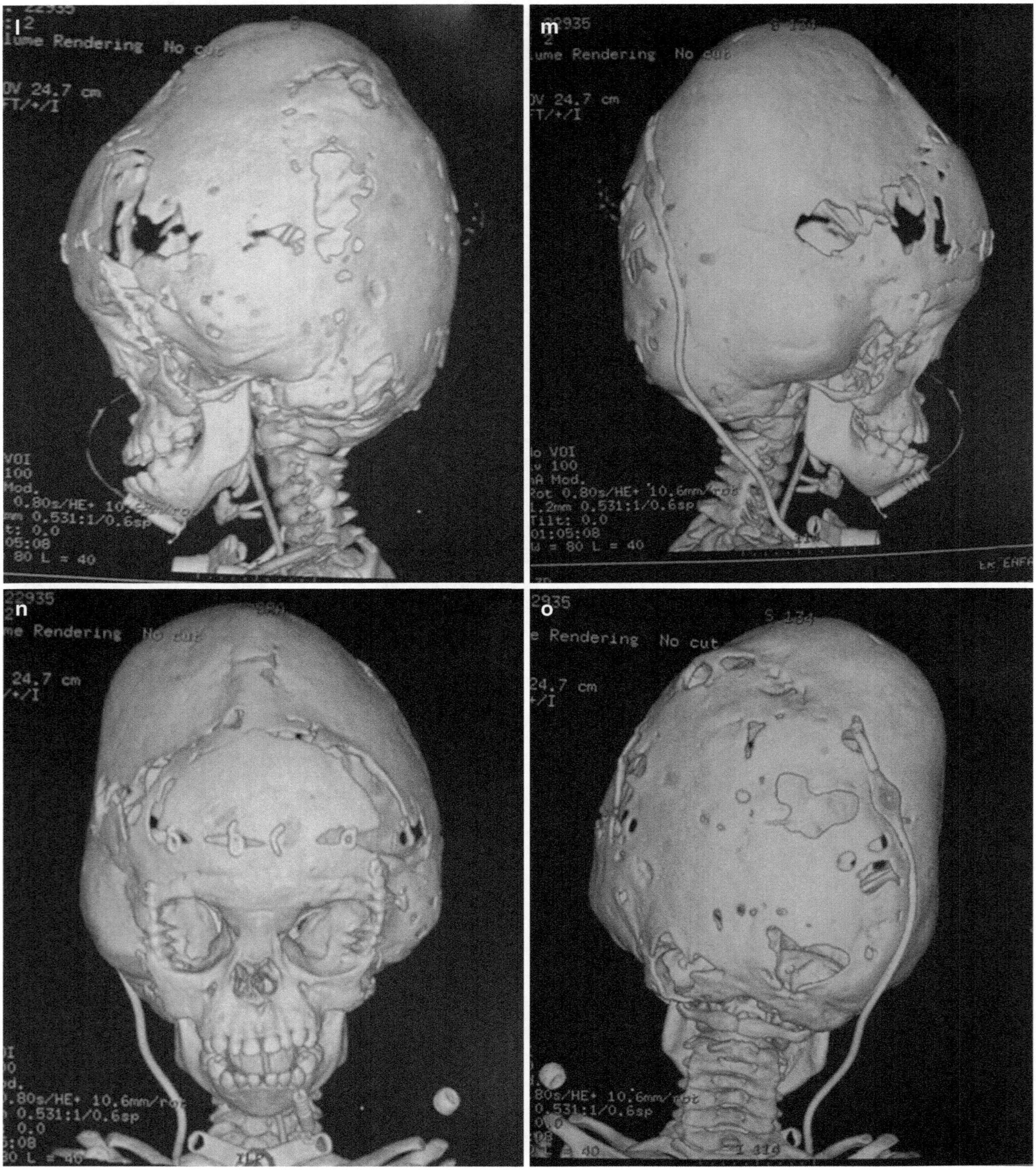

Fig. 6.2 (continued)

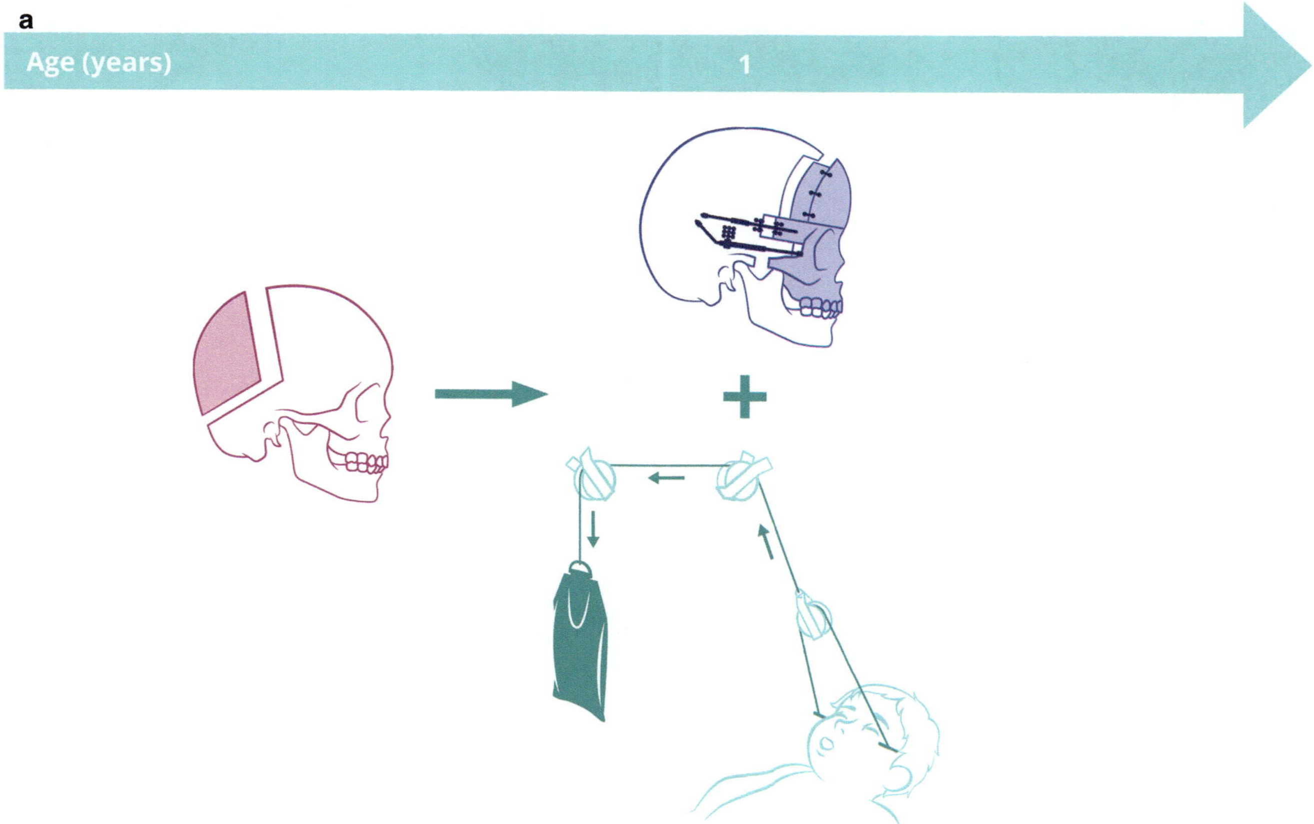

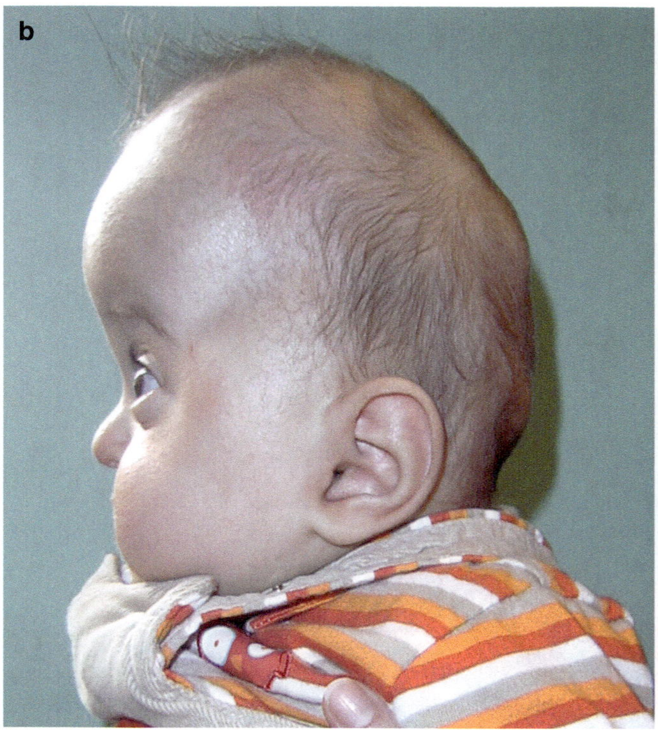

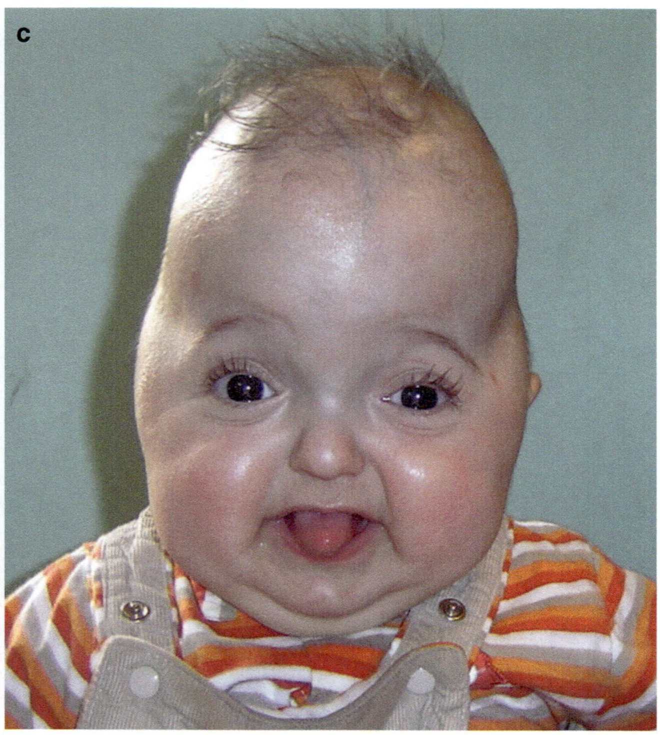

Fig. 6.3 (**a**, **b**, **c**) Patient with Crouzon—acanthosis nigricans (FGFR3 mutation) aged 9 months. ©Cassandra Vion. Cloverleaf skull and intracranial hypertension. (**d**, **e**) CT scan aspect before very early FFMBA at 14 months of age after PVE has been performed. (**f-i**) Very early FFMBA: osteotomies performed at 14 months of age. Notice a vertex distractor was inserted, actually used as a skull contractor to reduce turricephaly. (**j**) Very early FFMBA with traction in process. (**k**) Postoperative CT scan result at 18 months of age, 4 months after the procedure. (**l**, **m**) Postoperative result at 2,5 years of age, 15 months after the procedure. Progressive relapse of the maxillary hypoplasia. Observe correction of cloverleaf aspect and decrease of turricephaly. (**n**, **o**) Postoperative result at 4 years of age. Progressive relapse of the maxillary hypoplasia. (**p**, **q**) Postoperative result at 6 years of age, Progressive relapse of the maxillary hypoplasia. (**r**, **s**) Postoperative result at 8 years of age, 7 years after the procedure. Progressive relapse of the maxillary hypoplasia aggravated by noninvasive ventilation mask [3]. This clinical presentation typically indicates LF3 (see Fig. 5.8)

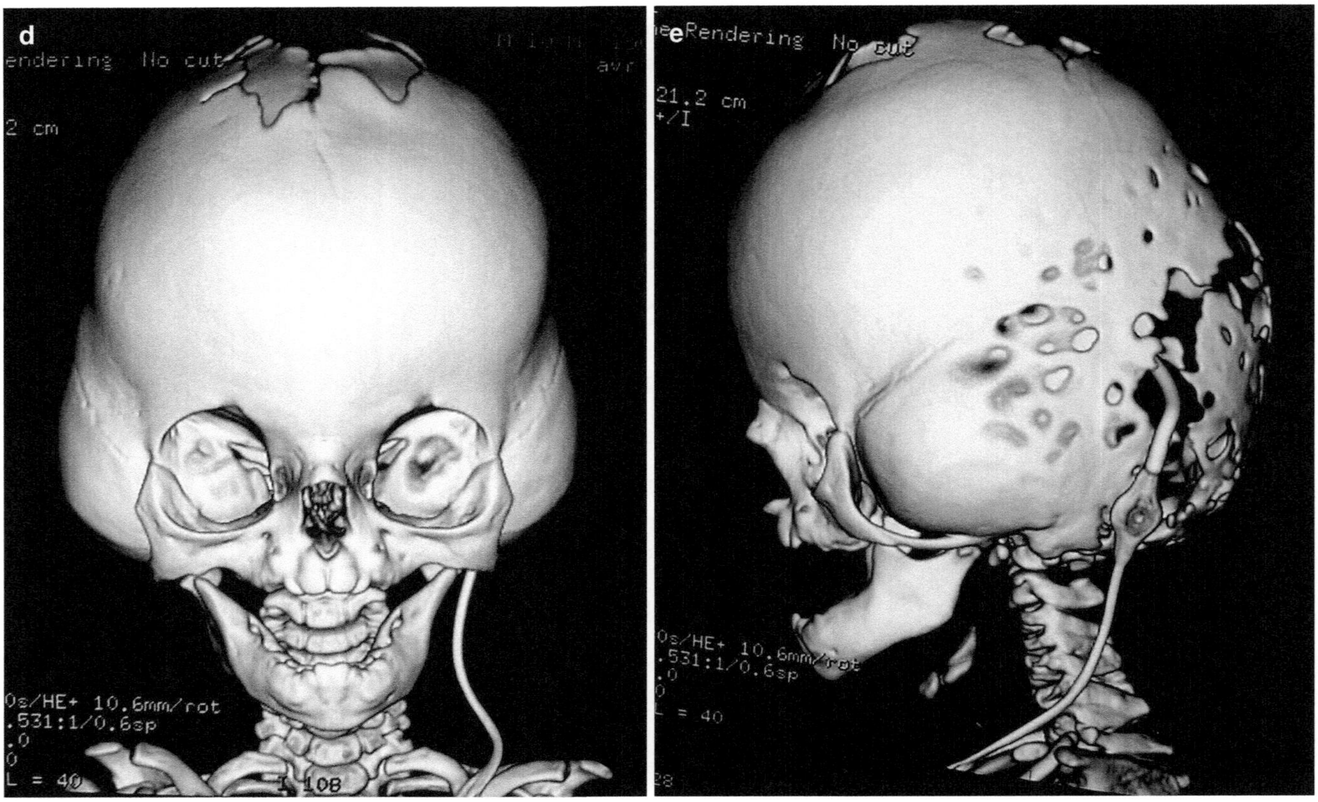

Fig. 6.3 (continued)

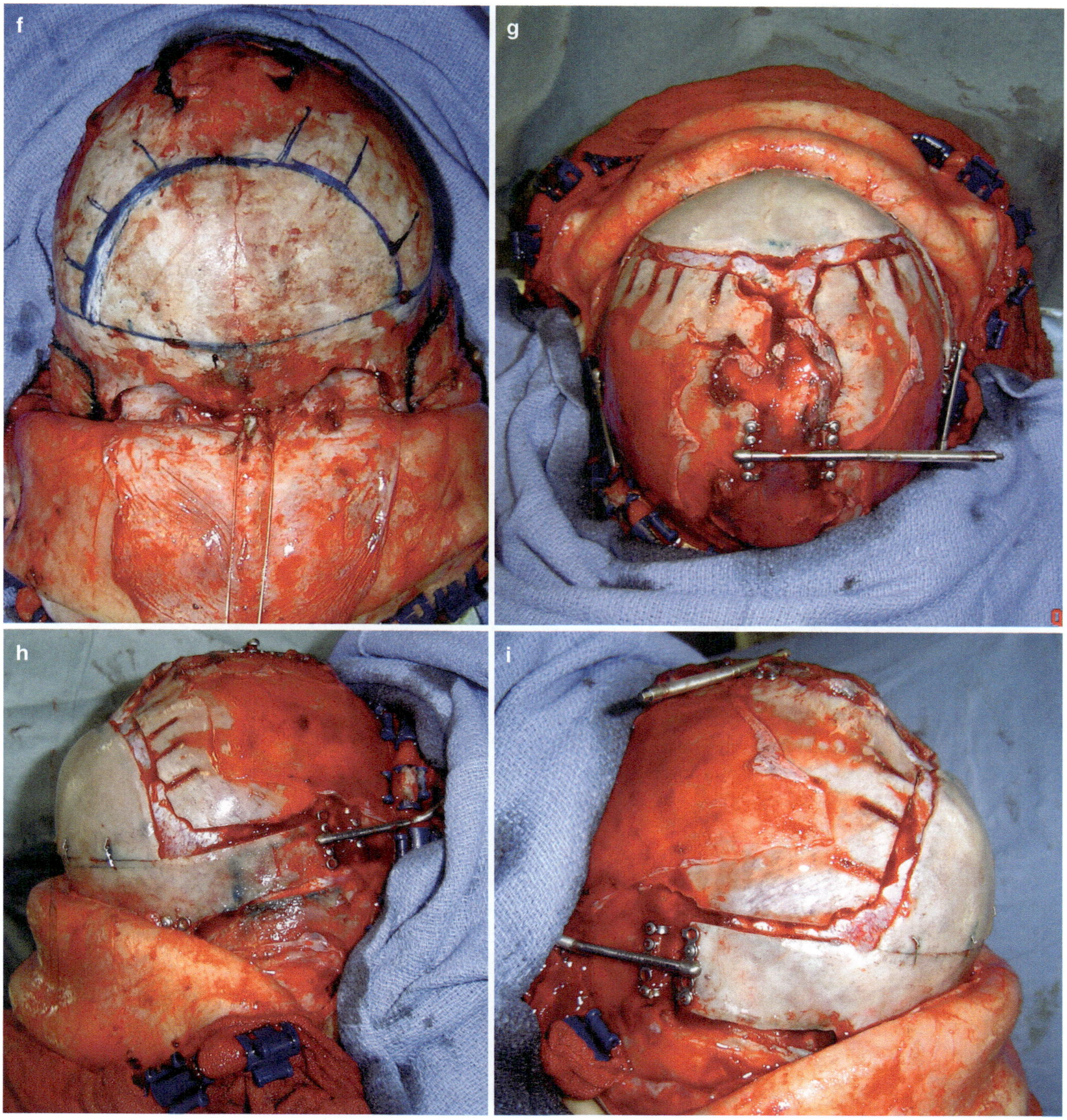

Fig. 6.3 (continued)

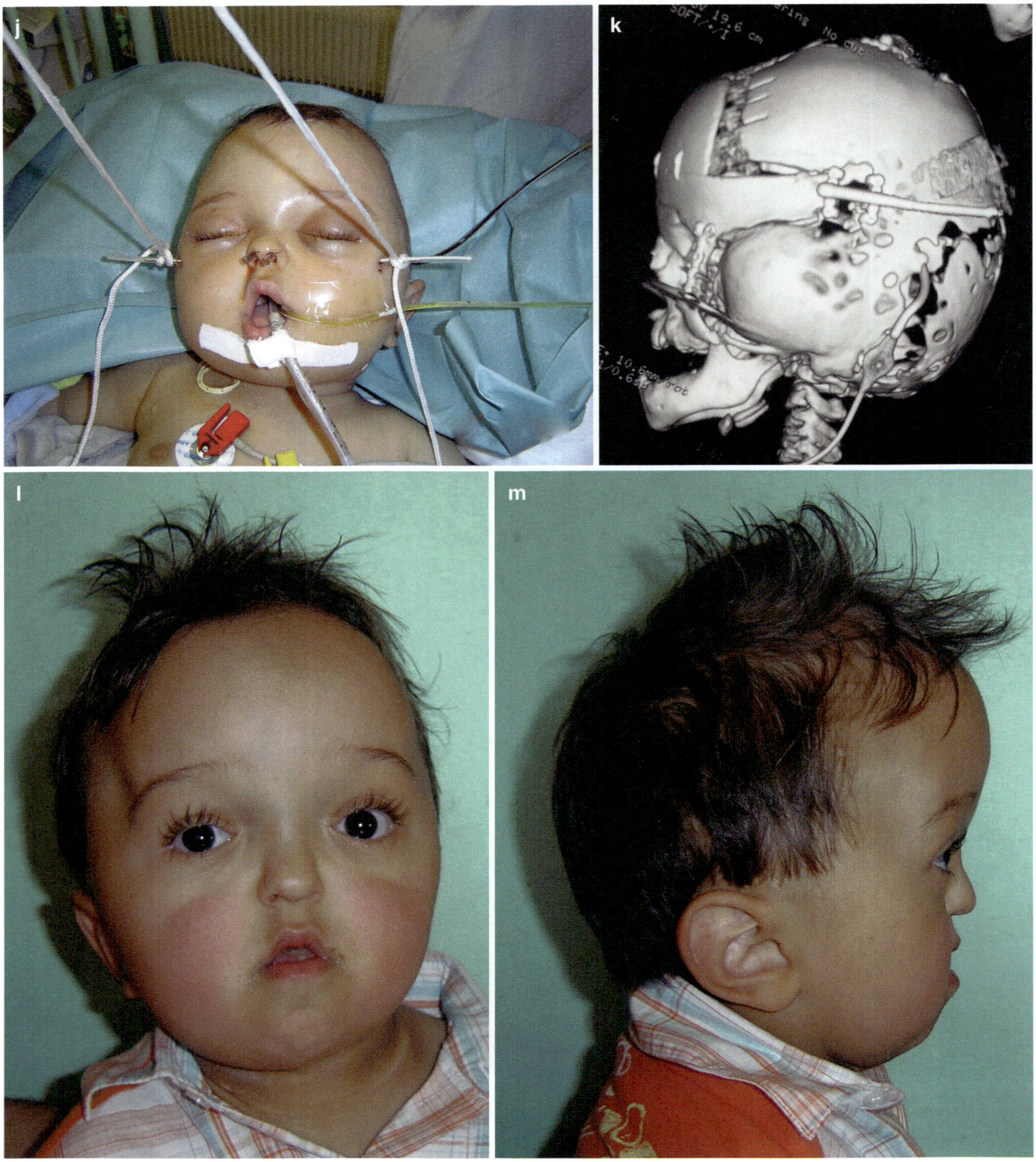

Fig. 6.3 (continued)

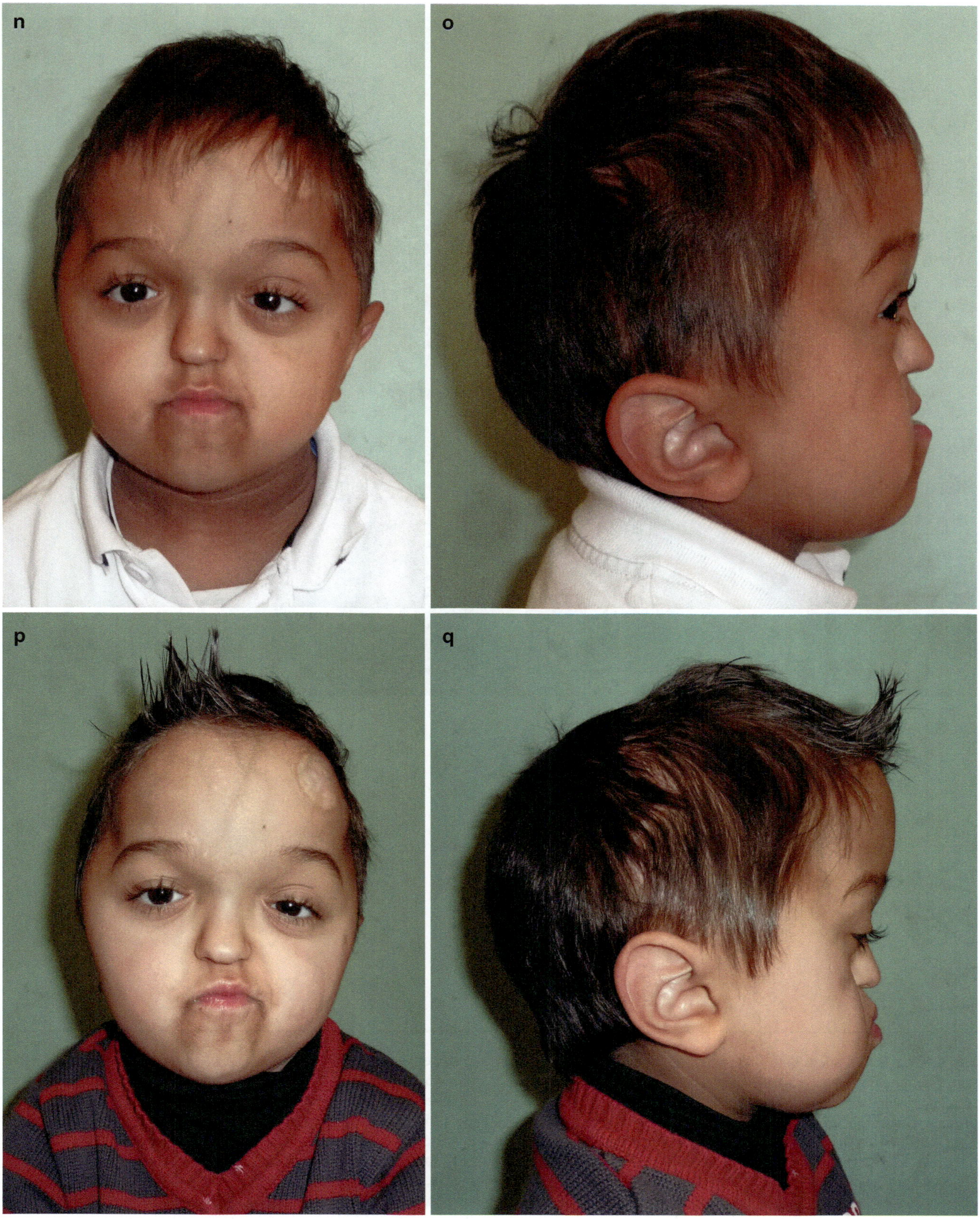

Fig. 6.3 (continued)

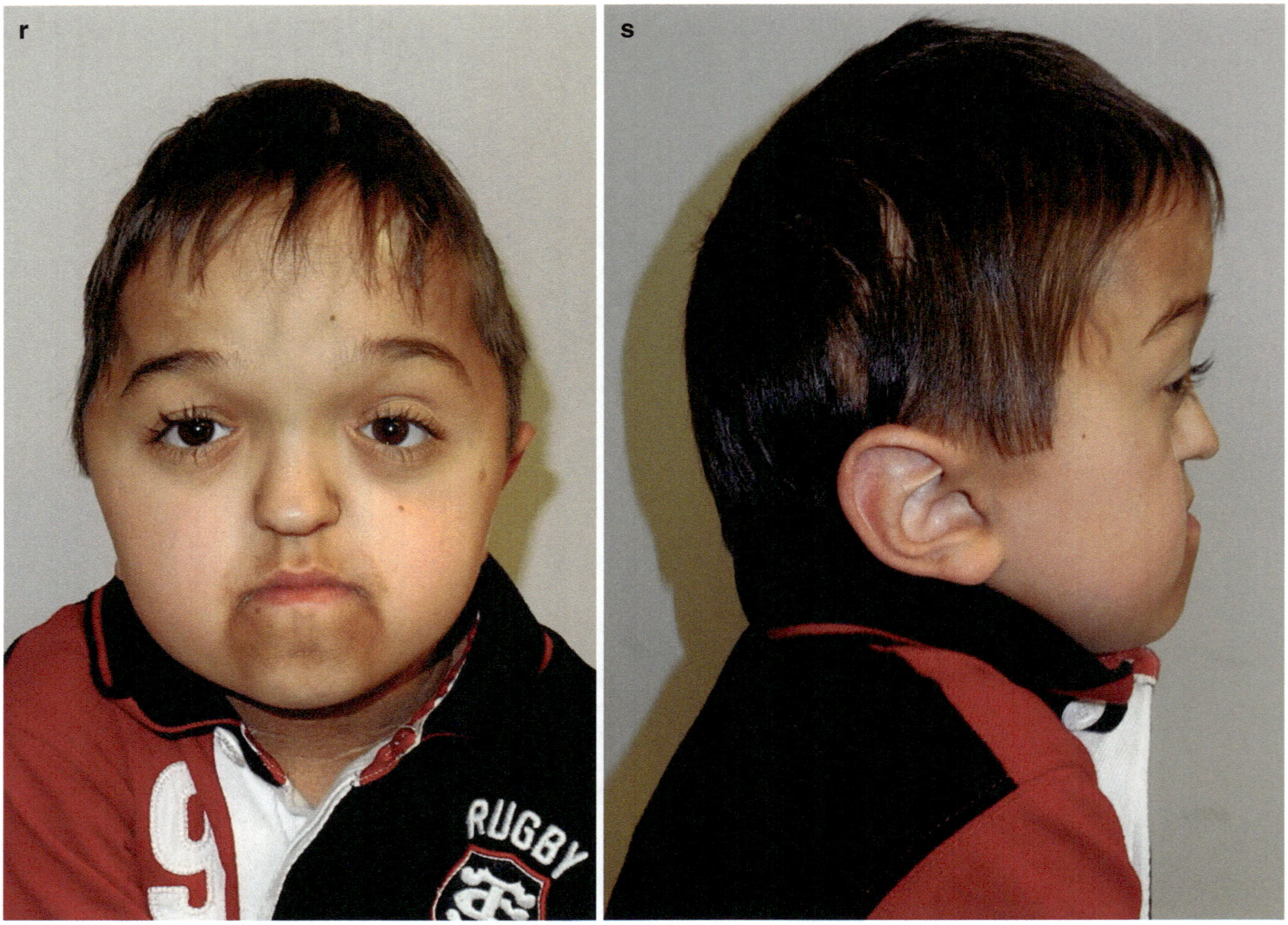

Fig. 6.3 (continued)

Fig. 6.4 (**a**, **b**, **c**) Patient with Pfeiffer syndrome at 12 months of age with previous history of posterior expansion (without distraction performed in another center). Severe exorbitism and tracheostomy are present. ©Cassandra Vion. (**d**) CT scan at 12 months of age, before FFMBA. (**e-h**) Very early FFMBA: osteotomies performed at 14 months of age. (**i**) Very early FFMBA with traction in process. (**j**) CT scan during distraction showing extreme advancement resulting in frontal intradural dead space (attachment of the dura was maintained) and severe class II malocclusion resulting in initial swallowing difficulties. (**k**) At the end of the distraction process, after 2 weeks of traction. (**l**, **m**) Immediate postoperative result with major overcorrection. (**n**, **o**) Postoperative result at 2 years of age, 10 months after the procedure. Moderate relapse of the maxillary hypoplasia. Tracheostomy has been removed. (**p-s**) Postoperative result at 3 years of age, 22 months after the procedure. Moderate relapse of the maxillary hypoplasia. (**t-v**) Postoperative result at 5 years of age, 38 months after the procedure. Moderate relapse of the maxillary hypoplasia. (**w**) CT scan at 5 years of age. (**x**, **y**, **z**, **a'**) Postoperative result at 6 years of age, Acceleration of the maxillary hypoplasia relapse. (**b'**) CT scan at 7 years of age, 6 years after very early FFMBA. (**c'**, **d'**) Postoperative result at 9 years of age, 8 years after the procedure. Acceleration of the maxillary hypoplasia relapse

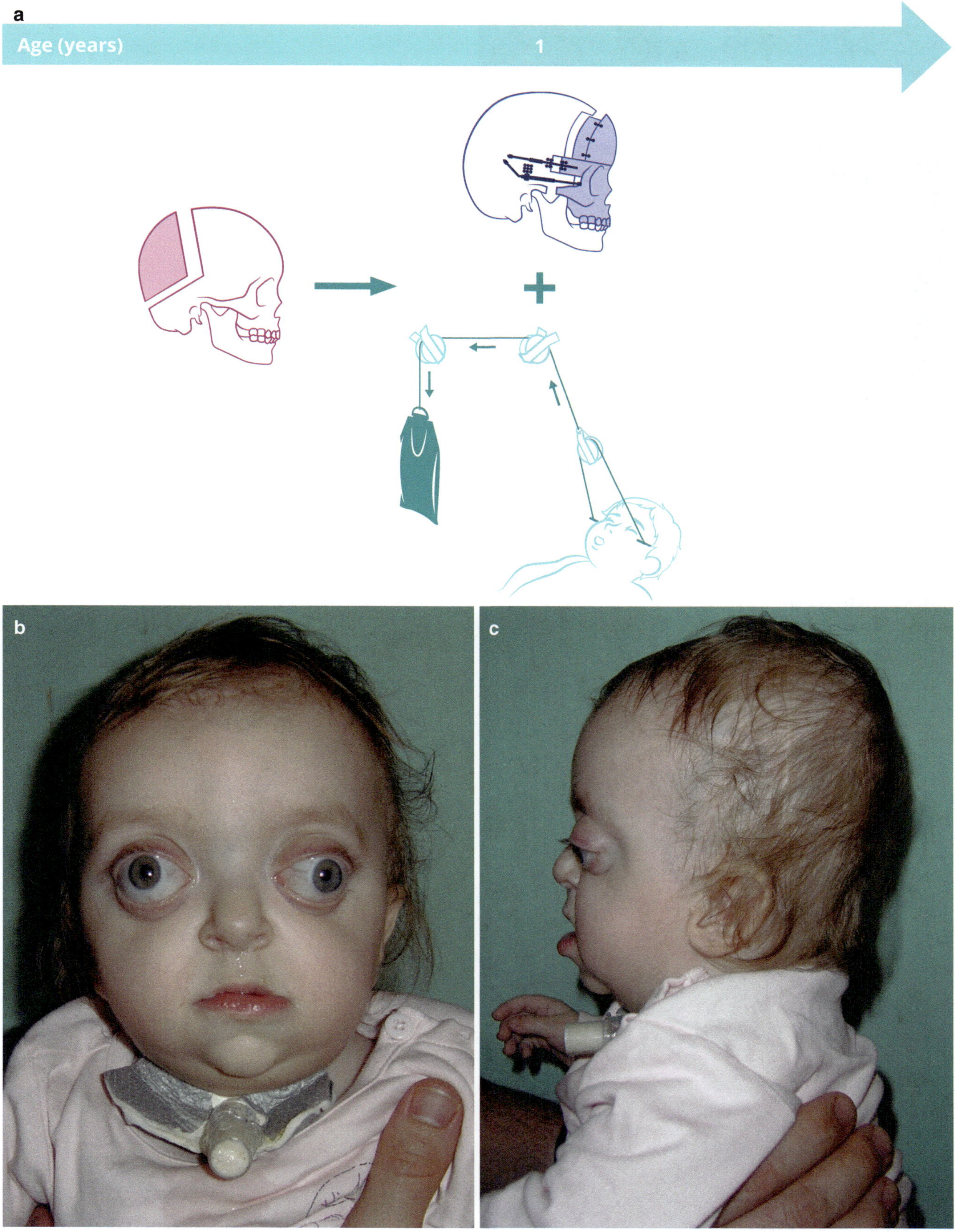
a
Age (years)
1
b
c

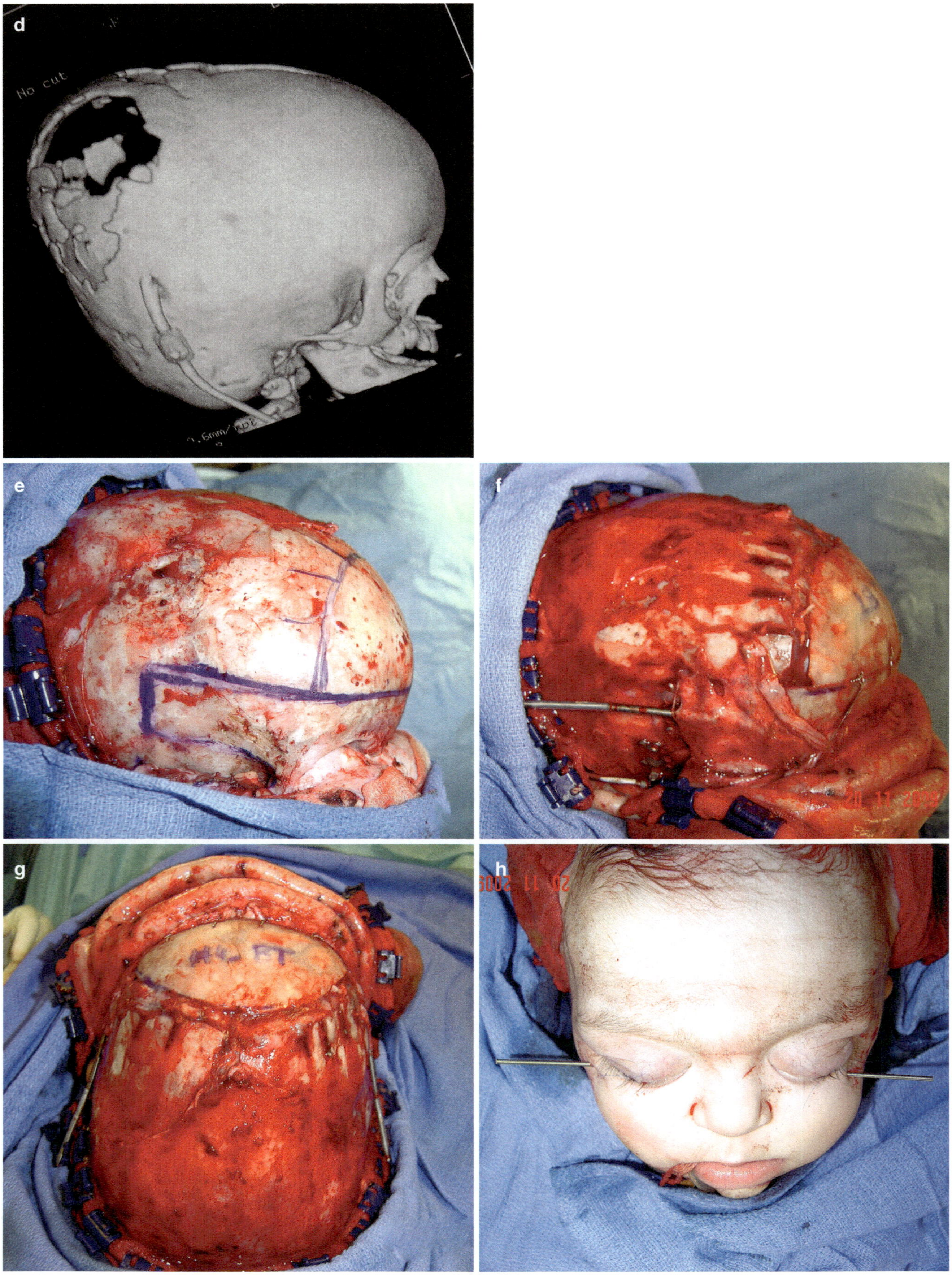

Fig. 6.4 (continued)

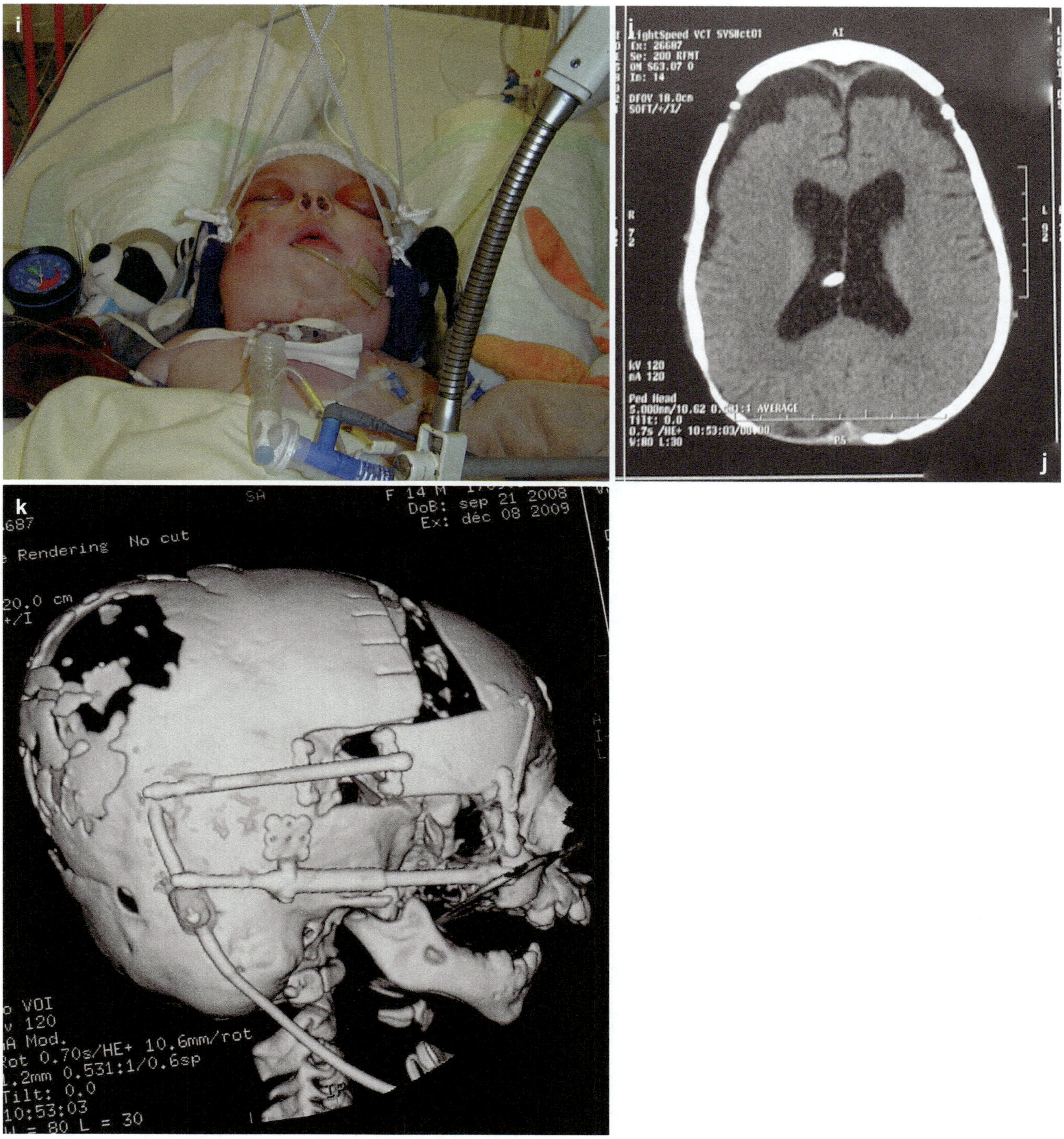

Fig. 6.4 (continued)

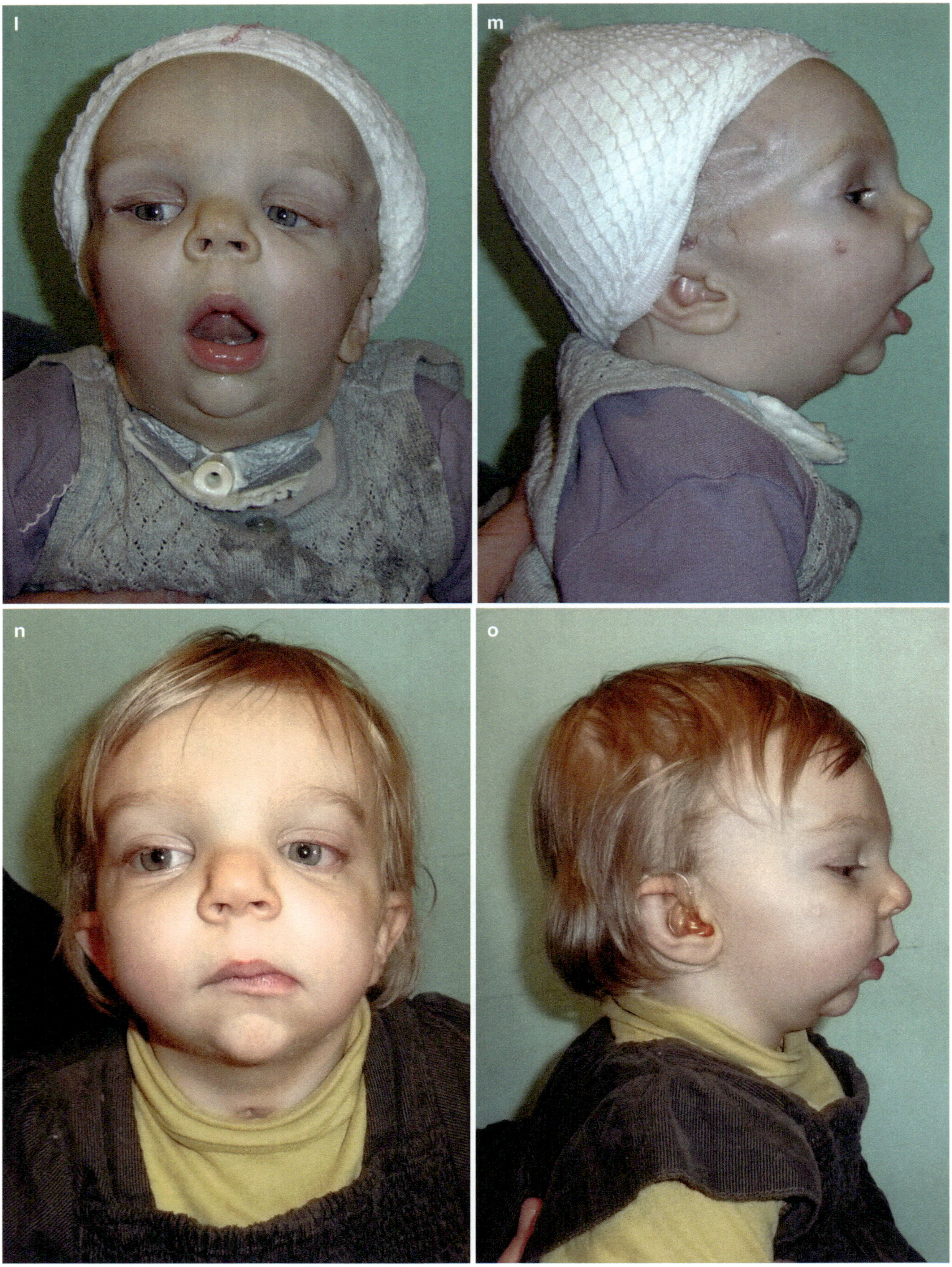

Fig. 6.4 (continued)

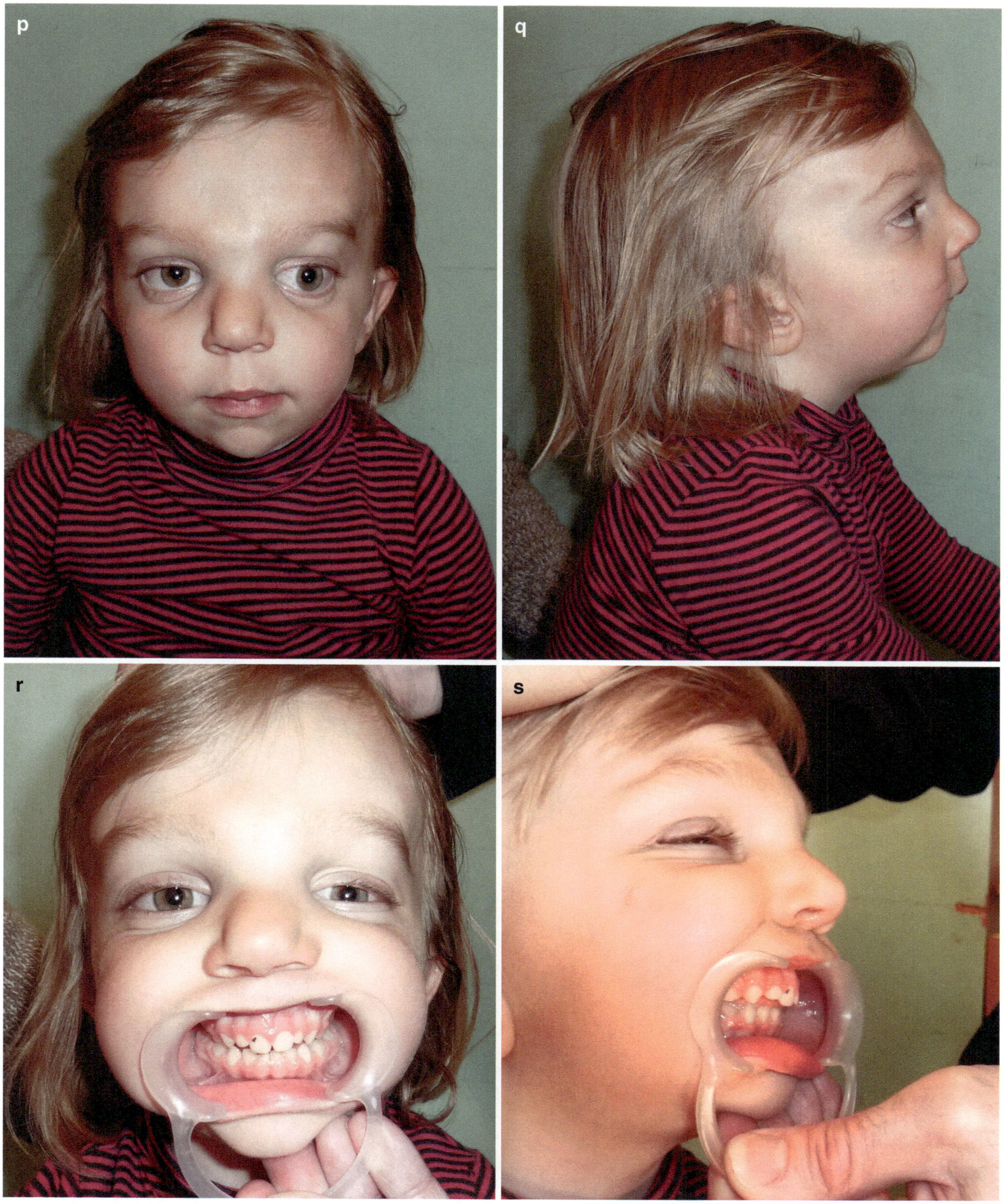

Fig. 6.4 (continued)

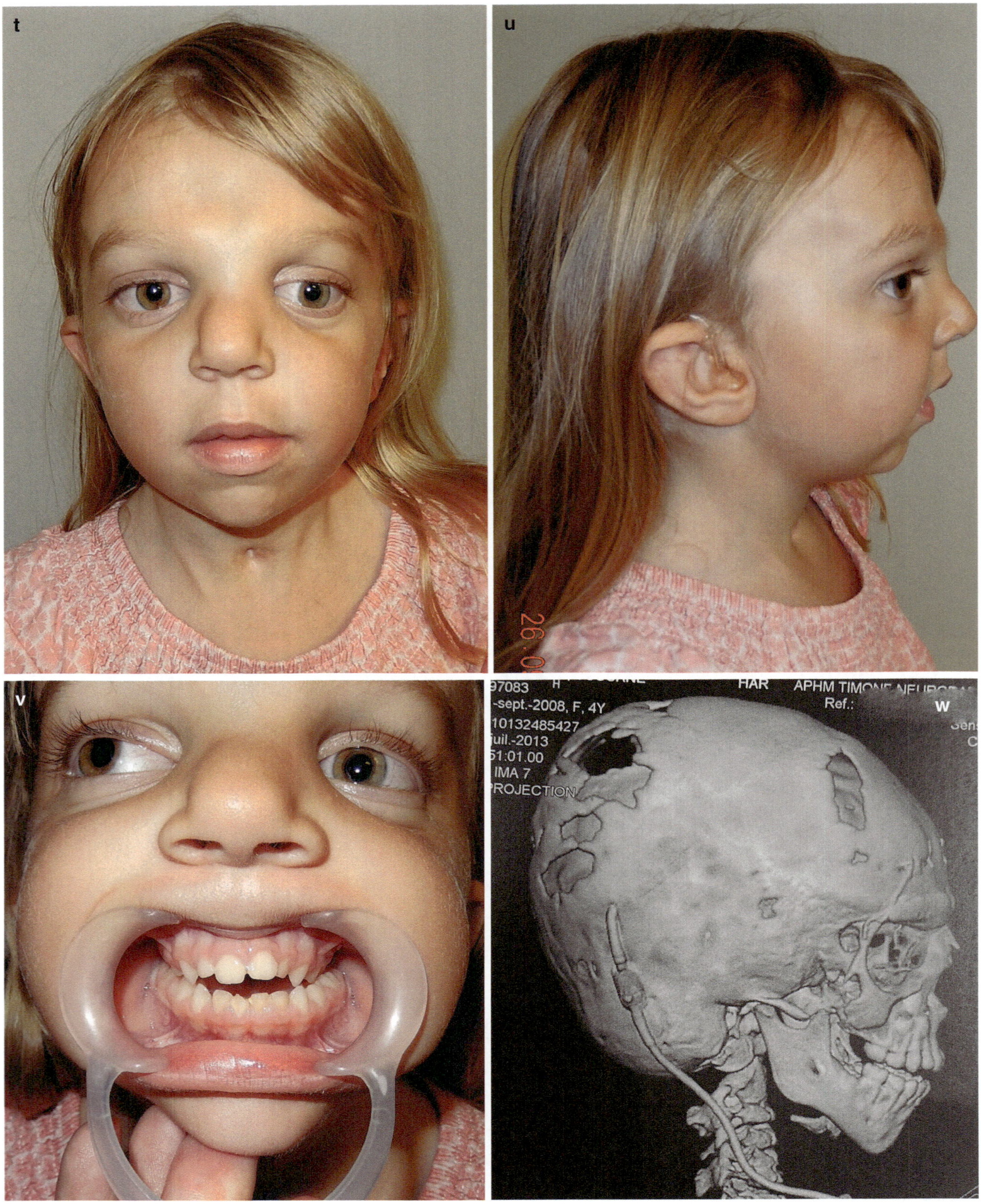

Fig. 6.4 (continued)

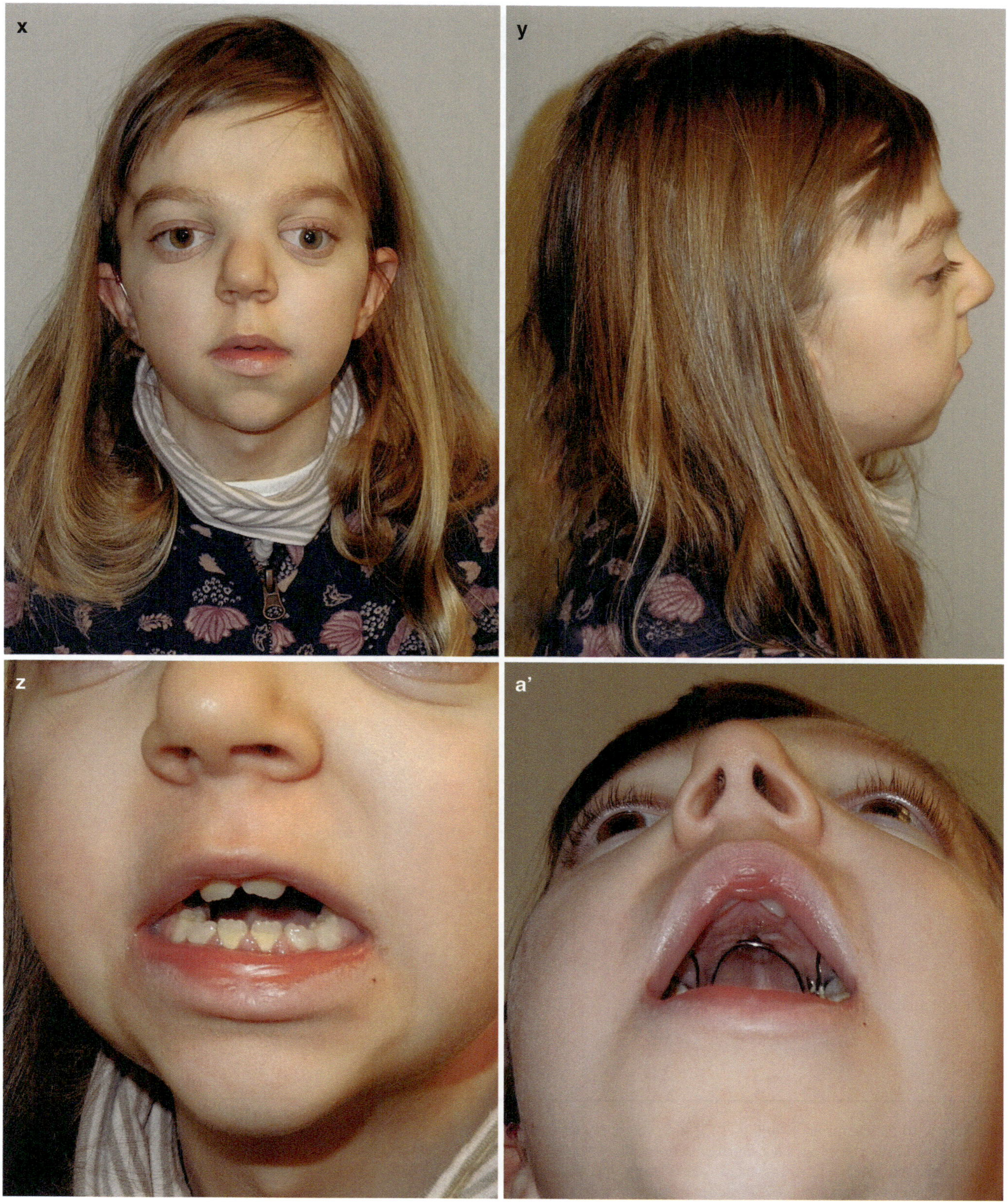

Fig. 6.4 (continued)

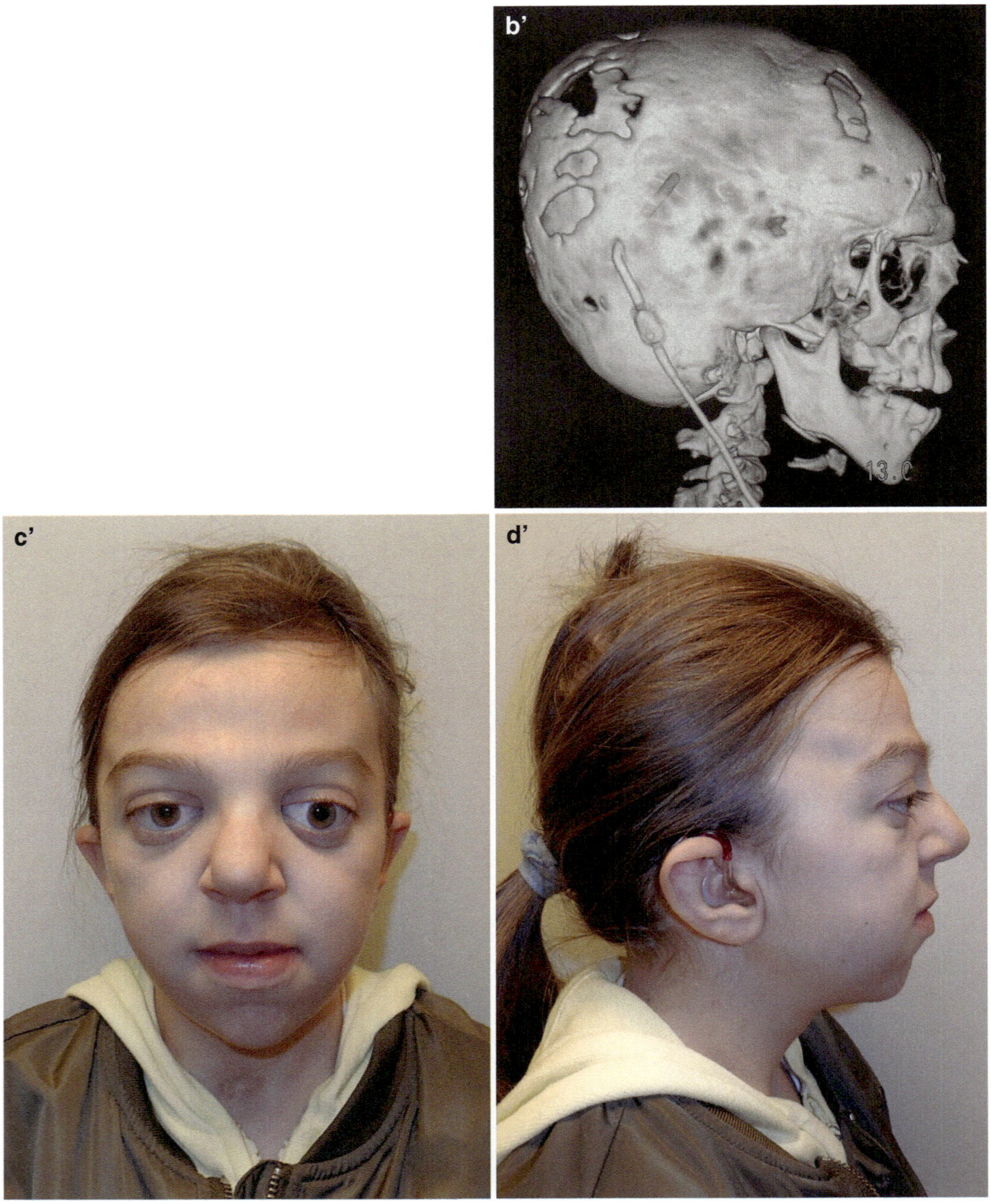

Fig. 6.4 (continued)

Fig. 6.5 (**a**, **d**) Patient (same as in Fig. 2.15) with very early monobloc performed at 12 months of age after initial posterior vault expansion performed at the age of 4 months. ©Cassandra Vion. (**c**) Immediate postoperative aspect with transfacial pin. (**d**) Postoperative sedation and external traction system applied on the transfacial pin. (**e**, **f**) Clinical and CT scan aspects at the end of the activation phase of distraction (4 weeks after FFMBA), with major overcorrection. (**g**, **h**) Clinical results after removal of the transfacial pin, 12 weeks after very early FFMBA. Major overcorrection. Tracheostomy was still in place. (**i**) CT scan 12 weeks after the end of the activation phase of distraction, showing major overcorrection. (**j**, **k**) Clinical results 6 months after very early FFMBA. Tracheostomy was still in place. (**l**) CT scan 6 months after very early FFMBA, showing the stability of midface advancement. (**m**, **n**) Clinical results 2 years after very early FFMBA, showing progressive relapse of midface hypercorrection reaching normality. A mandibular distraction had to be performed to remove the tracheostomy. (**o**, **p**) Clinical results 4 years after very early FFMBA, showing decannulation. (**q**, **r**) Clinical results at 6 years, 5 years after very early FFMBA. (**s**) CT scan 5 years after very early FFMBA, showing relapse of midface hypoplasia. (**t**, **u**) Clinical results at 10 years of age, 9 years after very early FFMBA. (**v**) CT scan 9 years after very early FFMBA, showing relapse of midface hypoplasia

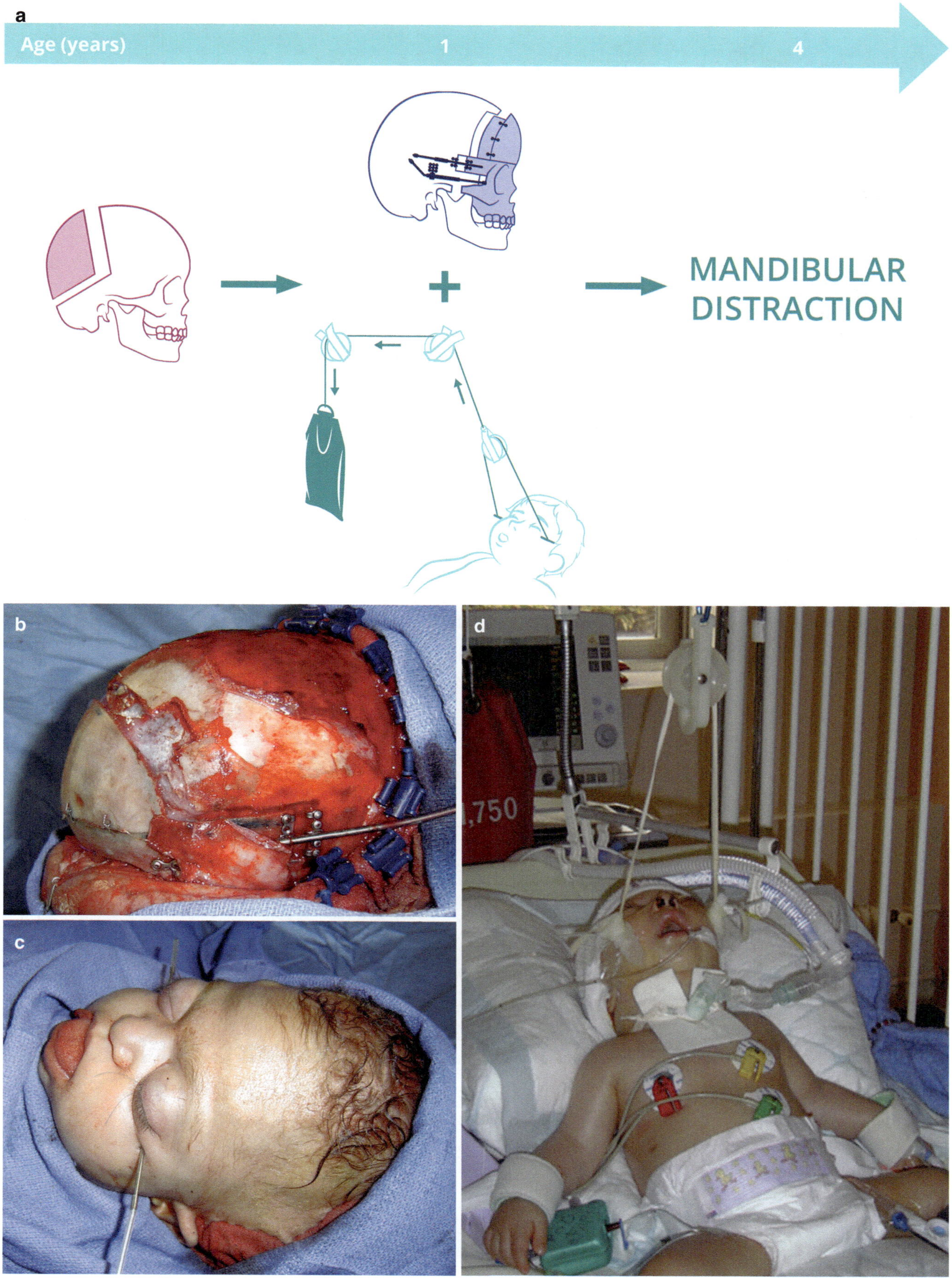
a
Age (years)
1
4
MANDIBULAR DISTRACTION
b
c
d

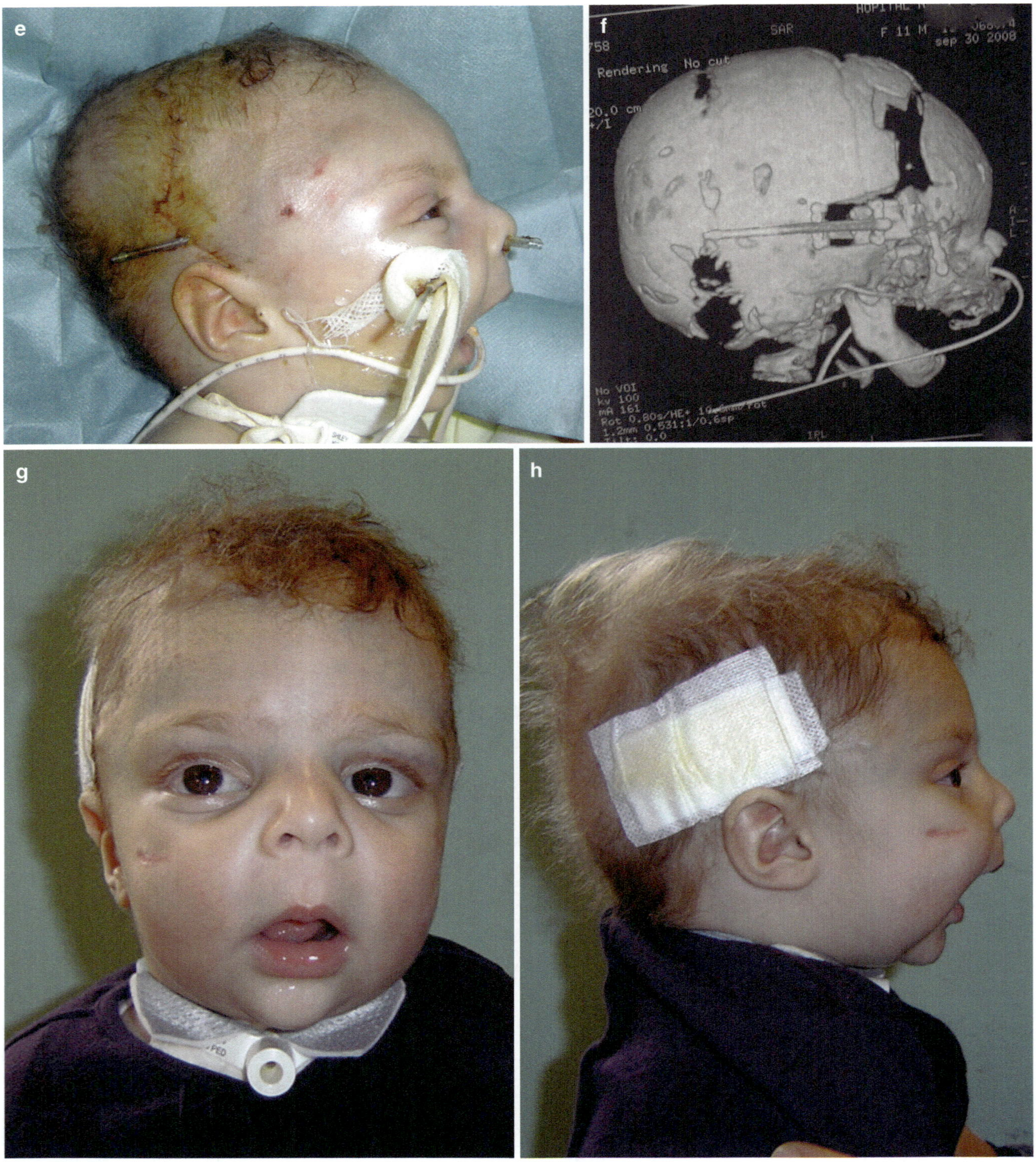

Fig. 6.5 (continued)

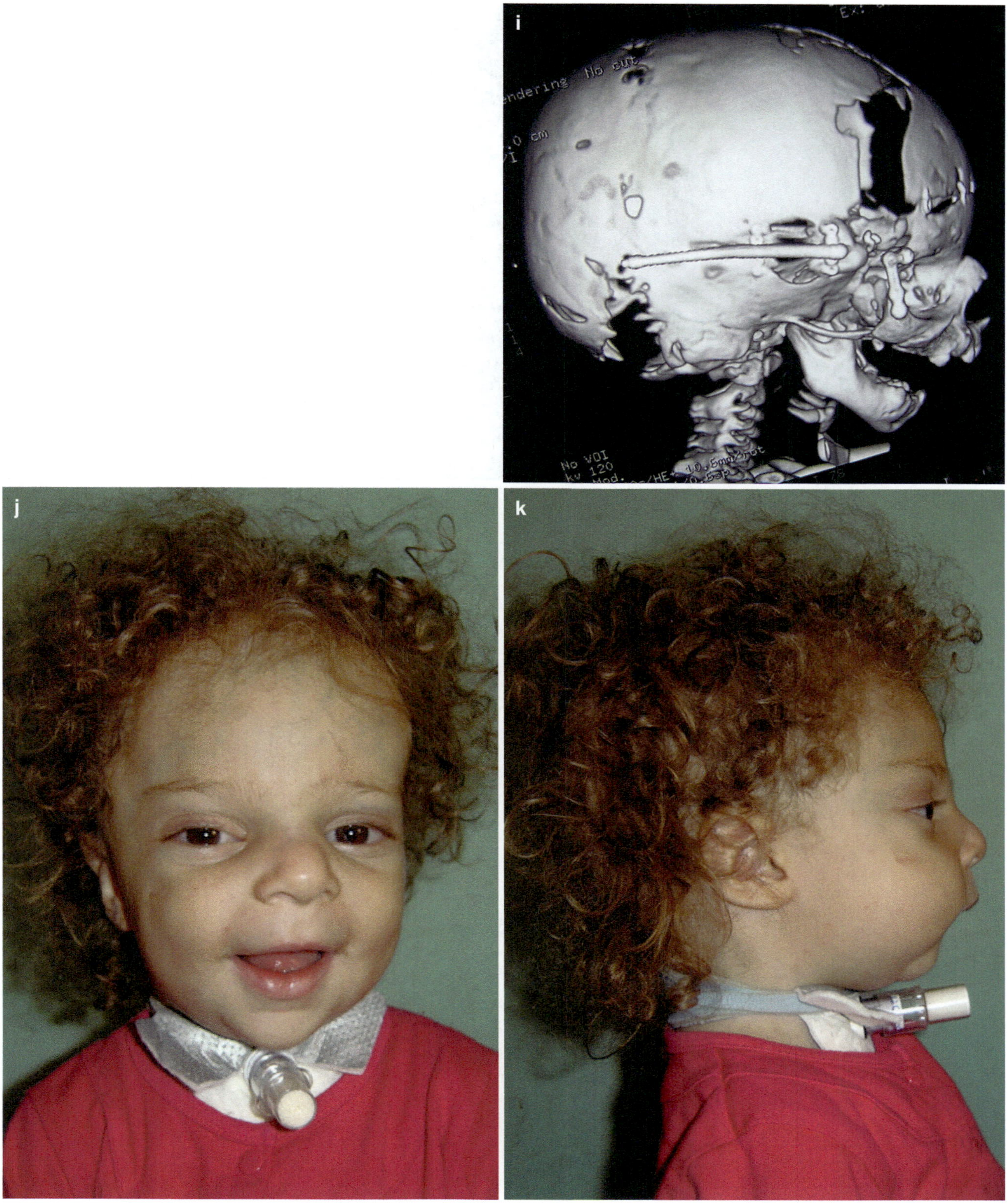

Fig. 6.5 (continued)

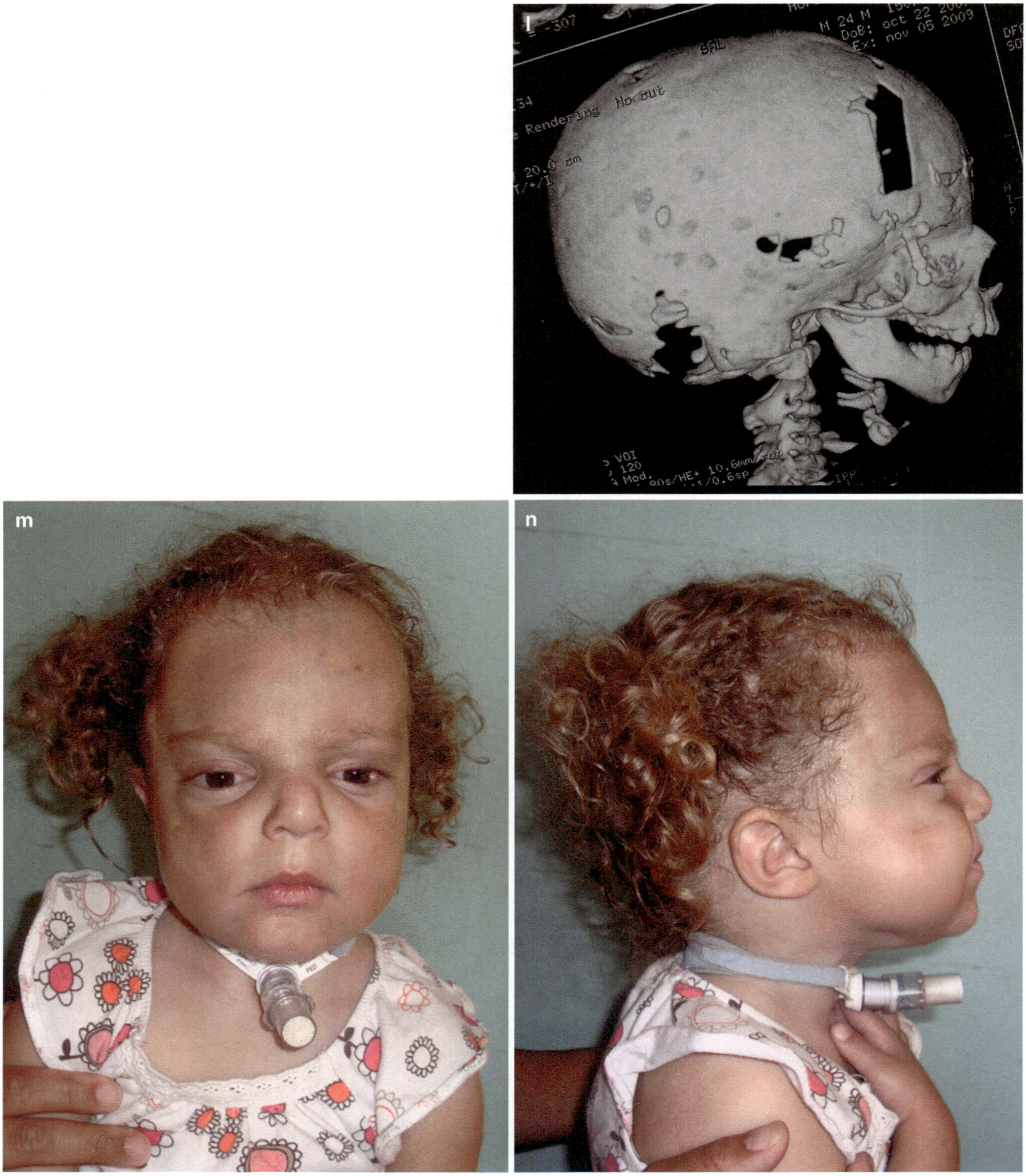

Fig. 6.5 (continued)

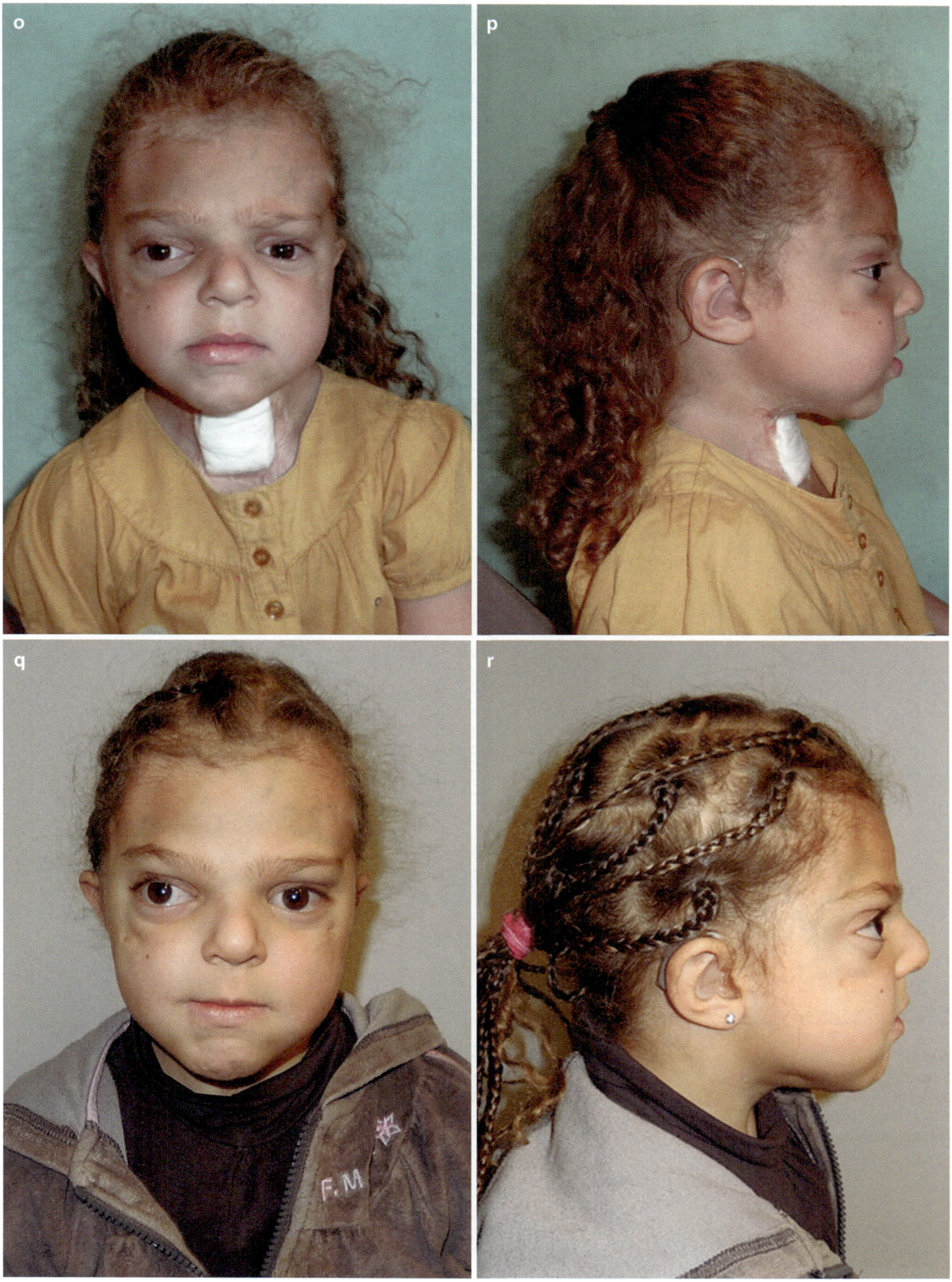

Fig. 6.5 (continued)

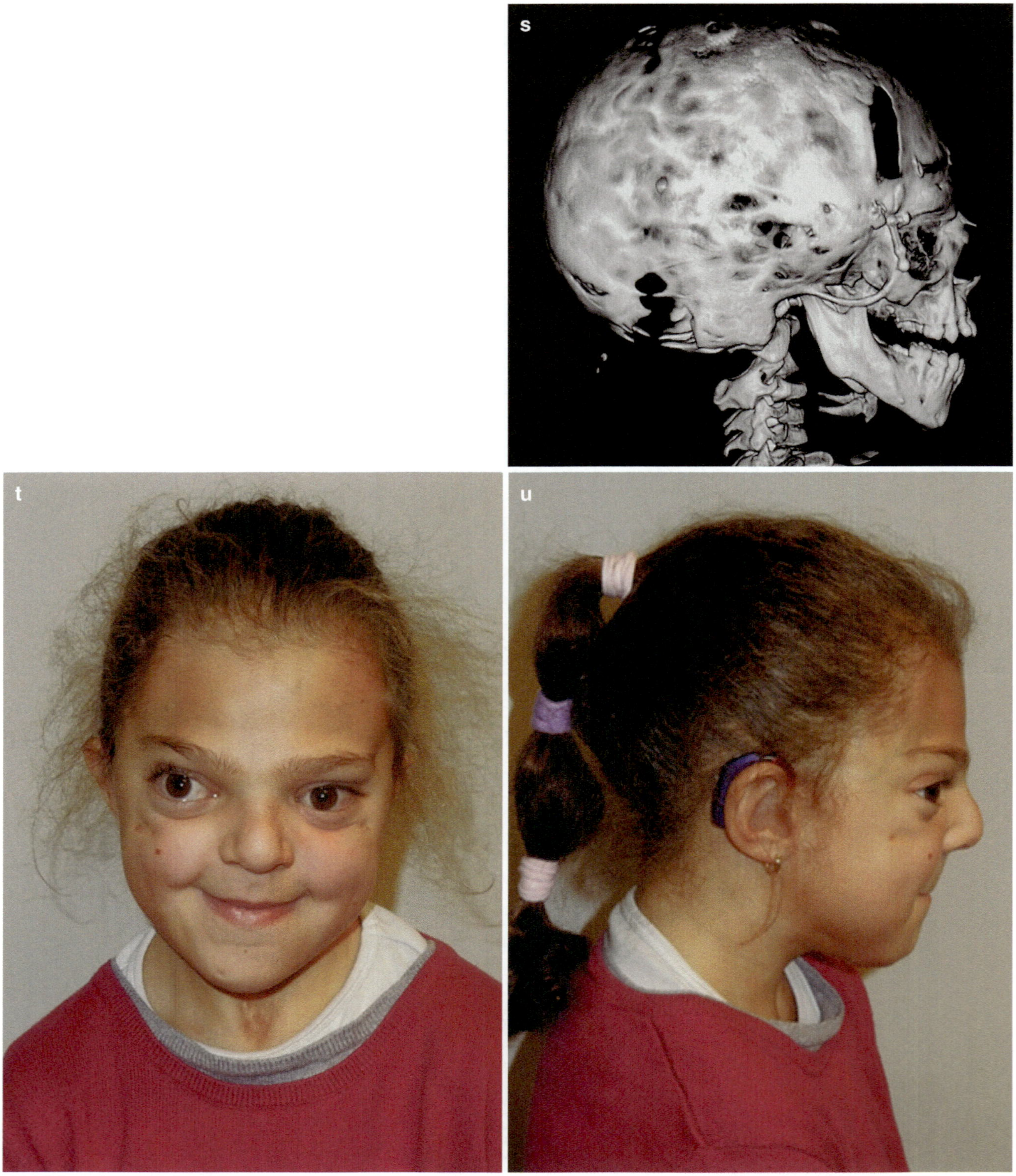

Fig. 6.5 (continued)

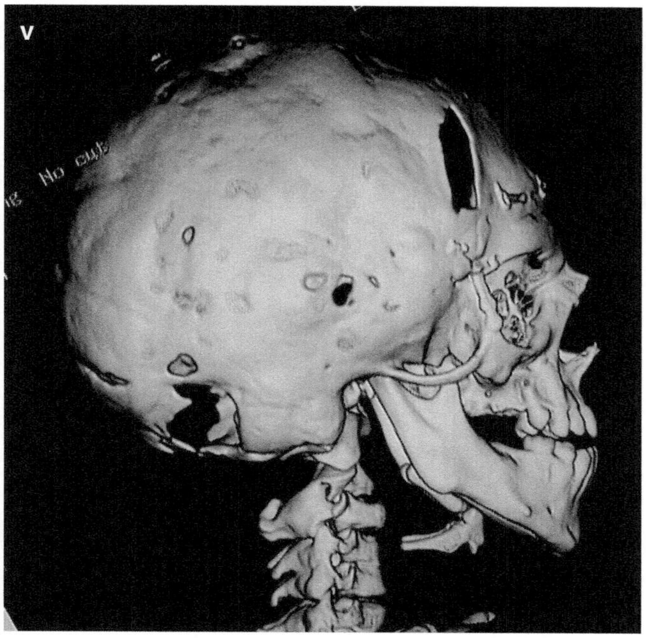

Fig. 6.5 (continued)

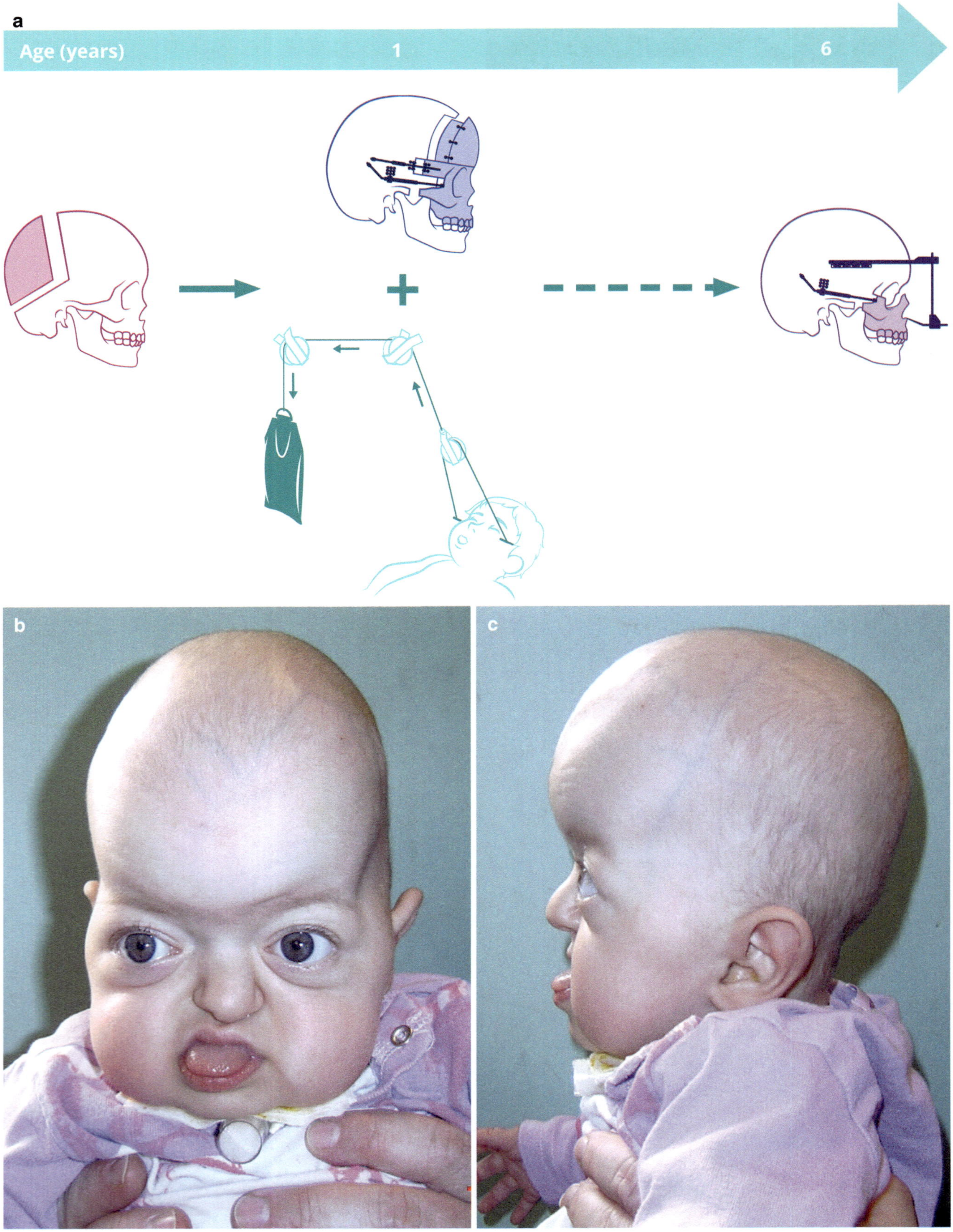
a
Age (years)
1
6
b
c

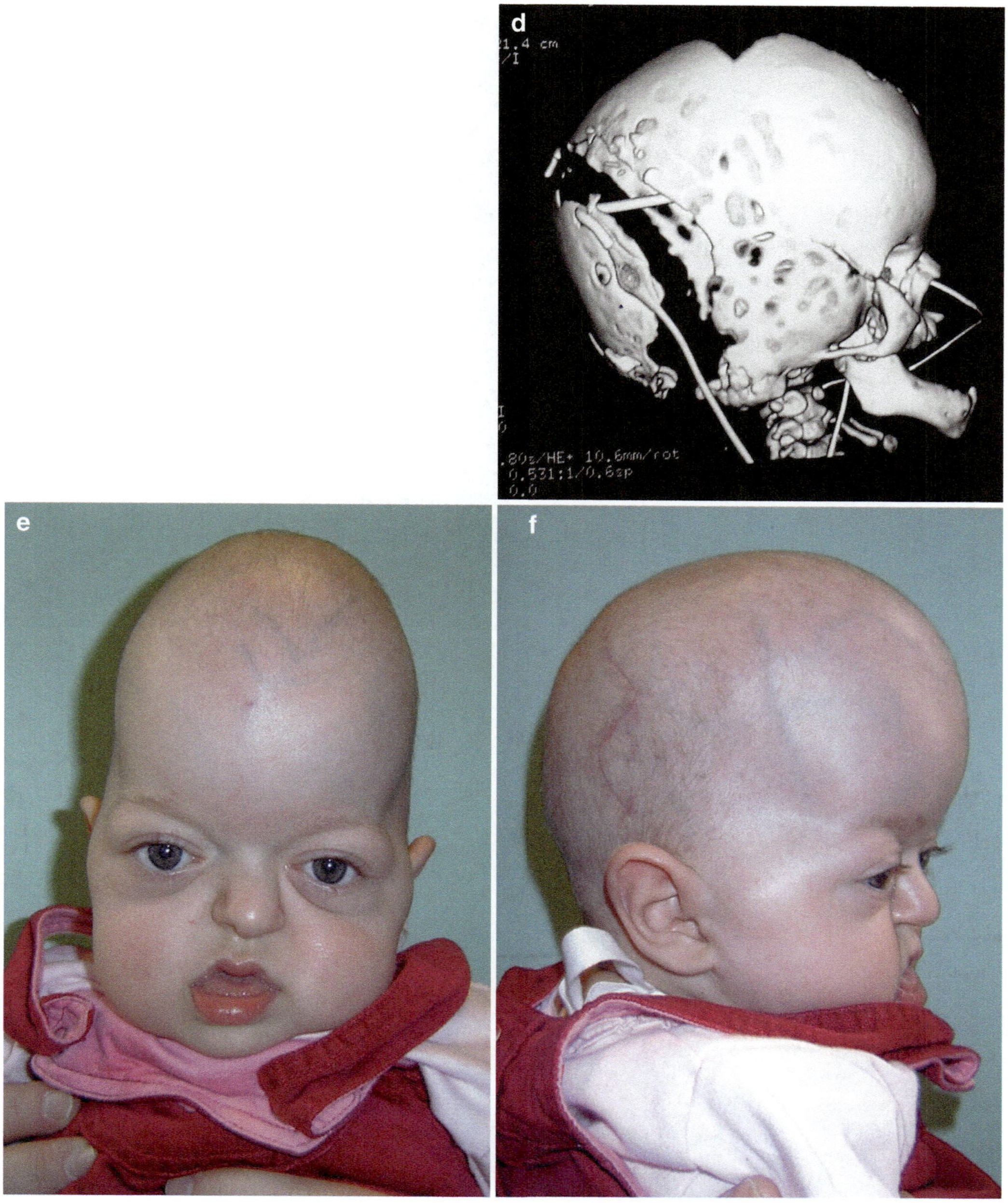

Fig. 6.6 (continued)

Fig. 6.6 (**a**, **b**, **c**) Patient with Crouzon syndrome with acanthosis nigricans at 6 months of age presenting with a cloverleaf aspect, posterior flattening, and turricephaly. Surgical history included ventriculoperitoneal shunting at another institution. ©Cassandra Vion. (**d**) CT scan demonstrating brain-mediated posterior vault expansion performed at 7 months of age. (**e**, **f**) Clinical result 12 weeks after posterior vault expansion. (**g**) CT scan 12 weeks after posterior vault expansion demonstrating improved posterior roundness and projection. Severe midface hypoplasia is evident. (**h**, **i**) Clinical result 6 months after posterior vault distraction, before very early FFMBA at age 18 months. (**j**) Intraoperative pictures during a very early monobloc at age 18 months demonstrating the osteotomies with the placement of a contractor on the vertex. (**k**) External traction system using the transfacial pin. (**l**) Effect of the contractor on device removal after 12 weeks of activation. (**m**, **n**) Clinical results 6 months after very early FFMBA, without overcorrection. (**o**, **p**) Clinical results 6 months after very early FFMBA. (**q**, **r**) Clinical results 24 months after very early FFMBA, with progressive relapse of the midface hypoplasia. (**s**, **t**) Clinical results 36 months after very early FFMBA, with progressive relapse of the midface hypoplasia. (**u**) CT scan 3 years after very early FFMBA, showing relapse of midface hypoplasia. (**v**, **w**) LF3 osteotomy performed at 6 years of age, 5 years after very early FFMBA, in order to correct the relapse in midface hypoplasia. (**x**, **y**) Clinical results 4 months after LF3, showing overcorrection in midface advancement. (**z**, **a'**) Clinical results 12 months after LF3, showing minimal relapse of midface hypoplasia. (**b'**) CT scan 4 years after LF3, showing relapse of midface hypoplasia. (**c'**, **d'**) Clinical results 48 months after LF3, showing relapse of midface hypoplasia. (**e'**) CT scan 4 years after LF3 at age 10

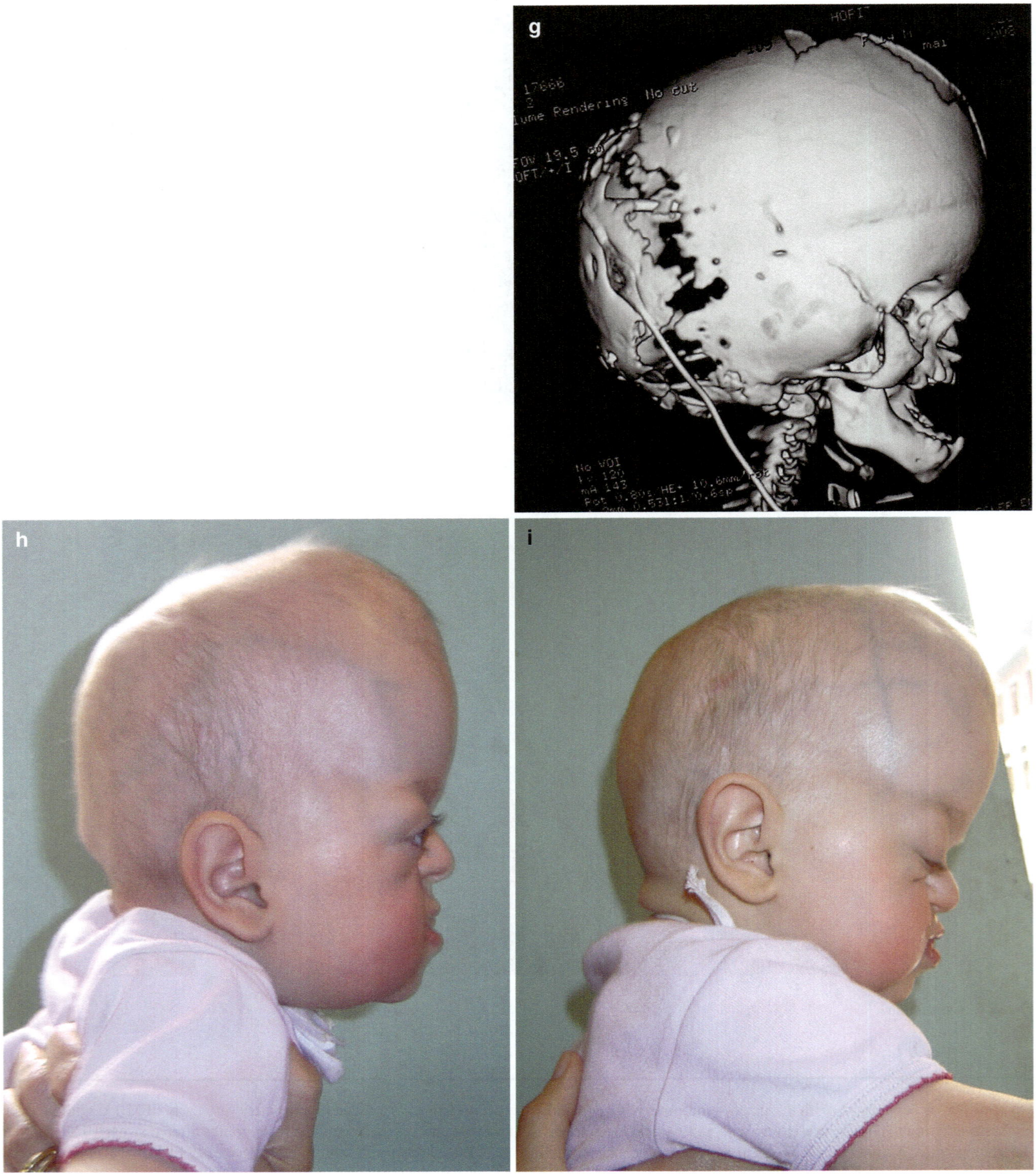

Fig. 6.6 (continued)

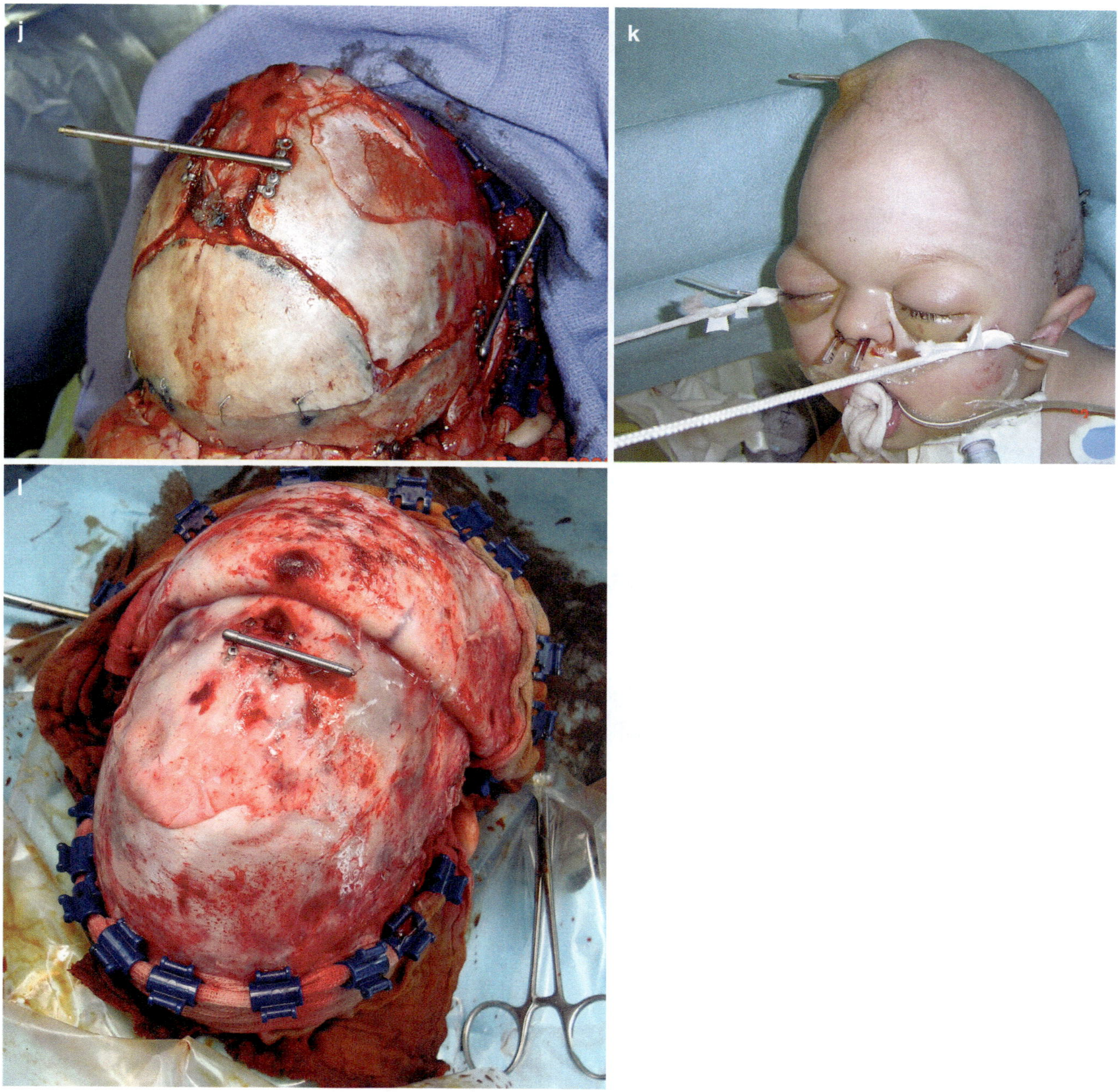

Fig. 6.6 (continued)

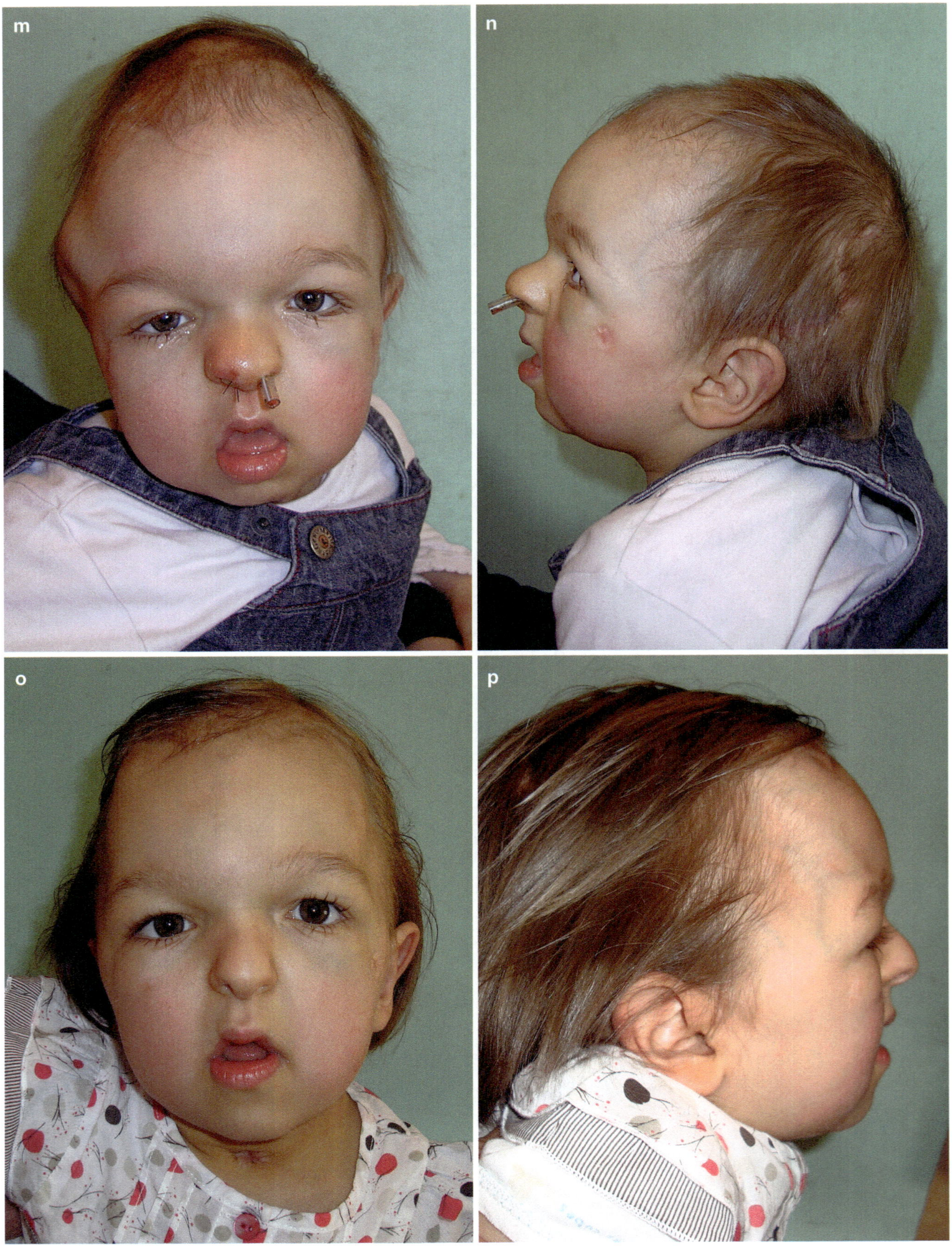

Fig. 6.6 (continued)

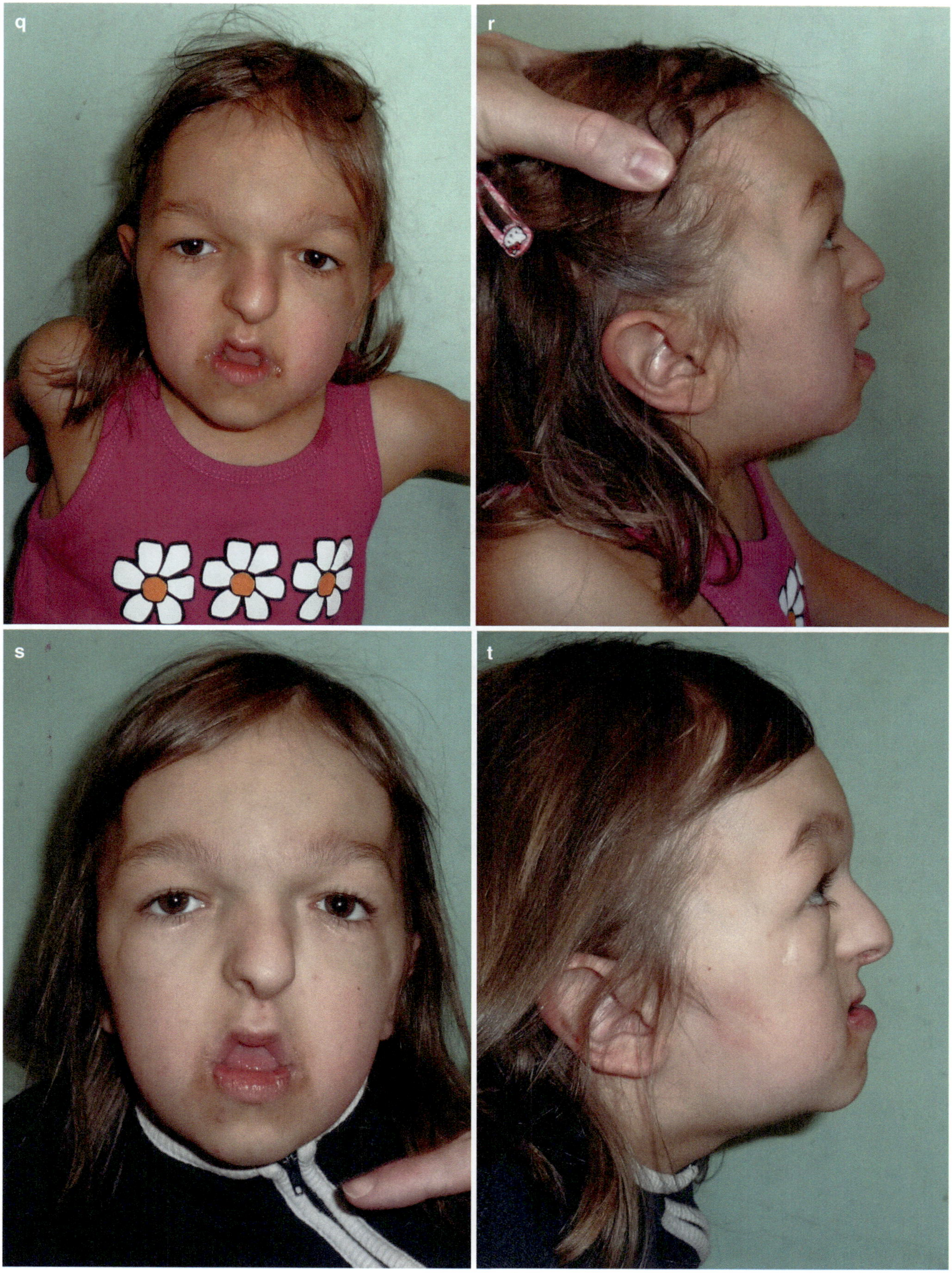

Fig. 6.6 (continued)

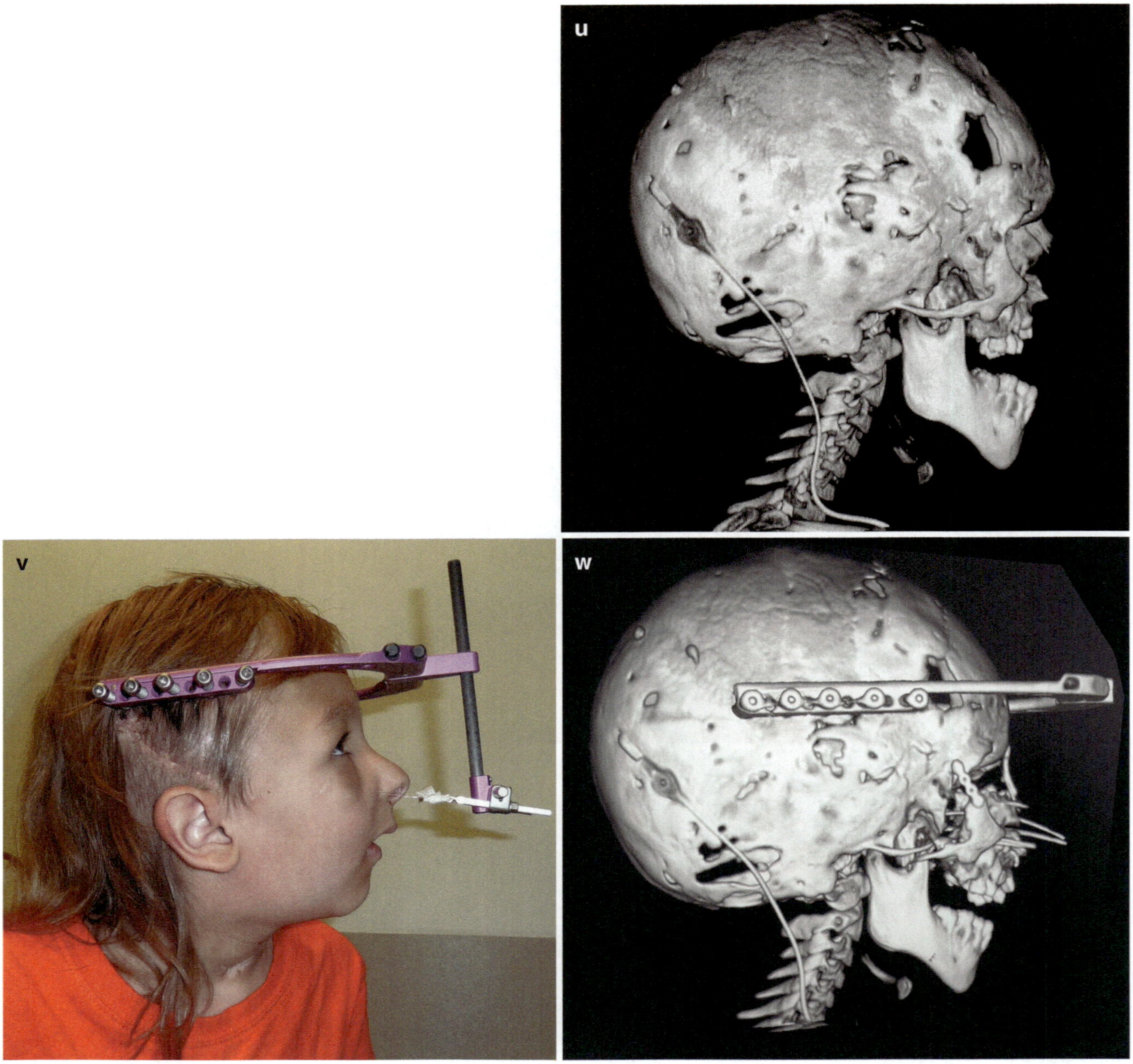

Fig. 6.6 (continued)

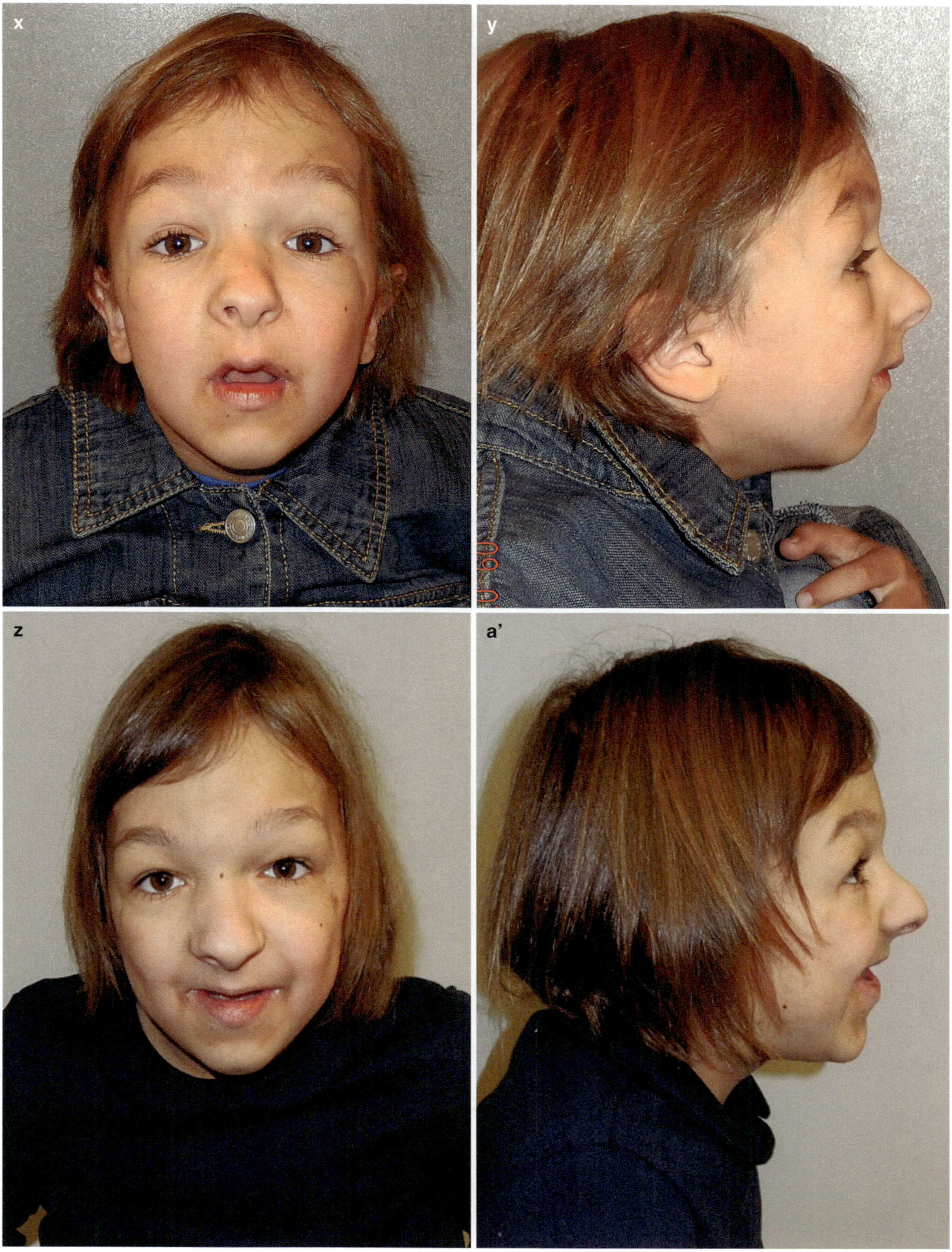

Fig. 6.6 (continued)

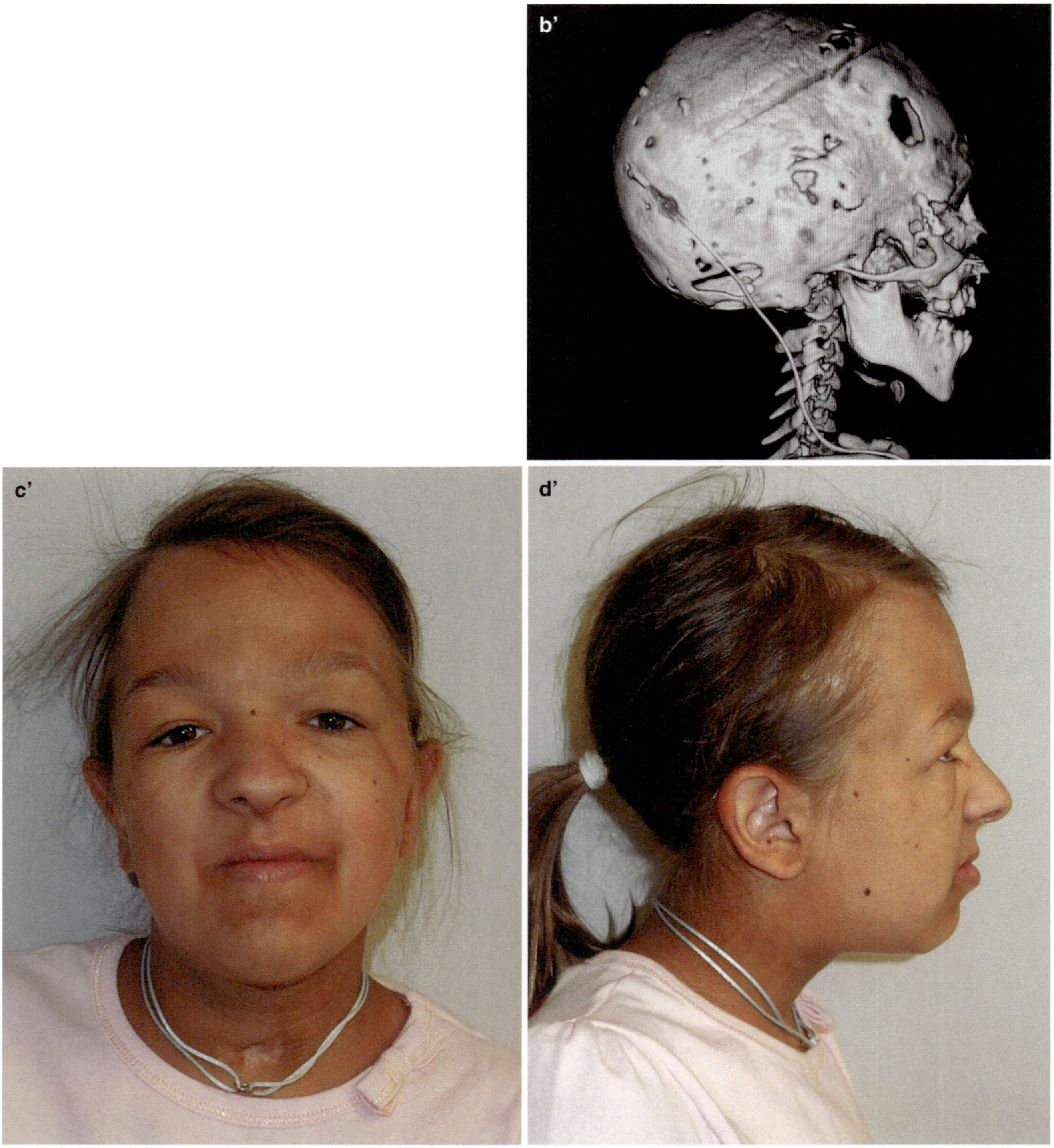

Fig. 6.6 (continued)

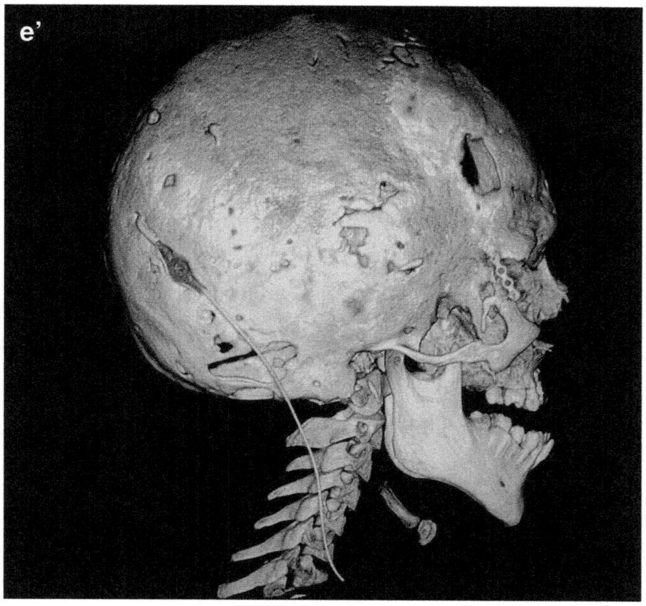

Fig. 6.6 (continued)

6.1 Alternative to External Traction with the Insertion of the Transfacial Pin Alone with 4 Internal Distractors

One example of an early monobloc with transfacial pin without external traction (Fig. 6.7) is provided when the facial skeleton was considered solid enough around 16 months of age.

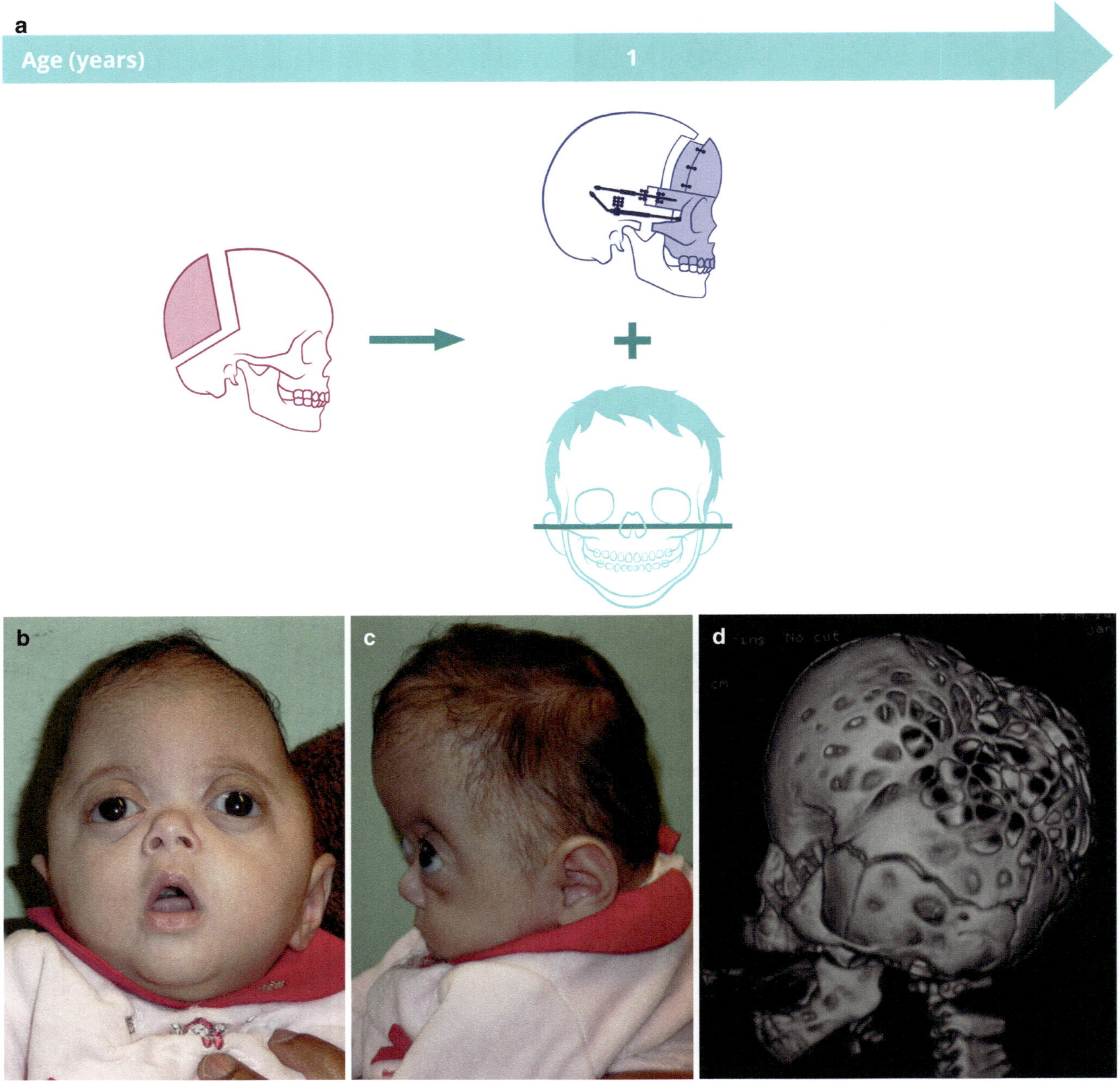

Fig. 6.7 (**a**, **b**, **c**, **d**) Patient with Crouzon syndrome at 5 months of age. ©Cassandra Vion. (**e**, **f**) Brain-mediated posterior vault distraction performed at 6 months of age. (**g**) Morphological result 8 weeks after posterior vault distraction. (**h**) Very early monobloc: osteotomies performed at 16 months of age, with insertion of 4 distractors and a transfacial pin. (**i**) Immediate postoperative result with transfacial pin, without external traction. (**j**, **k**) Clinical results after 4 weeks of distraction, showing maxillary overcorrection. (**l**, **m**) Clinical results 8 months after very early FFMBA, with persistence of the overcorrection. (**n**, **o**) Clinical results 12 months after very early FFMBA, with minor relapse. (**p**) Occlusion at 28 months of age, 12 months after very early FFMBA, showing the progressive relapse of midface hypoplasia. (**q**) CT scan performed at 28 months of age, 1 year after very early FFMBA, showing the relapse in midface hypoplasia. (**r**, **s**) Clinical results 2 years after very early FFMBA, showing relapse in midface hypoplasia. (**t**) Occlusion at 3,3 years of age, 2 years after very early FFMBA. (**u**) CT scan performed at 3.3 years of age, 2 years after very early FFMBA. (**v**, **w**) Clinical results 4 years after very early FFMBA. (**x**) Occlusion at 5 years of age, 48 months after very early FFMBA, showing the relapse of midface hypoplasia. (**y**, **z**, **a'**, **b'**) Clinical results 4 years after very early FFMBA, showing the relapse of midface hypoplasia

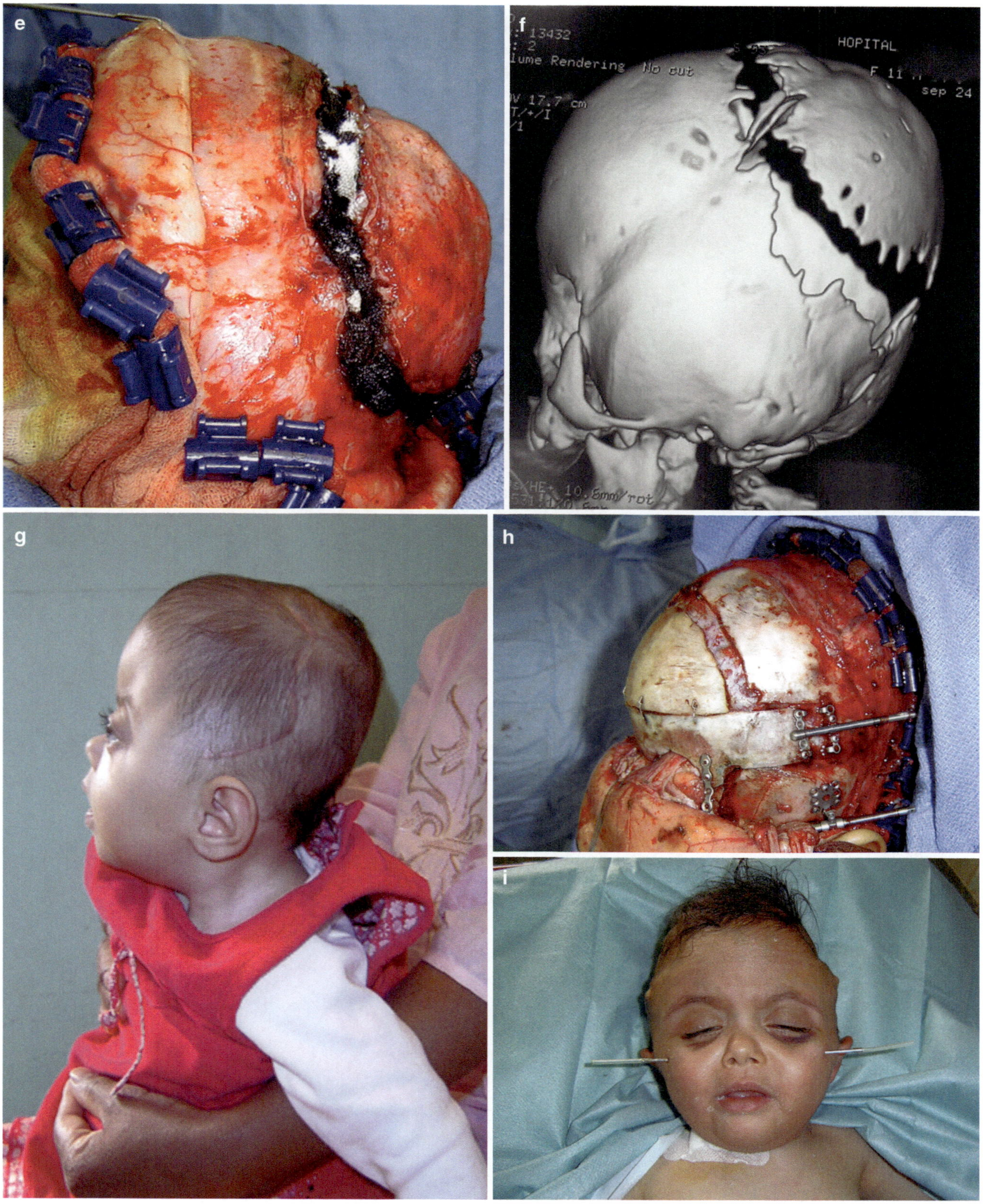

Fig. 6.7 (continued)

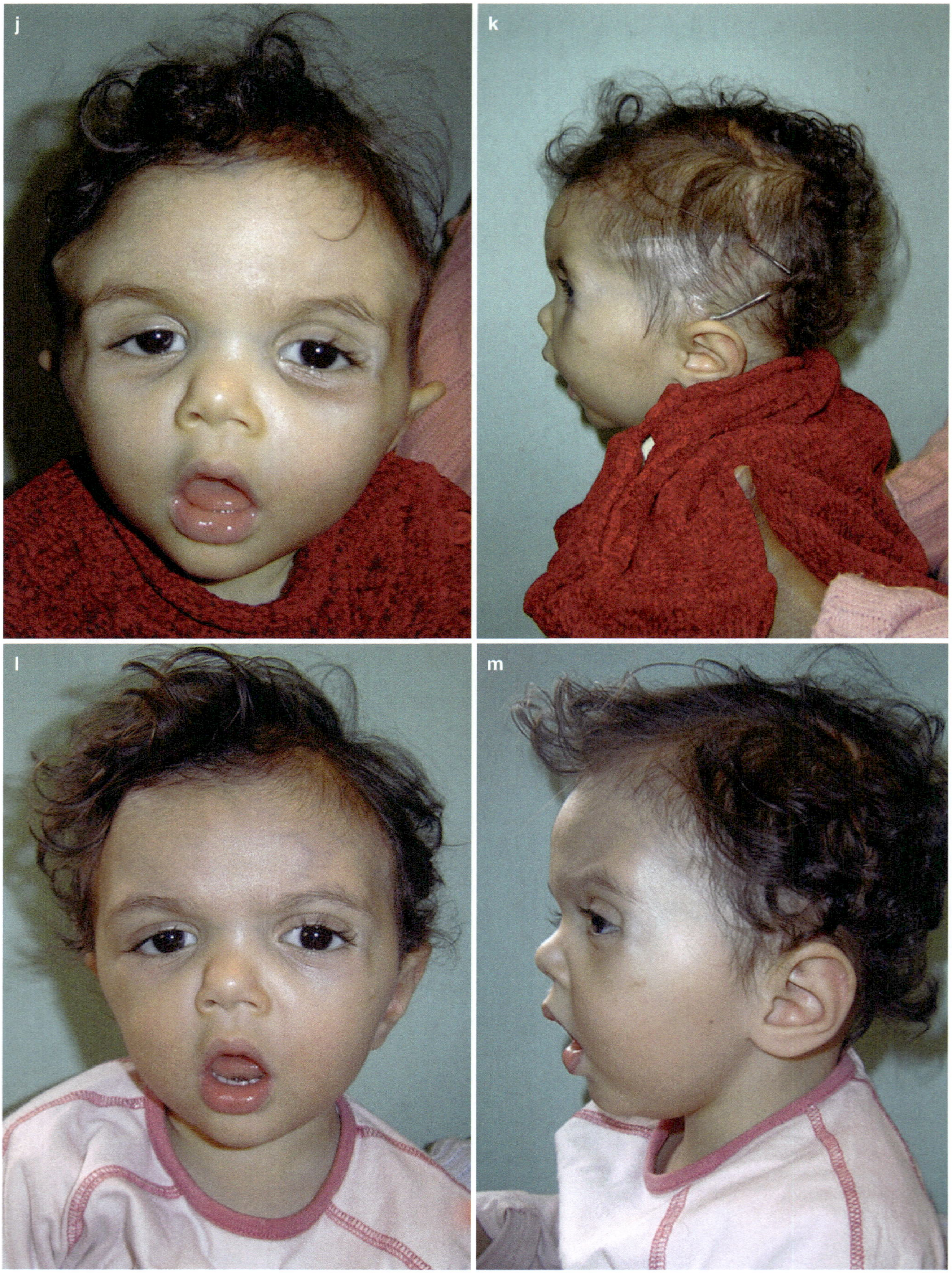

Fig. 6.7 (continued)

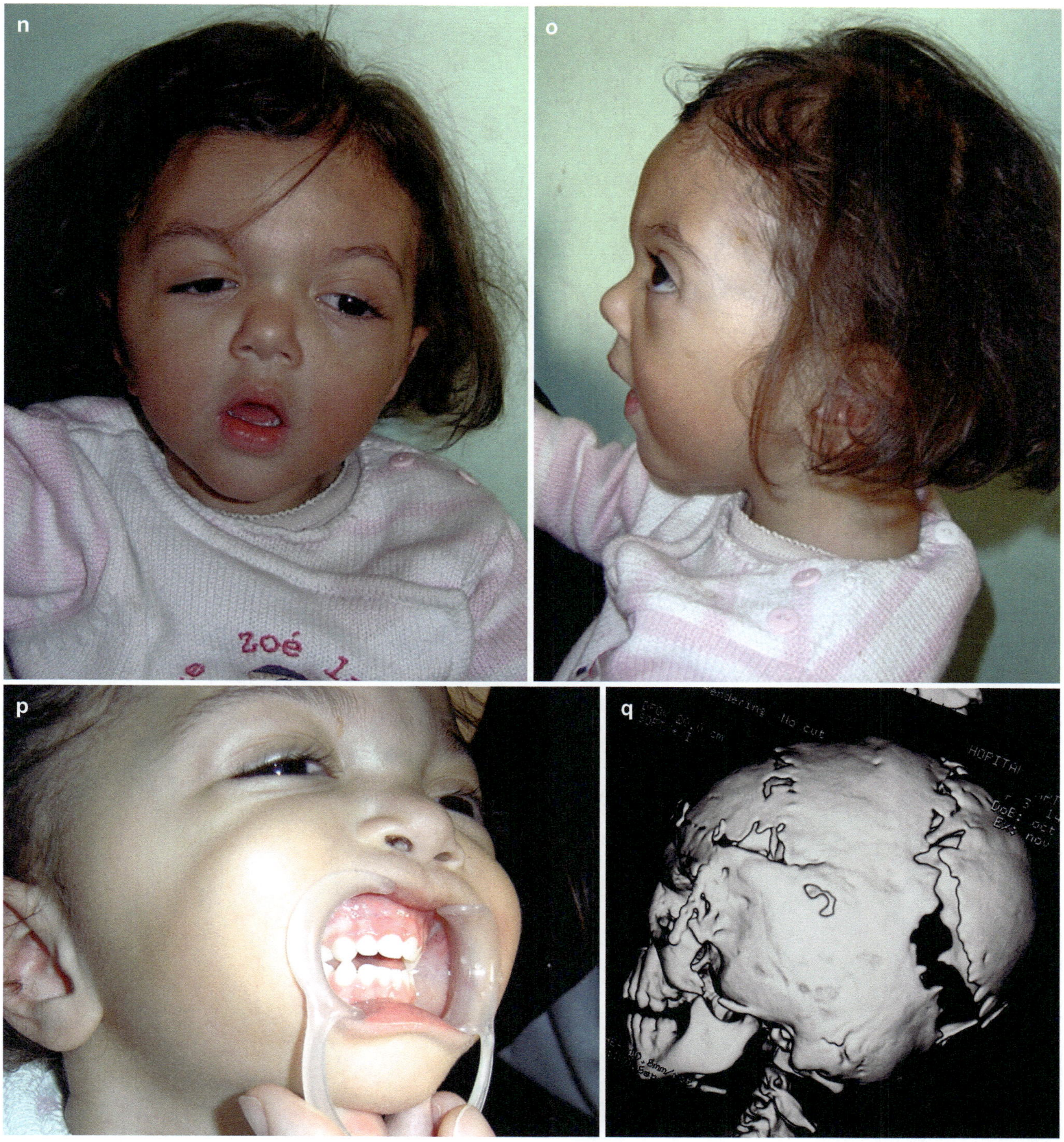

Fig. 6.7 (continued)

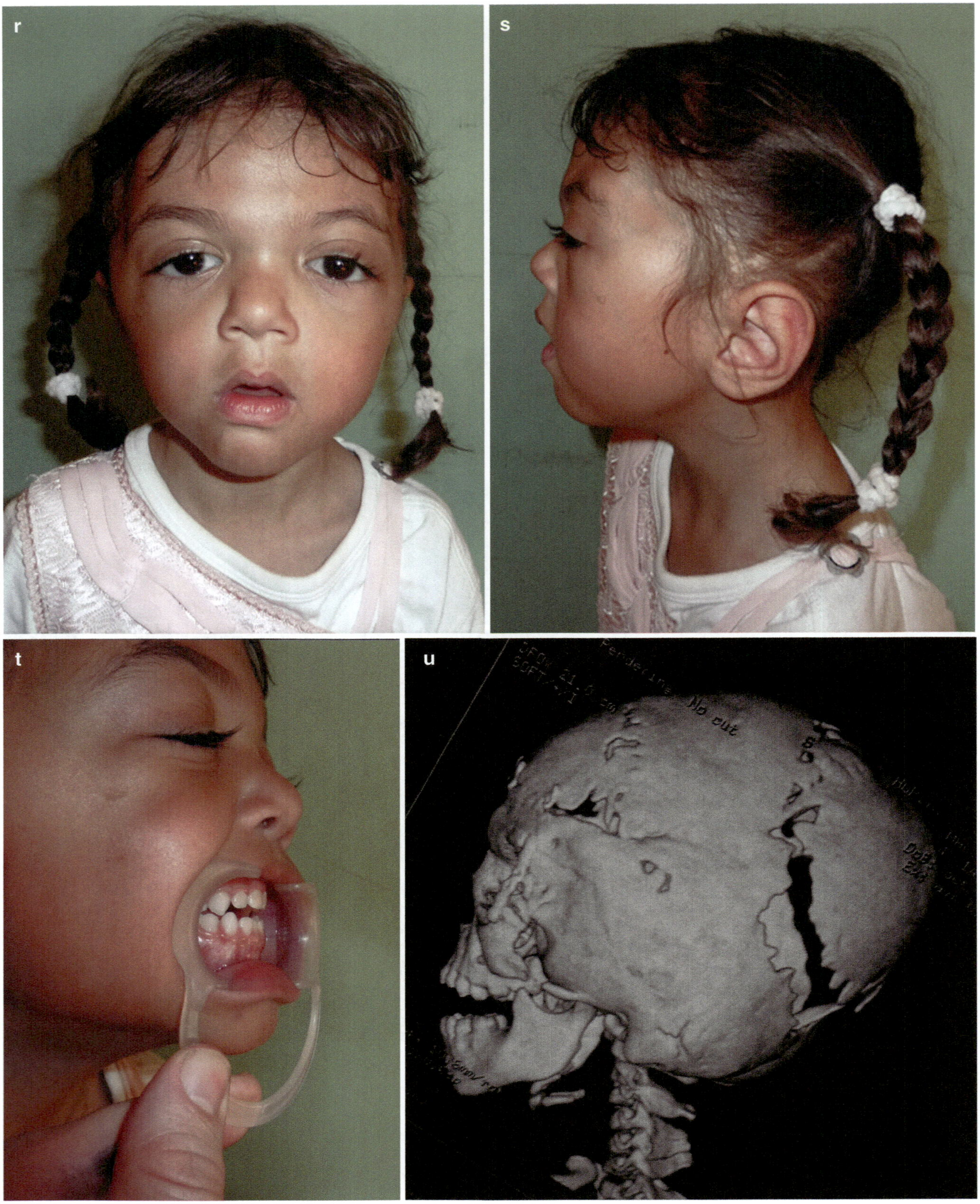

Fig. 6.7 (continued)

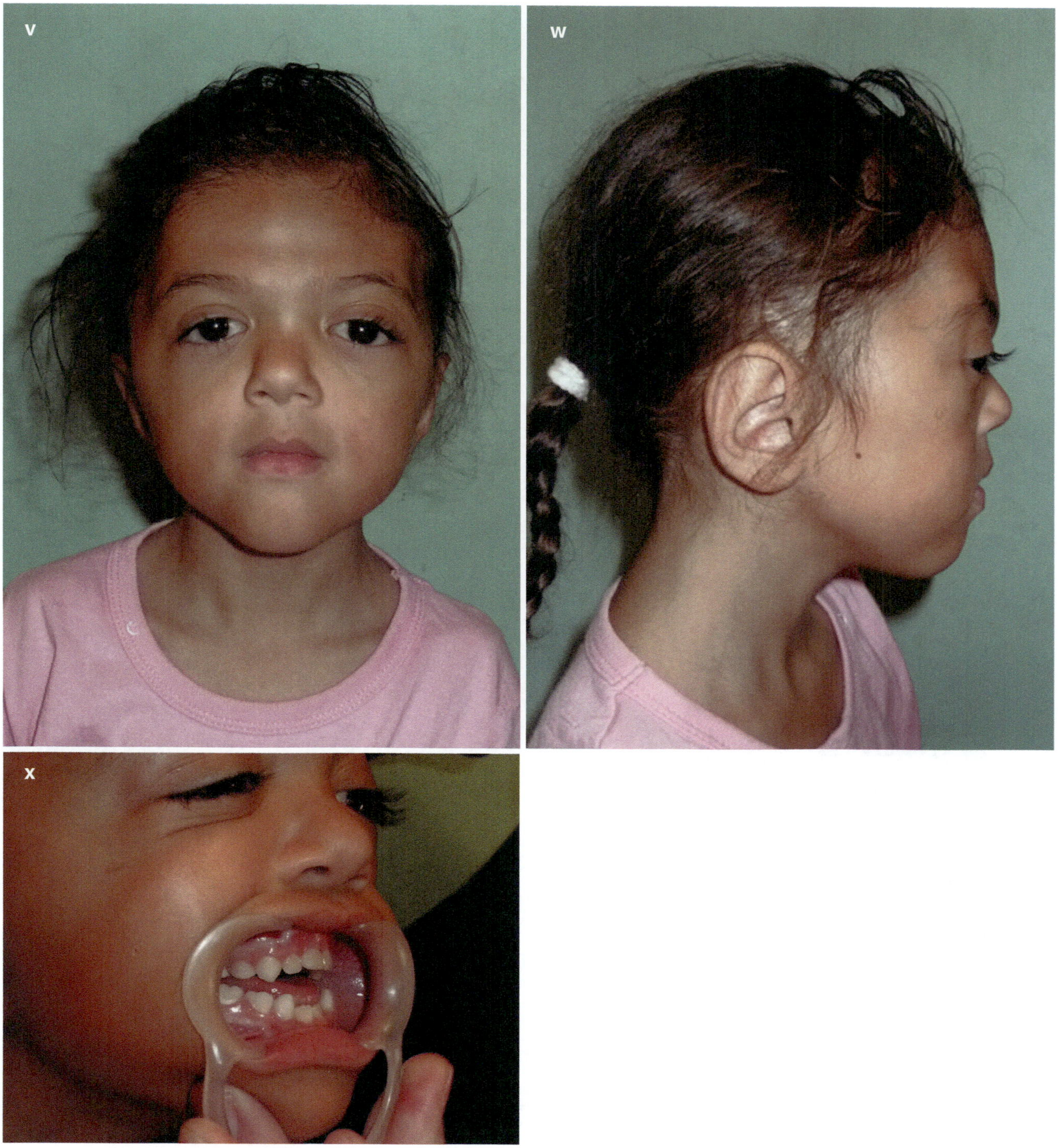

Fig. 6.7 (continued)

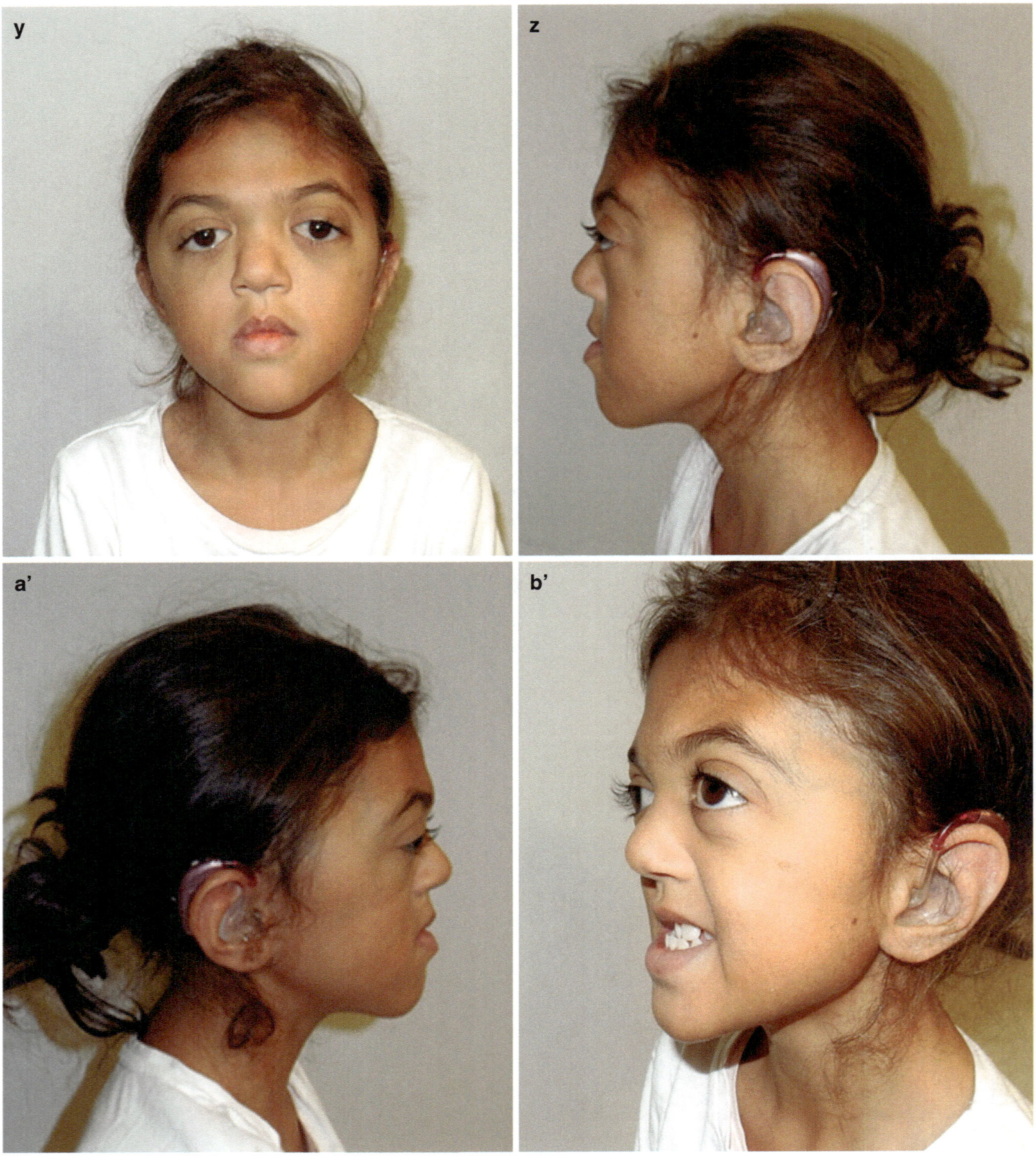

Fig. 6.7 (continued)

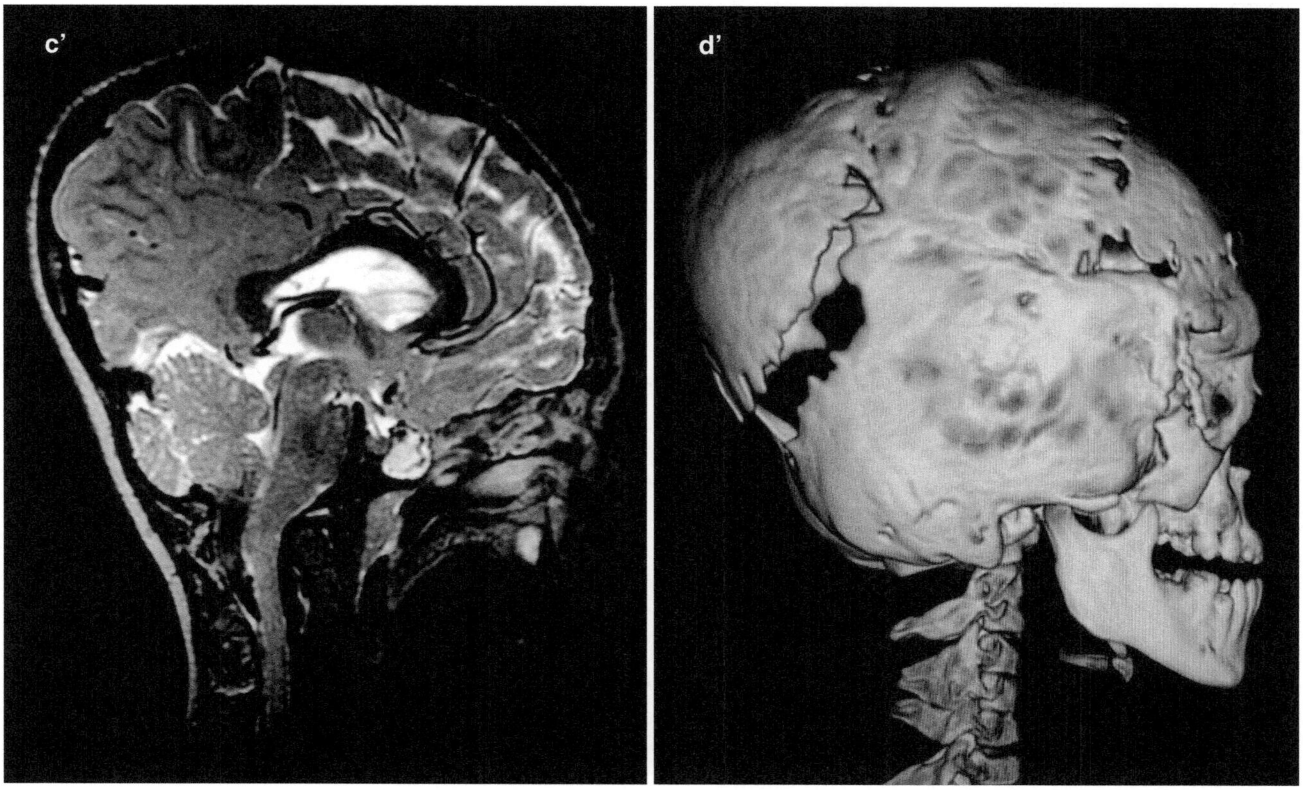

Fig. 6.7 (continued)

References

1. Paternoster G, Haber SE, Khonsari RH, et al. Craniosynostosis: Monobloc distraction with internal device and its variant for infants with severe syndromic Craniosynostosis. Clin Plast Surg. 2021 Jul;48(3):497–506.
2. Arnaud E, Antunez S, Khonsari H, et al. SYM9.9F Transfacial external traction and internal distraction for young and severe Faciocraniosynostoses: the very early Monobloc. Plast Reconstr Surg–Global Open. 2019 Aug;7(8S-2):9.
3. Fauroux B, Lavis J-F, Nicot F, et al. Facial side effects during noninvasive positive pressure ventilation in children. Intensive Care Med. 2005 Jul;31(7):965–9.

Tracheostomy Management: How FFMBA Contributes to the Removal?

7

1. Employ all available means to avoid the tracheostomy (ENT surgery such as choanal repermeation, nasopharyngeal, tubes, and CPAP).
2. Conduct a thorough airway evaluation including drug-induced sleep endoscopy (DISE) to assess laryngeal tonus.
3. If severe laryngomalacia is confirmed, tracheostomy is temporarily indicated until the child outgrows this condition.
4. FFMBA remains the best option to prevent or remove the tracheostomy in FCST.
5. LF3 with distraction, palatal transverse distraction, and mandibular distraction may follow to normalize the AHI.
6. CPAP is effective against obstructive sleep apnea but its prolonged use in children worsens facial retrusion. It is rather used temporarily until the upper airway is re-permeabilized.

Our FCST management protocol aims to avoid tracheostomy by all means, unless it is absolutely necessary [1–4]. As of the patient's birth, breathing assistance, ENT surgeries, and facial osteotomies act to prevent tracheostomy [5–7]. This strategy significantly decreases the proportion of patients requiring tracheostomy (Tables 7.1, 7.2, and 7.3). In those patients who actually do end up with a tracheostomy, our protocols aim at removing it as soon as surgery may effectively open the airway. This is where FFMBA (or its variant: the very early FFMBA (VEM)) comes into play.

In a consecutive series of 108 FCST patients who underwent FFMBA in our unit, 16 presented with tracheostomy. Among those patients, the decannulation rate seemed to be higher in patients operated on very early (before age 18 months). This was surprising because those were also the most severe cases. A technical variant had been systematically applied in this subgroup: a transfacial Kirschner wire to stabilize the maxillo-zygomatic sutures. The distraction system employed was either the usual FFMBA protocol with four internal distractors or the external traction system with two internal distractors, especially in Pfeiffer syndrome [7].

We, therefore, advocate for early craniofacial surgery to prevent or remove tracheostomy before school age. Figures 7.1 and 7.2 demonstrate how early aggressive surgery contributes to the removal of the tracheostomy.

Figure 7.2 is related to the case of our first very early FFMBA associated with external traction. It came evident, when an early relapse occurred, that the design of tongue and grove was mandatory to provide a point of upper ossification, as well as the necessity of an inferior distractor to maintain stability for further consolidation. Eventually in that case a subsequent LF3 allowed tracheostomy removal after the early relapse. Subsequently, four distractors were used in very young patients.

E. Arnaud et al., *Frontofacial Monobloc Advancement with Internal Distraction*, https://doi.org/10.1007/978-3-031-07574-2_7

Table 7.1 Population of patients with tracheostomy: 16/108 faciocraniosynostoses

Preop. tracheostomy—*n* = 16/108 (15%)		
Syndrome type		
Crouzon	5	31%
Pfeiffer	9	56%
Apert	2	13%
AHI range = 20–91 / h.		

Table 7.2 Decannulation rates after FFMBA in tracheotomized patients presenting to our unit

	Decannulation rate (*n* = 16 patients)	
Shortly after FFMBA (< 10 months)	4	Decannulation in 10/16 patients (62%)
Later after FFMBA (10–67 months)	2	
After ENT surgery	1	
After mandibular distraction	1	
After LF3	1	
After LF3 + mandibular distraction	1	
No decannulation after FFMBA	5/16 (31%)	
No follow-up after FFMBA	1/16 (7%)	

Table 7.3 Decannulation rate according to age at FFMBA

	Treatment	
	Very early FFMBA (<18 months)	Standard FFMBA (>18 months)
Patients presenting with tracheostomy	10	6
Decannulation shortly after FFMBA (<10 months)	3	1
Delayed decannulation (>10 months)	1	1
Decannulation after ENT surgery/LF3/mandibular distraction	3	1
No decannulation	2	3
Decannulation rate	70%	50%

Fig. 7.1 (**a**, **b**, **c**) Forty-two-month-old patient with Crouzon and Acanthosis Nigricans syndromes (FGFR3 mutation) with tracheostomy and gastrostomy (Same patient as in Fig. 2.13). Surgical history included ETV at 27 months of age and PVE with distraction at 32 months of age to treat obstructive hydrocephalus and tonsillar herniation. The clinical photographs at age 42 months demonstrate midface hypoplasia, class III malocclusion, and exorbitism. Polysomnography with a capped tracheostomy cannula showed OSA (AHI = 13 per hour). Tonsillectomy and adenoidectomy followed by FFMBA were indicated to attempt decannulation. (**d**) FFMBA performed at 45 months of age, 9 months after distractor removal for PVE, and 4 months after tonsillectomy and adenoidectomy. Distractors were removed after 3 months of consolidation. Polysomnography with capped tracheostomy cannula demonstrated the resolution of sleep apnea (AHI = 0 per hour). (**e**, **f**) Three-month-postoperative photographs demonstrating midface advancement. The tracheostomy cannula remained capped. (**g**, **h**) Clinical photographs at age 6 years, 2 years, and a half after FFMBA. The rehabilitation allowed decannulation. (**i**, **j**) Clinical photographs at age 8 years, 4 years after FFMBA demonstrating relapse of midface retrusion related to the FGFR3 mutation. Notice the worsening of acanthosis nigricans in the neck region. (**k**, **l**, **m**) Clinical photographs and CT scan at age 11 years, 7 years after FFMBA. OSA relapsed (AHI = 15 per hour). CPAP was initiated. She subsequently required a secondary Le Fort III facial advancement which successfully treated relapsing OSA. ©Cassandra Vion

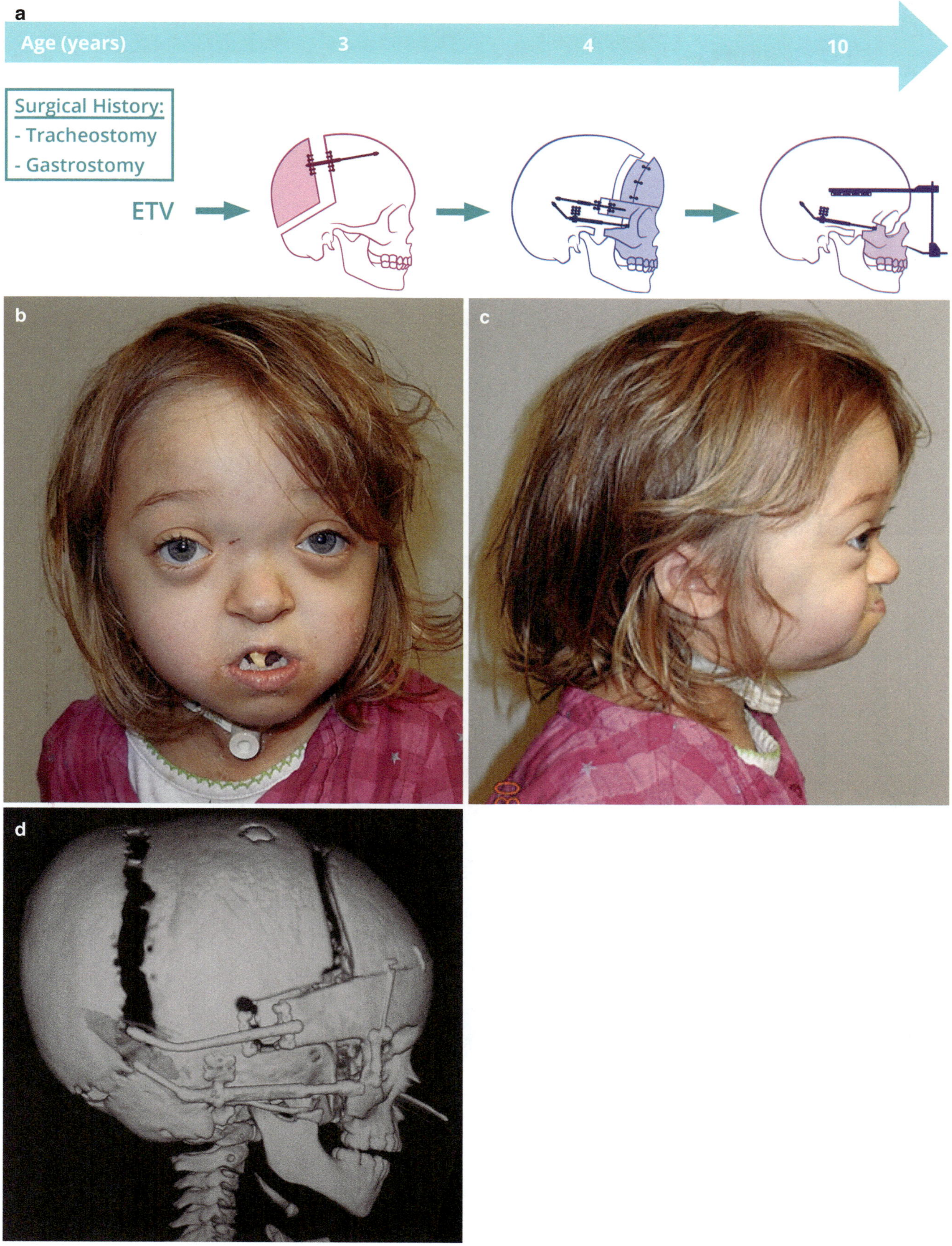
a
Age (years)
3
4
10
Surgical History:
- Tracheostomy
- Gastrostomy
ETV
b
c
d

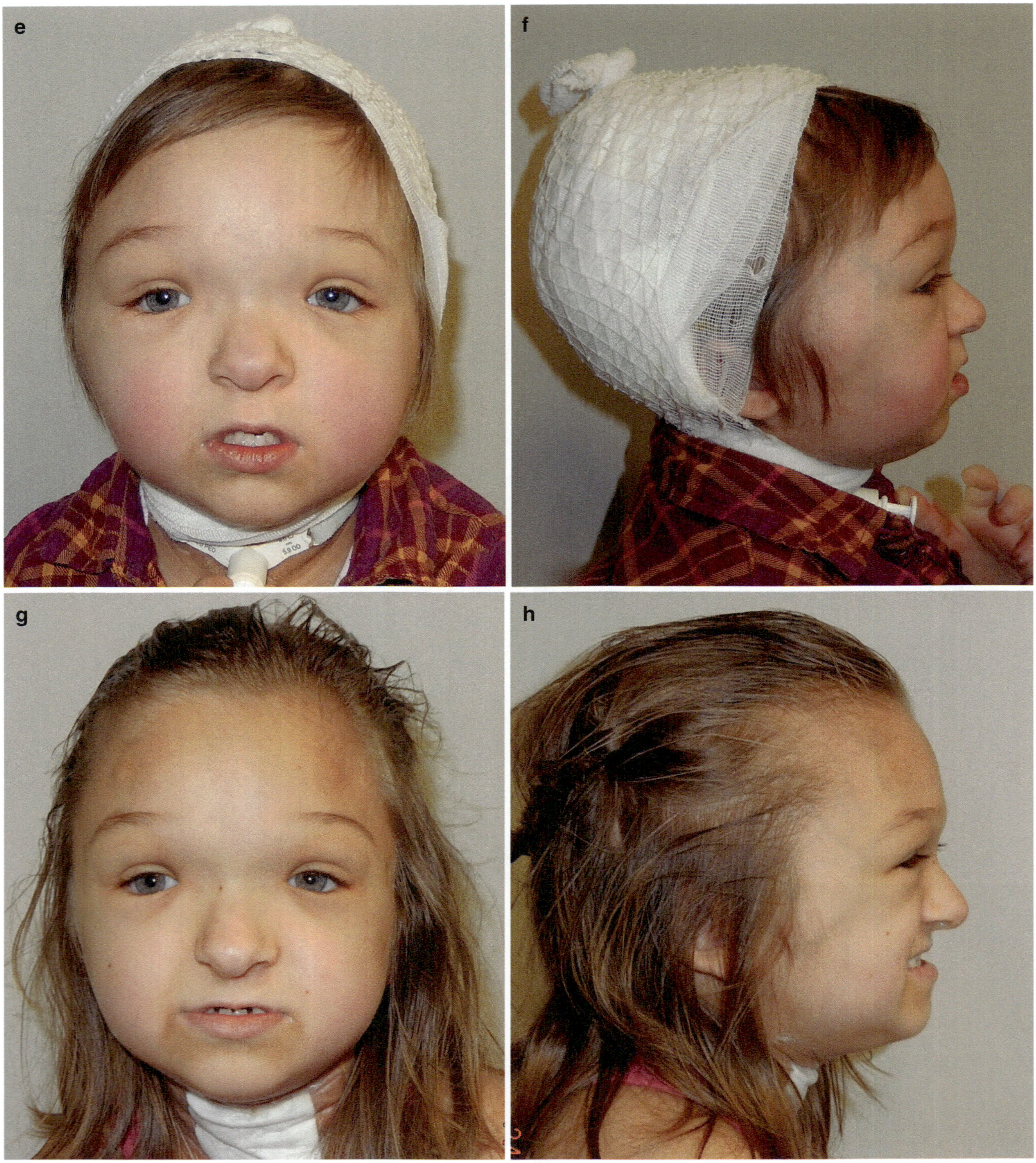

Fig. 7.1 (continued)

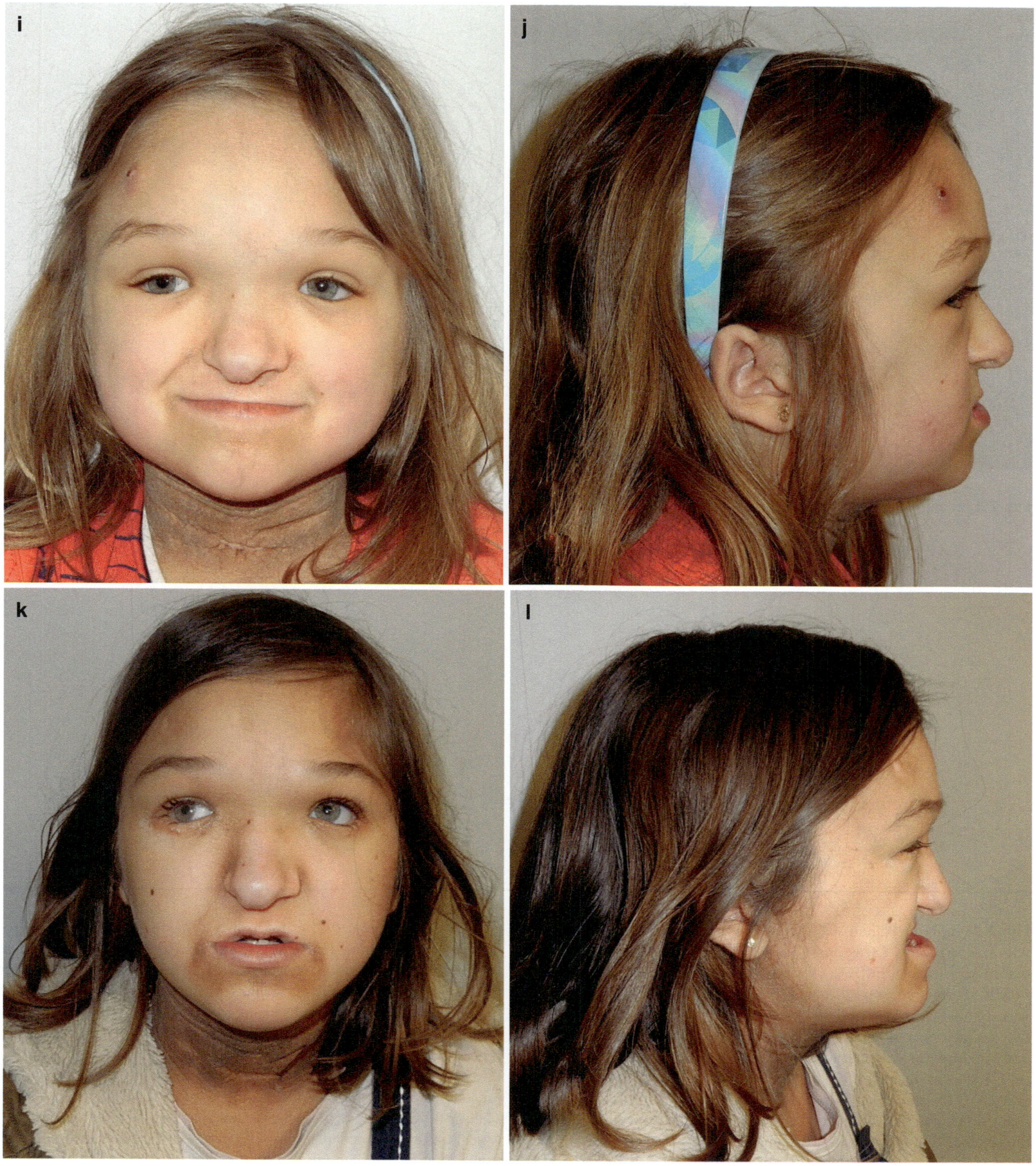

Fig. 7.1 (continued)

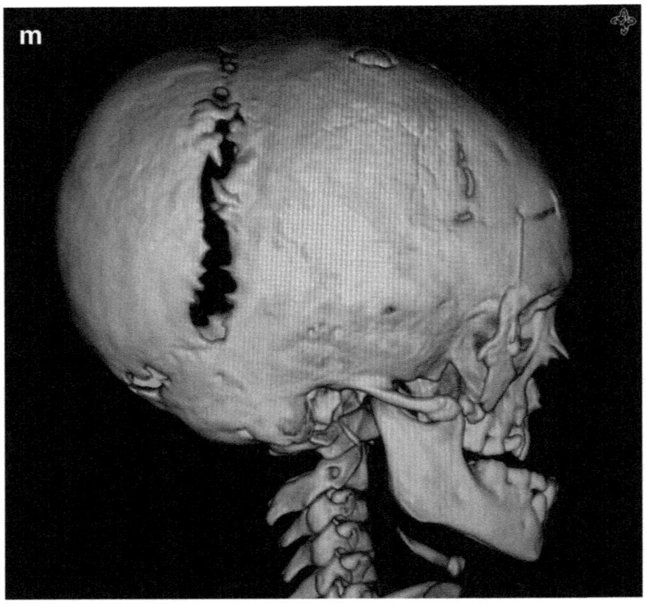

Fig. 7.1 (continued)

Fig. 7.2 (**a**, **b**, **c**) Patient with Crouzon syndrome at 4 months of age, with tracheostomy. ©Cassandra Vion. (**d**) CT scan at 4 months of age before very early FFMBA. Observe the tiny maxilla. (**e**) Very early FFMBA: osteotomies performed at 5 months of age. The temporal bone was so thin that tongue and groove osteotomy was impossible and only two distractors could be implanted. This subsequently caused a severe early relapse. (**f**) Very early FFMBA with external traction in process. (**g**) CT scan at the end of the distraction process, after 3 weeks of traction. (**h**) CT scan during distraction showing a large prefrontal subdural space filled with CSF. It reflects extreme forehead advancement. Notice the absence of dead space as the dura rapidly reattached to the frontal bone. (**i**, **j**) Six-month-postoperative result showing early relapse. (**k**, **l**) Twelve-month-postoperative result showing the removal of the tracheostomy but early relapse of the maxillary hypoplasia and exorbitism. (**m**) CT scan at 2 years of age, 19 months after very early FFMBA showing the early relapse of the midface hypoplasia despite complete mineralization of the zygomatic arch. (**n**, **o**) Secondary bibloc [4] (FOA + LF3): osteotomies performed at 2 years of age. A bandeau had to be reconstructed in order to allow forehead advancement. External distraction was performed using a rigid external distraction (RED) device. (**p**, **q**) Secondary bibloc showing progressive fronto-facial advancement based on a pair of internal distractors, a RED device and a transfacial pin placed in order to avoid maxilla-zygomatic disjunction. (**r**, **s**) Result immediately after removal of the rigid external device, with major overcorrection. (**t**, **u**) Result at 2 years of age, 6 weeks after the secondary Bibloc. (**v**) CT scan 2 months after secondary Bibloc showing satisfactory fronto-facial advancement. (**w**, **x**, **y**, **z**) Postoperative result at 4 years of age, 24 months after the secondary procedure. Appearance of a maxillary hypoplasia relapse. (**a'**-**d'**) Postoperative result at 6 years of age, 48 months after the secondary procedure. Acceleration of the maxillary hypoplasia relapse. (**e'**) CT scan at 6 years of age showing severe maxillary hypoplasia relapse, 4 years after the secondary procedure. (**f'**-**i'**) Postoperative result at 8 years of age, 6 years after the procedure. Recurrence of maxillary retrusion. (**j'**) CT scan at 8 years of age showing LF3 osteotomies performed to treat the relapsing midface hypoplasia. (**k'**, **l'**) Postoperative result 3 months after secondary LF3 performed after a very early FFMBA and a secondary bibloc (FOA + LF3): This case, the first one of our series, taught us the importance of the tongue and groove design and the importance of using 4 distractors rather than 2. (**m'**, **n'**) Postoperative result at 10 years of age, 24 months after secondary LF3. Stability of the midface advancement

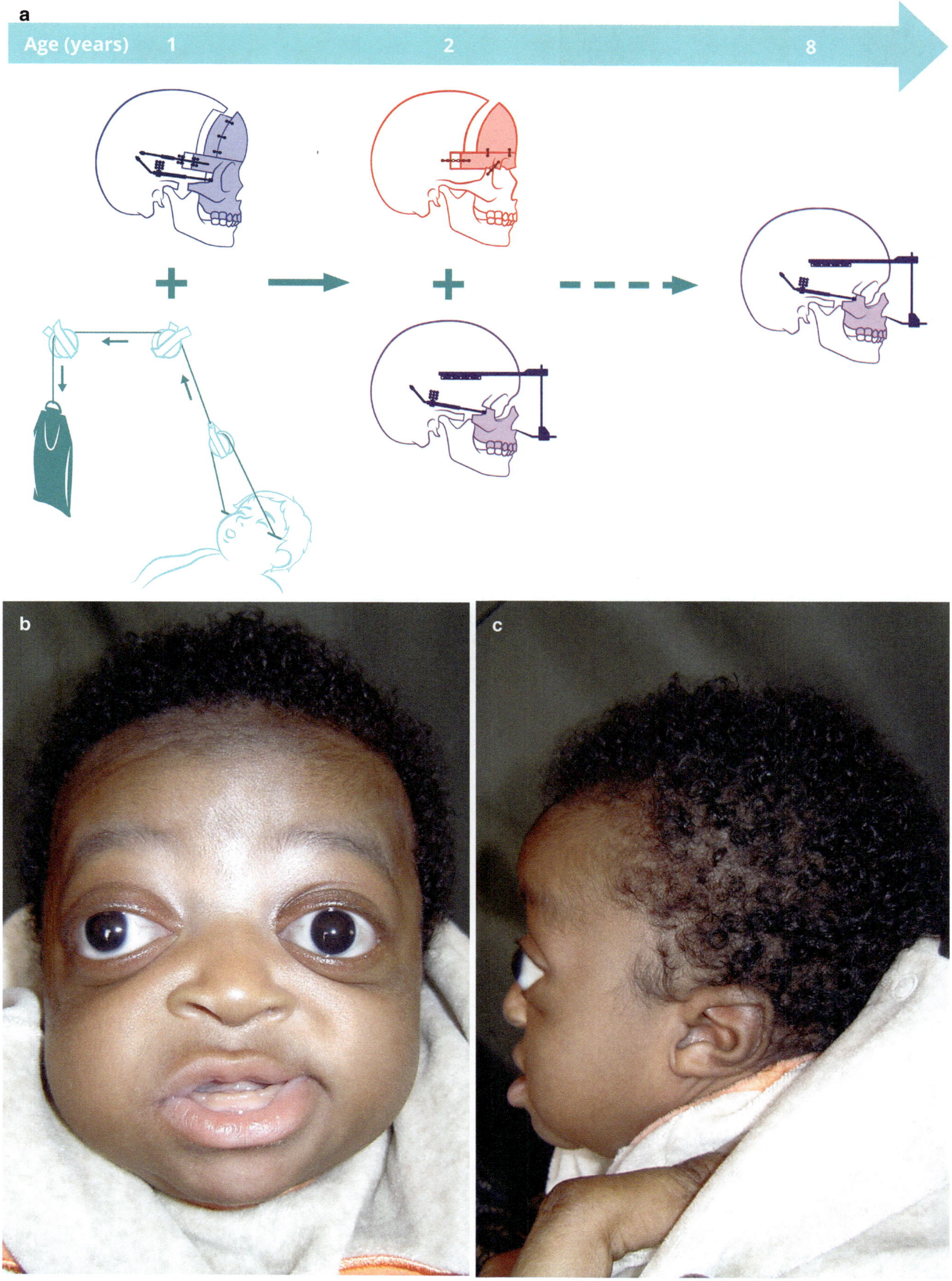
a
Age (years)
1
2
8
b
c

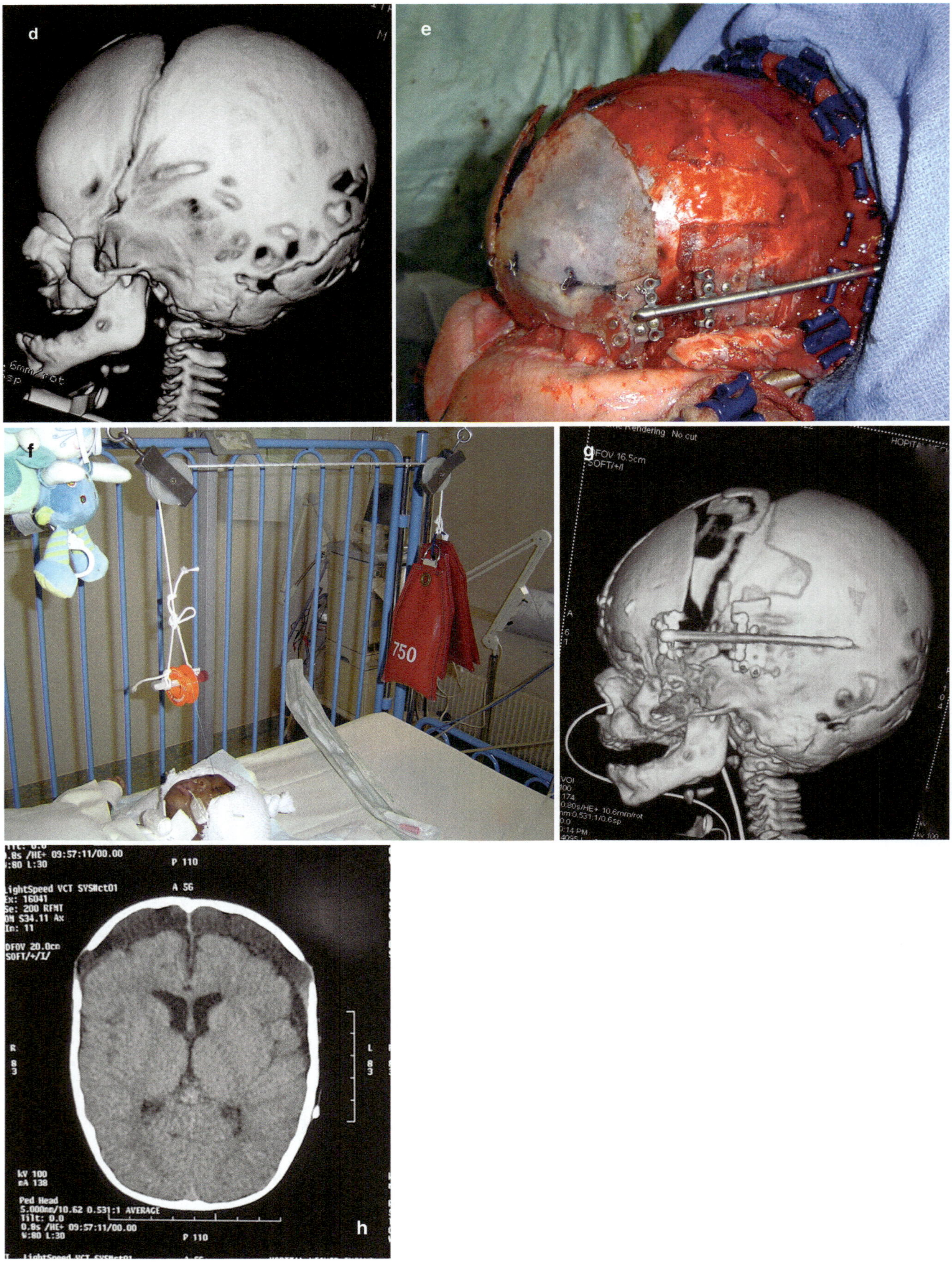

Fig. 7.2 (continued)

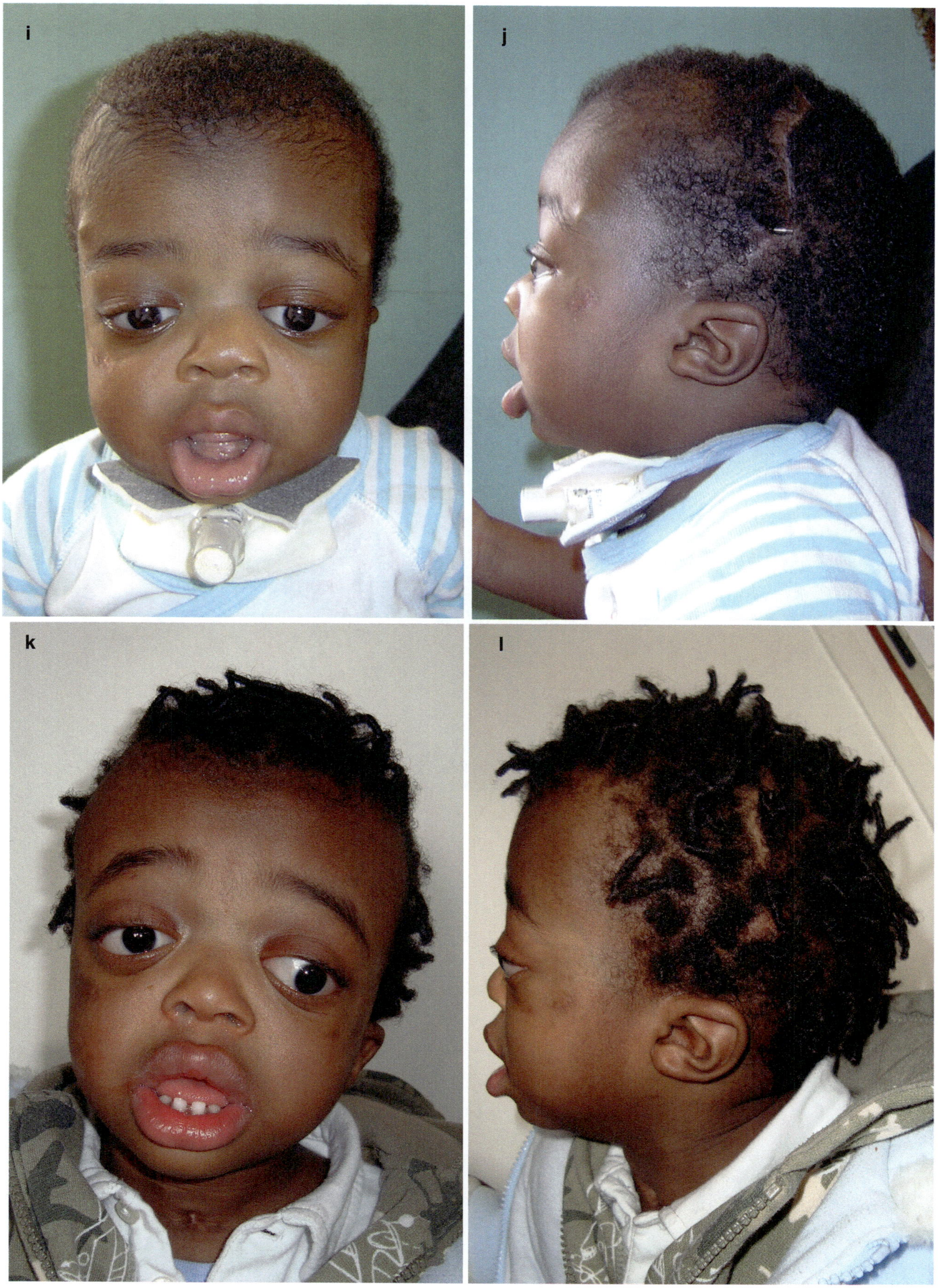

Fig. 7.2 (continued)

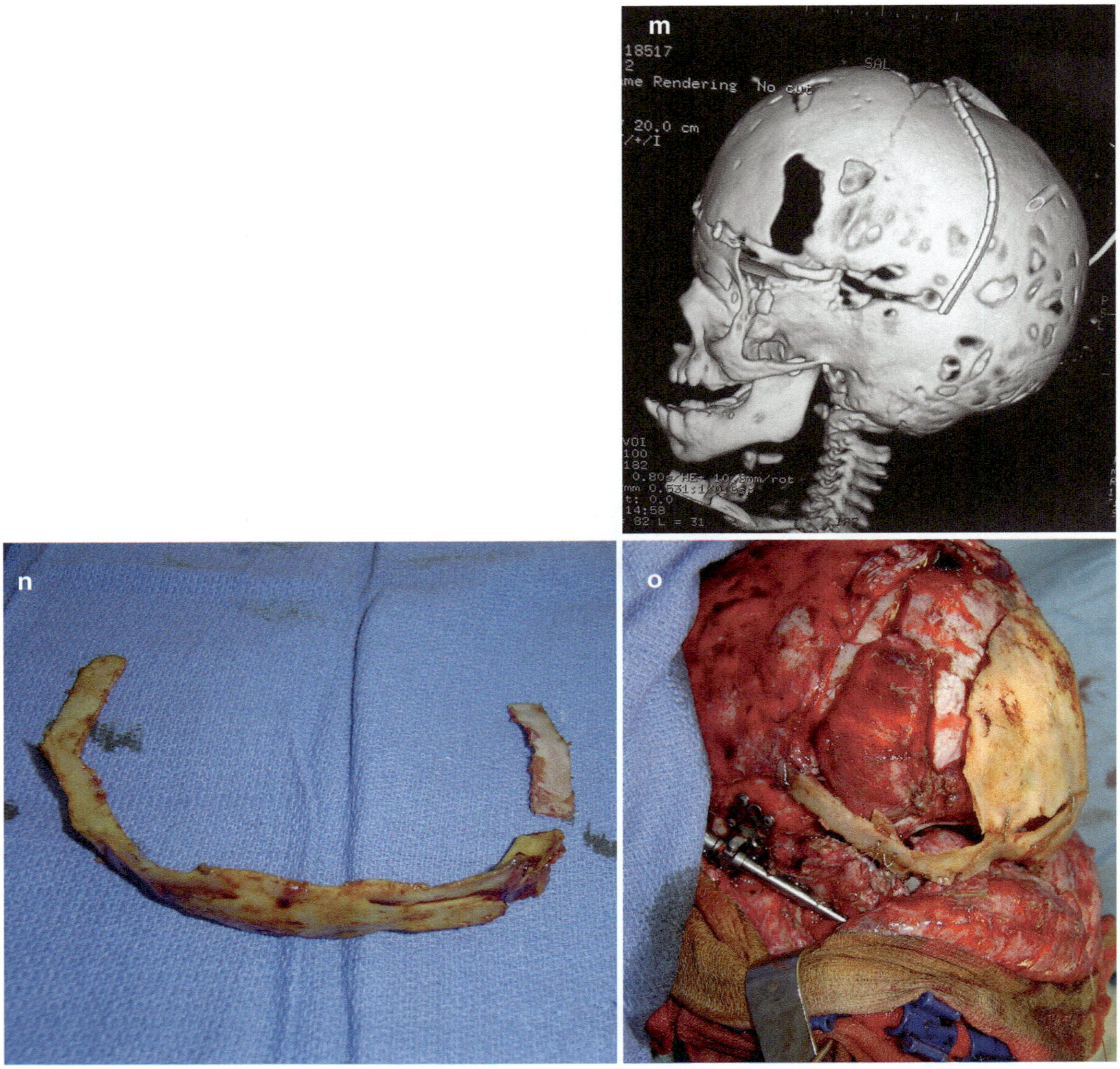

Fig. 7.2 (continued)

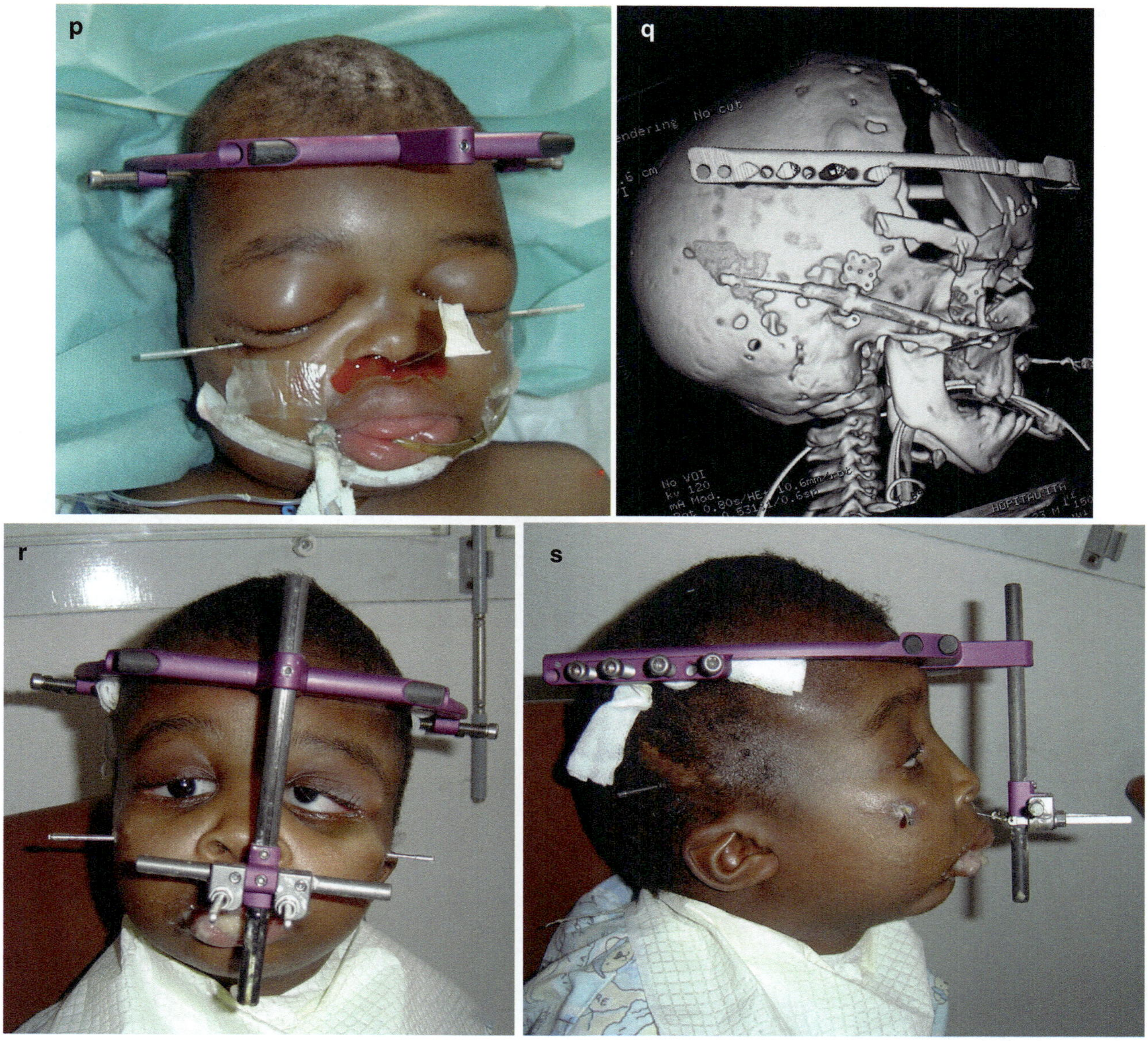

Fig. 7.2 (continued)

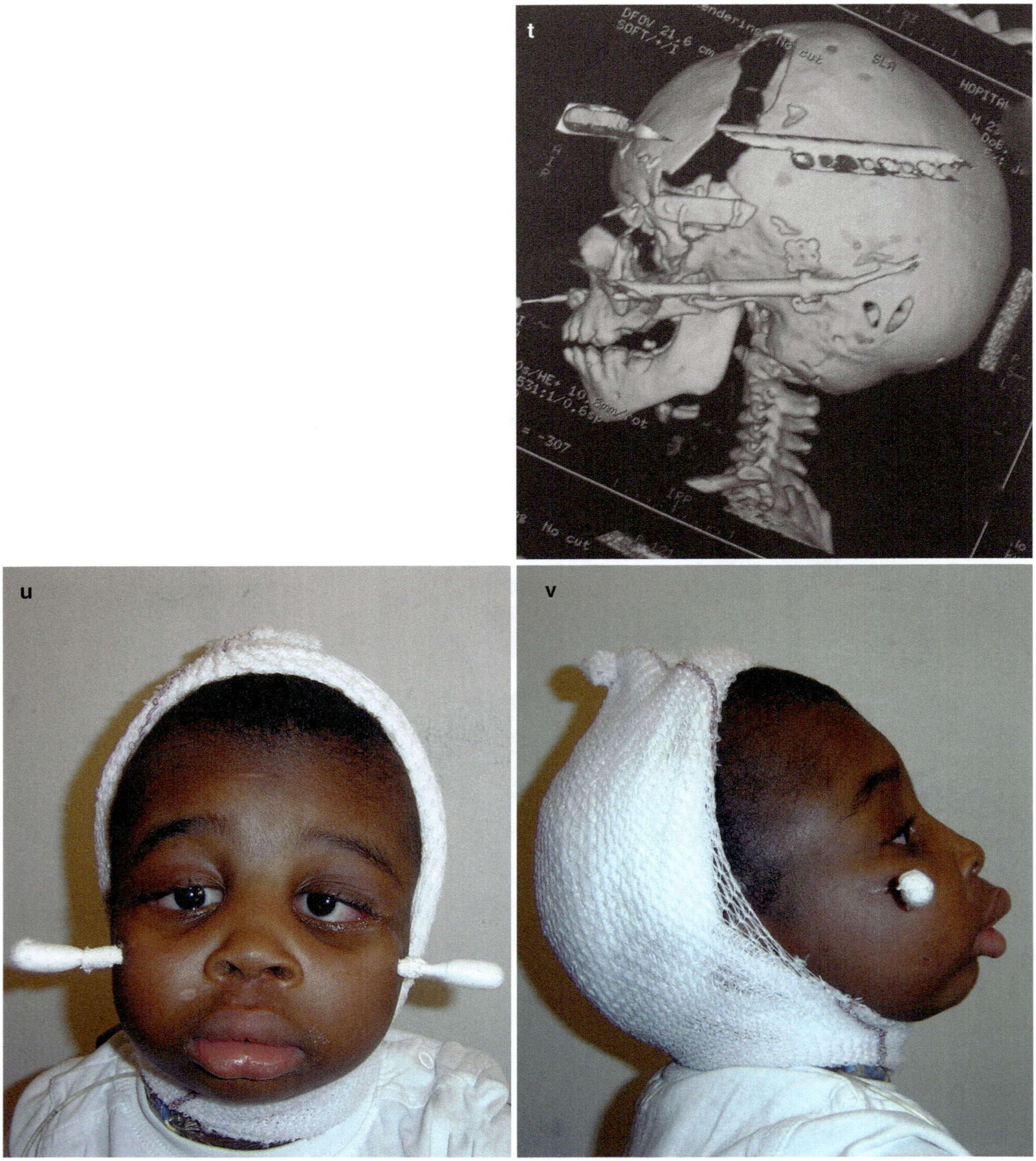

Fig. 7.2 (continued)

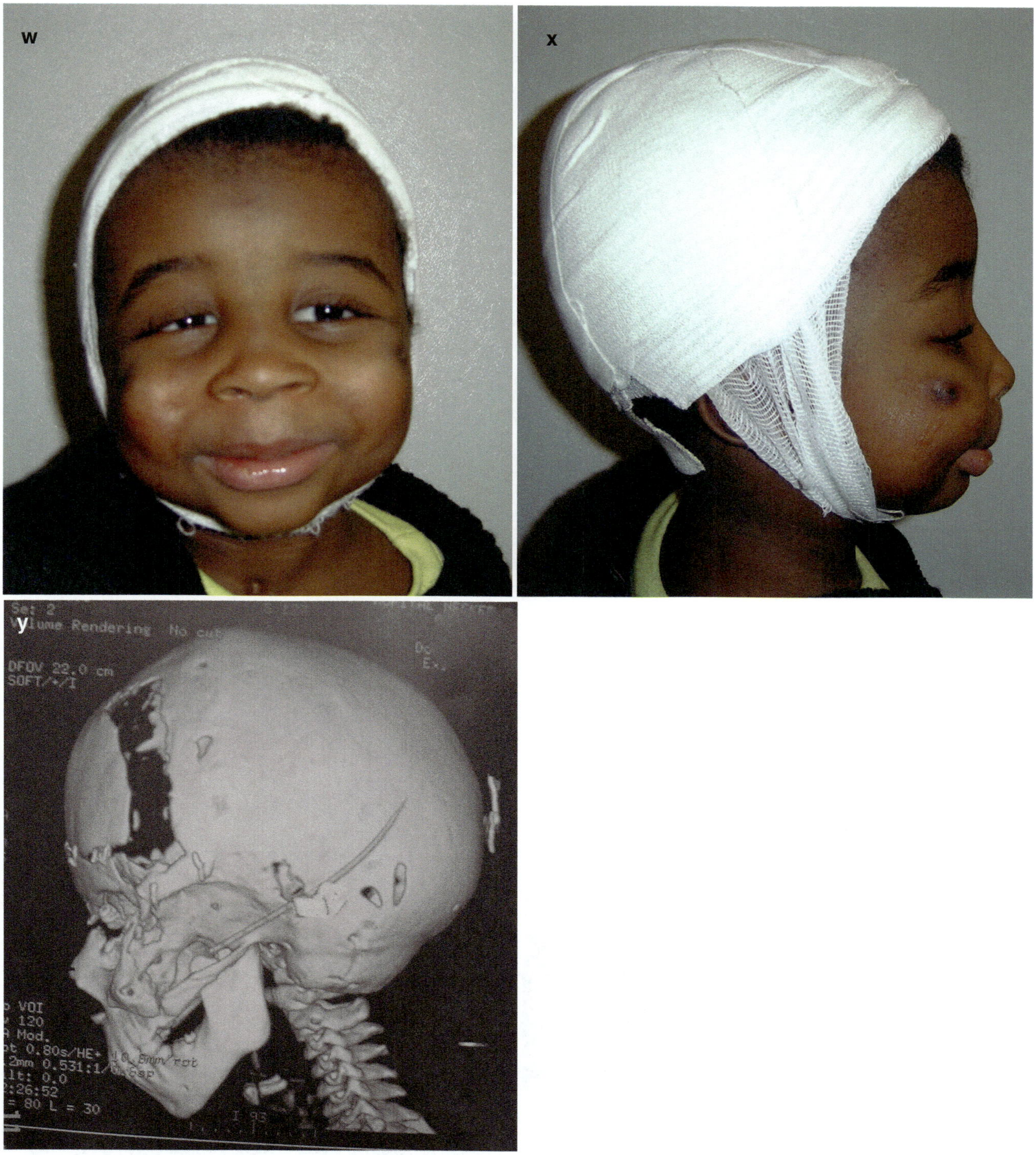

Fig. 7.2 (continued)

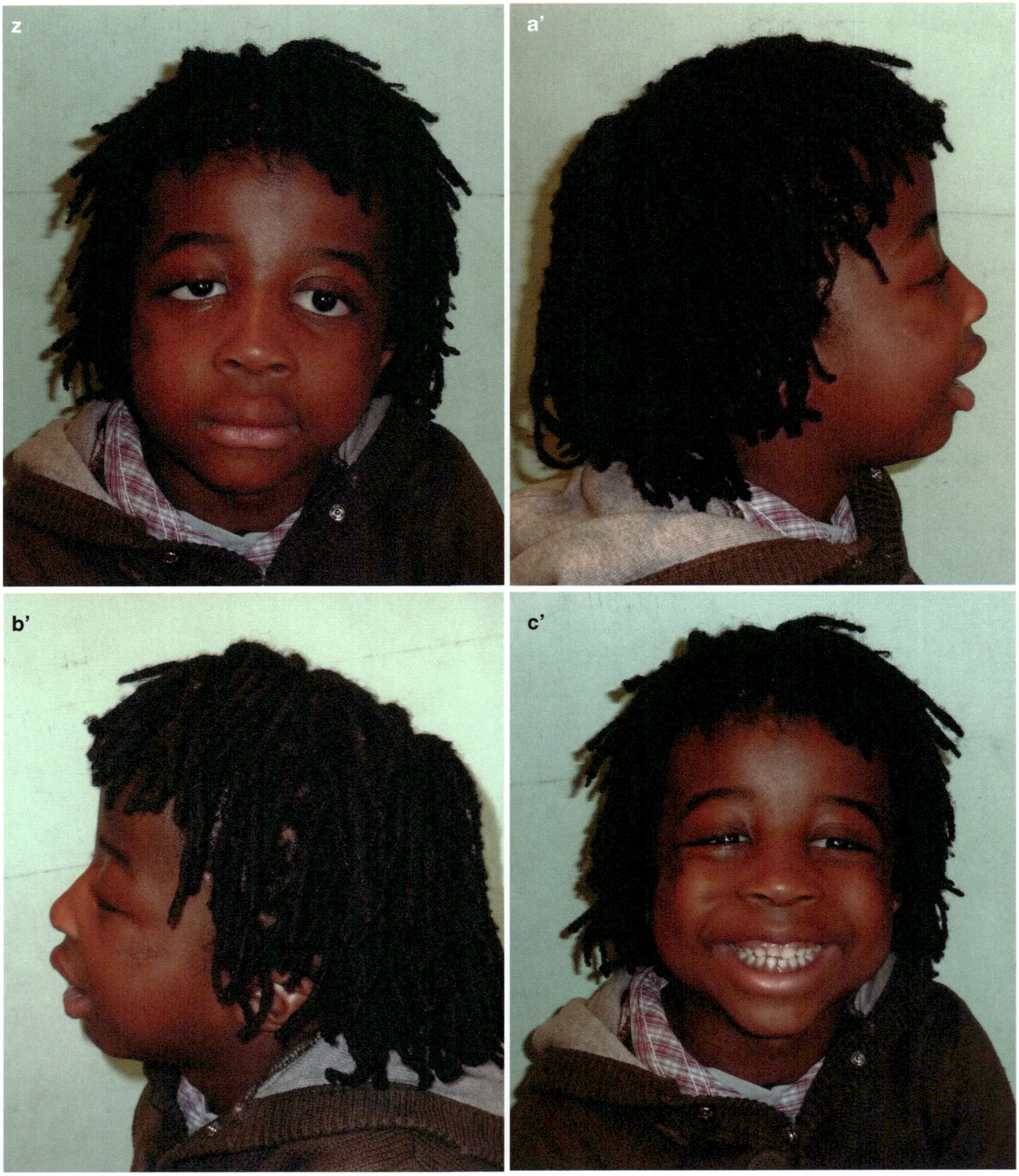

Fig. 7.2 (continued)

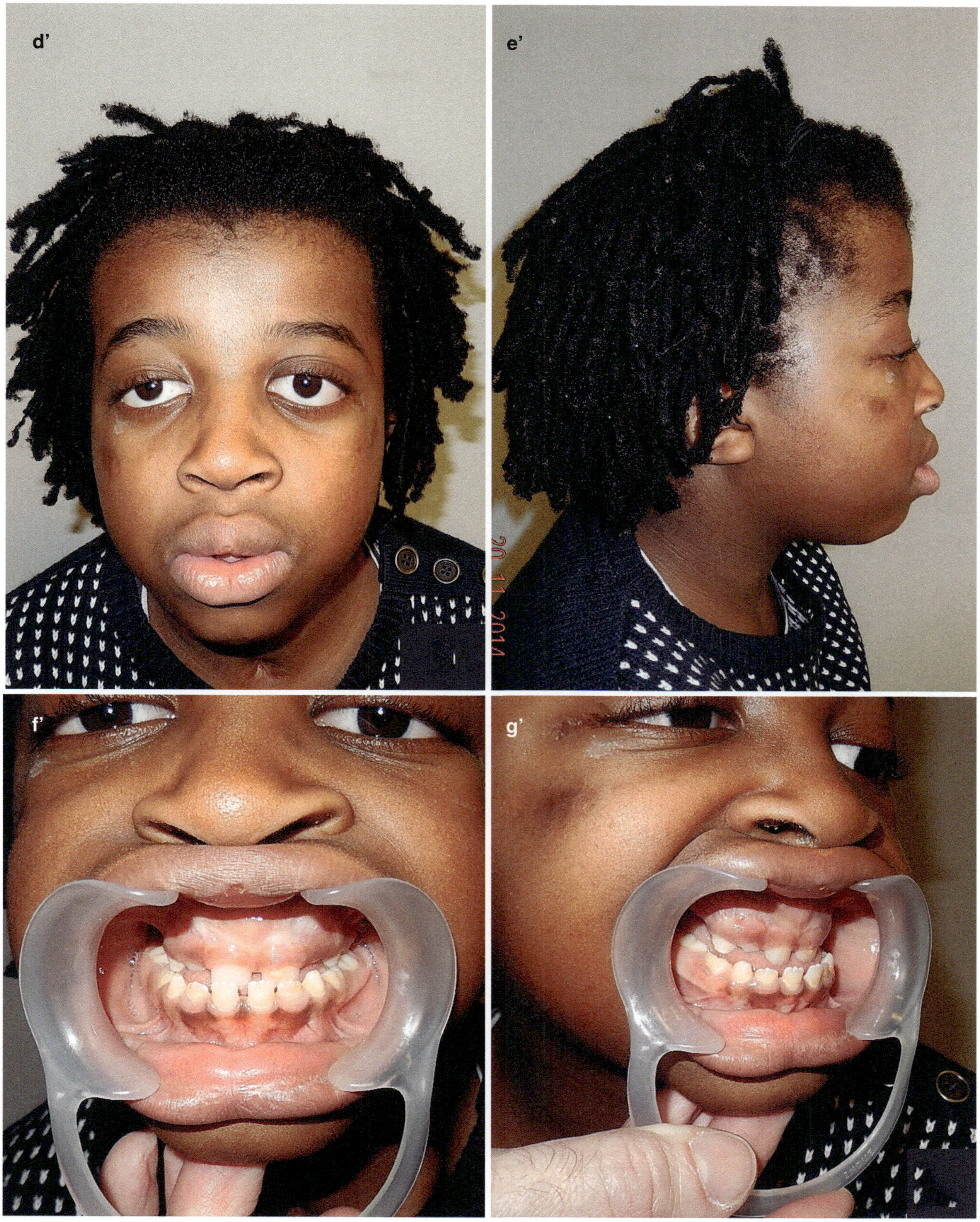

Fig. 7.2 (continued)

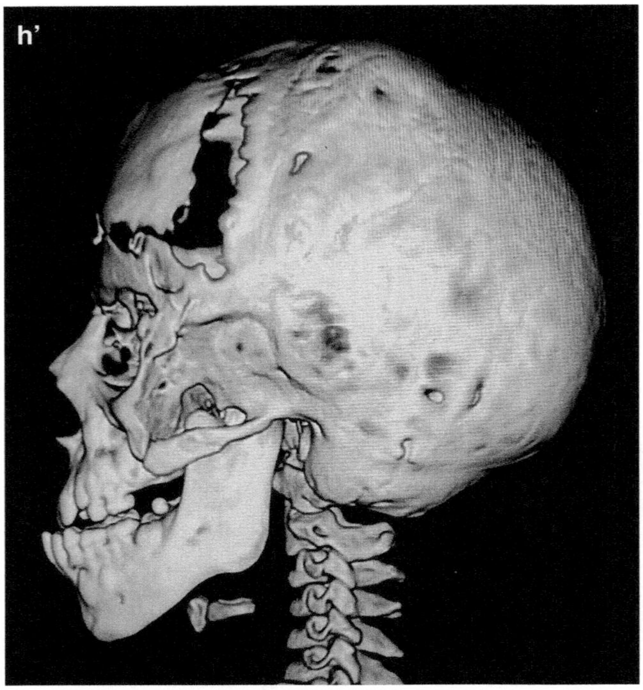

Fig. 7.2 (continued)

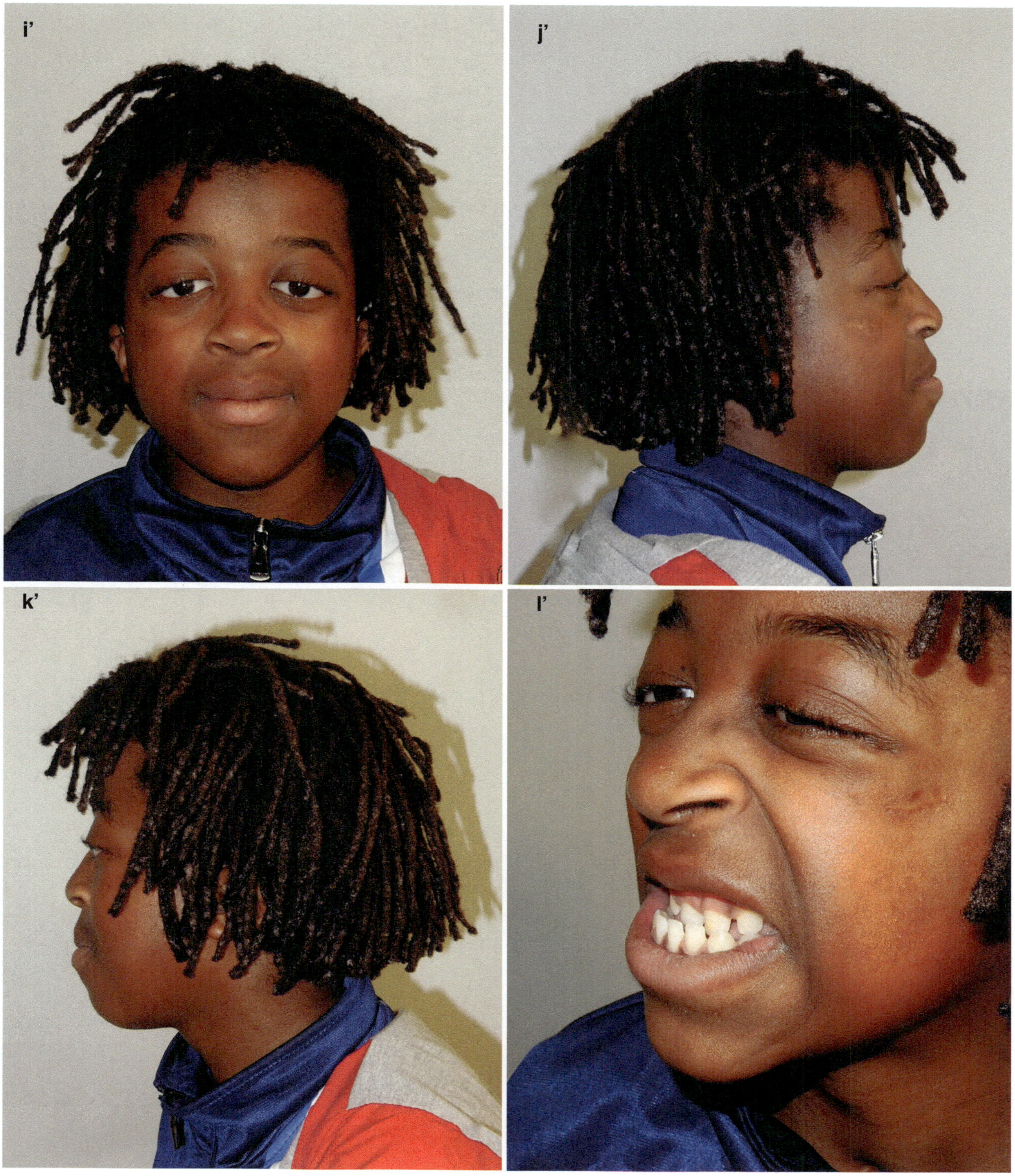

Fig. 7.2 (continued)

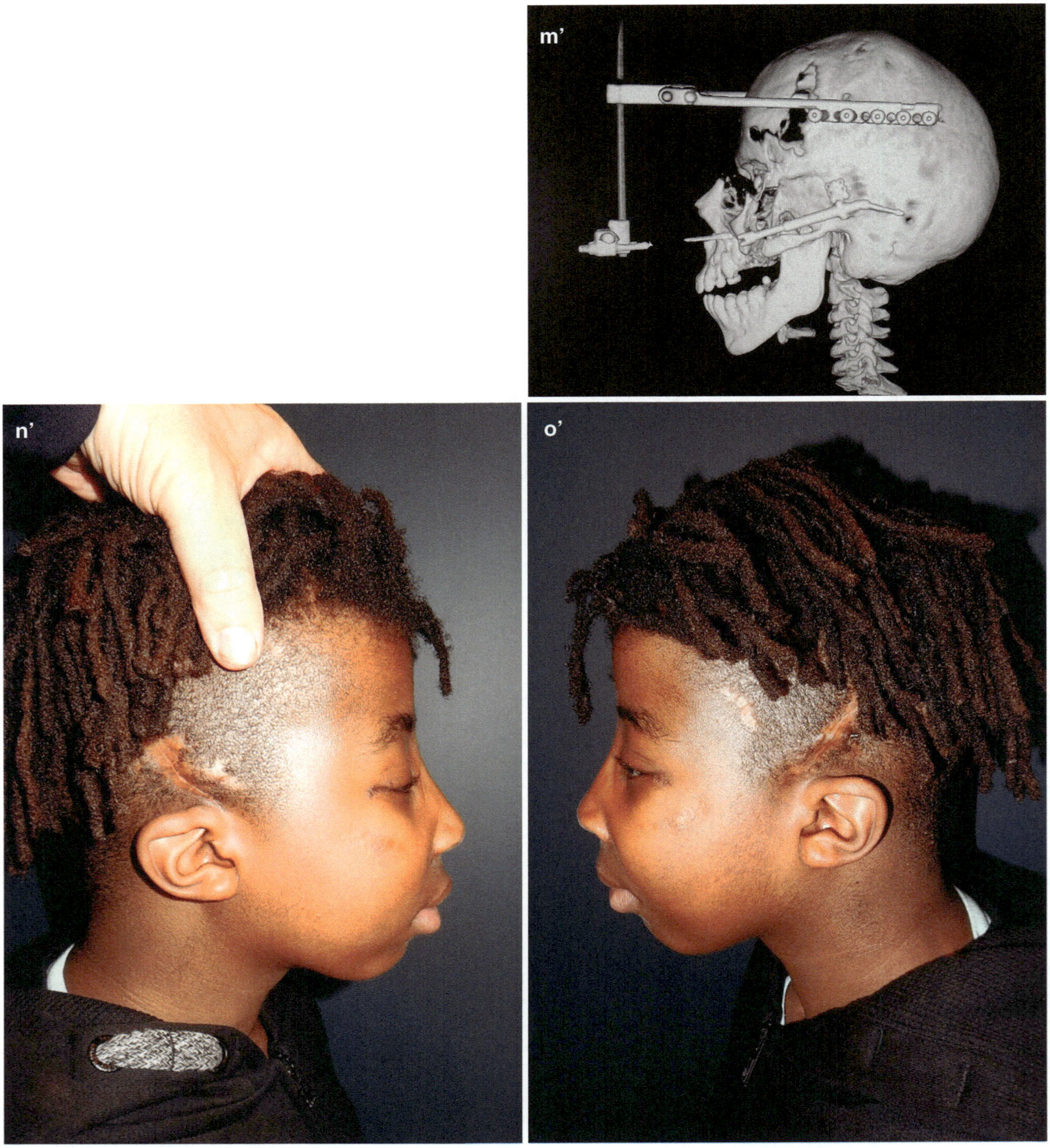

Fig. 7.2 (continued)

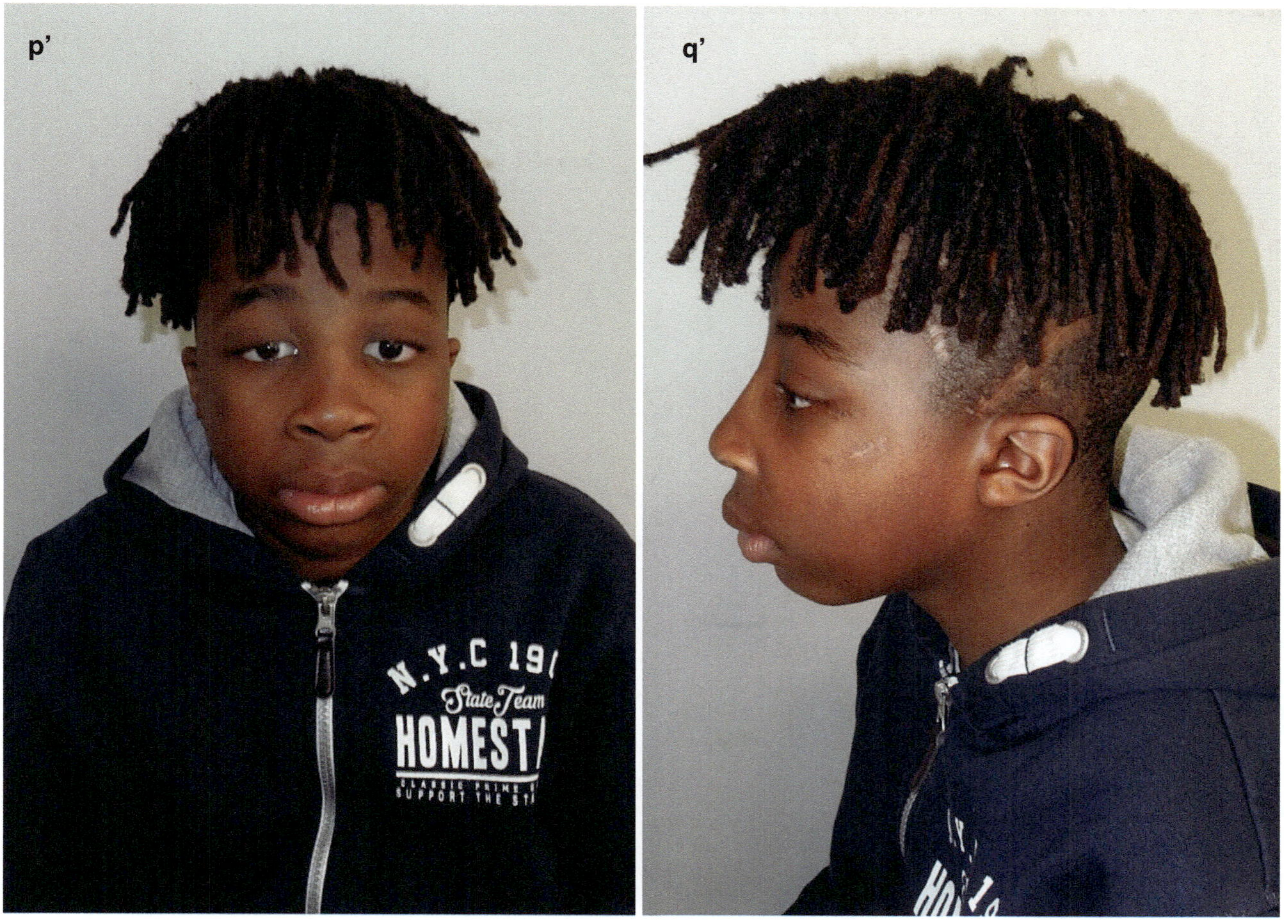

Fig. 7.2 (continued)

References

1. Kremer B, Botos-Kremer AI, Eckel HE, et al. Indications, complications, and surgical techniques for pediatric tracheostomies–an update. J Pediatr Surg. 2002 Nov;37(11):1556–62.
2. Cohen SR, Suzman K, Simms C, et al. Sleep apnea surgery versus tracheostomy in children: an exploratory study of the comparative effects on quality of life. Plast Reconstr Surg. 1998 Nov;102(6):1855–64.
3. Lo LJ, Chen YR. Airway obstruction in severe syndromic craniosynostosis. Ann Plast Surg. 1999 Sep;43(3):258–64.
4. Maunsell R, Avelino M, Caixeta Alves J, et al. Revealing the needs of children with tracheostomies. Eur Ann Otorhinolaryngol Head Neck Dis. 2018 Sep;135(5S):S93–7.
5. Arnaud E, Di Rocco F. Faciocraniosynostosis: monobloc frontofacial osteotomy replacing the two-stage strategy? Childs Nerv Syst. 2012 Sep;28(9):1557–64.
6. Arnaud E, Antunez S, Khonsari RH, et al. SYM9.9F Transfacial external traction and internal distraction for young and severe Faciocraniosynostoses: the very early Monobloc. Plastic and Reconstructive Surgery–Global Open. 2019 Aug;7(8S-2):9.
7. Paternoster G, Haber SE, Khonsari RH, et al. Craniosynostosis: Monobloc distraction with internal device and its variant for infants with severe syndromic Craniosynostosis. Clin Plast Surg. 2021 Jul;48(3):497–506.

Dental Consequences of FFMBA

8

1. Intrinsic dental anomalies in FCST are not clinically relevant.
2. FFMBA before 3 years of age can damage molar tooth buds during pterygo-zygomatic disjunction and trans-zygomatic wire positioning.
3. The risk to the teeth decreases with older age at surgery.
4. Molar tooth damage complicates orthodontic management and orthognathic surgery.

Dental concerns in patients undergoing FFMBA can be either intrinsic or due to the adverse effects of the procedure.

Intrinsic dental anomalies in patients with FCST are not clinically significant in early childhood. These anomalies are generally moderate [1, 2] with controversy regarding the prevalence of primary dental agenesis in patients with *FGFR2* mutations. In the rare type of *FGFR3*-related Crouzon with *acanthosis nigricans*, odontogenic tumors resembling odontoma have been reported and may require surgical removal at later ages [3, 4] (Fig. 8.1). In brief, intrinsic dental anomalies are not the primary concern in the early management of children with FCST.

In fact, the main dental issue in patients undergoing FFMBA, especially at early ages (<36 months) is the iatrogenic damage inflicted to the tooth buds of the third molars during the procedure. More precisely, tooth bud injuries occur during pterygo-maxillary disjunction and transfacial pinning [2] (Figs. 8.2, 8.3, 8.4, and 8.5).

Of note, central incisor damage can occur during midline osteotomies for facial bipartition and intermaxillary disjunction: the axes of the incisor roots have to be assessed before this procedure and piezosurgery can be used to minimize dental damage.

We have recently assessed this risk: in a population of 15 patients with Crouzon syndrome due to *FGFR2* mutations, children who benefited from a very early (<18 months) or an early FFMBA (< 36 months), had 71% of malposition of the first permanent maxillary molars and 58% of missing second permanent maxillary molars. Malpositioned teeth had frequent shape anomalies. The risk of dental damage significantly decreased with age at surgery, and increased with the use of transfacial pins [2].

Similar results had been previously reported [5] and a recent study has replicated our conclusions [6]. Missing maxillary molars complicate further orthodontic and orthognathic management of children with FCST. In fact, the vast majority of these patients require transversal maxillary expansion and double-jaw surgery to correct maxillary retrusion at the end of growth [6, 7].

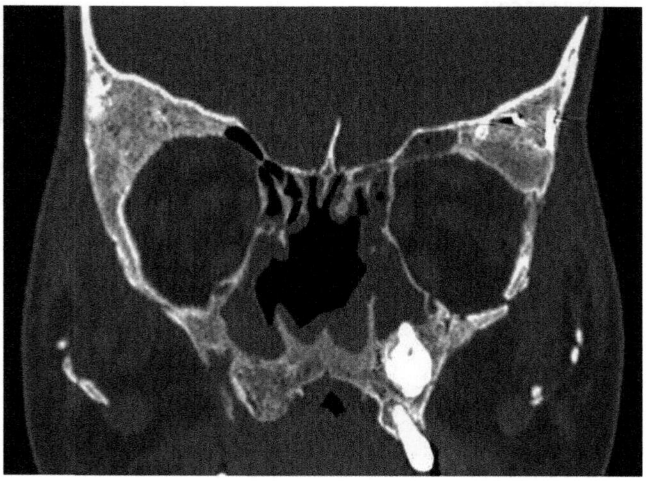

Fig. 8.1 Left maxillary odontoma in an 11-year-old patient with *FGFR3*-related Crouzon with *acanthosis nigricans*

E. Arnaud et al., *Frontofacial Monobloc Advancement with Internal Distraction*, https://doi.org/10.1007/978-3-031-07574-2_8

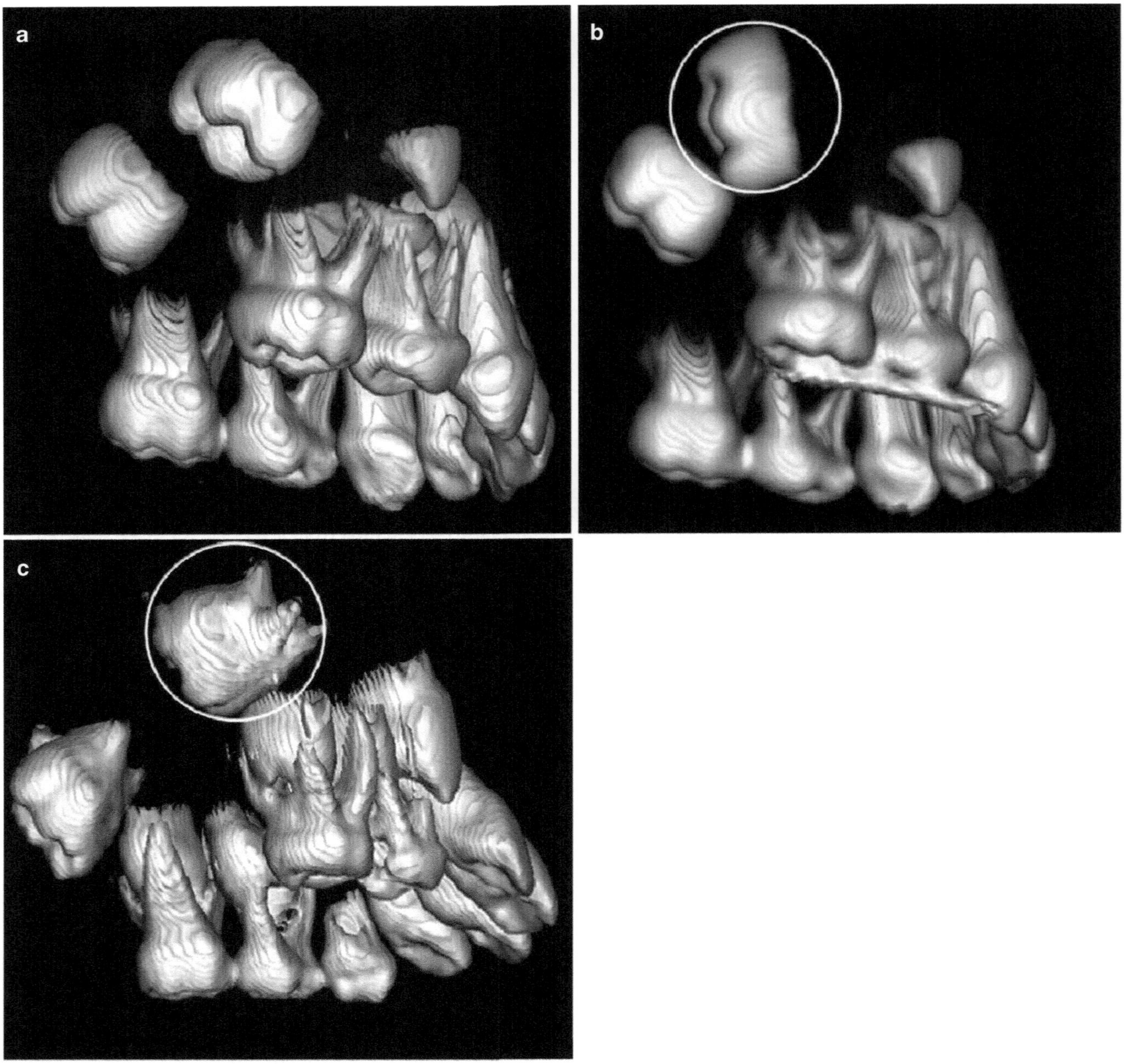

Fig. 8.2 (**a**) Before FFMBA in a 42-month-old patient. (**b**) After FFMBA, rotation of the germ of the first permanent molar. (**c**) Five years later, abnormal root erection with closed apex of the first permanent molar [2]

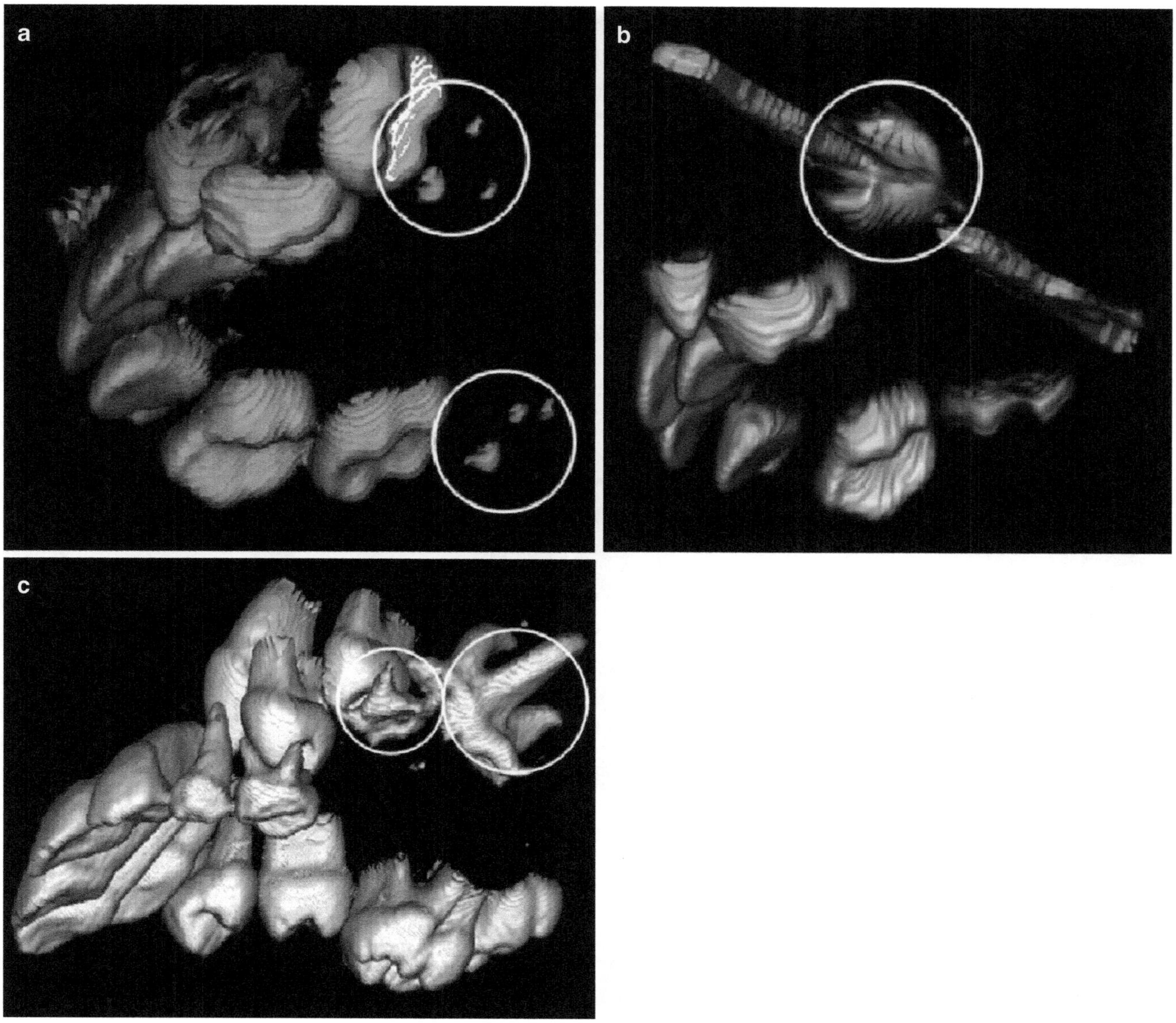

Fig. 8.3 (**a**) Before FFMBA in a 3-month-old patient. The mineralization of the cups of the first permanent molars has started. (**b**) After FFMBA with a transfacial pin skewering the second temporary molar. (**c**) Nine years postoperatively, first and second permanent molars are present on the right side. On the left side, persistence of an abnormal second deciduous molar (white circle), misshapen crown of the second permanent molar, and lack of the first permanent molar

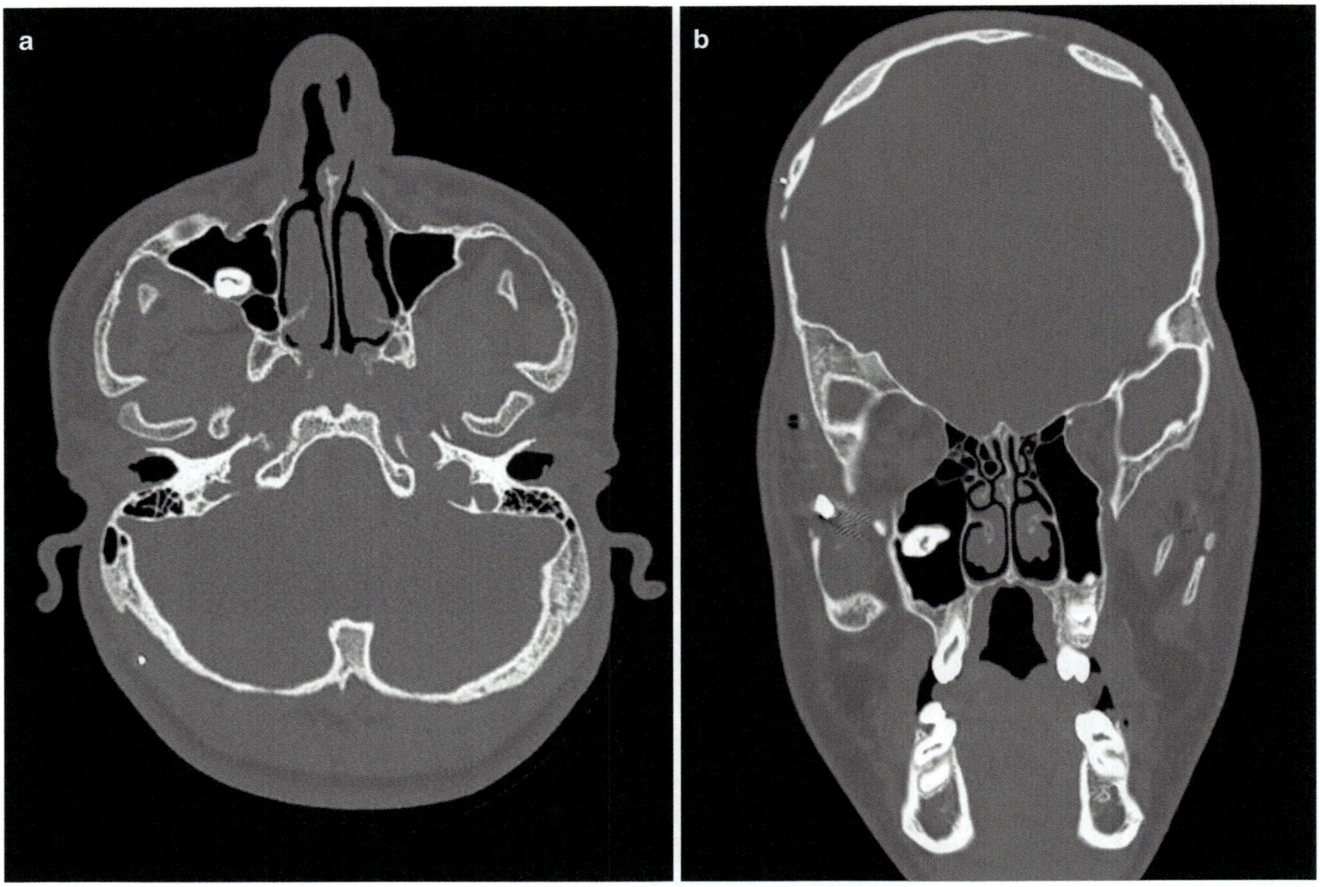

Fig. 8.4 (**a**, **b**) Molar odontoma in the right maxillary sinus in a 15-year-old patient with Crouzon syndrome who had benefited from very early FFBMA

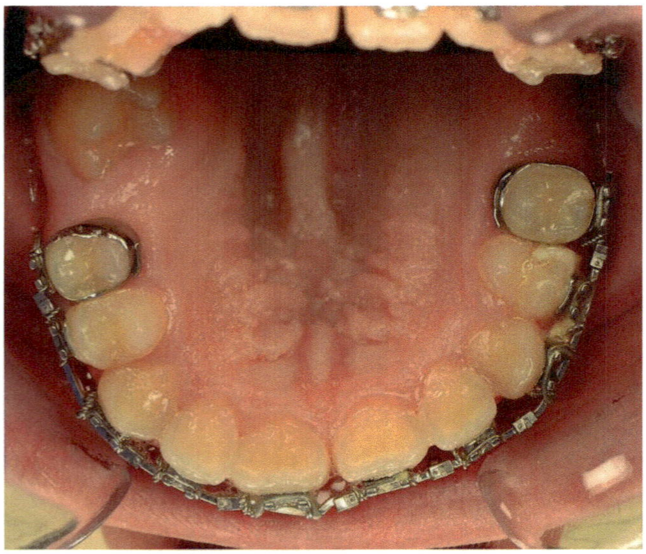

Fig. 8.5 Missing molars in a 17-year-old patient with Crouzon syndrome who underwent a very early FFMBA before age 36 months. The missing molars complicate orthodontic management and orthognathic surgery

References

1. Reitsma JH, Balk-Leurs IH, Ongkosuwito EM, et al. Dental maturation in children with the syndrome of crouzon and apert. Cleft Palate Craniofac J. 2014 Nov;51(6):639–44.
2. Sicard L, Hounkpevi M, Tomat C, et al. Dental consequences of pterygomaxillary dysjunction during fronto-facial monobloc advancement with internal distraction for Crouzon syndrome. J Craniomaxillofac Surg. 2018 Sep;46(9):1476–9.
3. Suslak L, Glista B, Gertzman GB, et al. Crouzon syndrome with periapical cemental dysplasia and acanthosis nigricans: the pleiotropic effect of a single gene? Birth Defects Orig Artic Ser. 1985;21(2):127–34.
4. Xu W, McDonald-McGinn DM, Melchiorre AJ, et al. Crouzon with acanthosis Nigricans and odontogenic tumors: a rare form of syndromic Craniosynostosis. Cleft Palate Craniofac J. 2018 Feb;55(2):296–300.
5. Sant'Anna EF, de Cury-Saramago A, Figueroa AA, et al. Evaluation of maxillary permanent molars in patients with syndromic craniosynostosis after monobloc osteotomy and midface advancement with rigid external distraction (RED). Cleft Palate Craniofac J. 2010 Mar;47(2):109–15.
6. Yang R, Shakoori P, Lanni MA, et al. Influence of Monobloc/Le fort III surgery on the developing posterior maxillary dentition and its resultant effect on Orthognathic surgery. Plast Reconstr Surg. 2021 Feb 1;147(2):253e–9e.
7. Vargervik K, Rubin MS, Grayson BH, et al. Parameters of care for craniosynostosis: dental and orthodontic perspectives. Am J Orthod Dentofac Orthop. 2012 Apr;141(4 Suppl):S68–73.

9 Complications After Fronto-facial Monobloc Advancement

1. Complications after FFMBA range from severe (rare) to benign (frequent), and decrease with the learning curve.
2. Lethal complications come from acute raised intracranial pressure associated with untreated tonsillar herniation and/or vascular related abnormalities.
3. Severe infections are associated with secondary FFMBA performed after FOA, and/or when a ventriculoperitoneal shunt was present.
4. Device-related dysfunctions decrease with completeness of osteotomies.
5. Minor inflammations around distractors are common and decrease with early removal of activation rods.
6. Limitation of buccal opening after FFMBA can be avoided by early postoperative physiotherapy.
7. Insufficient maxillary advancement is associated with incompleteness of osteotomies.
8. Worsening of respiratory status after FFMBA might result from the lack of resection of the tonsils/adenoids prior to FFMBA.
9. Early relapse can be avoided by a long tongue and groove design and a consolidation period of 5-6 months.
10. Lack of calvarial re-ossification is more frequent in Pfeiffer syndrome.

Between 2000 and 2015, 149 patients with faciocraniosynostosis underwent FFMBA in Necker Hospital. Two subgroups were identified according to age at surgery:

- < 18 months: 25 patients (17%),
- 18 months: 124 patients (83%).

Their previous surgical history included:

- Ventriculoperitoneal shunting in 27 patients (18%),
- Posterior vault expansion with +/− distraction in 70 patients (49%),
- Foramen magnum decompression in 26 patients (17%).

The strategy and the surgical planning for these patients drastically changed over the last 20 years (Fig. 9.1).

Before 2004, fronto-facial monobloc advancement was either performed primarily (primary FFMBA) or secondarily after fronto-orbital advancement or subtotal vault remodeling. In this last subgroup, patients had been operated previously of a FOA with an insufficient result and were reoperated with a FFMBA (secondary FFMBA).

Between 2004 and 2011, given the morbidity of the secondary FFMBA, the intervention was reserved for primary cases without previous fronto-orbital interventions, in patients with intact pericranium that could be pedicled to seal the anterior cranial fossa from the underlying sinuses and nasal cavities. Biparietal expansion was considered the first-line intervention before FFMBA when urgent intracranial decompression was indicated. Foramen magnum decompression could also be indicated before FFMBA in case of cerebellar tonsillar hernia.

As of 2011, we finally adopted our current protocol consisting of beginning with posterior cranial expansion with—whenever possible—internal distractors. Compared to biparietal expansion, posterior expansion gives better morphological improvement of the brachycephaly as it directly corrects the anteroposterior shortening of the cranium. PVE is capable of more cranial expansion, especially when distraction osteogenesis can be performed. PVE directly augments posterior fossa volume with adequate cerebellar decompression and radiological improvement of cerebellar tonsillar hernia on MRI. PVE also presents better localization of the temporal osteotomy lines which prepares for the upcoming FFMBA several years later. PVE facilitates simul-

E. Arnaud et al., *Frontofacial Monobloc Advancement with Internal Distraction*, https://doi.org/10.1007/978-3-031-07574-2_9

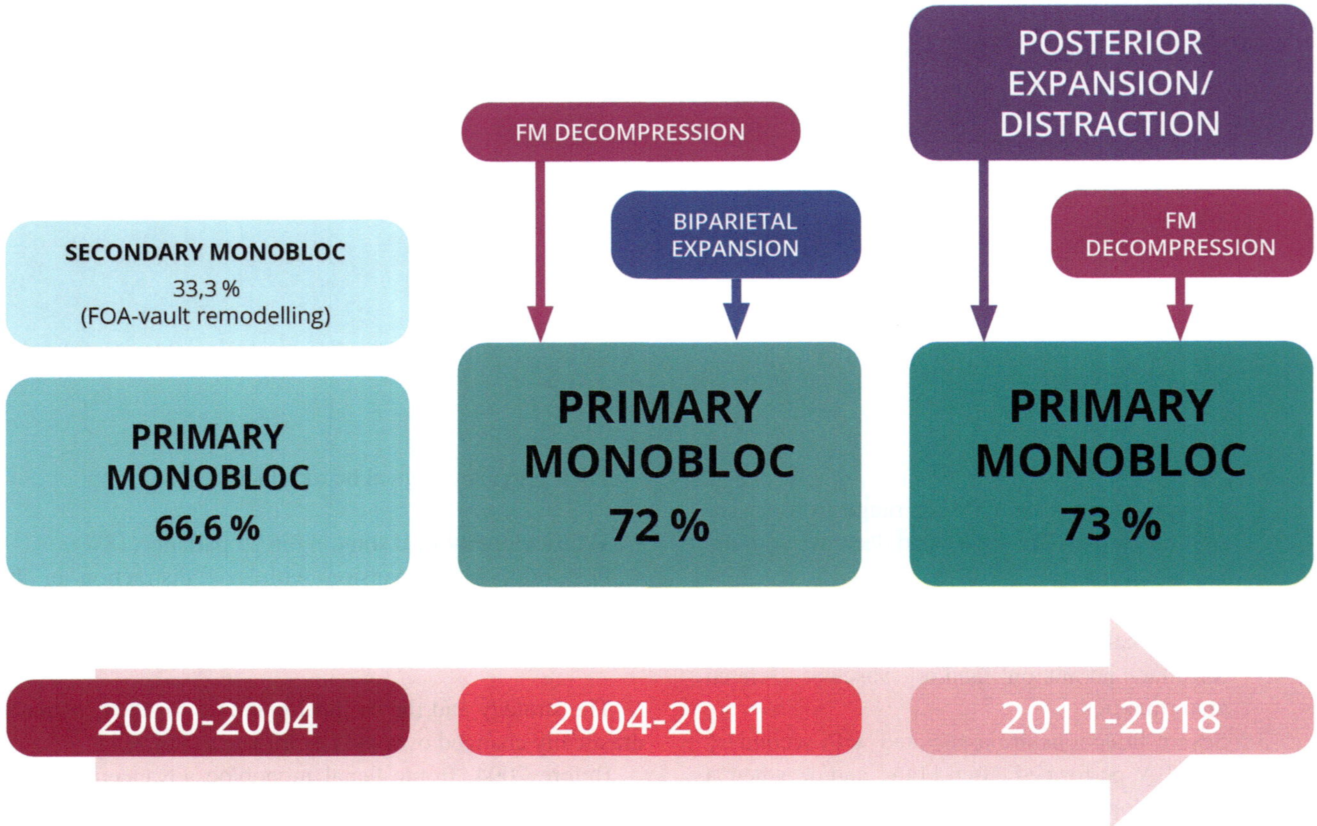

Fig. 9.1 Progressive steps toward the definition of the current management protocol for faciocraniosynostosis (similar figure as Fig. 2.1)

taneous foramen magnum decompression when needed in the prone intraoperative positioning.

Despite this standardized protocol with PVE creating good surgical conditions for fronto-facial advancement, FFMBA remains a risky procedure. Complications can be classified as such:

1. Surgical problems
   - Communications between brain cavity and anterior fossa/nasal cavity via skull base osteotomies.
   - Retrofrontal dead space.
2. Device problems
   - Fixation/screws/malpositioning
3. Early age at surgery (<18 months)
   - Transfacial pin.
4. Previous surgery (FOA/PVE).
5. ICP/CHIARI management.

In our distraction protocol, we can identify four consecutive periods: (1) immediate postoperative, (2) distraction, (3) consolidation, and (4) late follow-up (Fig. 9.2).

Each period is associated with specific complications (Fig. 9.3).

In the immediate postoperative period, three patients from our cohort died (3/149–2%):

- Two patients died in the immediate postoperative period from venous sinus thrombosis (abnormal venous pattern) (Fig. 9.4).
- One patient died from acute tonsillar herniation (neglected untreated tonsillar herniation) (Fig. 9.5 and 5bis).

To reduce these lethal risks, we included in the preoperative imaging, systematic brain, and medullary MRI with venous flow sequences (Inhance 3D velocity/2D TOF).

In the distraction period, we observed mostly device-related issues: 3.3% of distractor displacement (5/149) and 2% of plate extrusion (3/149). The reinforcement of the fronto-zygomatic junction by metallic miniplates prevents disjunction at this level. The use of resorbable plates at the FZ junction was not strong enough (Fig. 9.6).

Furthermore, in 2% of cases (3/149), the weakness of the maxillary bone was responsible for maxillo-zygomatic disjunction that required the secondary insertion of transfacial pins or miniplates. This disjunction was mainly due to incomplete osteotomies (Figs. 9.7 and 9.8).

In 27% of cases, we detected CSF leaks (40/149), treated with repetitive subtractive lumbar puncture or external lum-

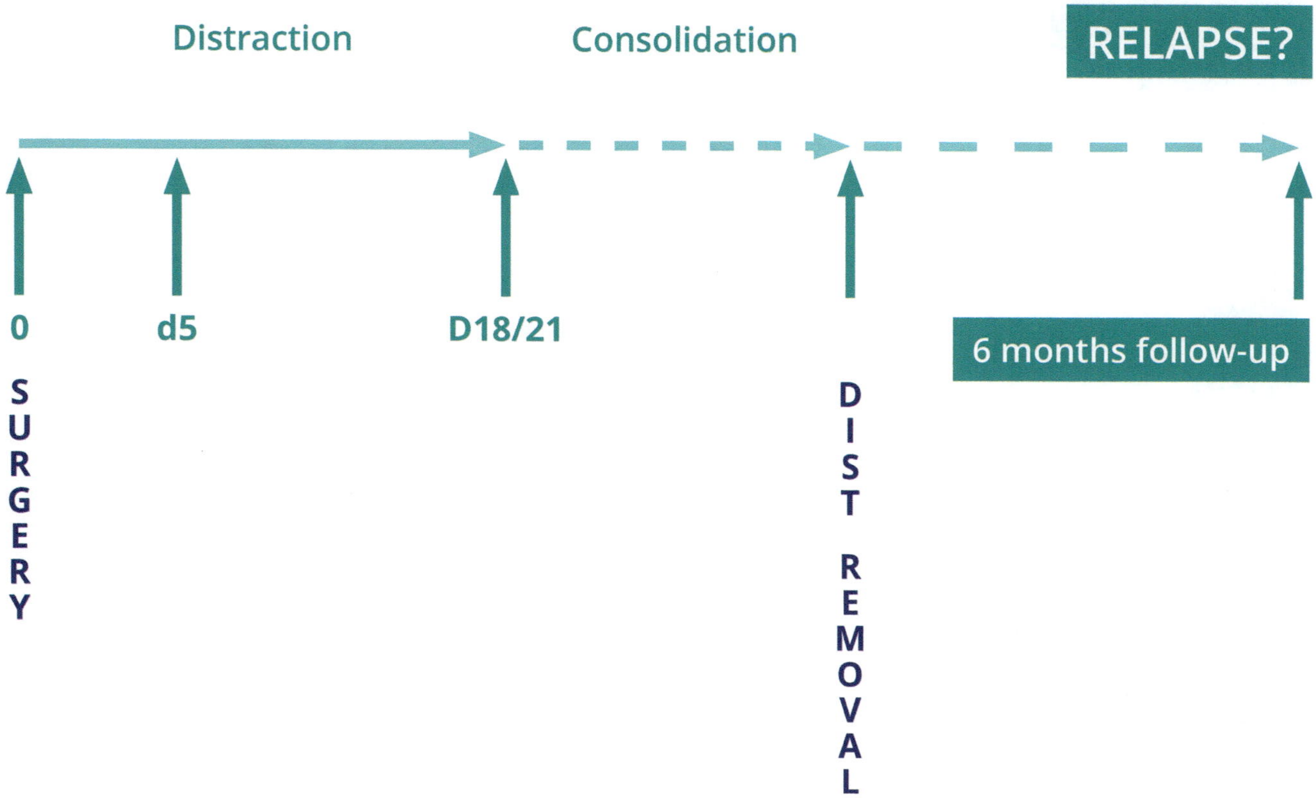

Fig. 9.2 Four periods after FFMBA: Immediate postoperative, distraction, consolidation, and late follow-up

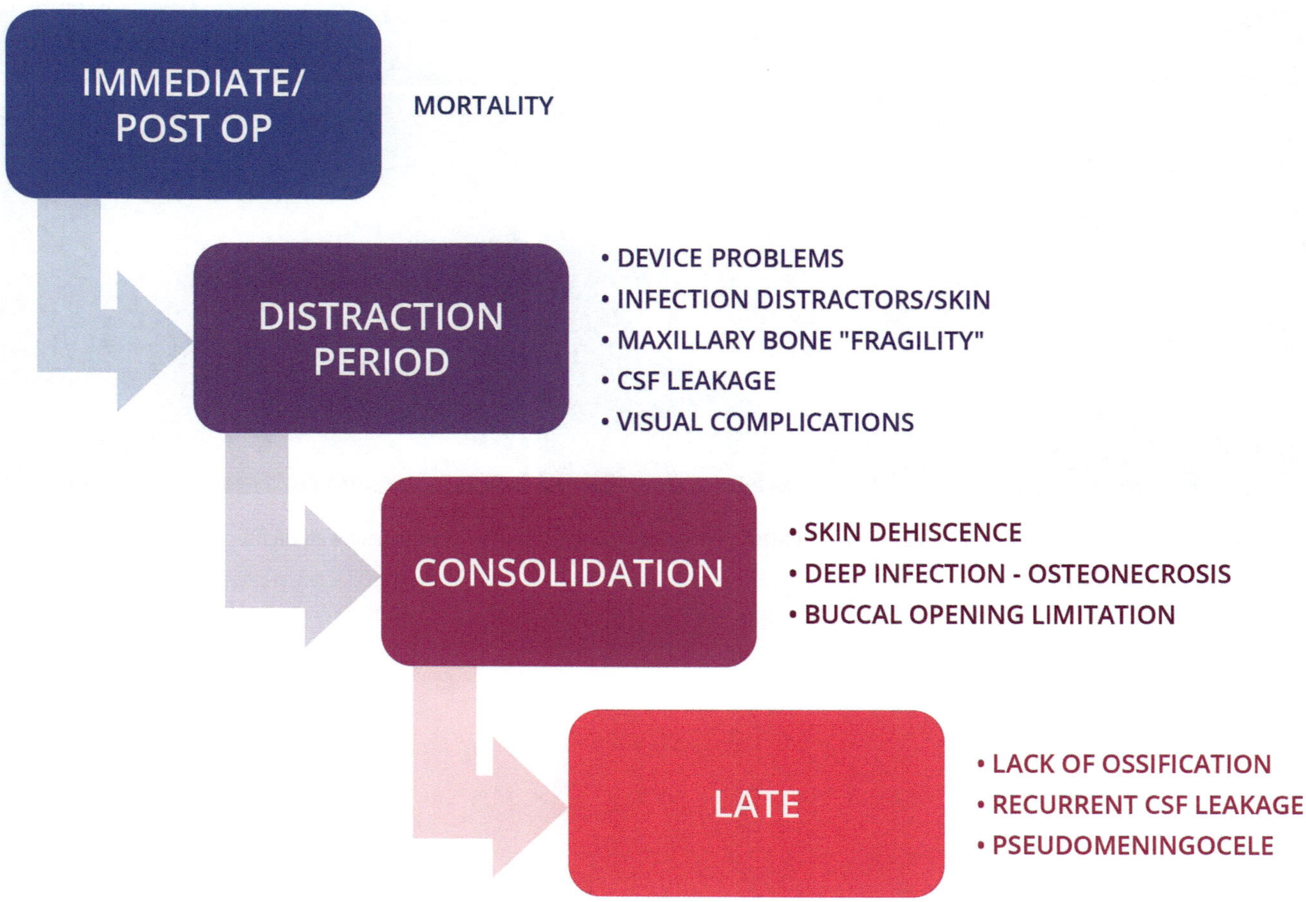

Fig. 9.3 Specific complications associated with each of the four postoperative periods: (1) immediate postoperative, (2) distraction, (3) consolidation, and (4) late follow-up

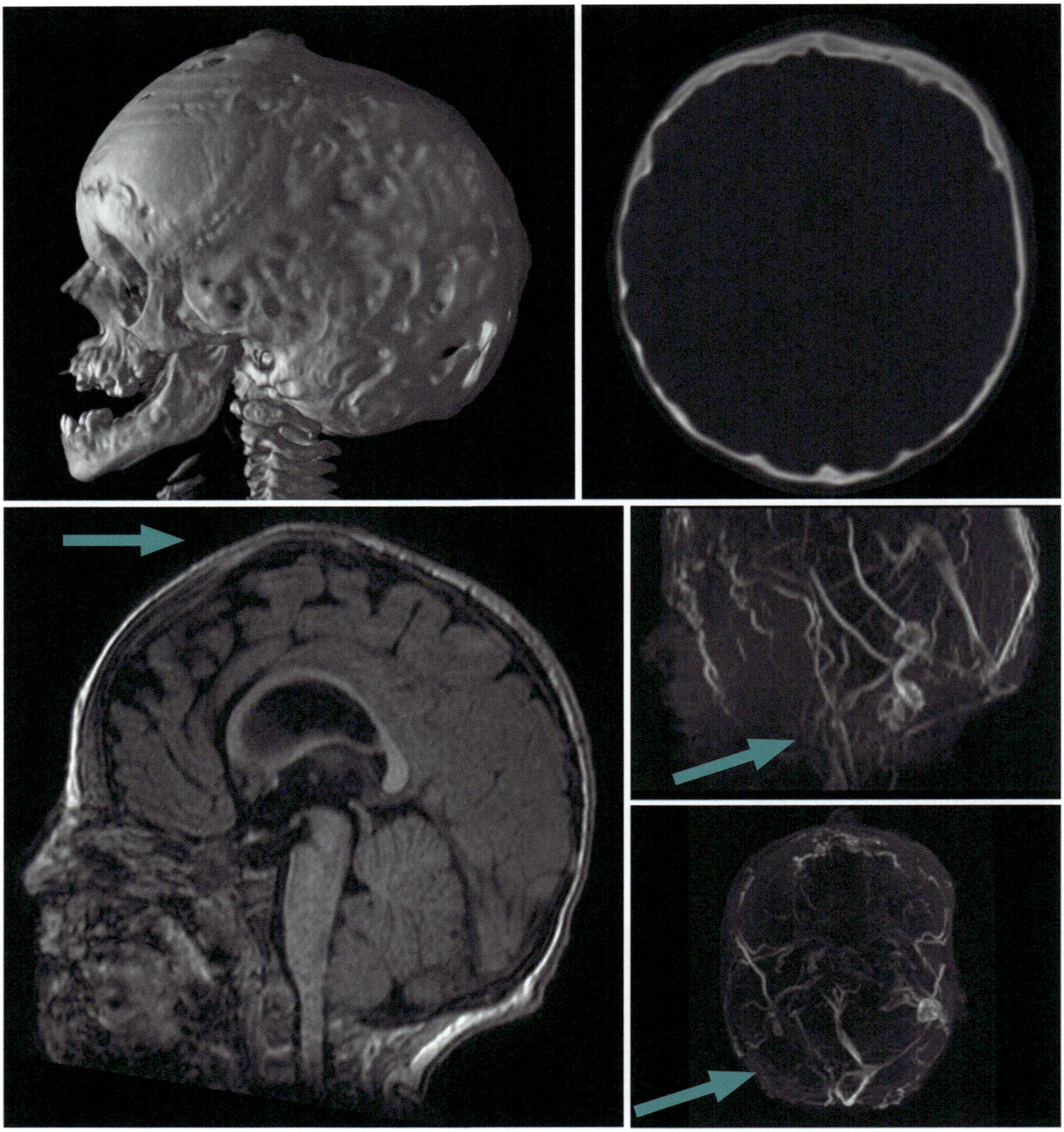

Fig. 9.4 Lethal venous thrombosis immediately after FFMBA performed at 18 months of age in a patient with Pfeiffer syndrome

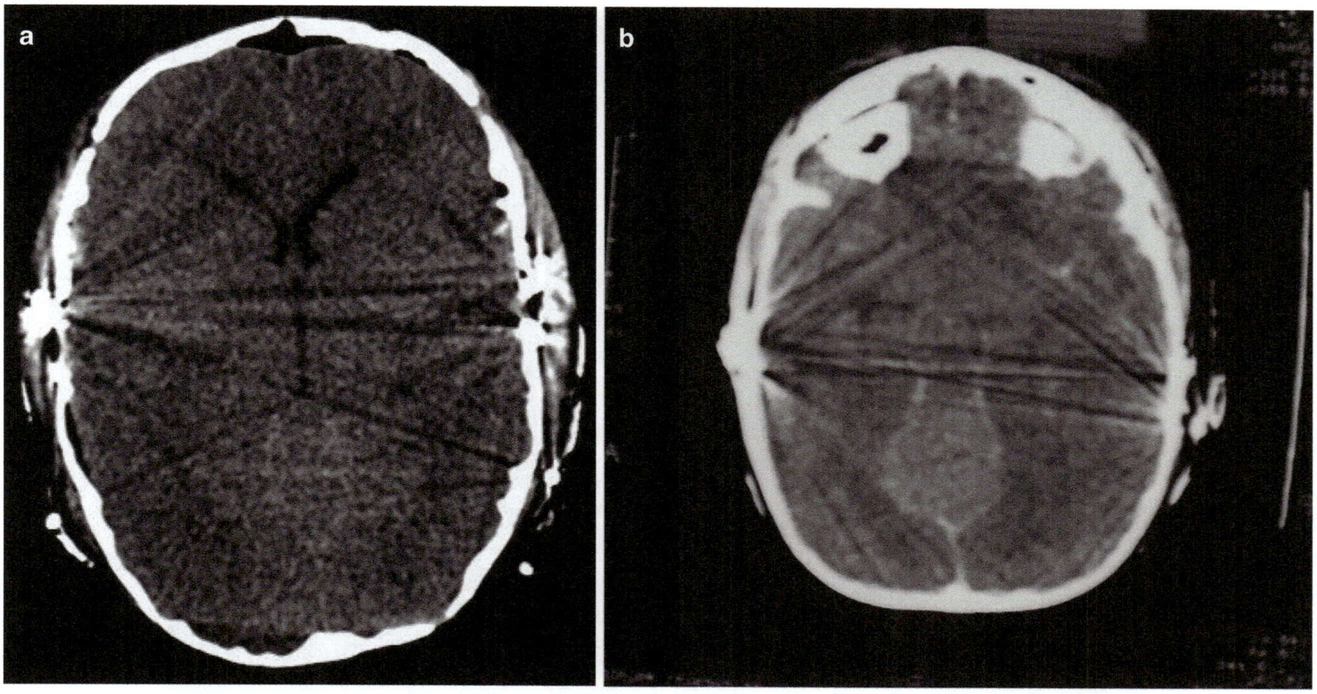

Fig. 9.5 Acute cerebral edema causing tonsillar herniation and death at day 1 after FFMBA in a 3-year-old patient with Crouzon syndrome

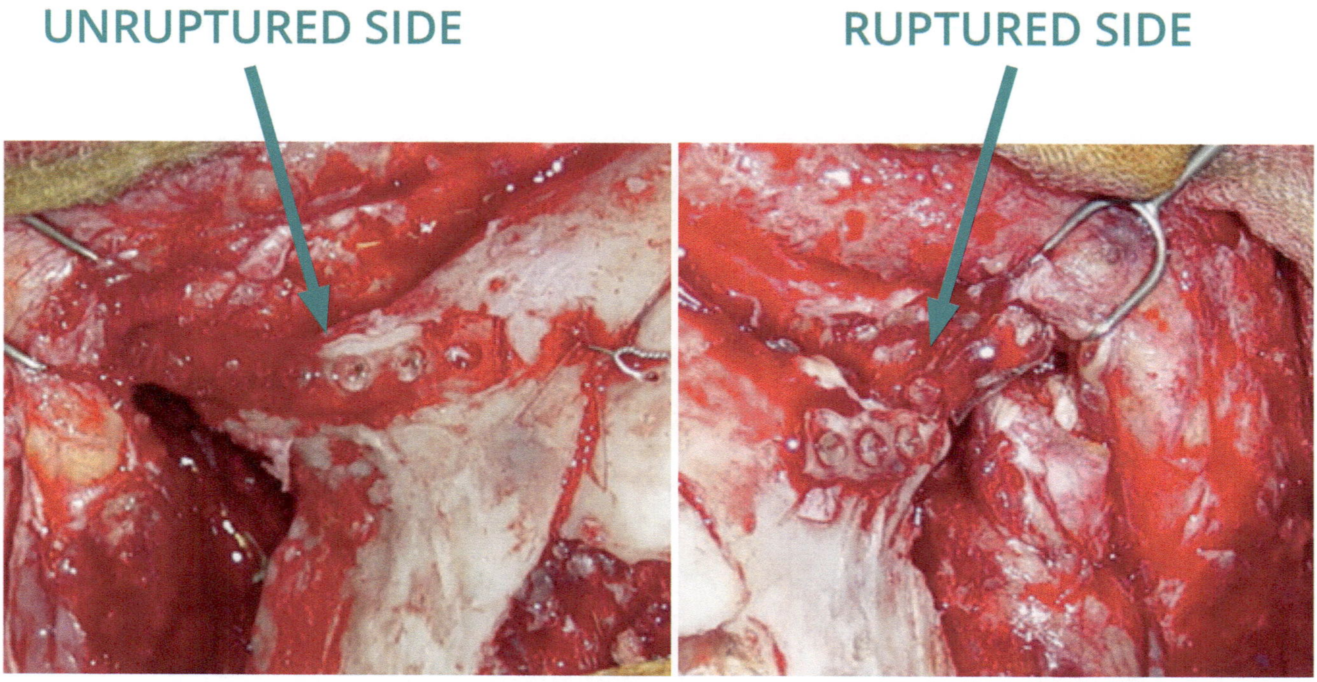

Fig. 9.6 Ruptured osteosynthesis plate at FZ junction in a 3-year-old patient with Crouzon syndrome

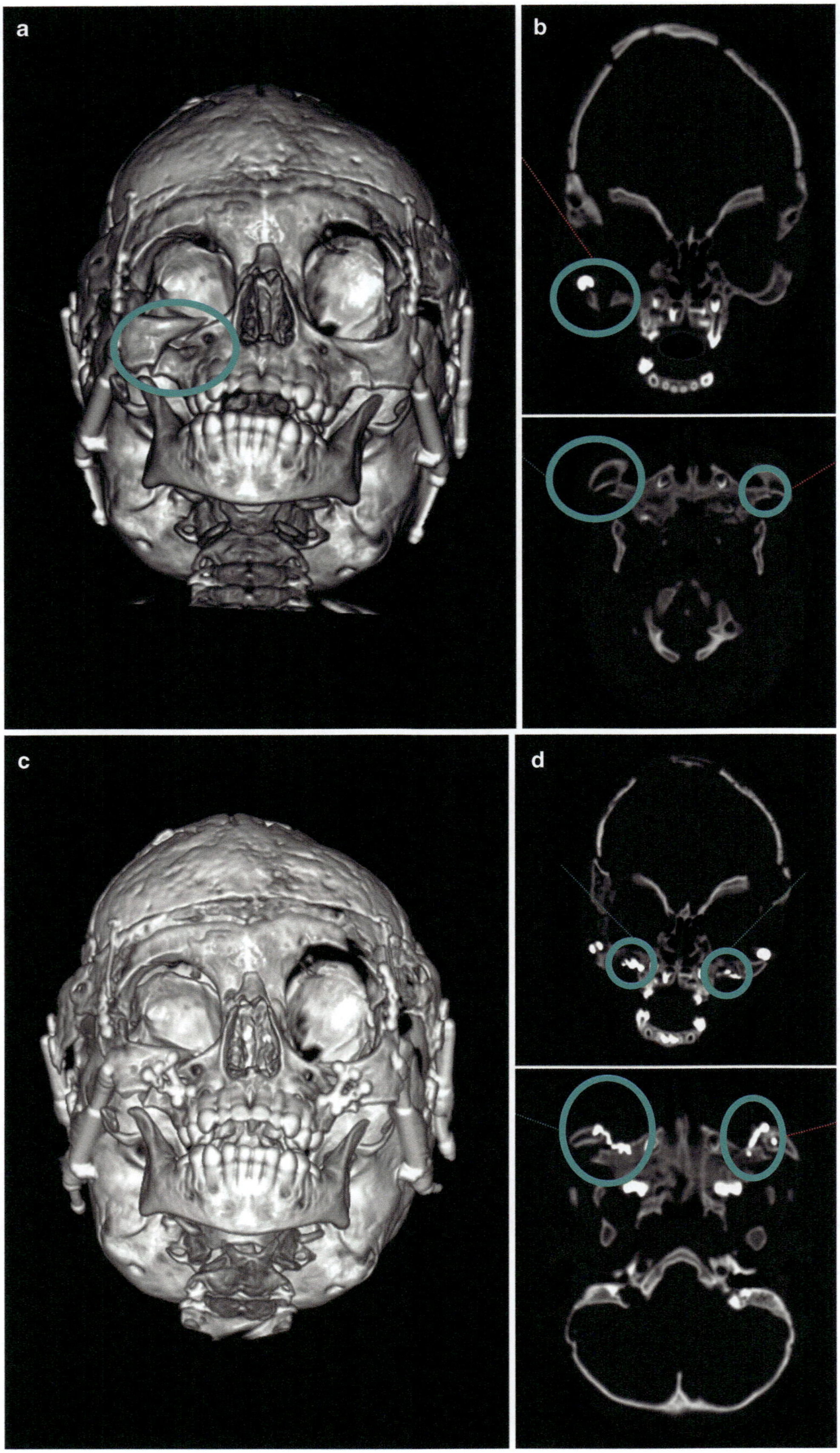

Fig. 9.7 (**a**, **b**) Secondary FFMBA performed at 2.5 years of age in a patient with Crouzon syndrome. Right maxillo-zygomatic disjunction on day 10 after surgery, during the distraction period. (**c**, **d**) Bilateral maxillo-zygomatic osteosynthesis using titanium plates and screws. (**e**) Ossification of the fracture sites 5 months after surgery

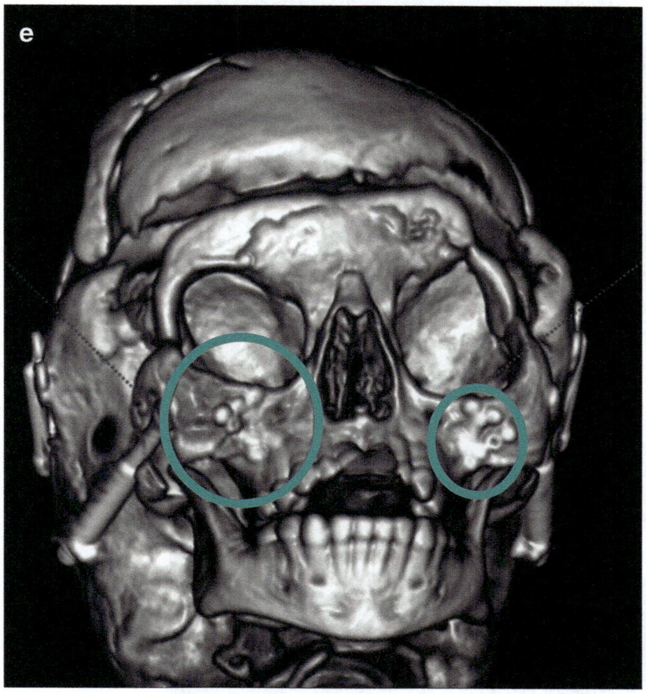

Fig. 9.7 (continued)

bar drainage. Finally, very rarely, we observed visual issues: transient loss of vision (3/149) in 2% of cases; transient diplopia (6/149) in 4%. All visual complications were resolved in 3 months.

In the consolidation period, 35% of patients, mostly younger ones, presented transient infection/dehiscence of the skin at the entry point of distractors (Fig. 9.9). This complication is benign and requires local care without the need for an early removal of the distractors. In fact, only 2% of patients required surgical drainage with at least partial bone loss due to osteitis. The presence of tracheostomy and previous surgery is most probably a risk factor for frontal bone loss: this complication was observed in 1/124 primary FFMBA cases (0.8%) vs 3/25 secondary FFMBA cases (12%). Furthermore, we believe that the introduction of bilateral pericranial flaps to obturate anterior fossa has highly reduced the rate of this complication.

FFMBA is followed by severe limitation in mouth opening. We have tackled this issue by establishing a standardized physiotherapy protocol starting in ICU, with passive maneuvers, followed by active exercises during the distraction period.

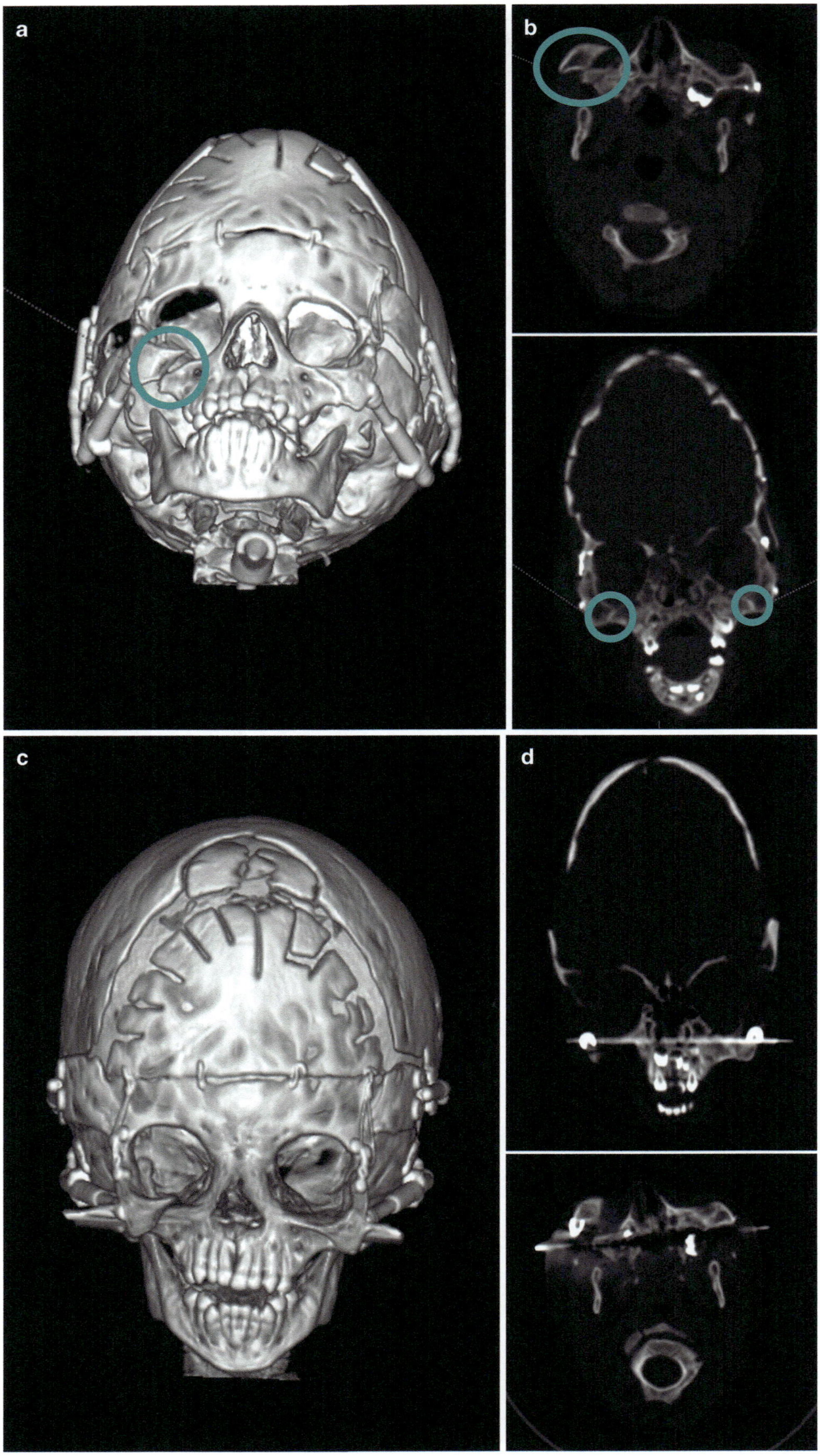

Fig. 9.8 (**a**, **b**) Primary FFMBA in a 2-year-old patient with Pfeiffer syndrome, tracheostomy, and a history of PVE. Right maxilla-zygomatic disjunction at day 12 of distraction. (**c**, **d**) Insertion of a transfacial pin. (**e**, **f**) Satisfactory ossification of the fracture site 18 months after surgery with mild asymmetry due to right midface retrusion

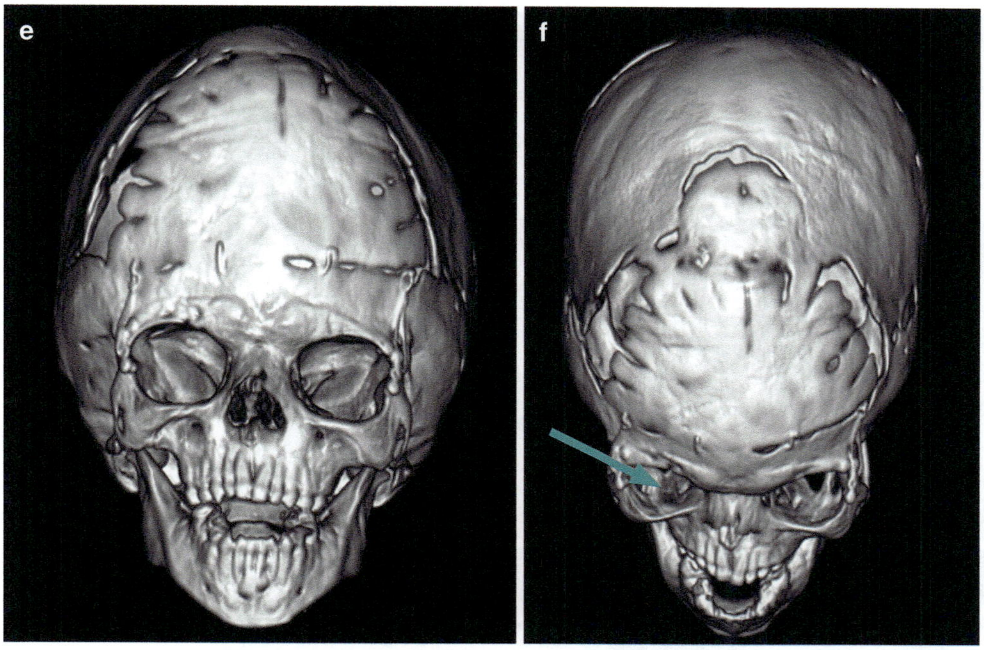

Fig. 9.8 (continued)

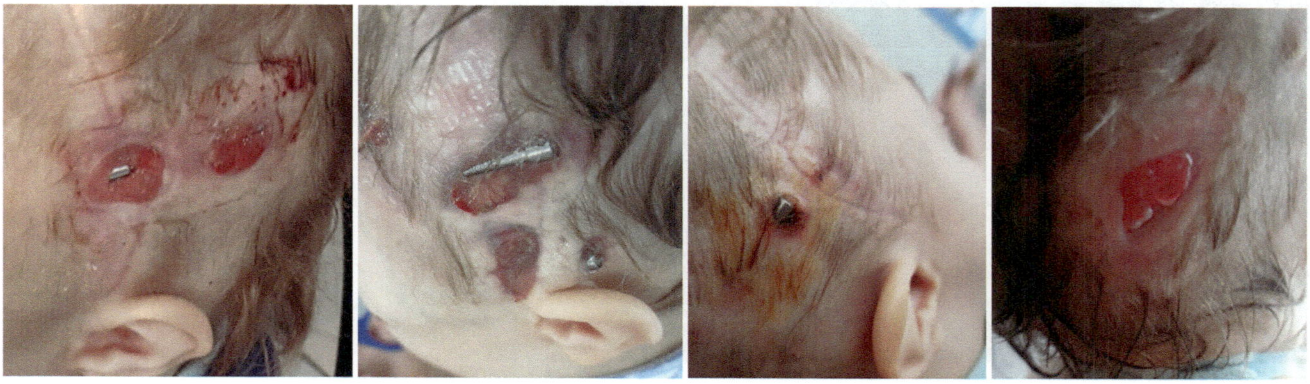

Fig. 9.9 Skin dehiscence at the entry points of the distractors during the consolidation period

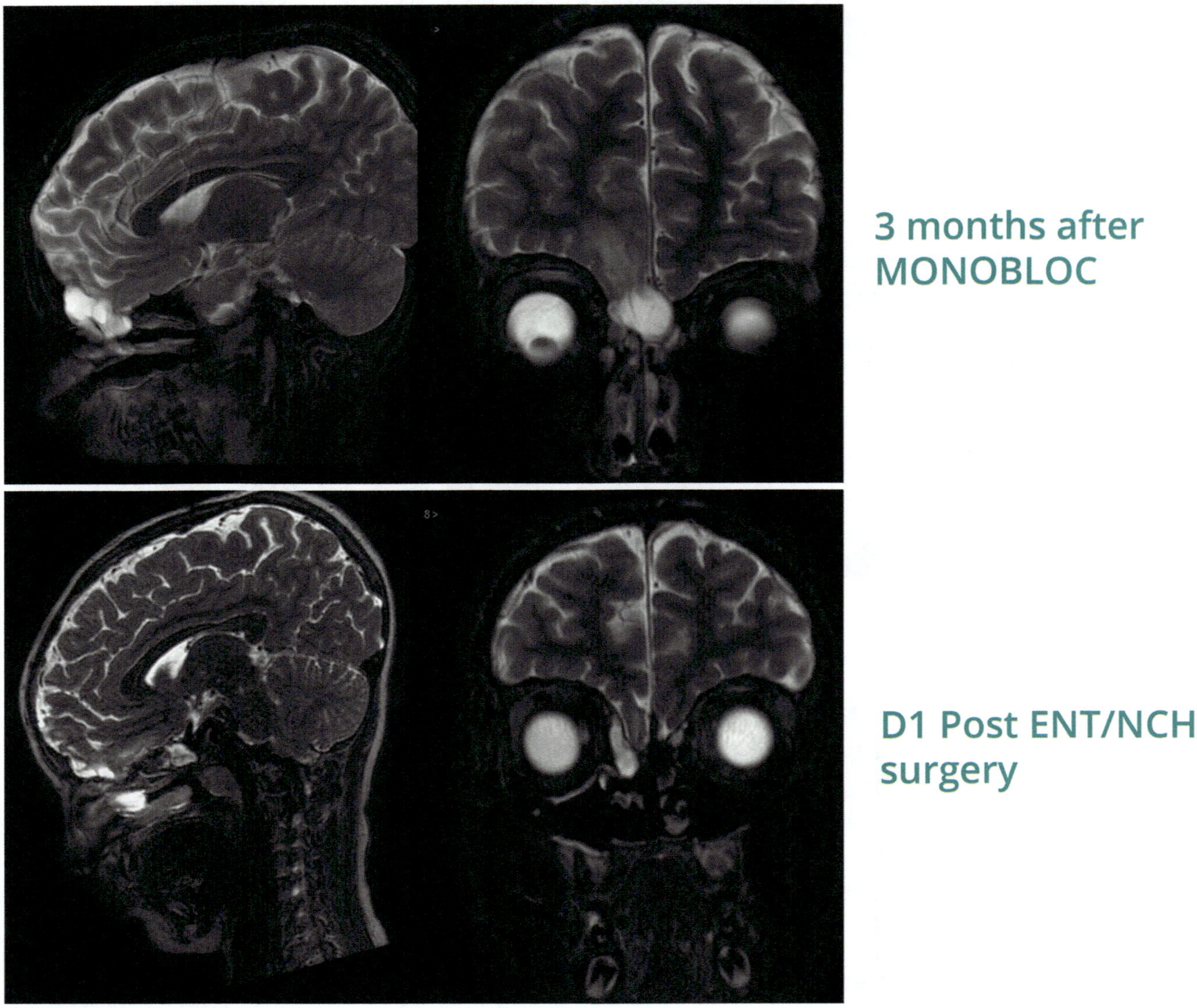

Fig. 9.10 Patient with Crouzon syndrome—FFMBA performed at 7 years of age. Pseudomeningocele on MRI 3 months after surgery, successfully treated by an endonasal skull base bone graft

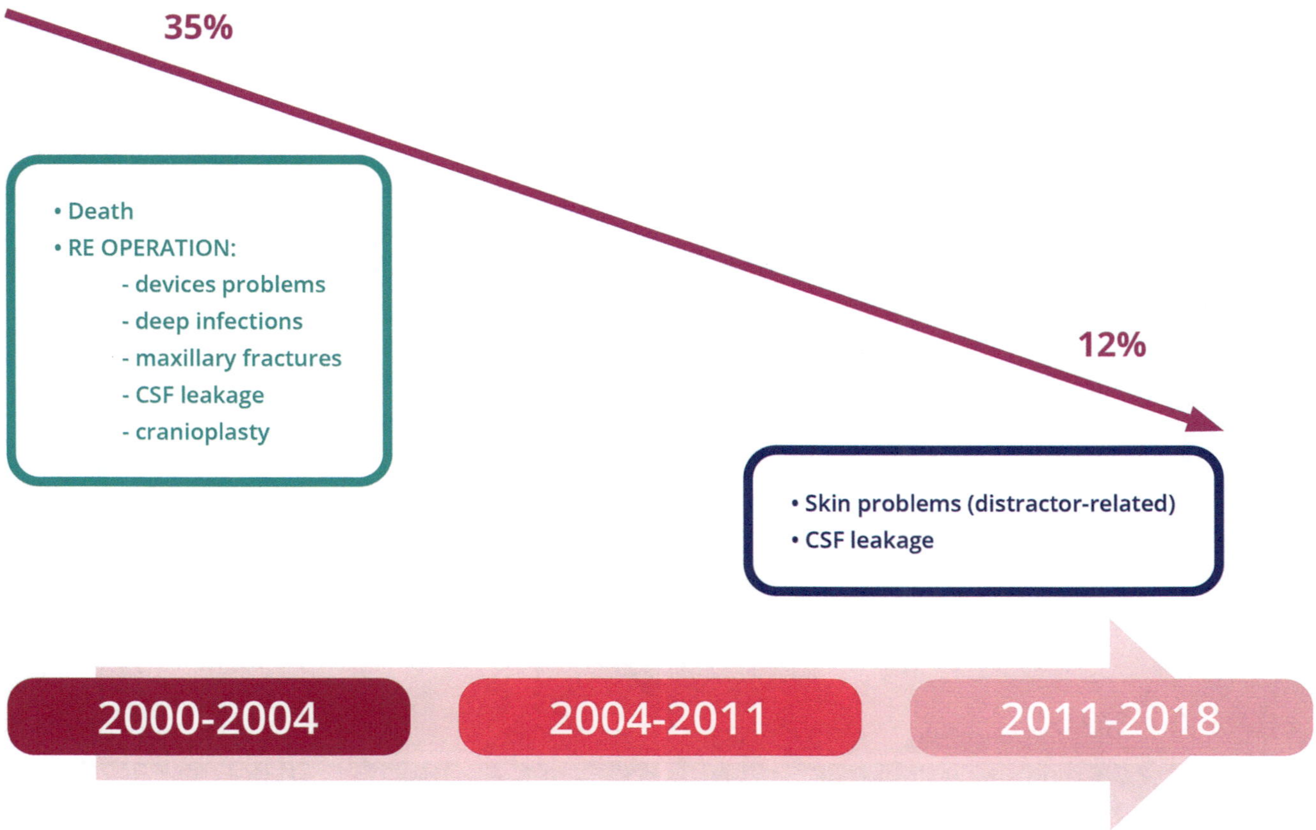

Fig. 9.11 Decrease of complication rates and complication severity with time and gain of experience of the craniofacial team

In the late follow-up period, 17% of patients presented with a lack of coronal ossification and a persisting gap (25/149) (Figs. 9.12, 9.14, and 9.15).

In less than 2%, a persisting CSF leakage or pseudomeningocele has been described and successfully treated by endonasal/endoscopic procedures (Fig. 9.10).

Asymmetric facial advancement was observed in 2% of cases (Fig. 9.13). Lacrymal duct obstruction was observed in 2% of cases (Fig. 9.16).

In conclusion, in our experience a learning curve can be identified, with a progressive reduction of the rate and the severity of complications. The safety of monobloc clearly increases with experience and older age at operation (Figs. 9.11, 9.12, 9.13, 9.14, 9.15, and 9.16).

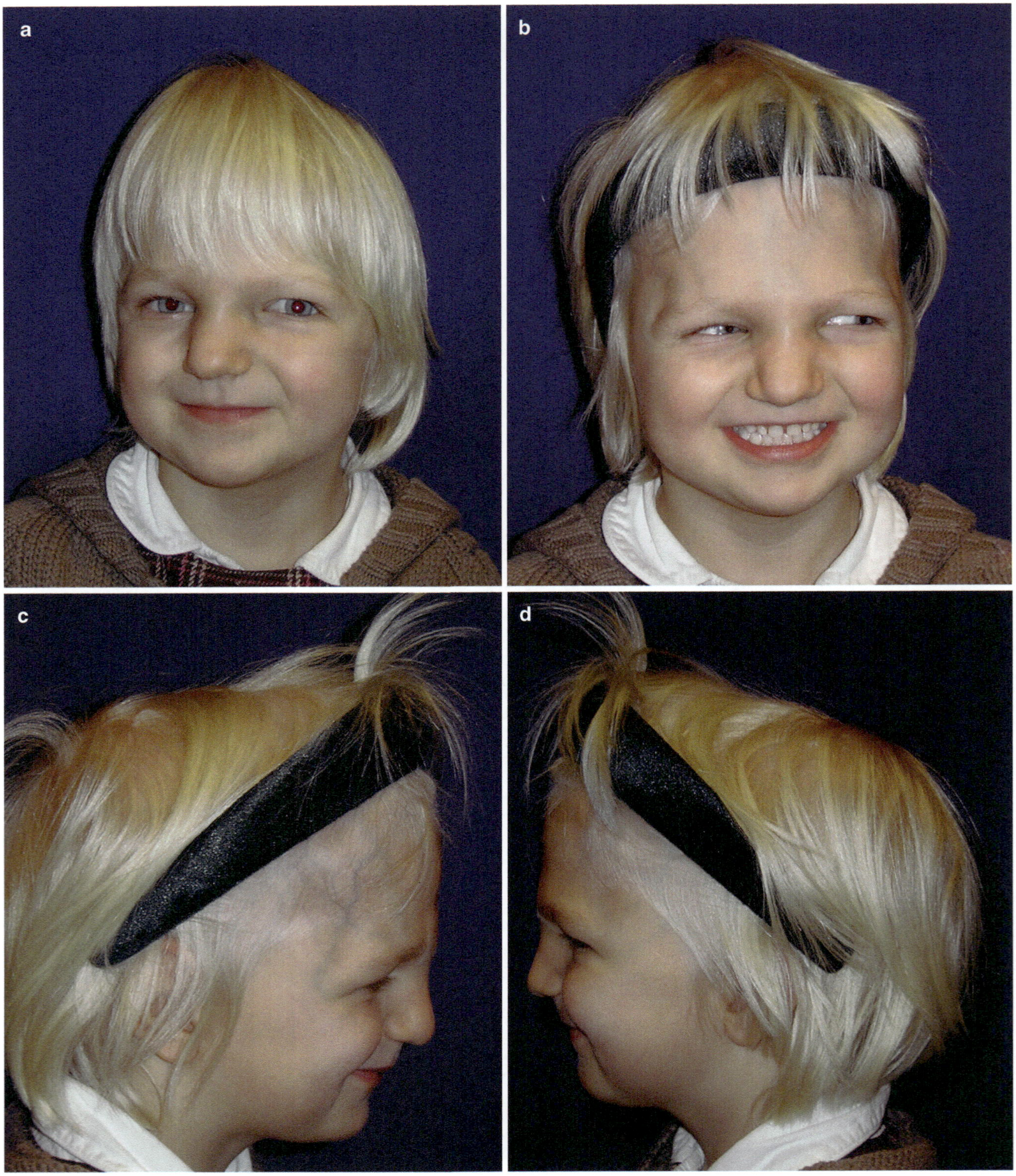

Fig. 9.12 (**a-d**) Patient with Crouzon syndrome aged 3 years, 18 months after FFMBA, presenting with large bony defects of the skull vault corresponding to the gaps in the coronal region which did not re-ossify. (**e**, **f**, **g**) CT scan at 3 years of age showing the large bony defects requiring reconstruction. (**h**) Intraoperative view of the defect zones. (**i**, **j**) Reconstruction of the defects using bone cement (polymethyl methacrylate) as a temporary reconstruction. (**k, l**) Postoperative result after reconstruction at 8 years of age. (**m**) LF3 osteotomy after vault reconstruction at 12 years of age. (**n**, **o**) Position of the internal distractors and the rigid external device relative to the reconstructed zones of the vault. (**p**, **q**) Clinical results at 14 years of age, 2 years after the LF3. (**r**, **s**) CT scan results of the LF3, 24 months after the procedure, at 14 years of age. (**t**) Definitive reconstruction of the vault defects using custom-made PEEK implants. (**u**, **v**) Clinical result at 16 years of age before rhinoplasty and temporal fat grafting

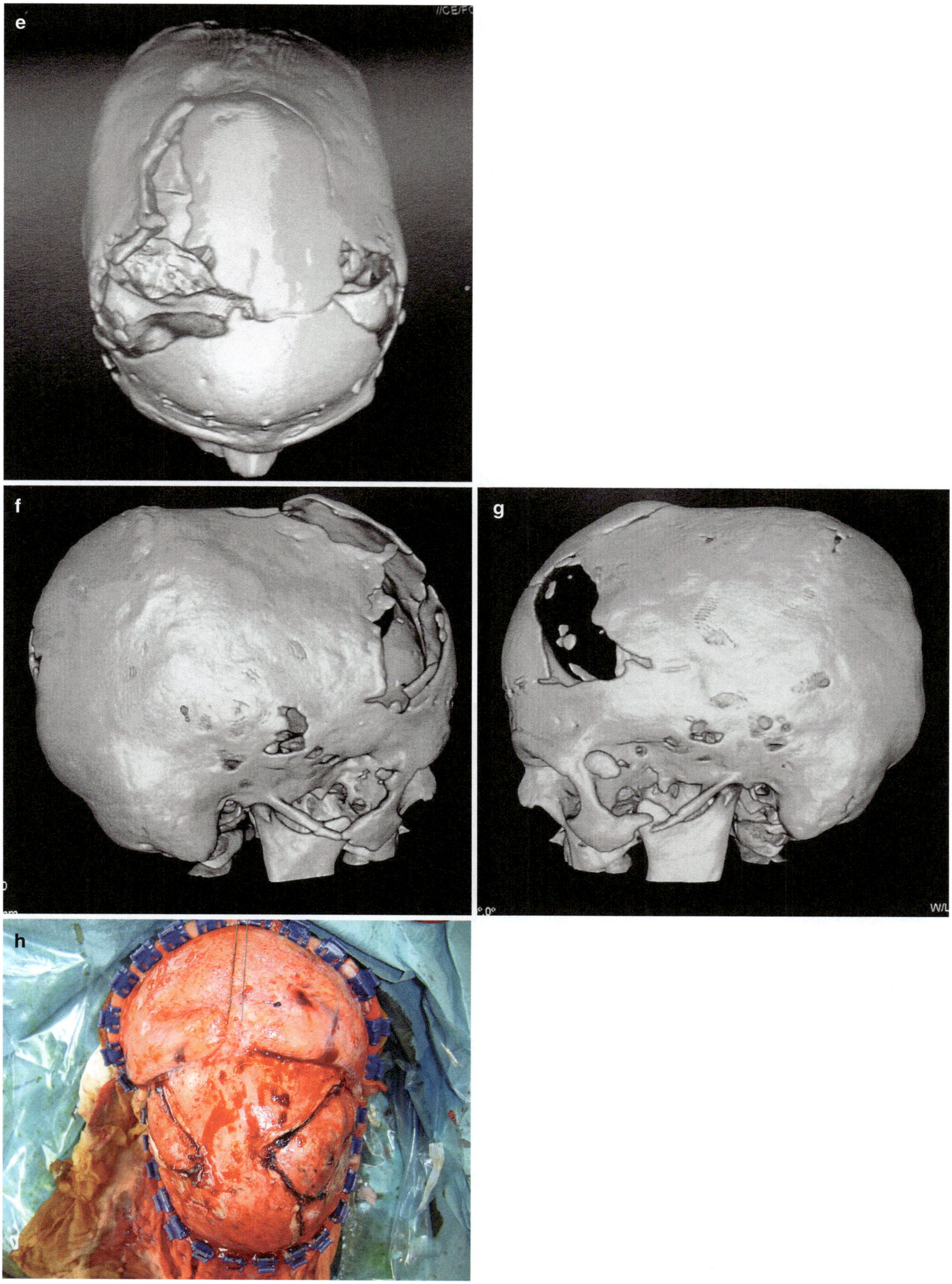

Fig. 9.12 (continued)

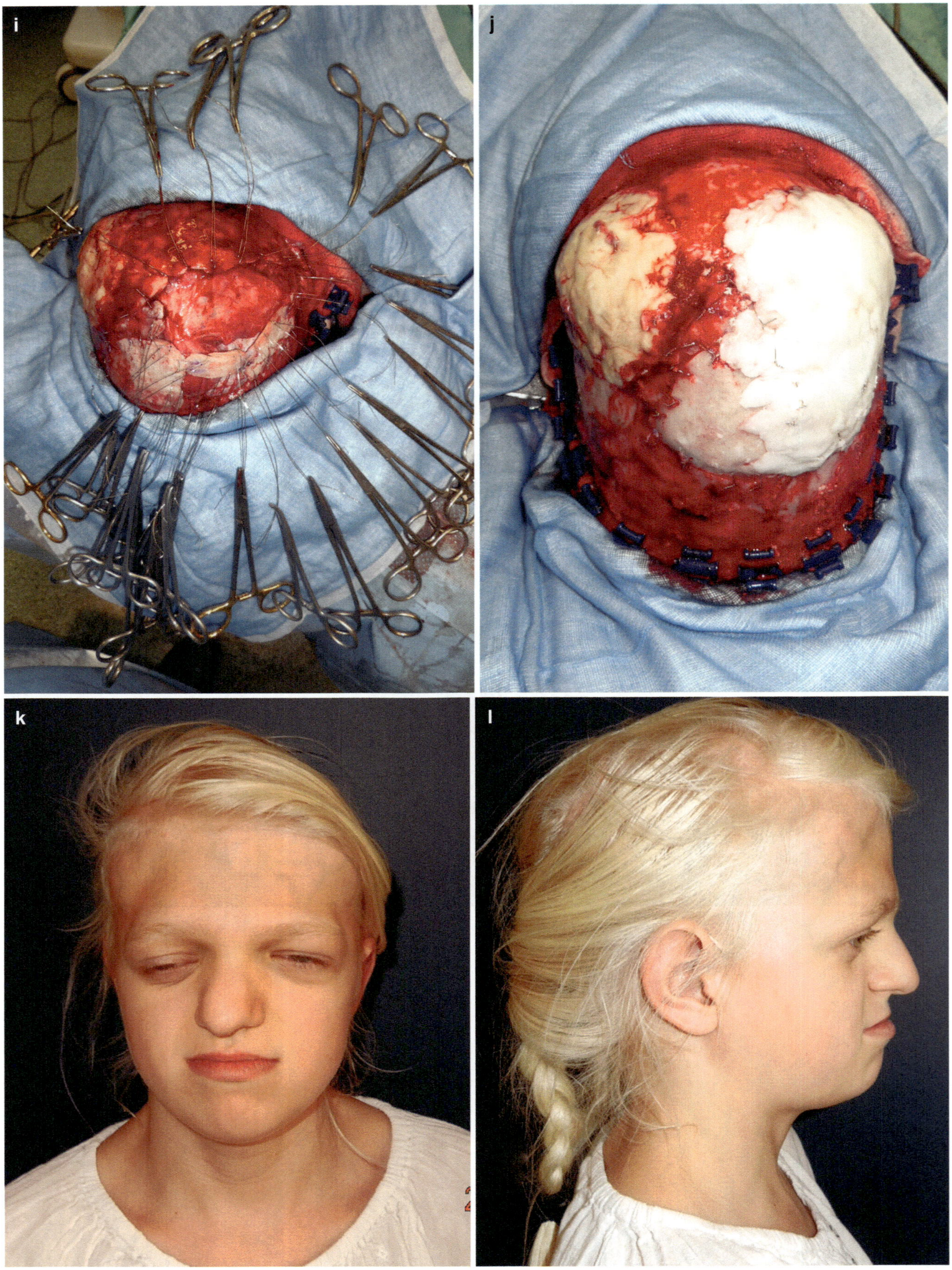

Fig. 9.12 (continued)

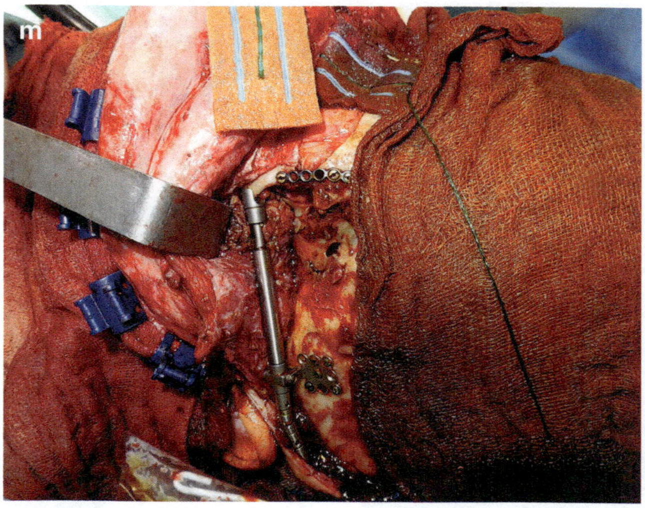

Fig. 9.12 (continued)

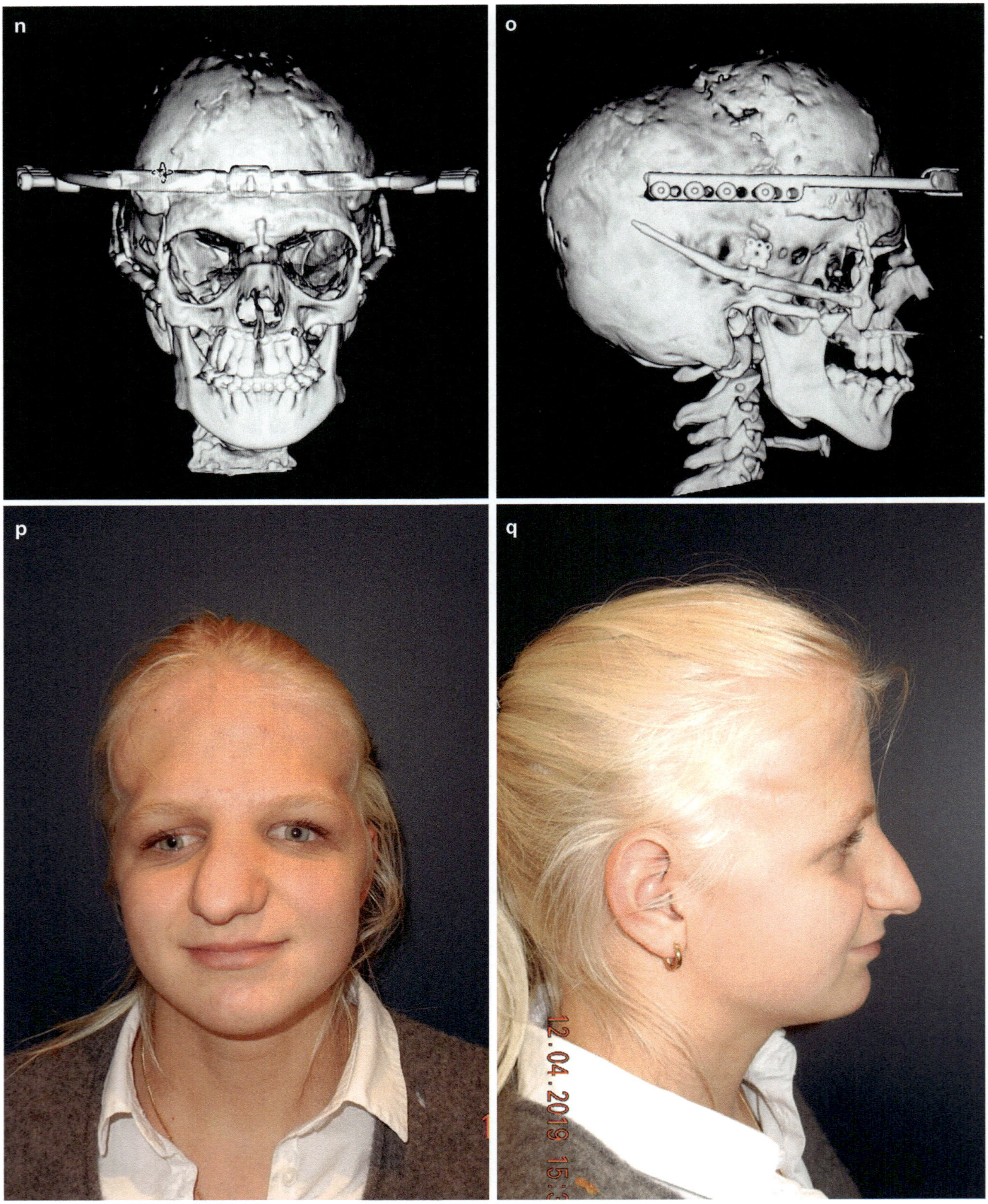

Fig. 9.12 (continued)

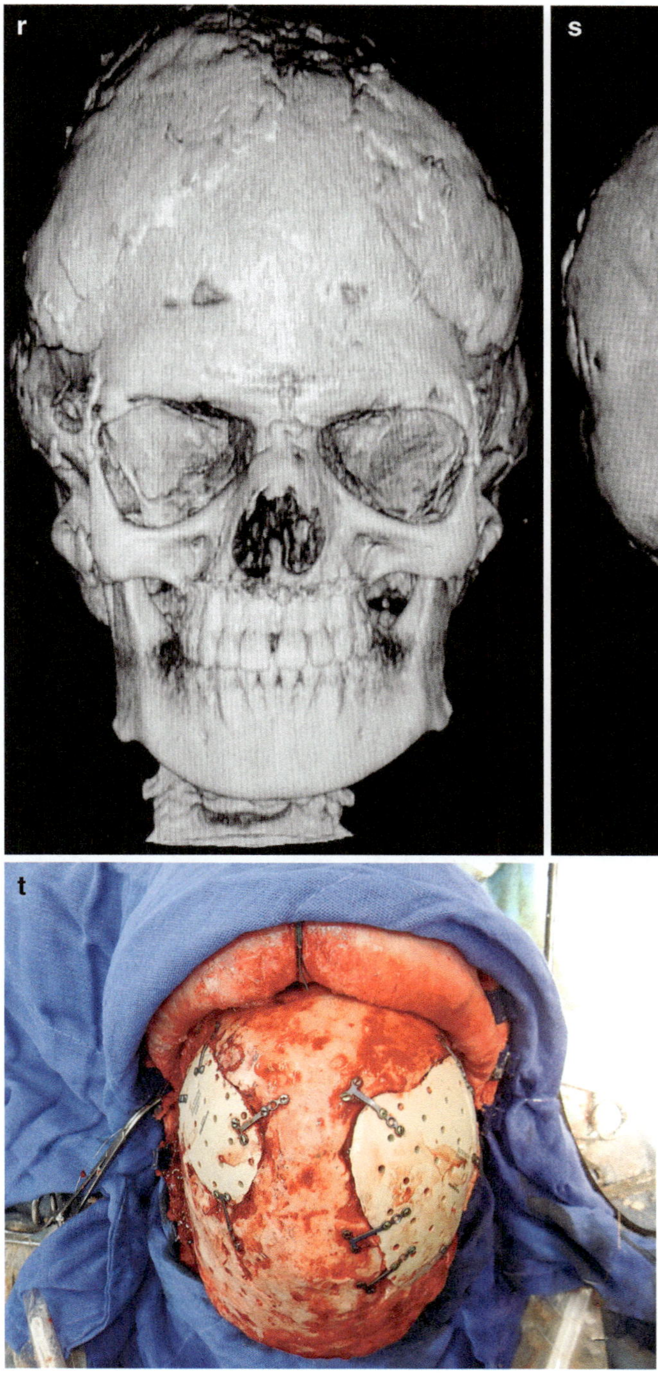

Fig. 9.12 (continued)

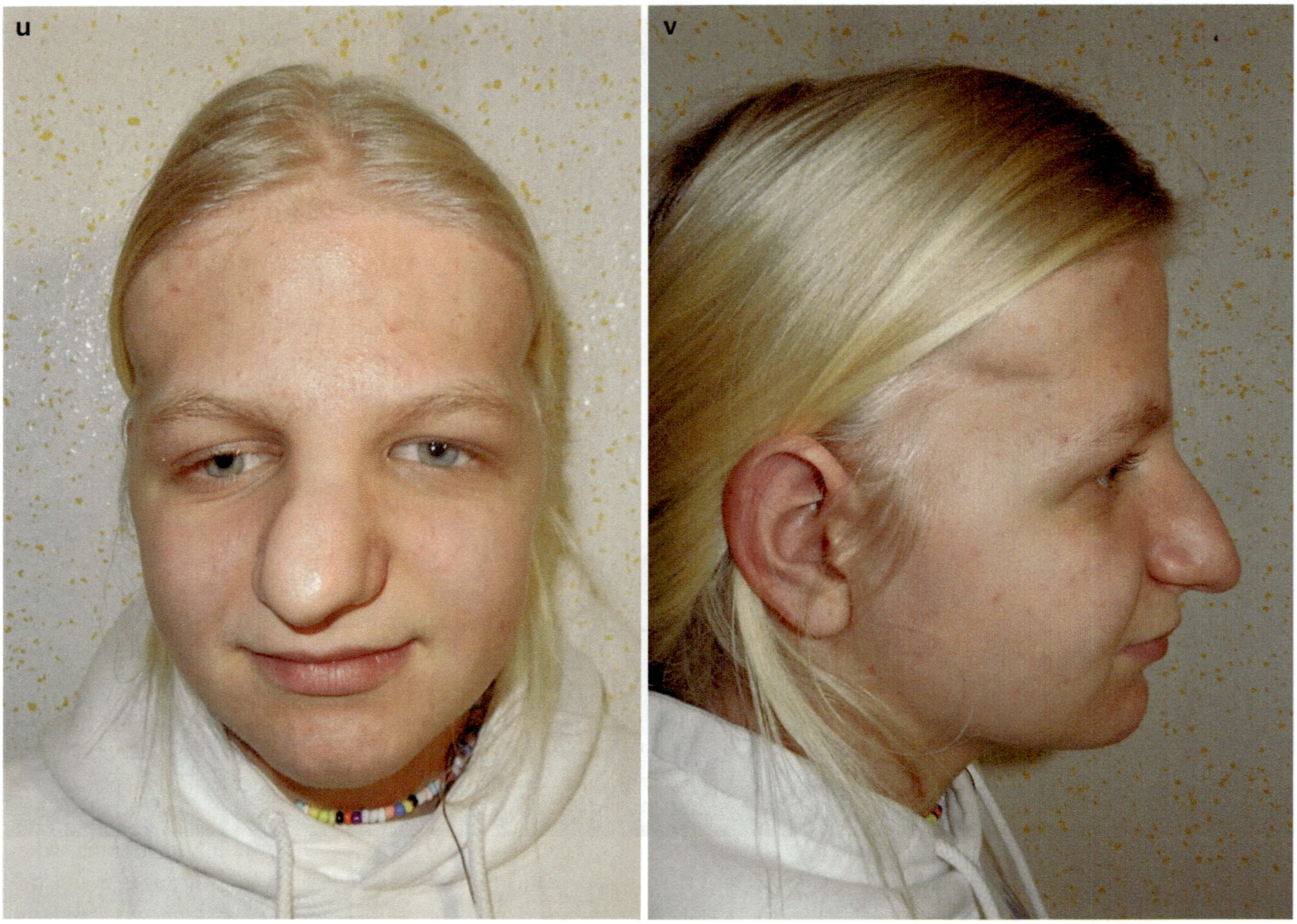

Fig. 9.12 (continued)

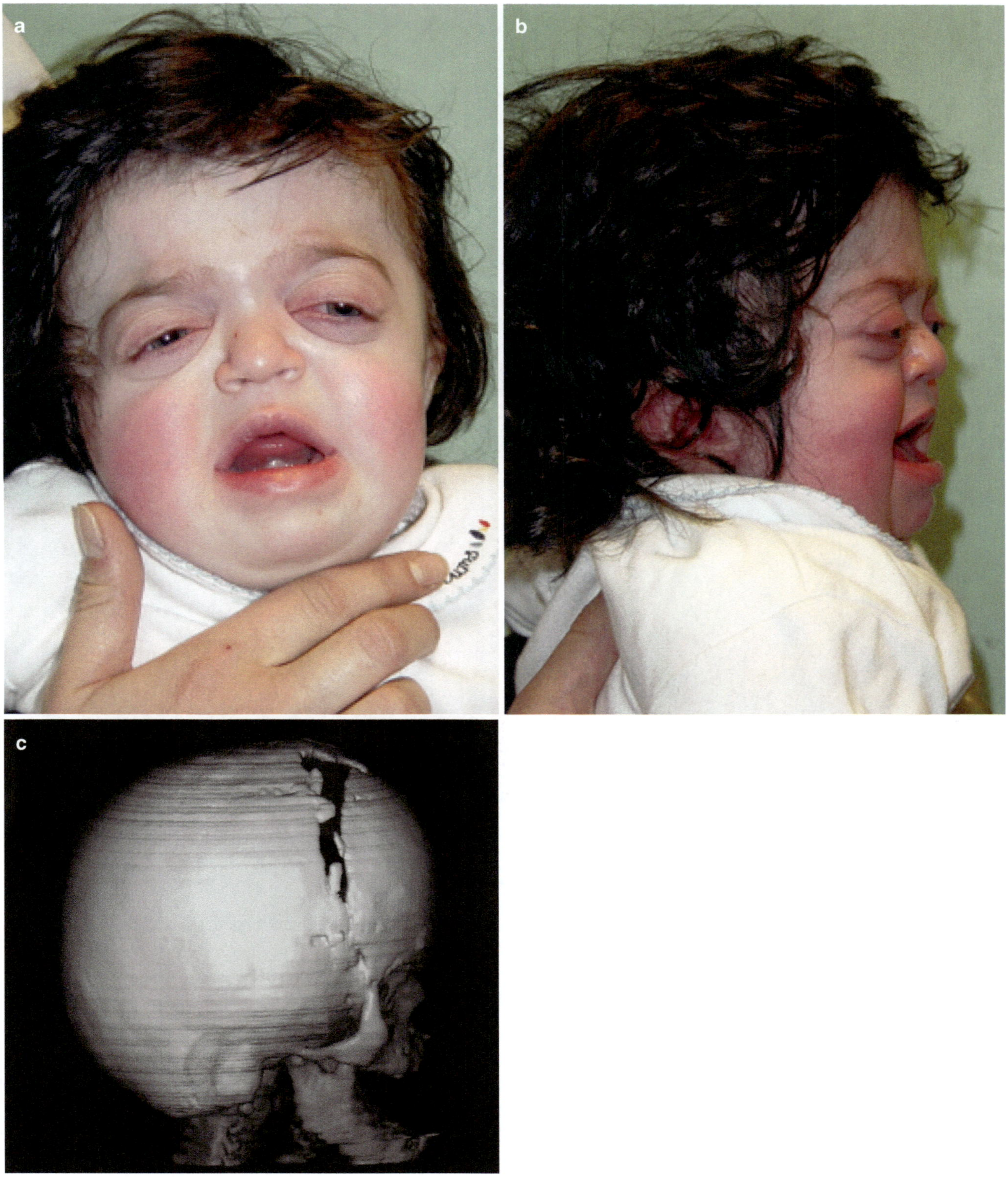

Fig. 9.13 (**a**, **b**) Patient with Pfeiffer syndrome aged 10 months after unsuccessful FOA (**c**) CT scan after FOA and before early FFMBA (**d**, **e**, **f**) Intraoperative view of FFMBA performed at 2 years of age. A transfacial pin was inserted to stabilize the 2 hemifaces (**g**) Clinical aspect at 3 months after FFMBA. Despite transfacial pin, asymmetric advancement provoked left enophthalmos. (**h**) early removal of osteosynthesis material and attempt of symmetrization. (**i**, **j**) Clinical aspect at 3 years of age, 1 year after FFMBA, showing residual asymmetry, as well as insufficient facial advancement (**k**) CT scan aspect of early Le Fort 3, at 3 years of age to improve breathing and resolve OSAS. (**l**) Clinical aspect at 4 years of age, 1 year after early Le Fort 3. (**m**, **n**) Clinical aspect at 5 years of age, 2 years after LF3. (**o**) Clinical aspect at 16 years of age after secondary LF3 and before correction of left zygomatic asymmetry. (**p**) Preoperative 3D reconstruction in rapid prototype. (**q**, **r**) Postoperative clinical result at 17 years of age after maxillary osteotomy

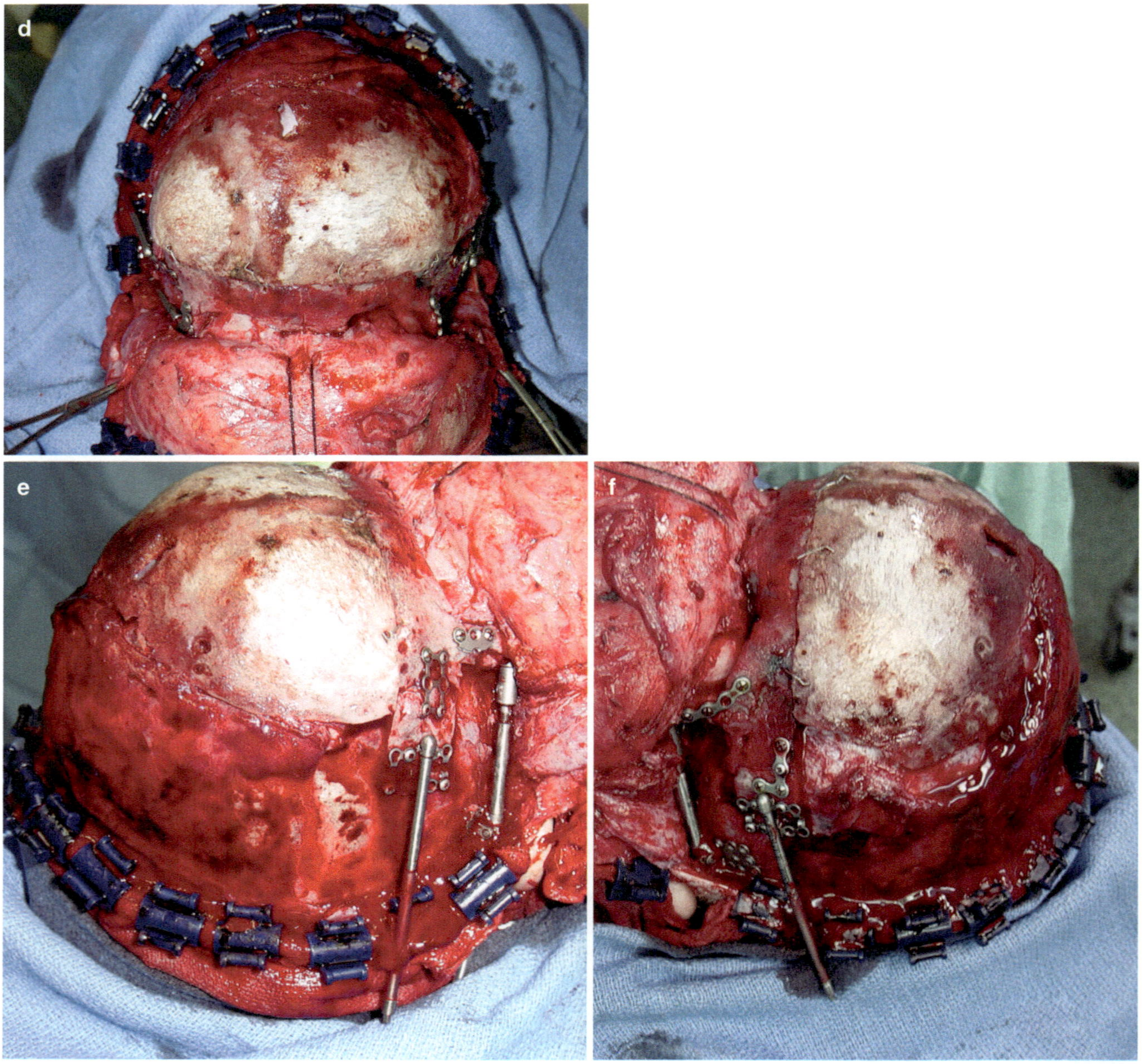

Fig. 9.13 (continued)

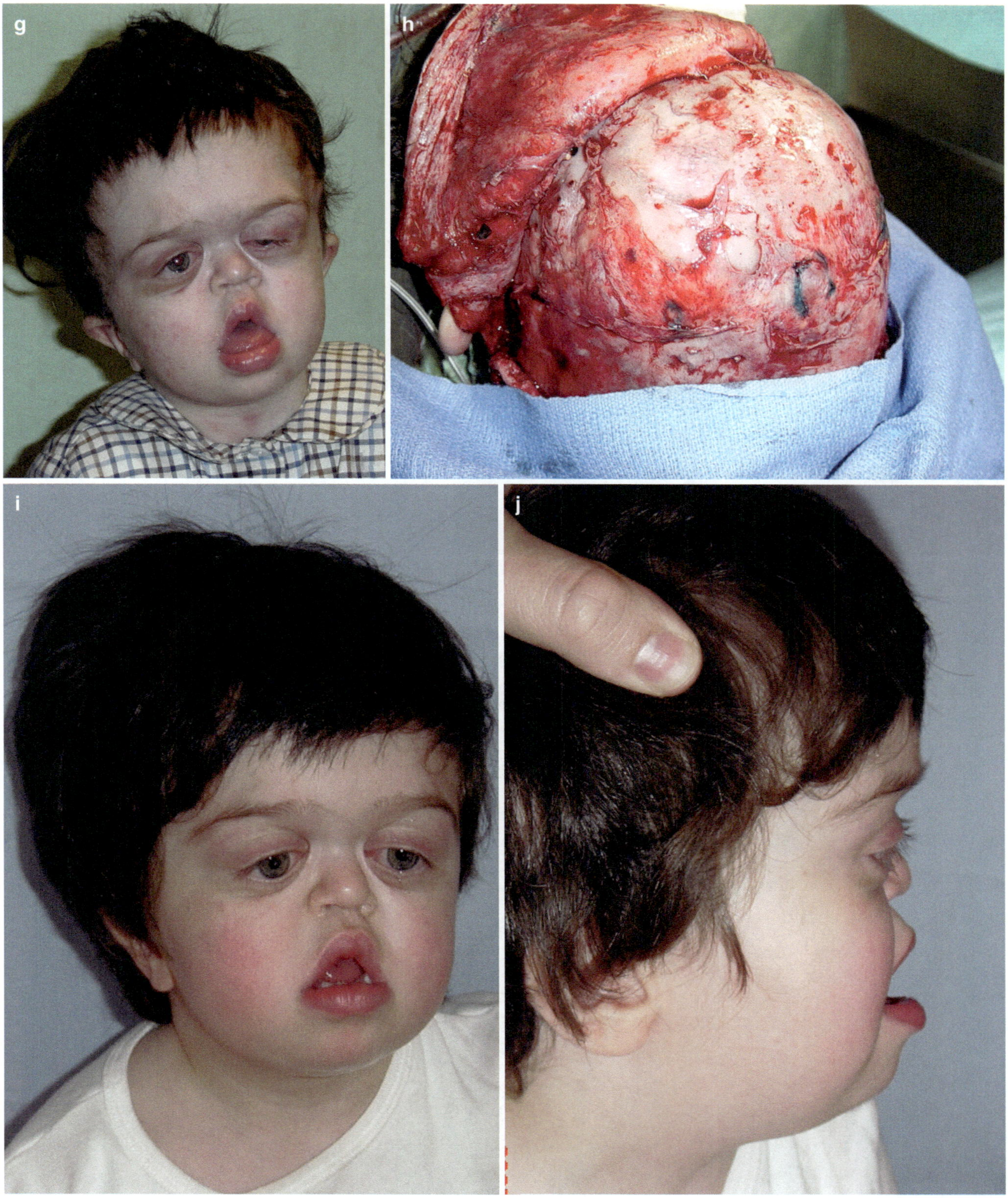

Fig. 9.13 (continued)

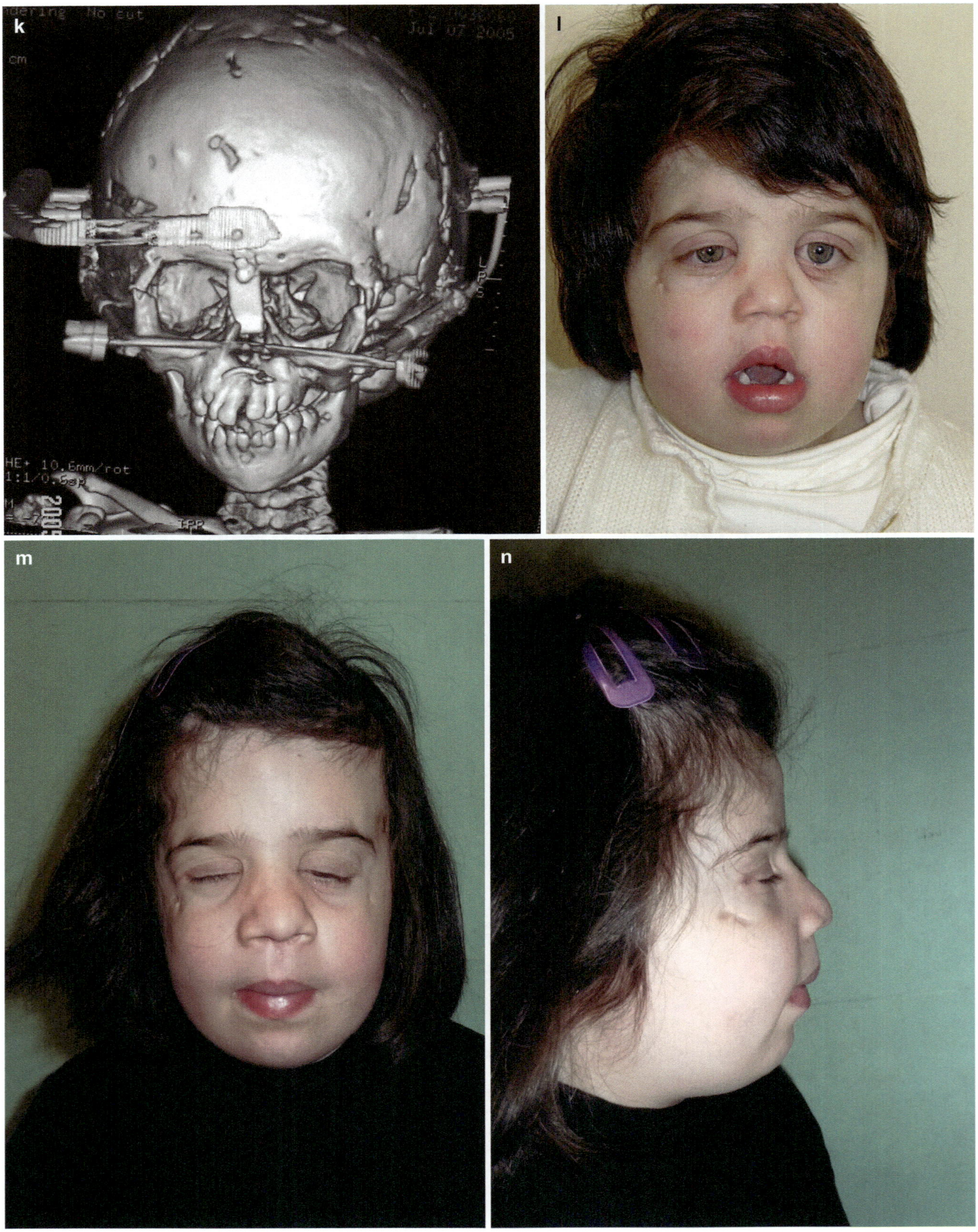

Fig. 9.13 (continued)

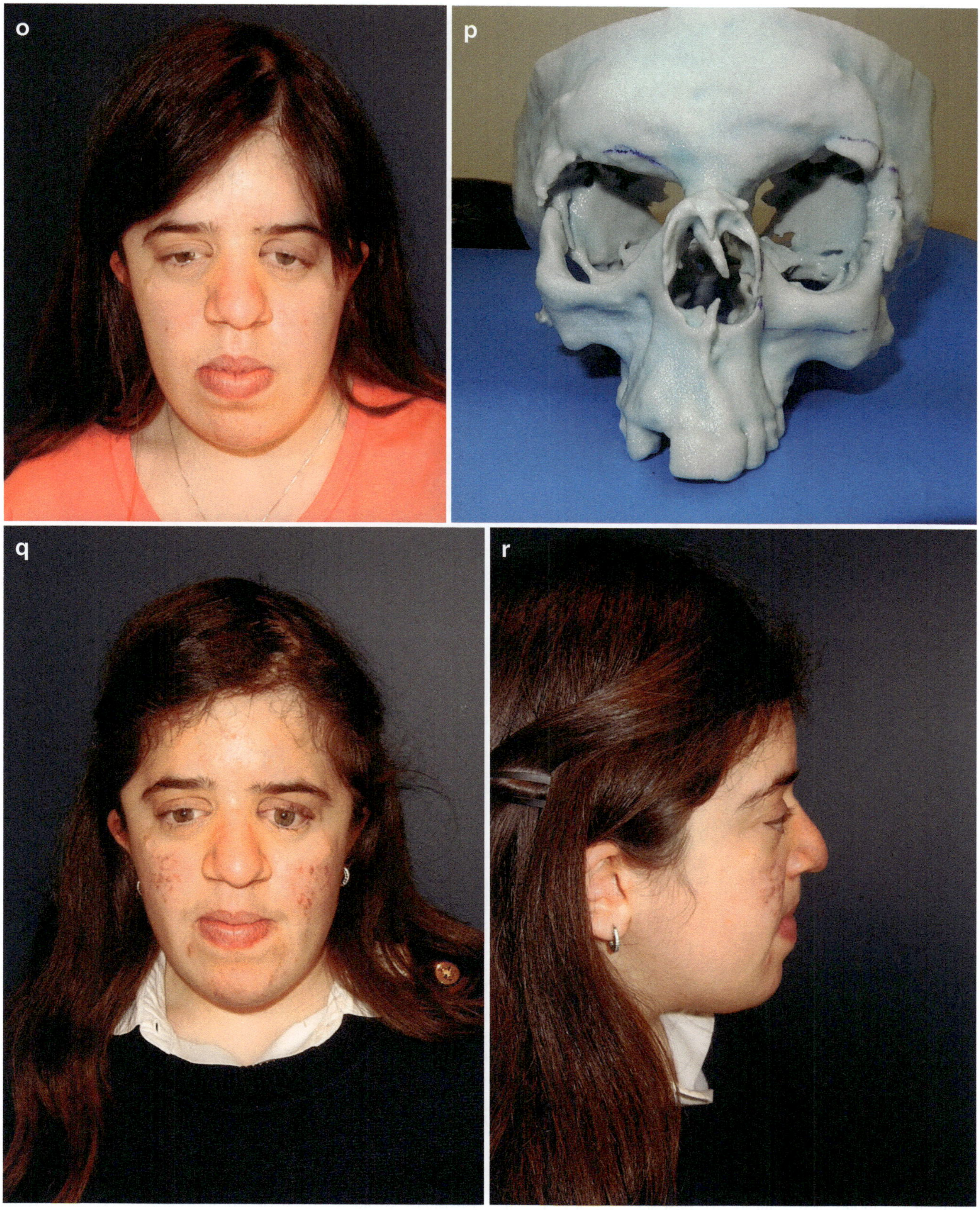

Fig. 9.13 (continued)

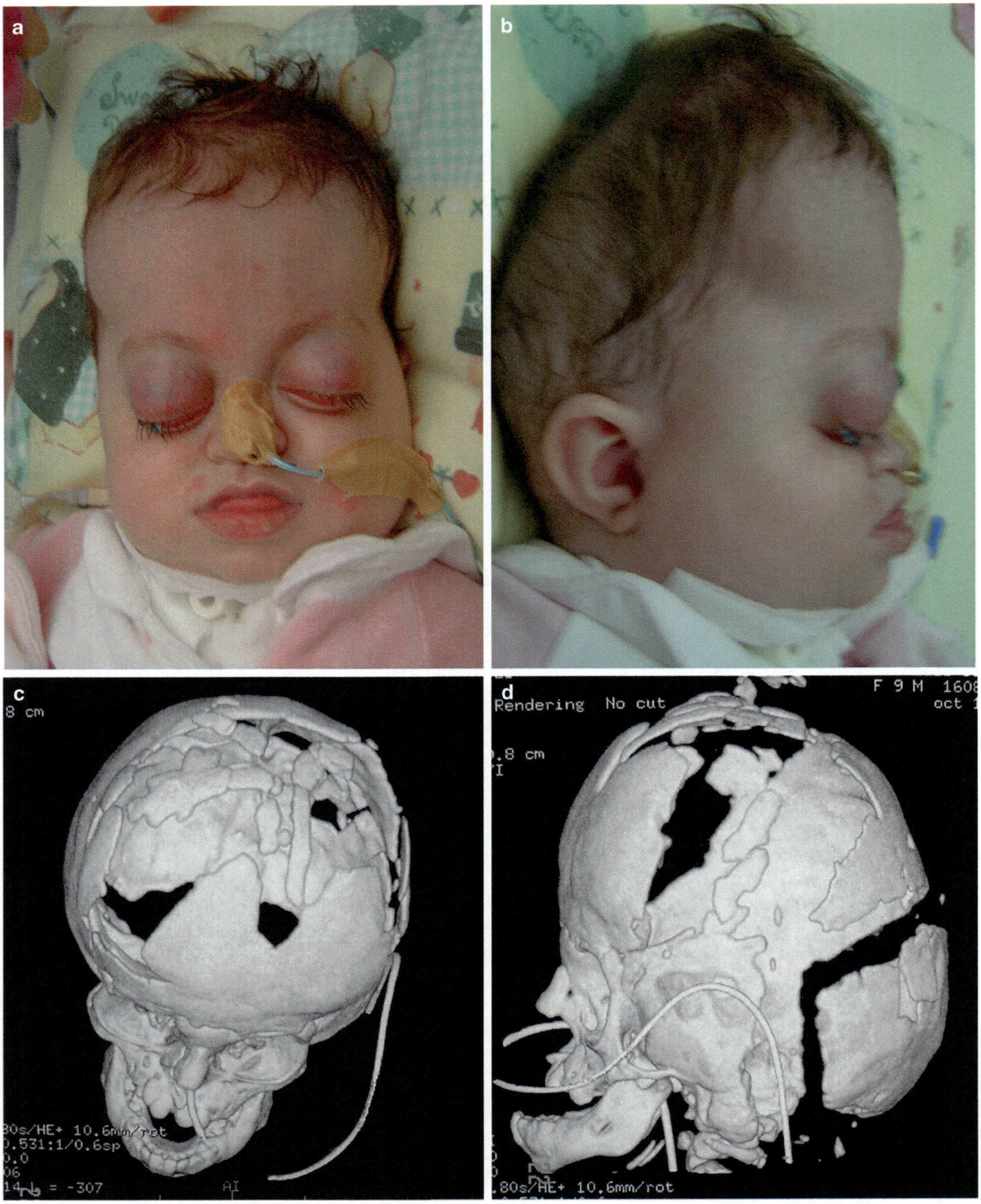

Fig. 9.14 (**a**, **b**): Severe patient with Pfeiffer syndrome aged 9 months already treated elsewhere of a fronto-calvarial remodeling. Severe exorbitism, tracheostomy, and shunt. (**c**, **d**): First stage was a PVE with brain-mediated expansion and retrieval of the shunt. (**e**) Immediate postoperative aspect after 2 weeks. Please observe the re-expansion (**f**, **g**): 3 months after PVE, before modified Bibloc (**h**) (**i**) (**j**) (**k**): Intraoperative view of Bibloc, necessitating reconstruction of bandeau at age 12 months. Transfacial pin is mandatory with external traction. (**l**, **m**): Postoperative aspect at age 14 months, 2 months after monobloc—Exorbitism correction is obtained (**n**, **o**): Postoperative aspect at 18 months, 6 months after Bibloc at time of removal of distractors (**p**) (**q**) (**r**) (**s**): First attempt of transient polymethylmethacrylate cranioplasties on multiple scarred scalp. (**t**, **u**) Clinical result at 4 years: tracheostomy cannot be removed. (**v**, **w**) Clinical aspect at 6 years: tracheostomy cannot be removed (**x**, **y**) Clinical aspect at 8 years: tracheostomy cannot be removed (**z**) Multiple scarred scalp before final cranioplasty necessitating staged autonomization procedures (delay phenomenon). (**a'**) After last delay staged procedure, recovery of partial ischemia confirms the need for previous autonomization. (**b'**, **c'**) Removal of transient cranioplasty and insertion of a custom-made PEEK implant (KLS Martin) (**d'**, **e'**): Final clinical aspect at 12 years. Tracheostomy was not removed

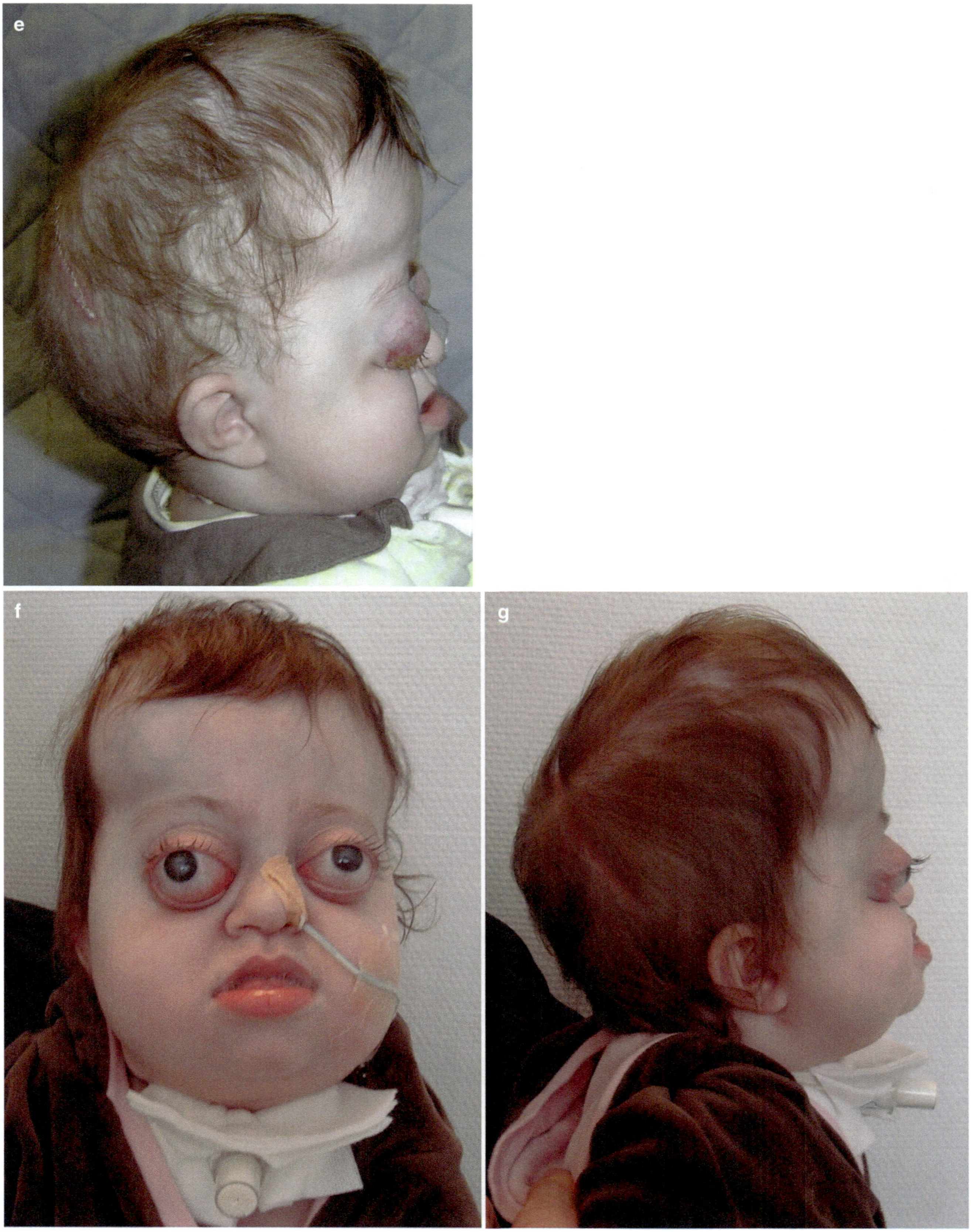

Fig. 9.14 (continued)

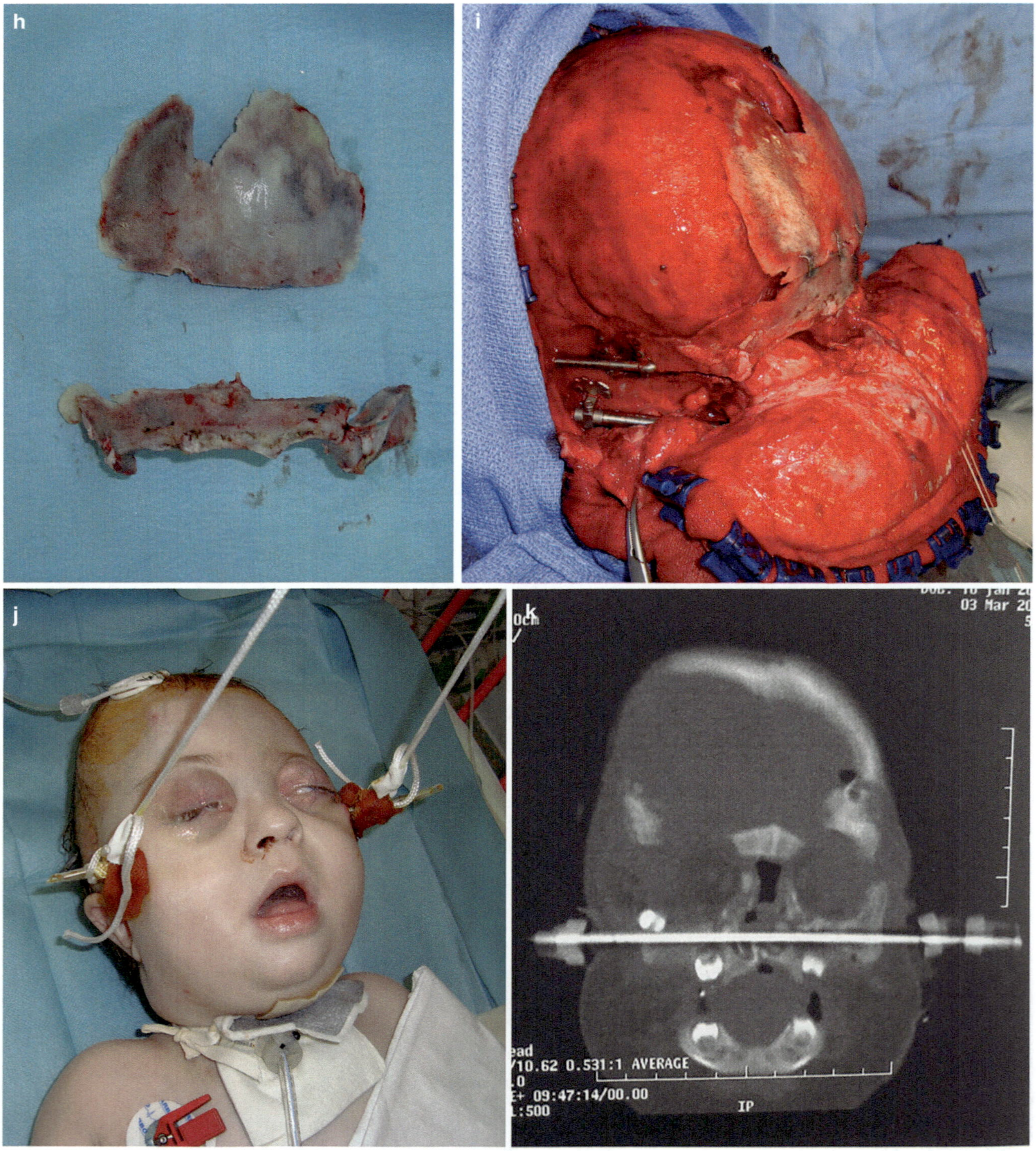

Fig. 9.14 (continued)

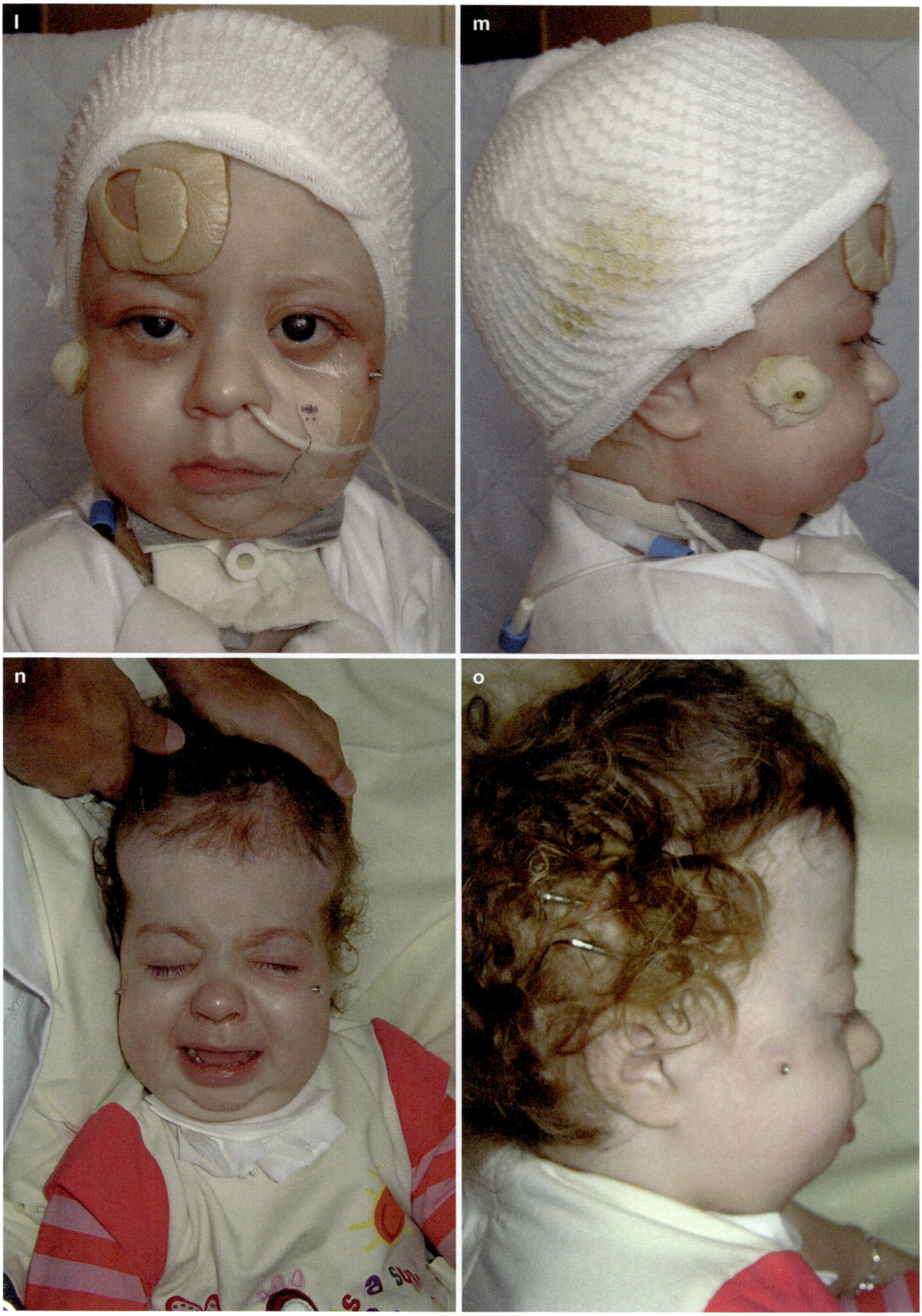

Fig. 9.14 (continued)

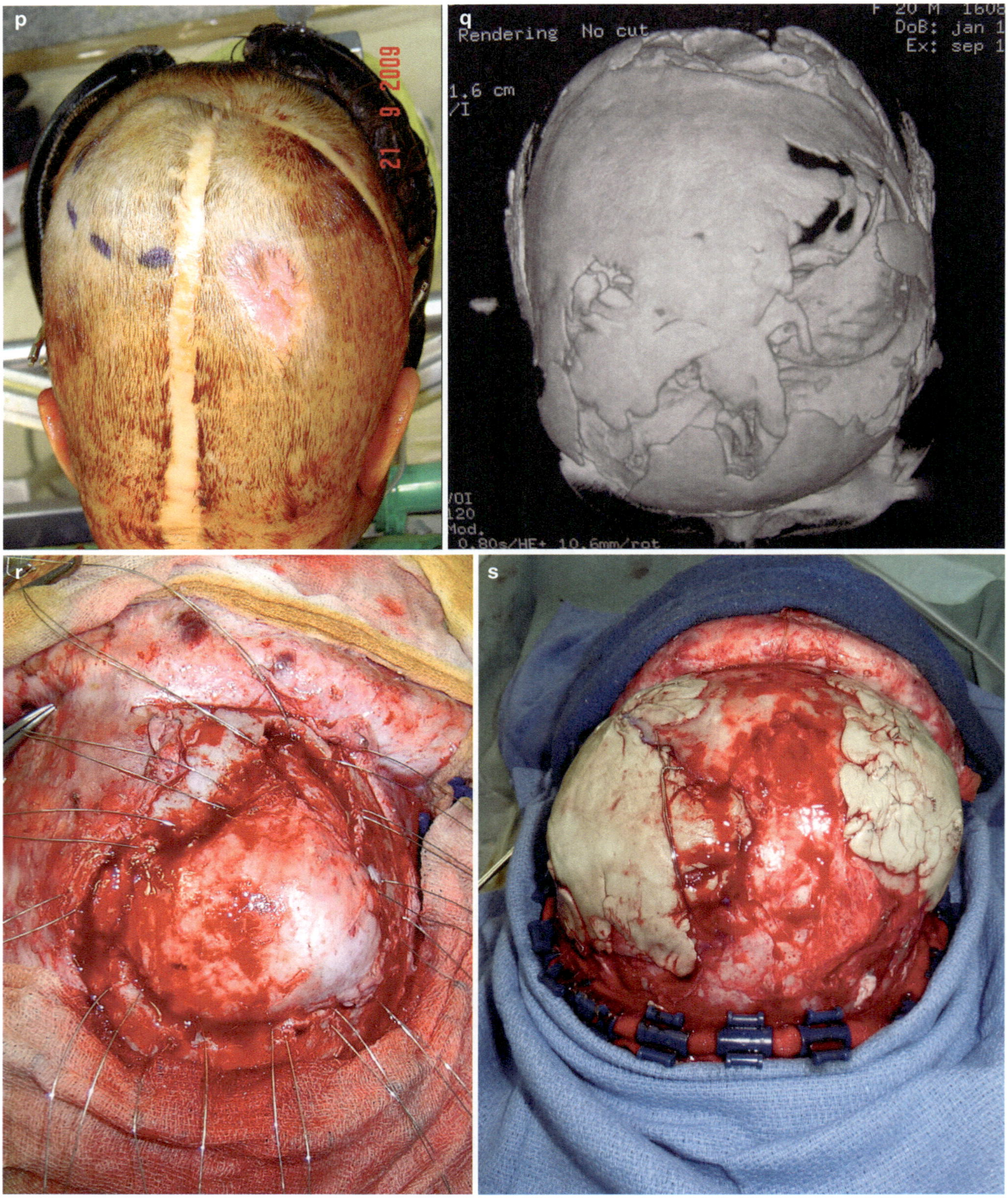

Fig. 9.14 (continued)

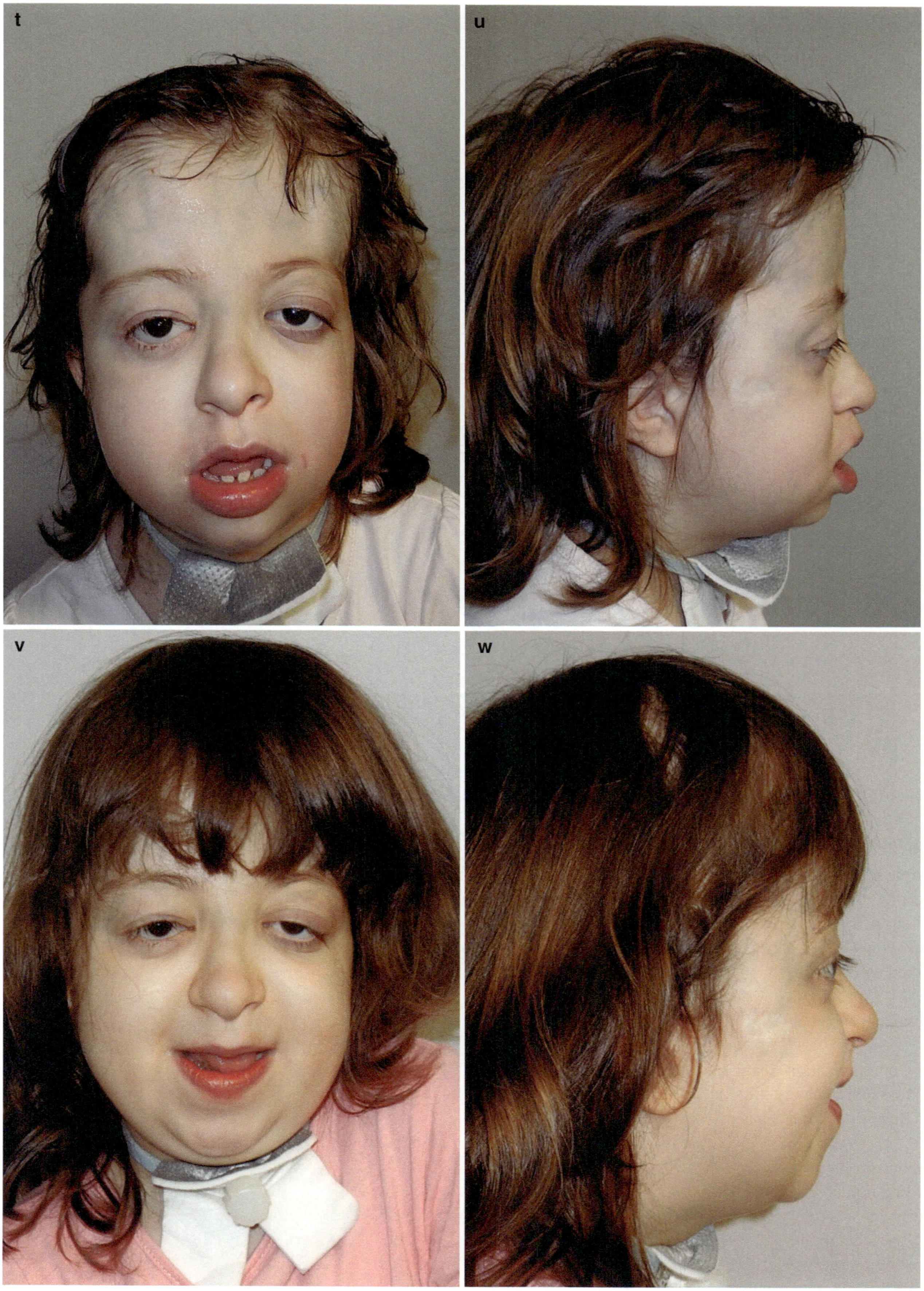

Fig. 9.14 (continued)

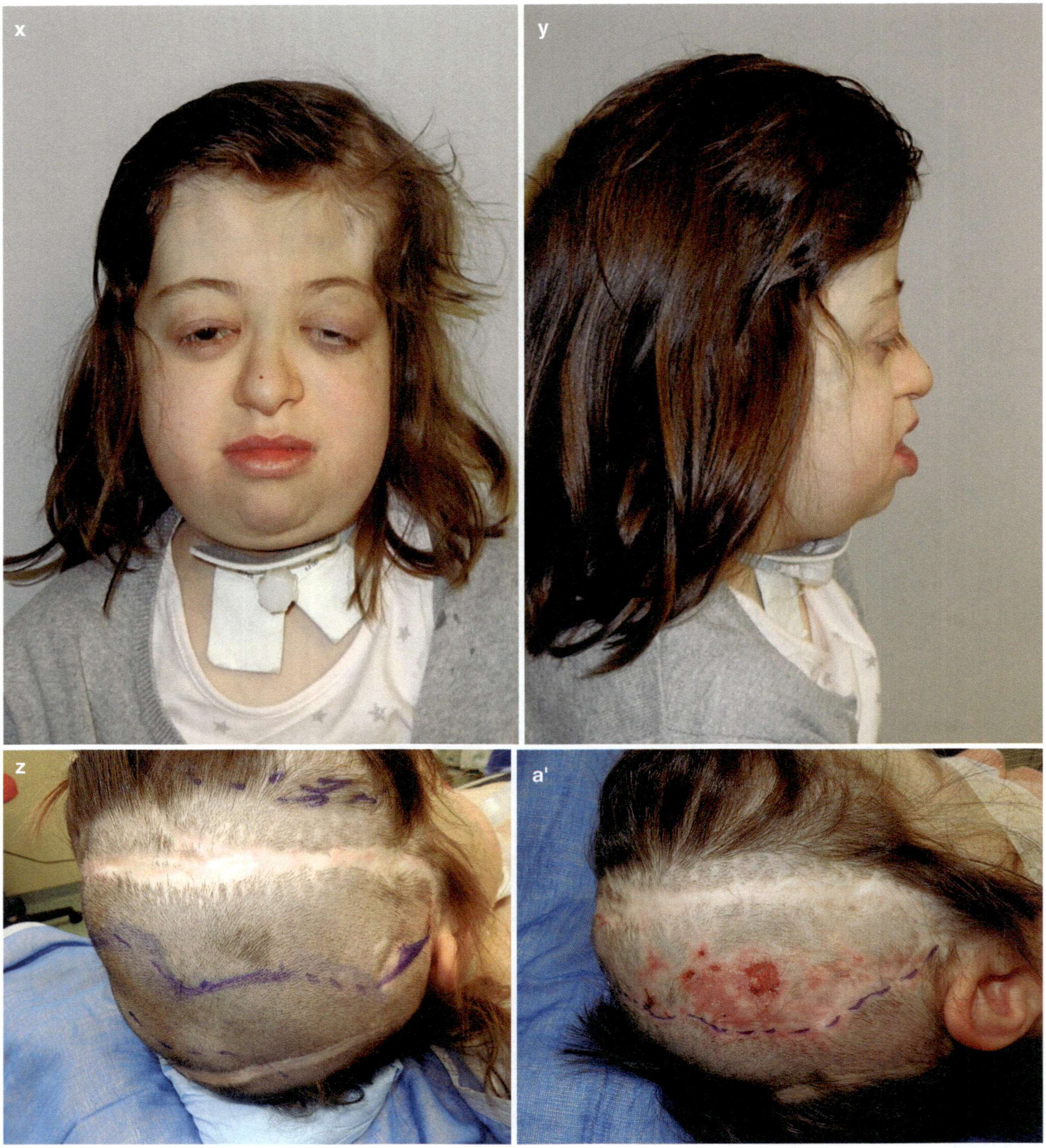

Fig. 9.14 (continued)

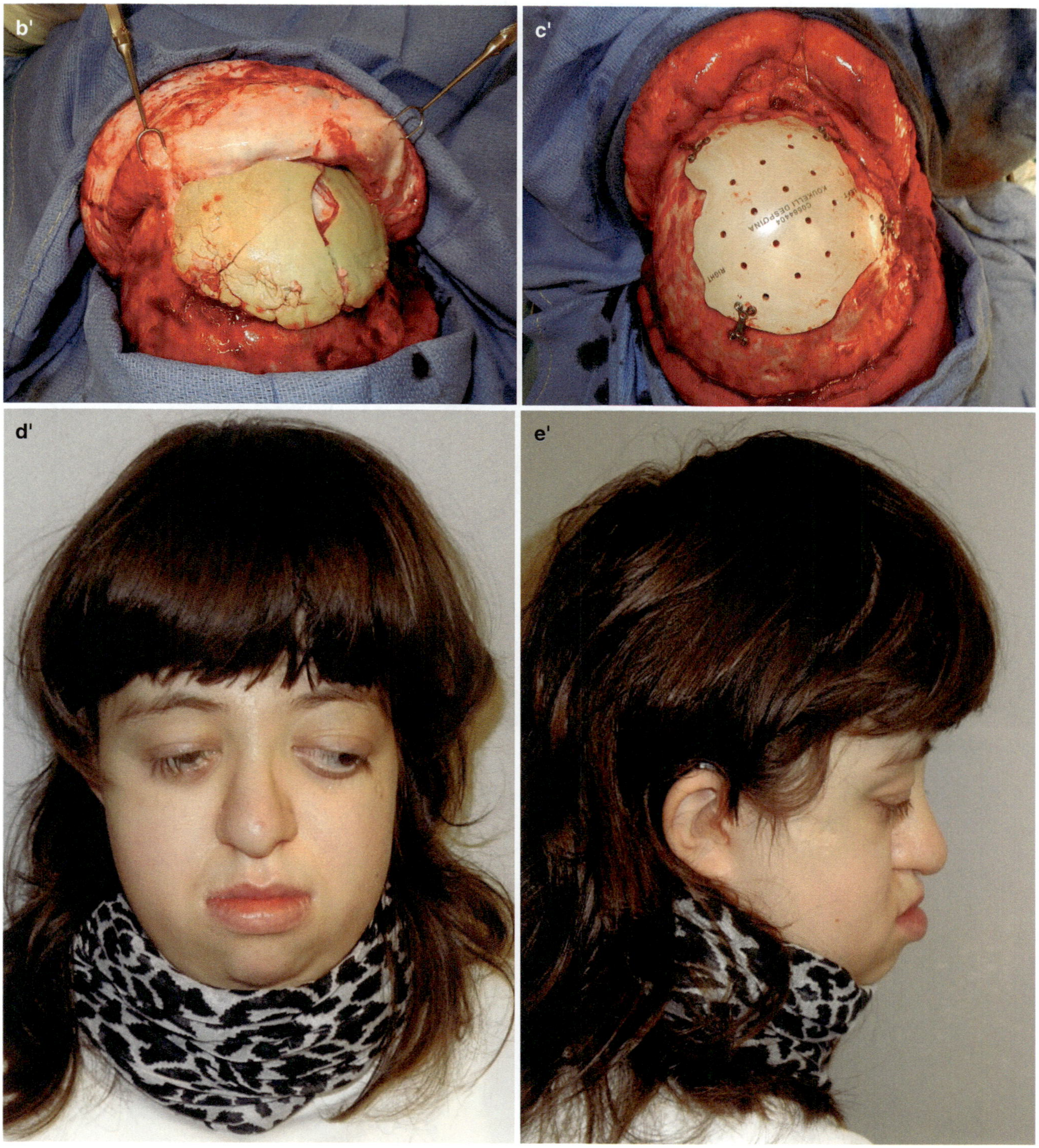

Fig. 9.14 (continued)

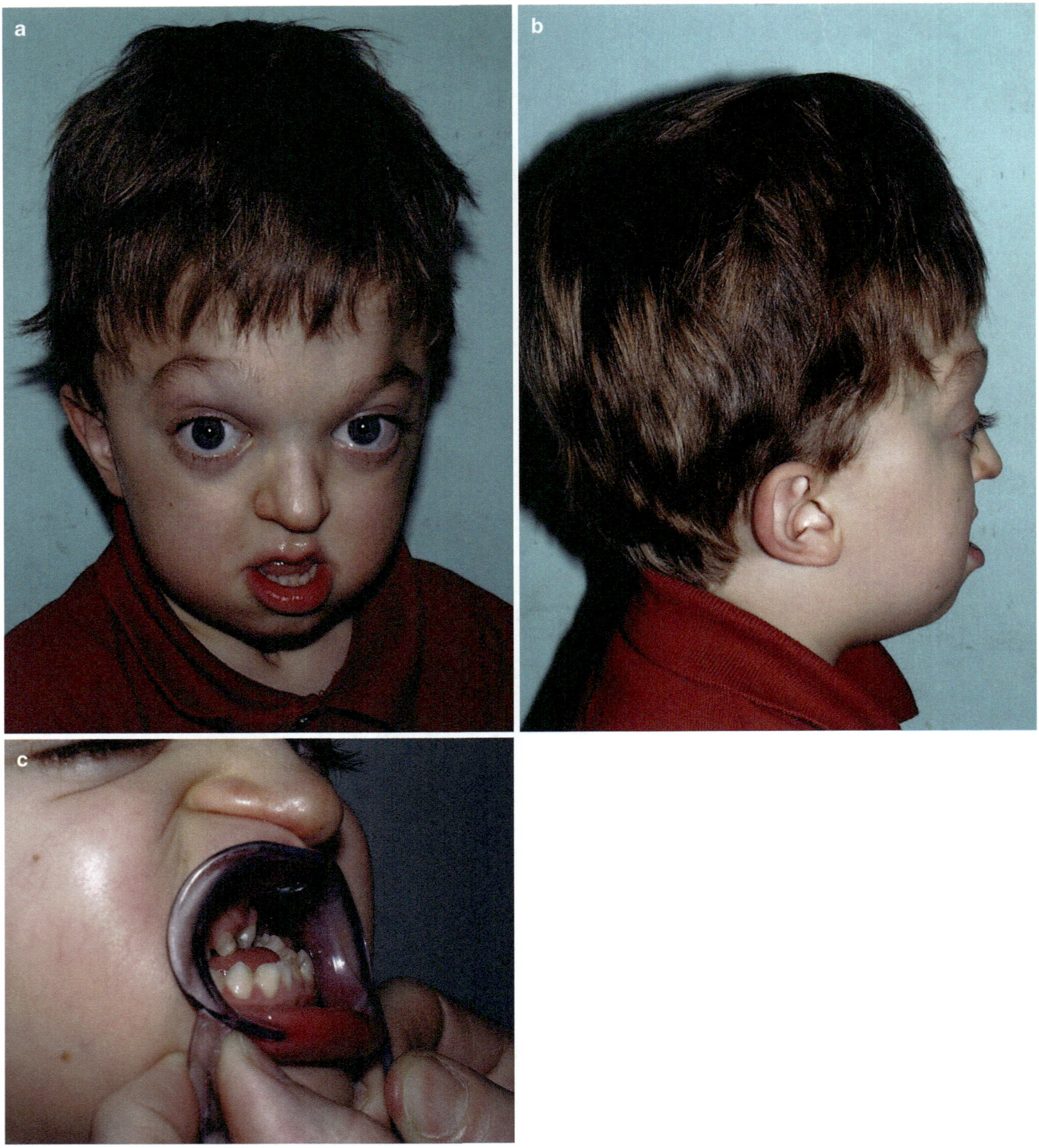

Fig. 9.15 (**a**, **b**, **c**) Patient with Crouzon syndrome aged 5 years previously operated of a FOA and early LF3. (**d**) Secondary FFMBA after FOA and LF3 at age 5. (**e**, **f**): Post FFMBA osteonecrosis of forehead, after 2 months. (**g**, **h**) Postoperative clinical aspect after FFMBA and forehead removal—Consolidation period. (**i**). CT scan of skull with missing forehead after removal of distractors. (**j**, **k**) At age 7, 1 year after FFMBA, before reconstruction of forehead. (**l**, **m**) Transient cranioplasty with PMMA for complete forehead reconstruction. (**n**, **o**) Postoperative aspect at age 12 with transient cranioplasty. Custom-made implant was used for definitive reconstruction at end of growth, requiring coverage with a *latissimus dorsi* free flap

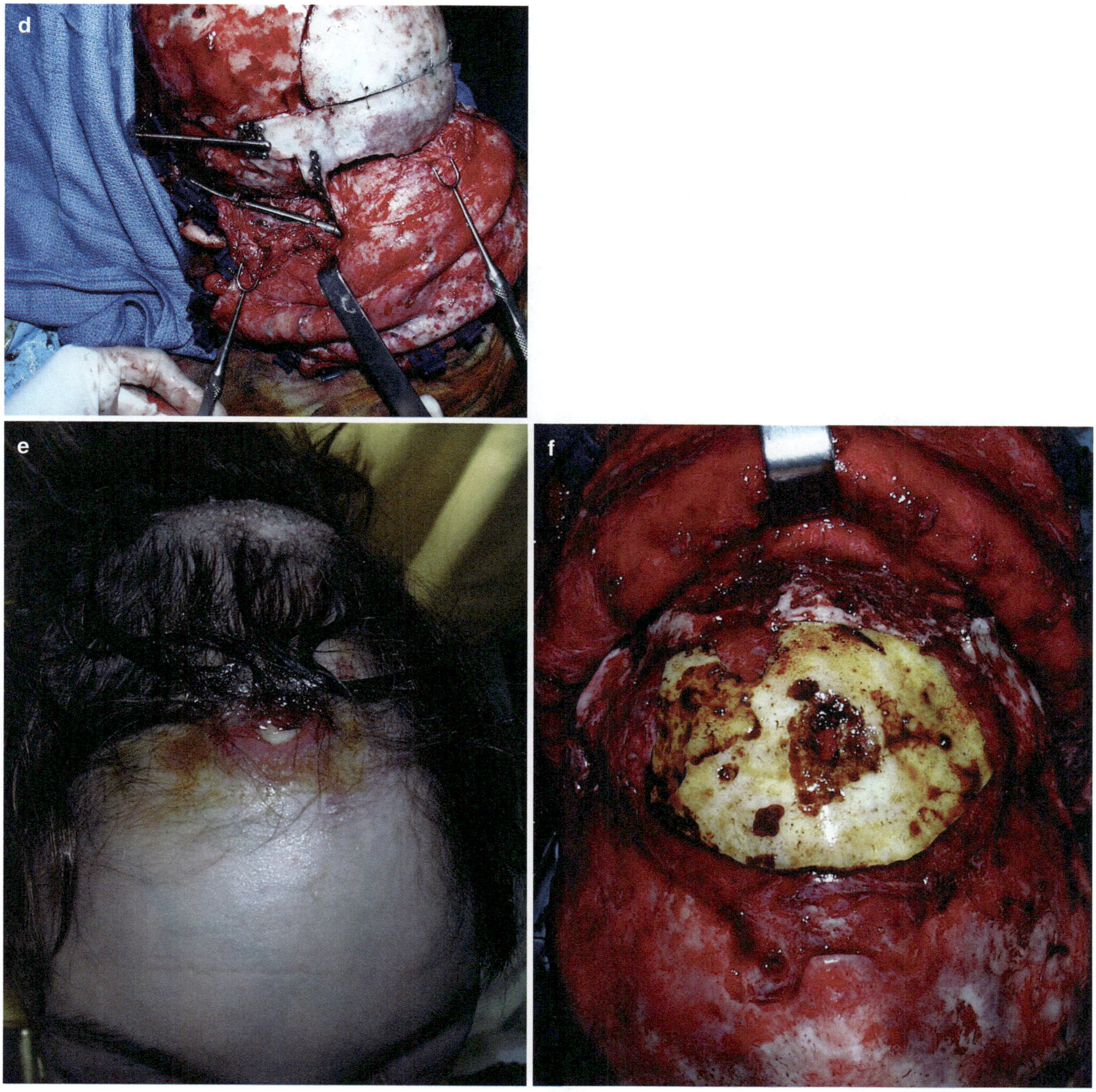

Fig. 9.15 (continued)

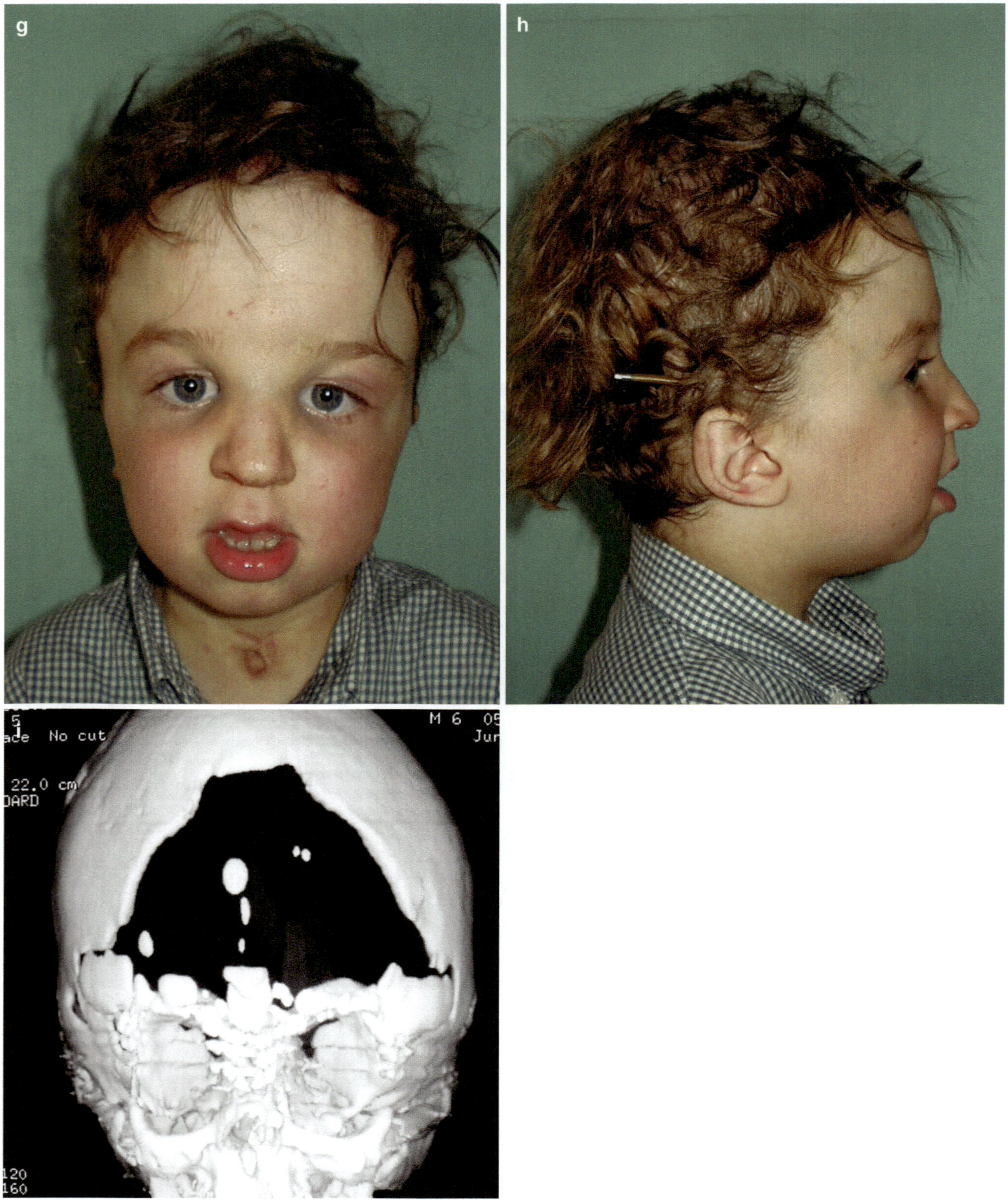

Fig. 9.15 (continued)

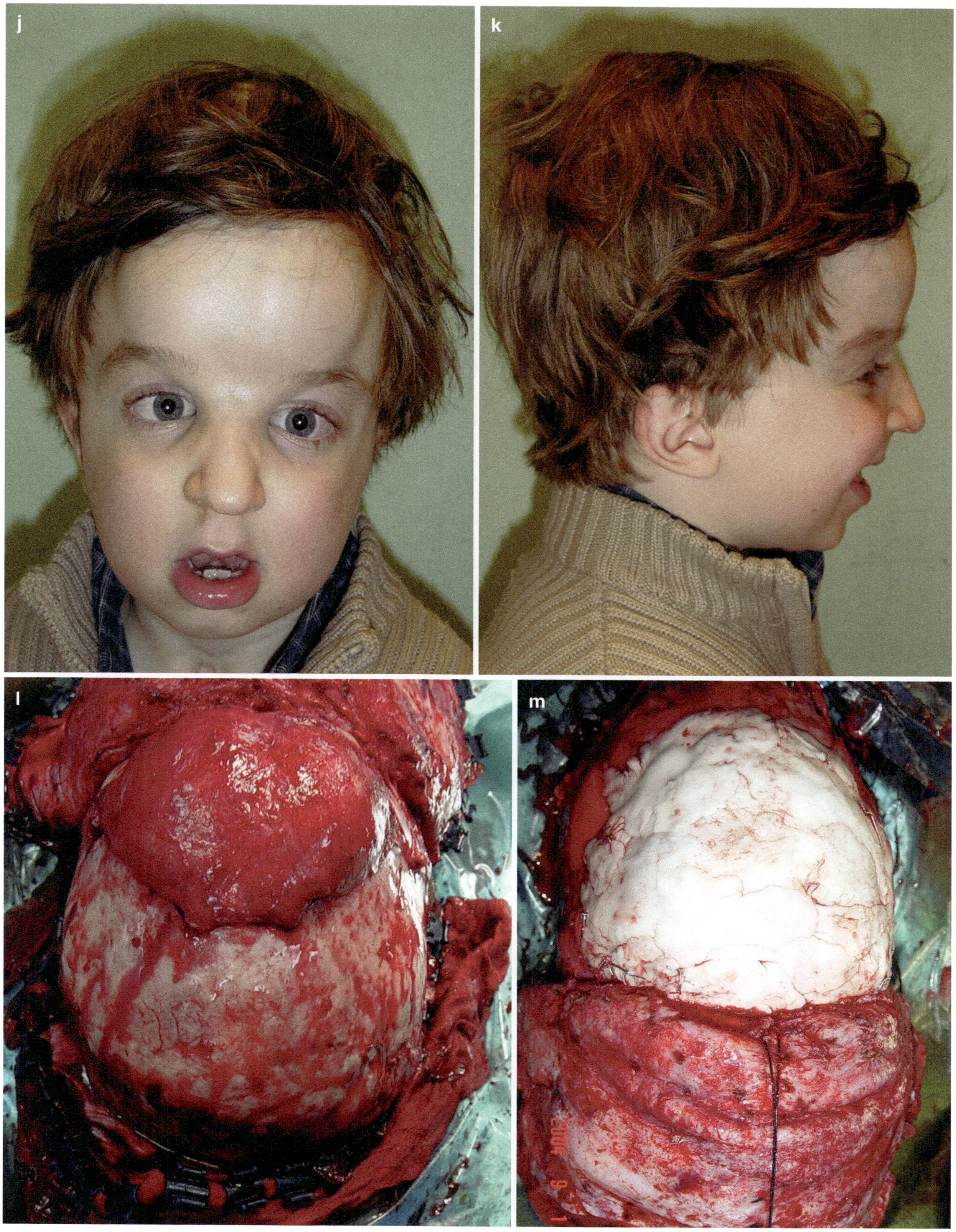

Fig. 9.15 (continued)

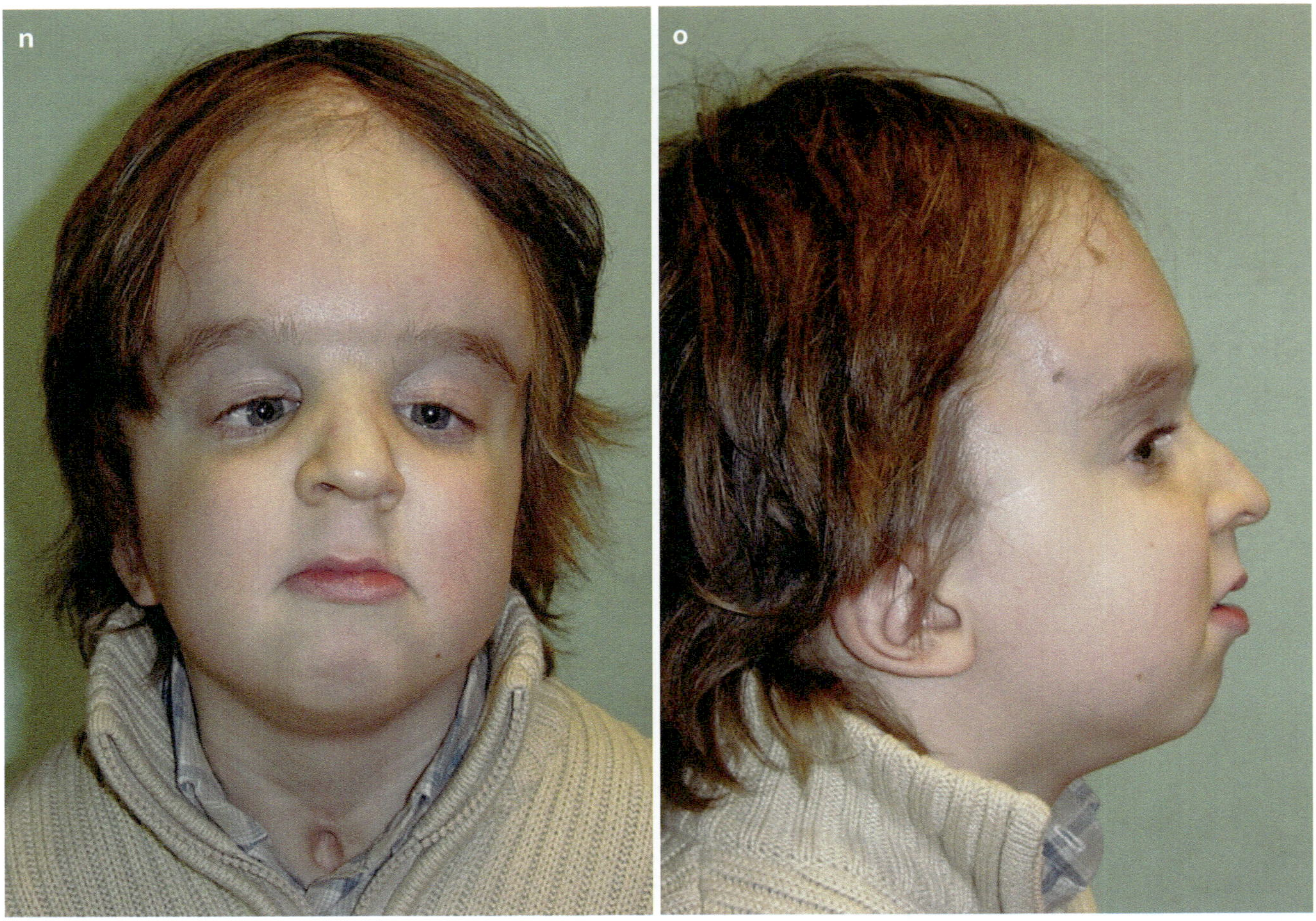

Fig. 9.15 (continued)

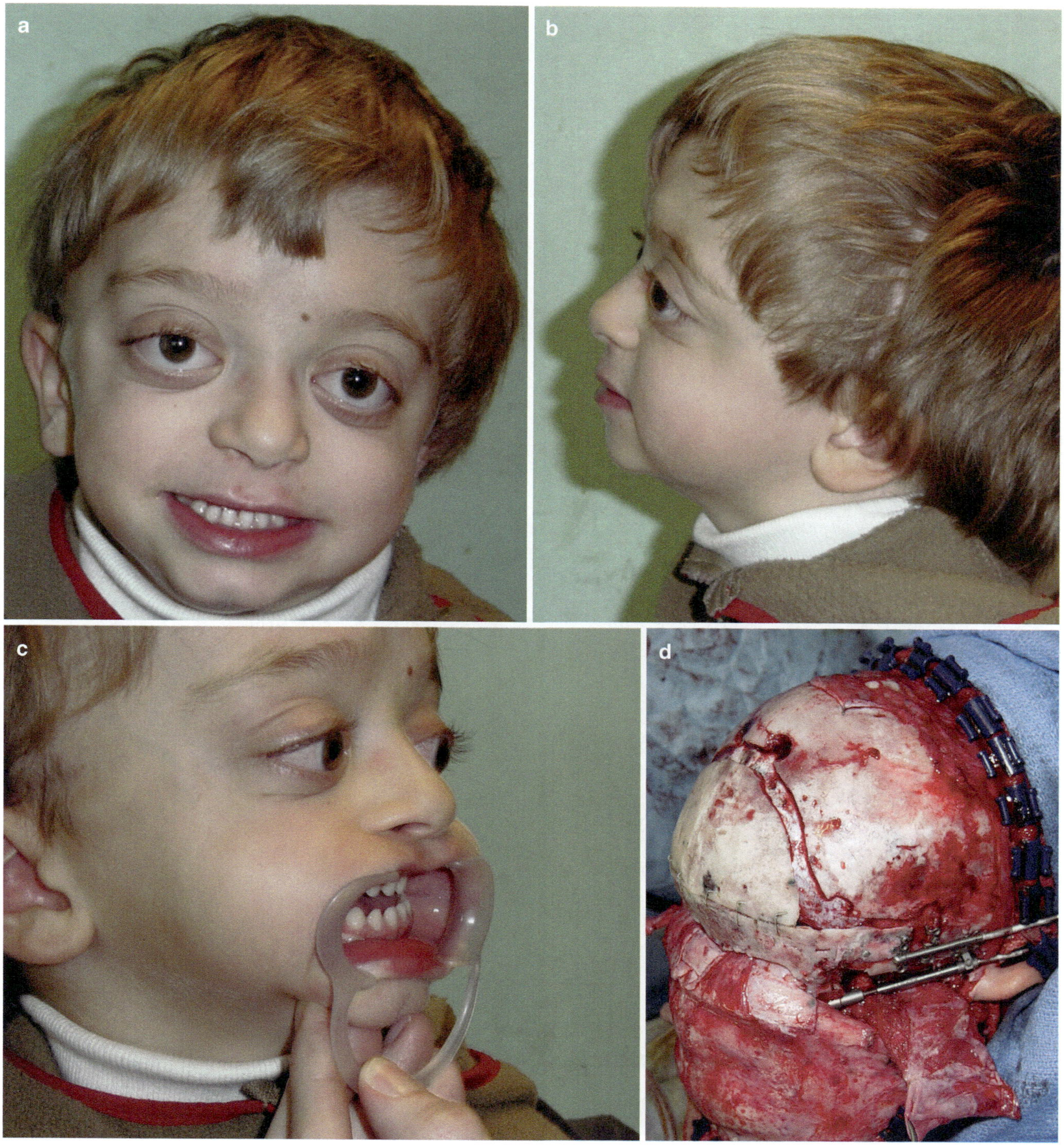

Fig. 9.16 (**a**, **b**, **c**) Patient with Crouzon syndrome aged 4 years having been operated elsewhere (FOA and attempt of early LF3). (**d**) Reoperation at age 4,5 years of a secondary FFMBA. (**e**) Immediate result after FFMBA, with fragilization of maxillary-zygomatic junction. (**f**, **g**) Clinical result after FFMBA during consolidation phase. (**h**, **i**, **j**) Clinical result at age 5.5, 1 year after FFMBA. Class I occlusion was not achieved. (**k**) Early LF3 1 year after FFMBA with internal and external distraction for respiratory reasons at age 6. (**l**, **m**, **n**) Clinical result at age 7 with hypercorrection obtained. (**o**, **p**) Clinical result at age 10, 4 years after FFMBA. (**q**, **r**) Clinical result at age 12 after fat grafting in inferior eyelids and zygoma, and lacrymal obstruction on the right side. (**s**) Attempt of advancement of right medial canthus. (**t**, **u**) At age 12, after correction of lacrymal duct on the right side. (**v**, **w**) At age 15 before tertiary LF3 with distraction. (**x**) CT scan during distraction of tertiary LF3. (**y**, **z**) Final result at age 19 after orthognathic surgery, and zygomatic implants. (**a'**, **b'**) Final occlusal view at age 19

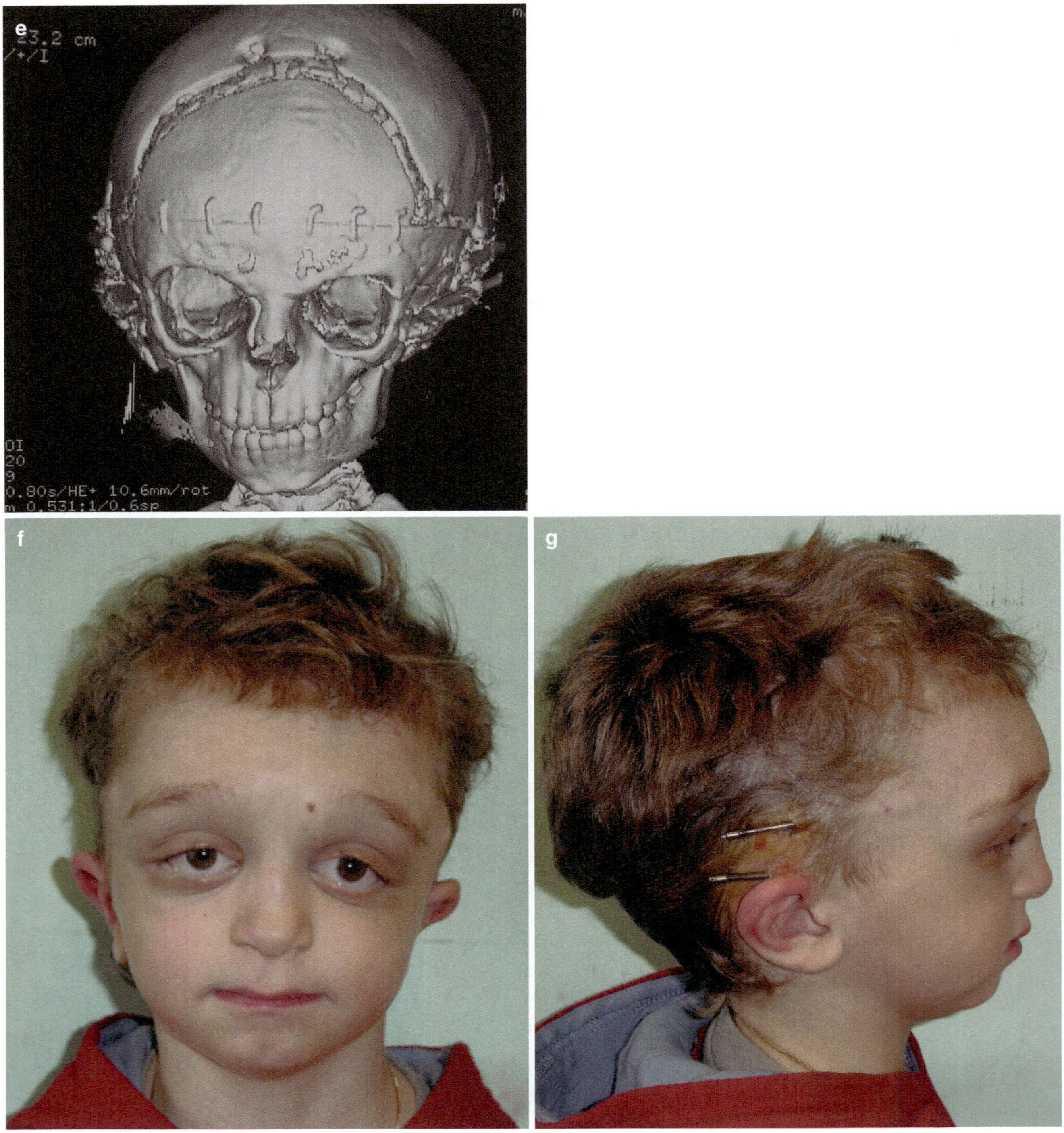

Fig. 9.16 (continued)

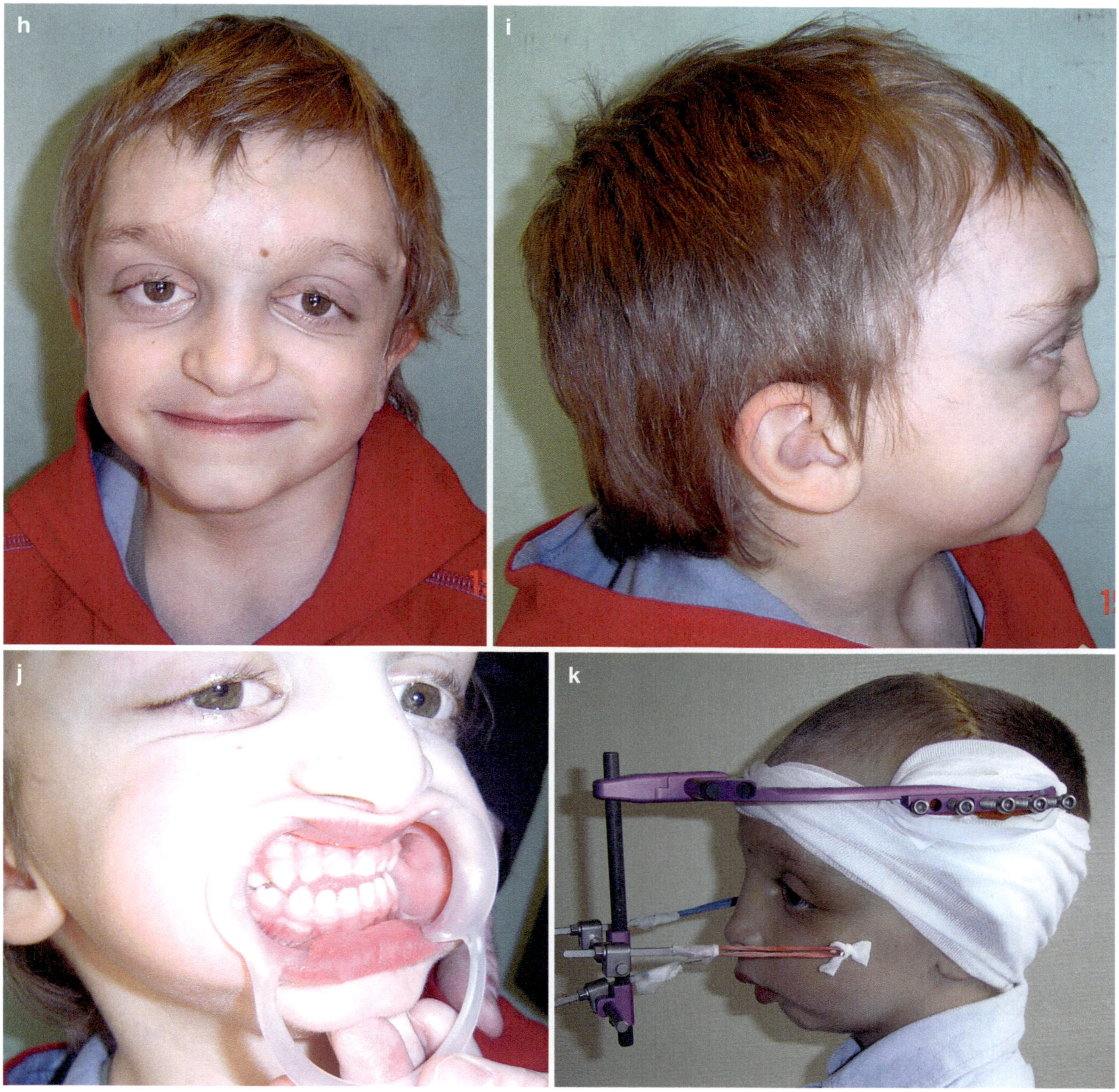

Fig. 9.16 (continued)

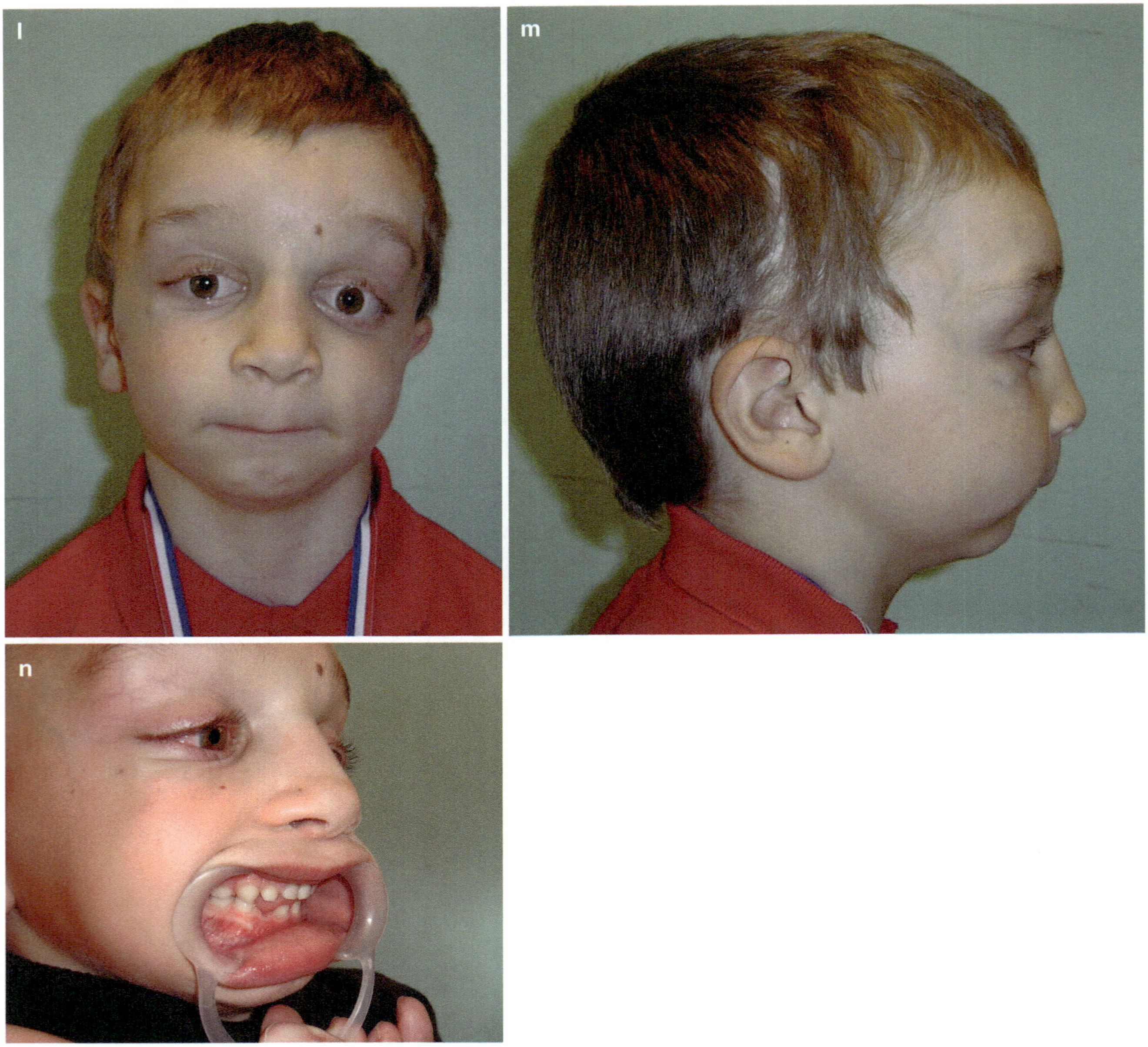

Fig. 9.16 (continued)

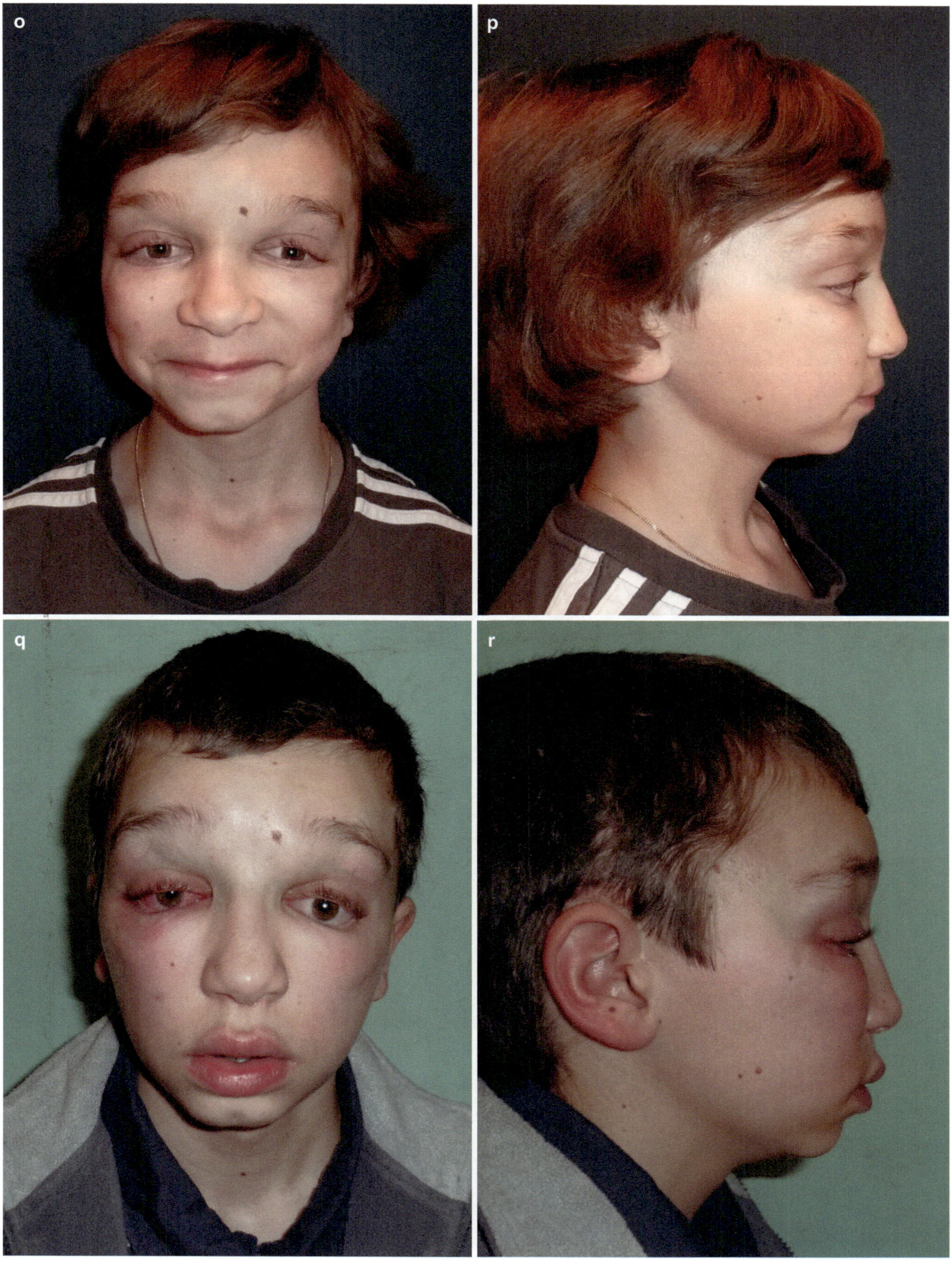

Fig. 9.16 (continued)

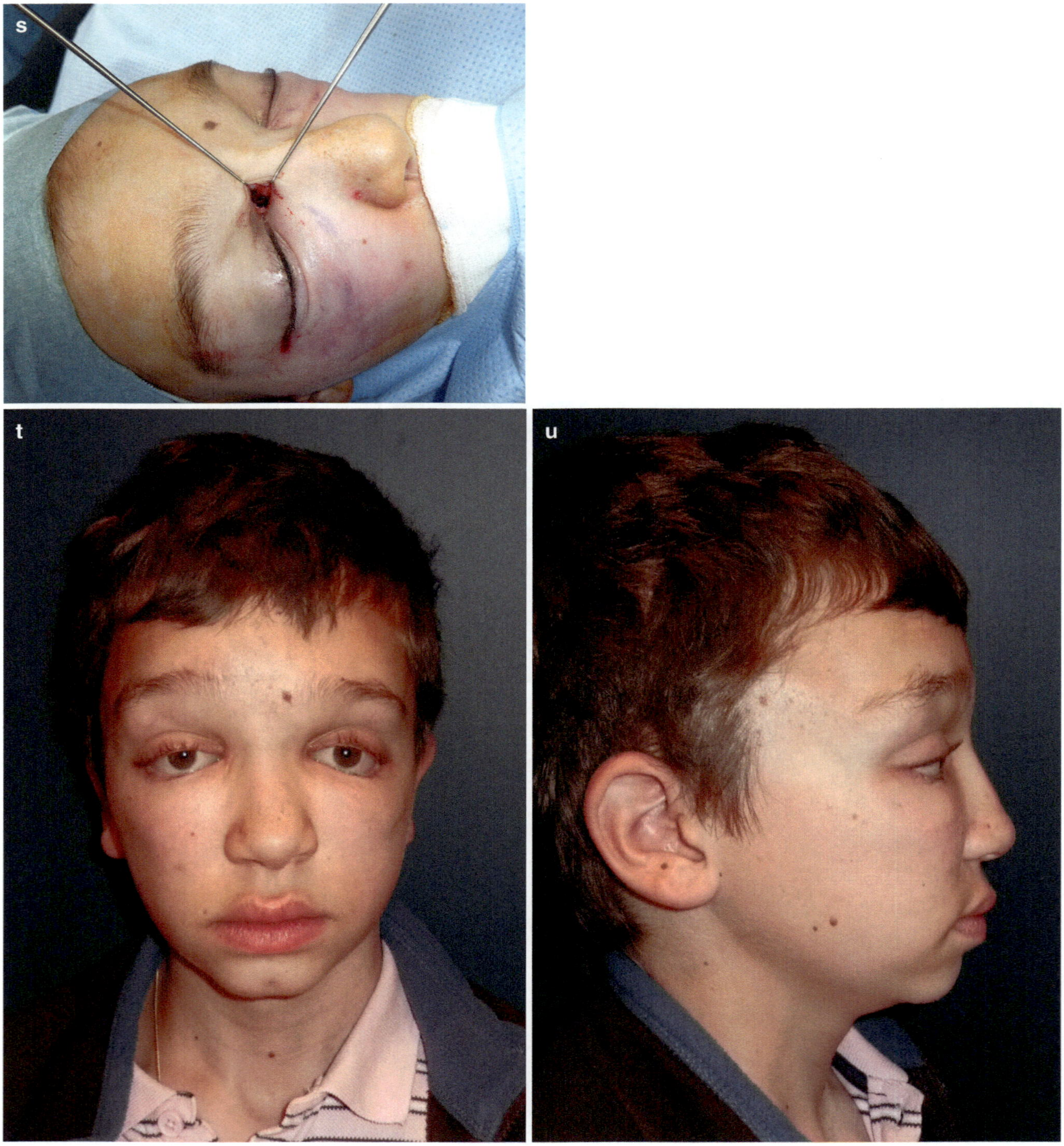

Fig. 9.16 (continued)

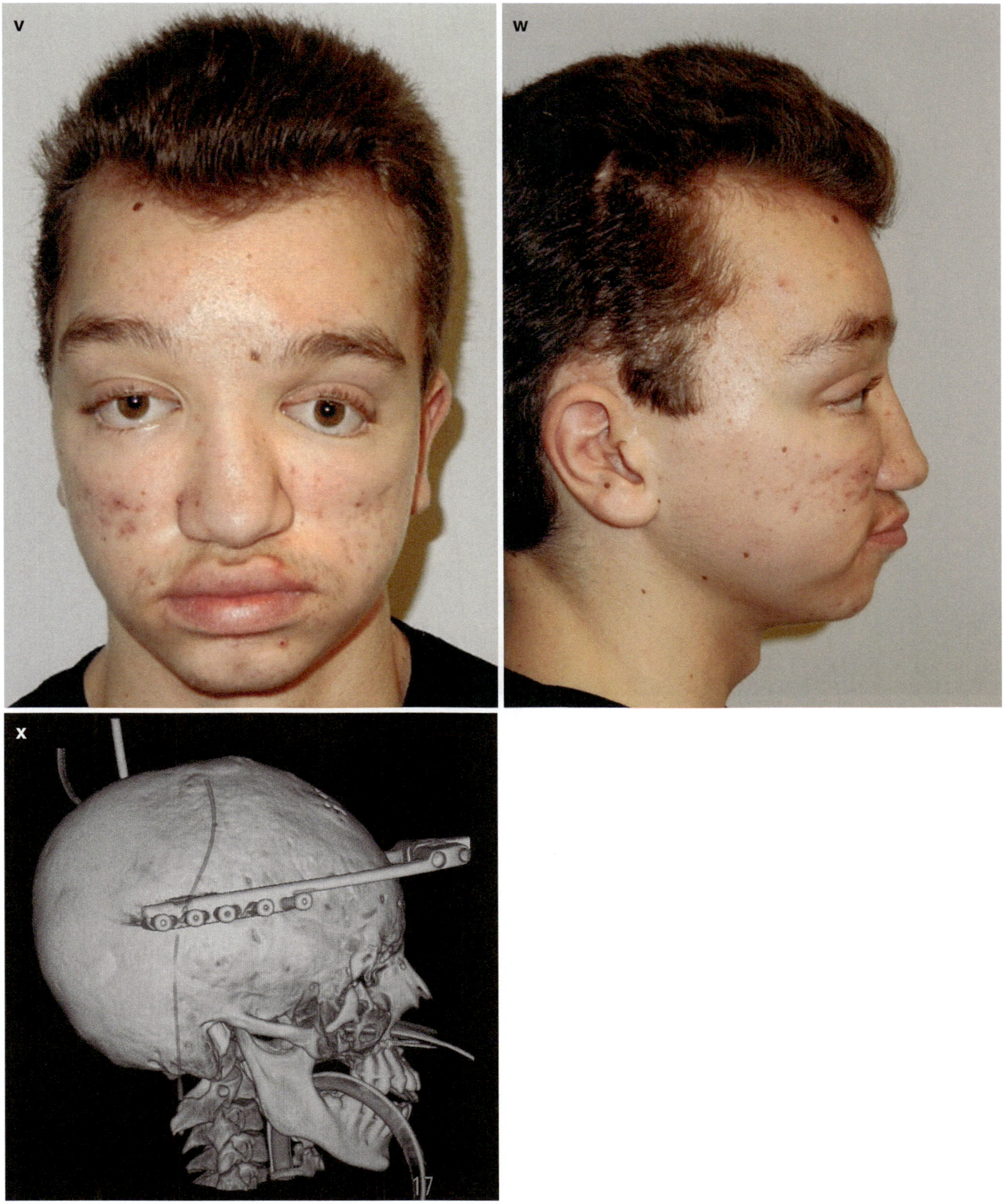

Fig. 9.16 (continued)

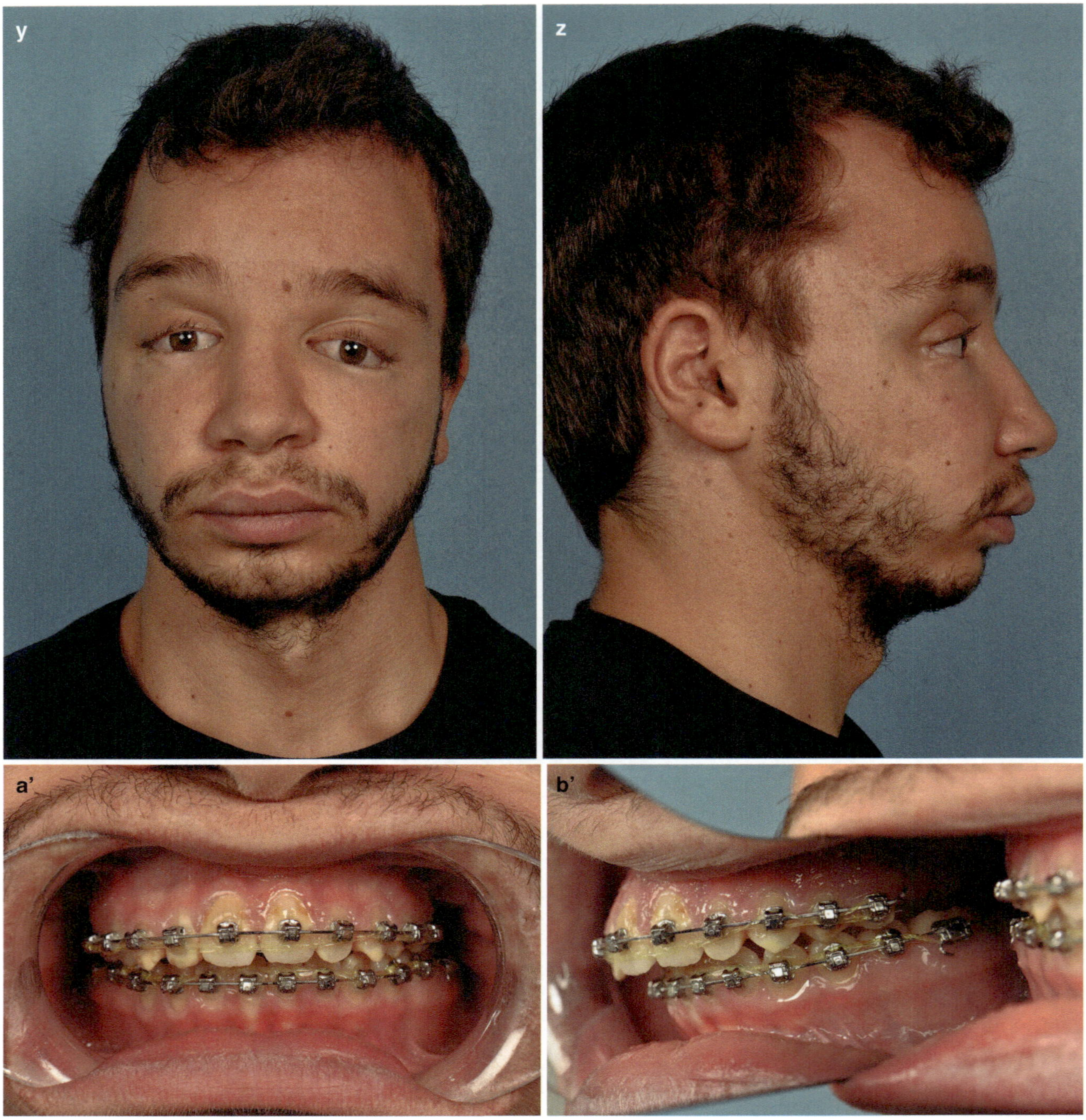

Fig. 9.16 (continued)

10 Treatment Strategies in Faciocraniosynostosis

After having detailed previously the techniques and consequences of FFMBA, we propose some examples of strategies for each of the three main FCST: Crouzon, Pfeiffer, and Apert syndromes. Each sequence of treatment relies on one or several of the various steps detailed in Fig. 10.1.

Even if we advocate the recourse to a sequence including FFMBA leading usually to a period of 10 years without any need for further procedures until the age of 10–14 years, we nevertheless give some examples of staged procedures in which the early LF3 is performed around 5–6 years (Fig. 10.2).

10.1 Treatment Strategies in Crouzon Syndrome

The rationale behind performing PVE before either one of these strategies is to start by solving the brain-related problems during its fast growth phase (first year of life). In fact, the (frequently) fused lambdoid sutures block posterior skull growth in Crouzon and Pfeiffer syndromes [1]. This causes turricephaly as brain growth pushes the skull upward. PVE corrects this deformity and provides the growing brain with plenty of intracranial space posteriorly [2–4]. In doing so, PVE expands the posterior fossa volume to accommodate the cerebellum and prevents/improves cerebellar tonsillar herniation through the foramen magnum. Moreover, PVE contributes to solve the problem of intracranial venous hypertension due to venous outflow obstruction [5–8].

Once PVE is completed, our "ideal" strategy is the one-step scenario. It addresses most aspects of the Crouzon deformity before irreversible neurological damage occurs: PVE around 6 months of age followed by FFMBA around 30 months of age [9, 10].

FFMBA also expands the intracranial volume, but should be delayed as much as possible for the following reasons. First, if performed too early, FFMBA has a high relapse risk. PVE "buys time" until the child gets old enough to reap long-lasting benefits from FFMBA [11, 12]. Second, the frontal bandeau develops thicker bone when FFMBA is delayed [13–16].

When the midfacial deformity is minimal without OSA, the potential morbidity of FFMBA cannot be justified by the expected aesthetic improvement alone. In this situation, FOA is indicated with osteosynthesis using absorbable hardware. The ideal age for FOA is between 8 and 13 months, when bone malleability allows remodeling through greenstick fractures. This is referred to as the classical two-step strategy, because the maxillary retrusion usually needs to be addressed secondarily by a LF3 at dental maturity [17–20].

Here, several illustrated examples of management strategy are given for Crouzon syndrome (Figs. 10.3, 10.4, 10.5, 10.6, 10.7, 10.8, 10.9, and 10.10), Pfeiffer syndrome (Figs. 10.11, 10.12, 10.13, and 10.14), and Apert syndrome (Fig. 10.15, 10.16, and 10.17).

E. Arnaud et al., *Frontofacial Monobloc Advancement with Internal Distraction*, https://doi.org/10.1007/978-3-031-07574-2_10

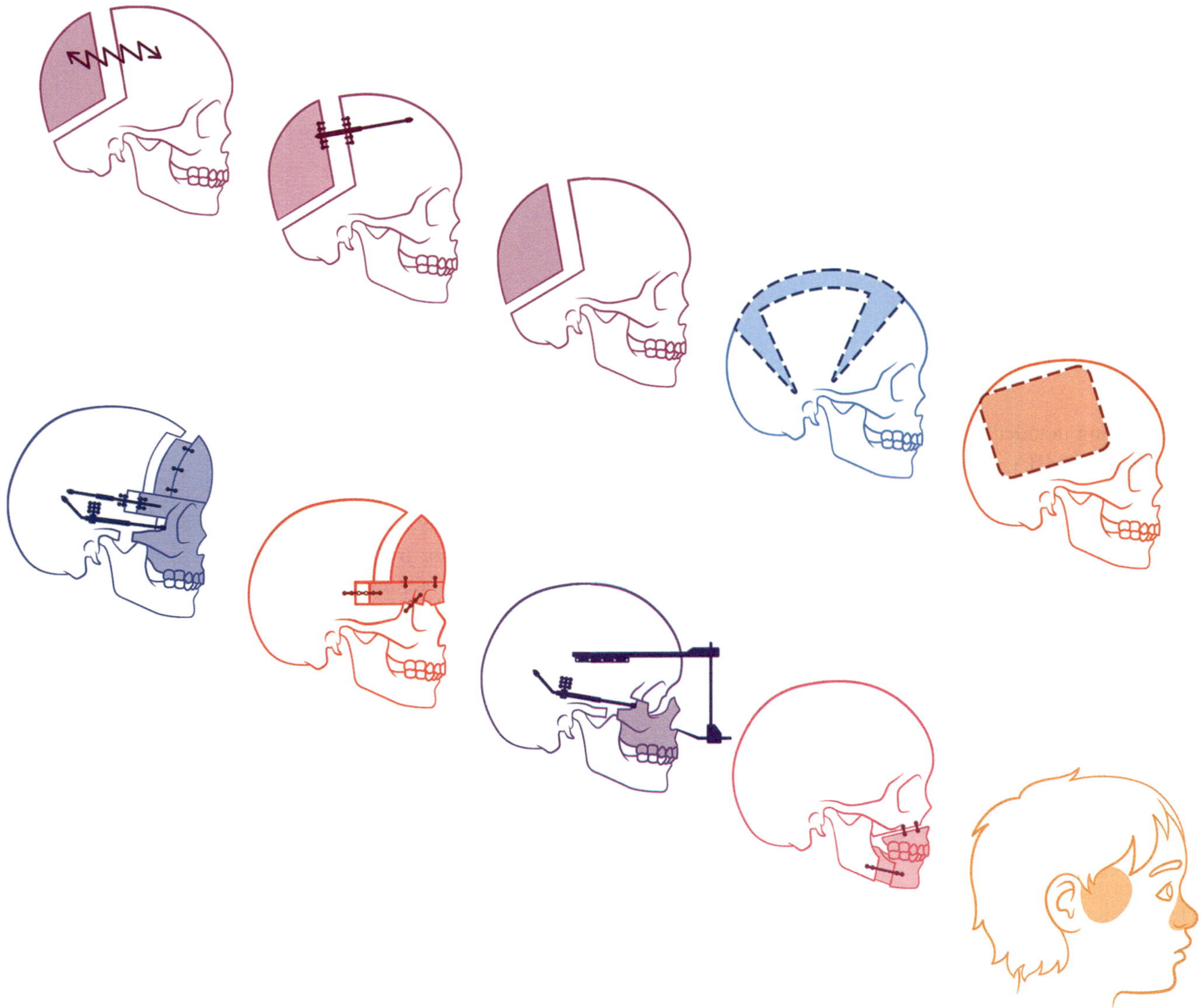

Fig. 10.1 Panorama of surgical strategies for faciocraniostenoses. Upper diagonal (from left to right): spring-mediated PVE, distractor-mediated PVE, brain-mediated PVE, H craniectomies, and biparietal decompression. Lower diagonal (from left to right): FFMBA, FOA, LF3, orthognathic surgery, and aesthetic surgery (similar to Fig. 1.2). ©Cassandra Vion

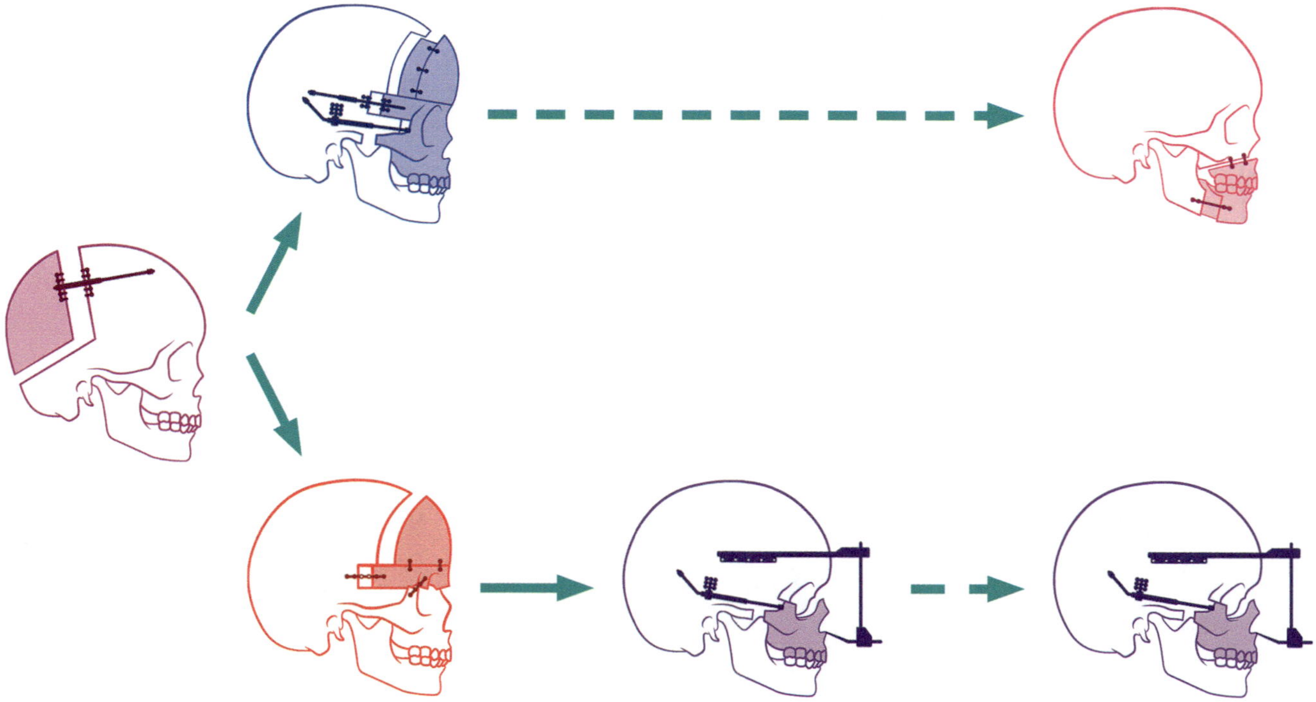

Fig. 10.2 Treatment strategies in Crouzon syndrome: PVE around age 6 months followed by:—(upper row) the single-step scenario with FFMBA (age 2–4 years), or—(lower row) the "classical" two-step scenario with FOA (age 11–18 months) and LF3 (age 6–10 years) (see Fig. 1.4). ©Cassandra Vion

10.1.1 Example №1 of Management Strategy in Crouzon Syndrome

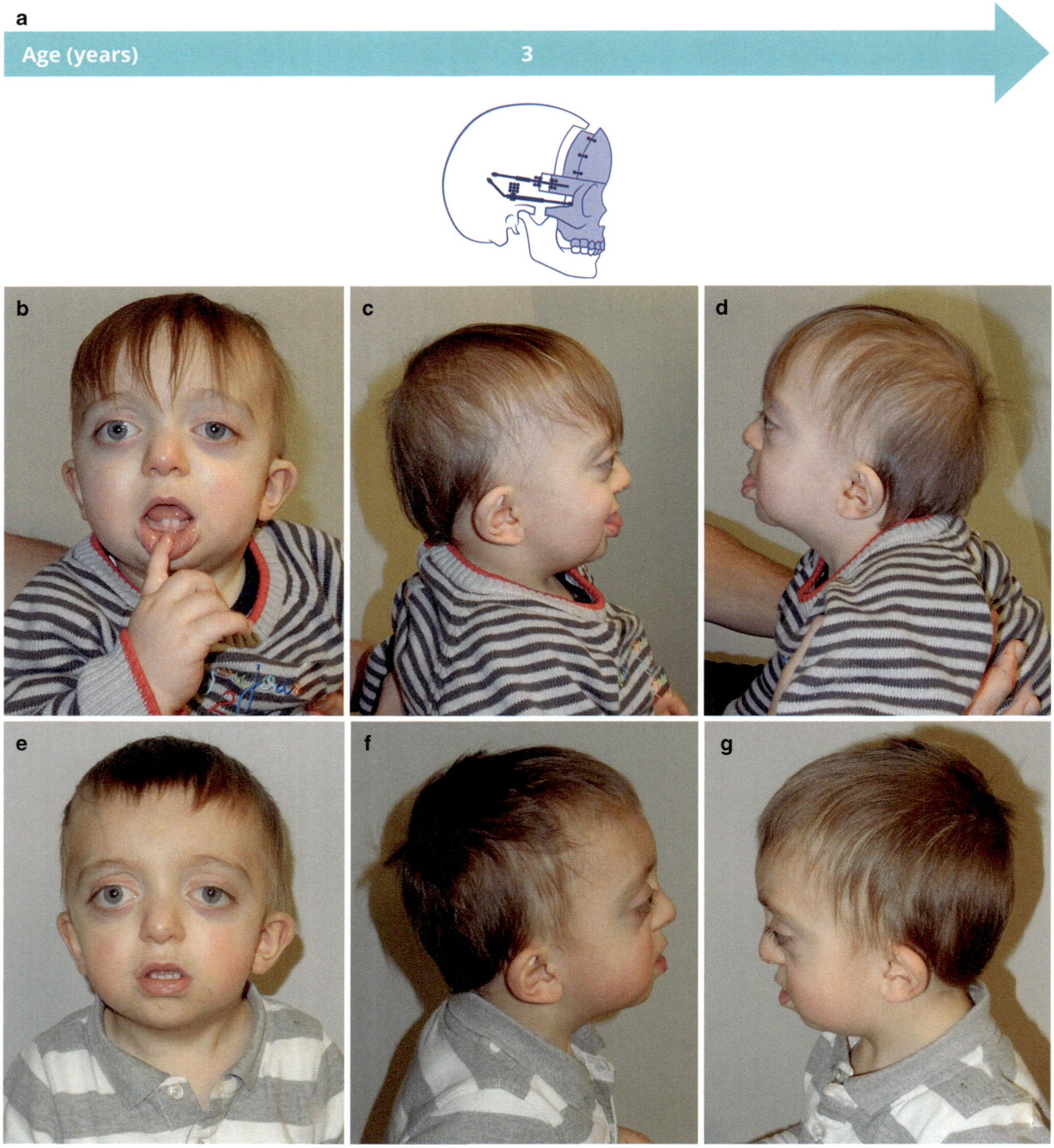

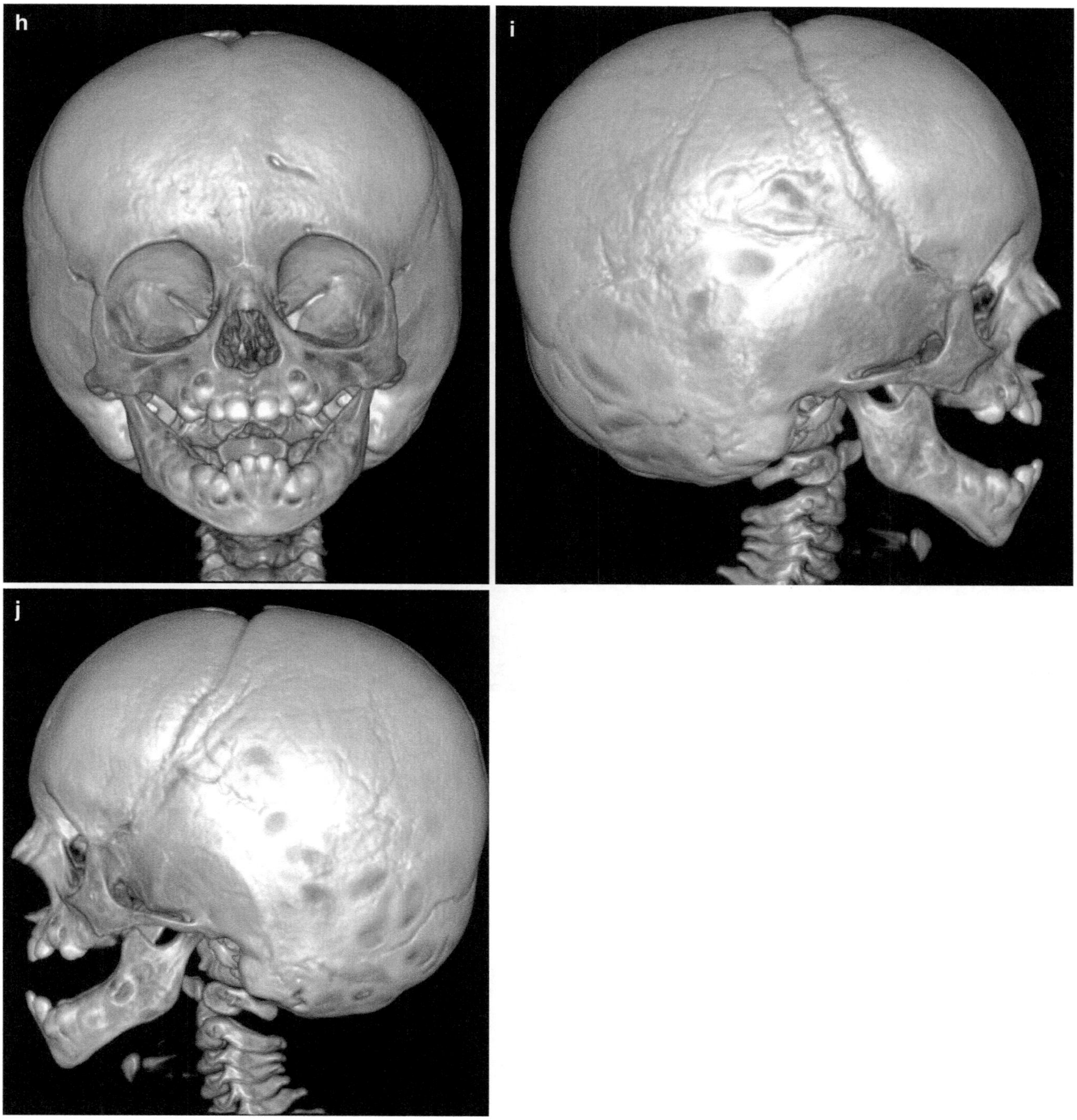

Fig. 10.3 (continued)

Fig. 10.3 (**a**-**d**) One-year-old patient with familial Crouzon syndrome presenting with exorbitism and maxillary hypoplasia. Fundoscopy confirmed the absence of papilledema and polysomnography was normal. (**e**, **f**, **g**) Clinical pictures at age 2 years. The patient developed snoring. Polysomnography showed severe OSA (AHI = 18.5 per hour). CPAP was initiated until FFMBA was performed at age 3 years. (**h**, **i**, **j**) Preoperative CT scan demonstrating maxillary hypoplasia partial bicoronal craniosynostosis. (**k**, **l**) Preoperative MRI demonstrating the absence of tonsillar herniation on T2-weighted images and a complex network of collateral venous circulation on Inhance 3D velocity MRI images. (**m**, **n**) Two-day postoperative CT scans demonstrating the osteotomy lines and the position of the distractors and the lateral orbital plates. Titanium plates were exceptionally used to stabilize the forehead without complications so far, but we subsequently changed this practice to use only resorbable material at this location with lateral bony wings for stability as detailed in Chap. 4. (**o**, **p**) Three-week-postoperative CT scan demonstrating fronto-facial advancement at the end of the activation phase of distraction. The distractors were removed after 3 months of consolidation. (**q**, **r**, **s**) One-year-postoperative clinical photographs demonstrating the resolution of exorbitism and midface hypoplasia. Polysomnography demonstrated the resolution of OSA (AHI = 0.8 per hour). (**t**, **u**, **v**) One-year-postoperative CT scan typically demonstrating satisfactory ossification at the tenon level and only partial ossification of the coronal defect

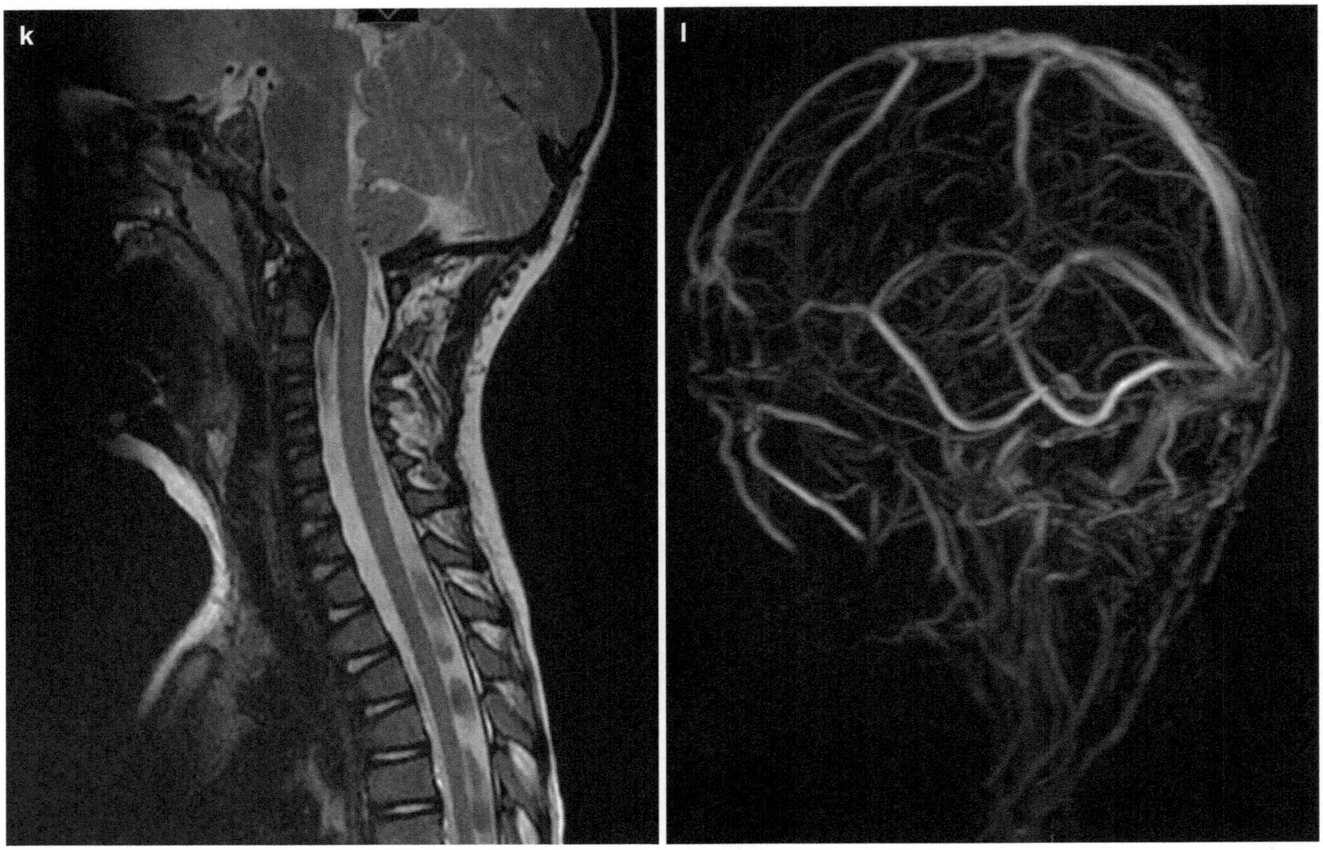

Fig. 10.3 (continued)

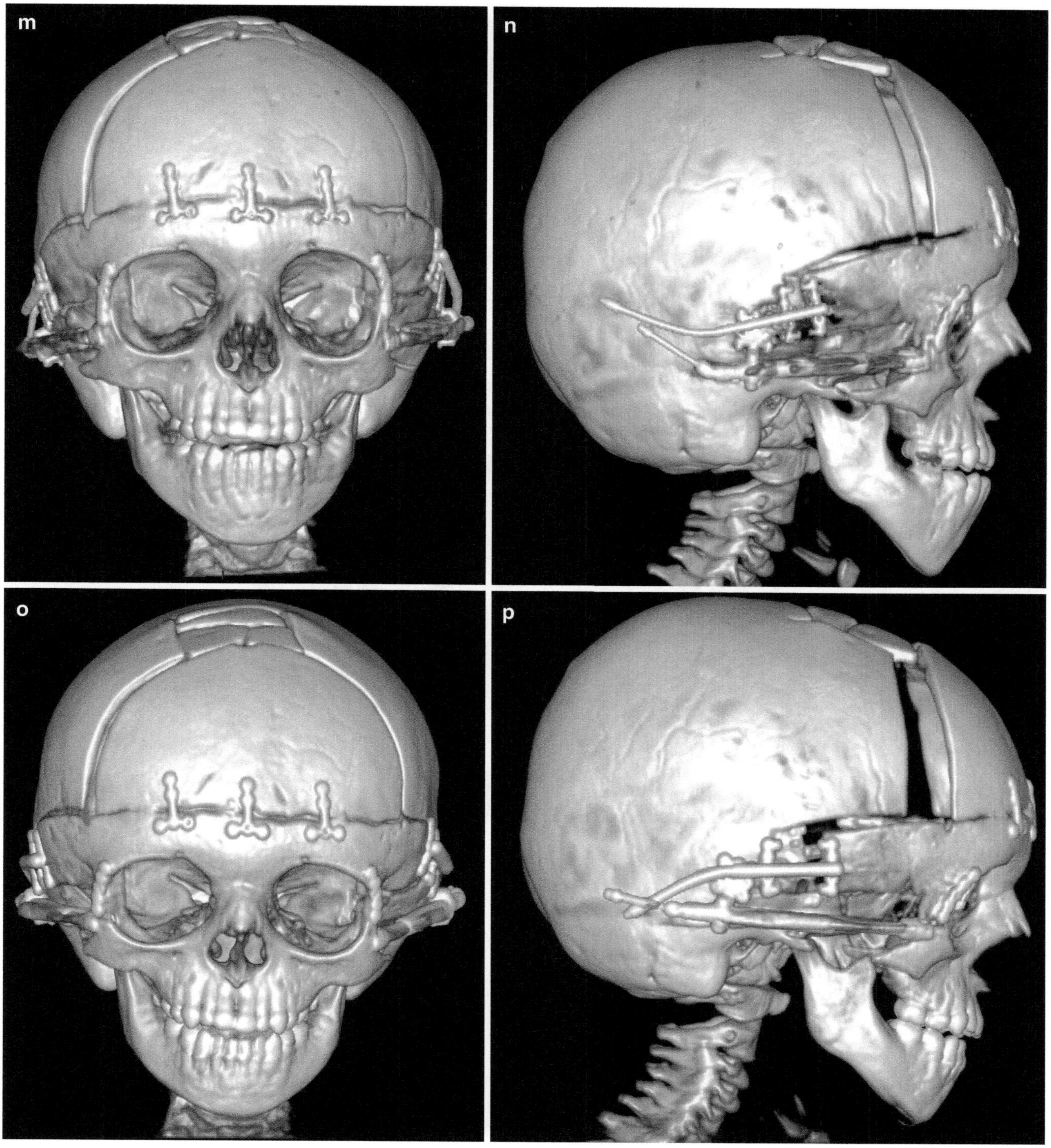

Fig. 10.3 (continued)

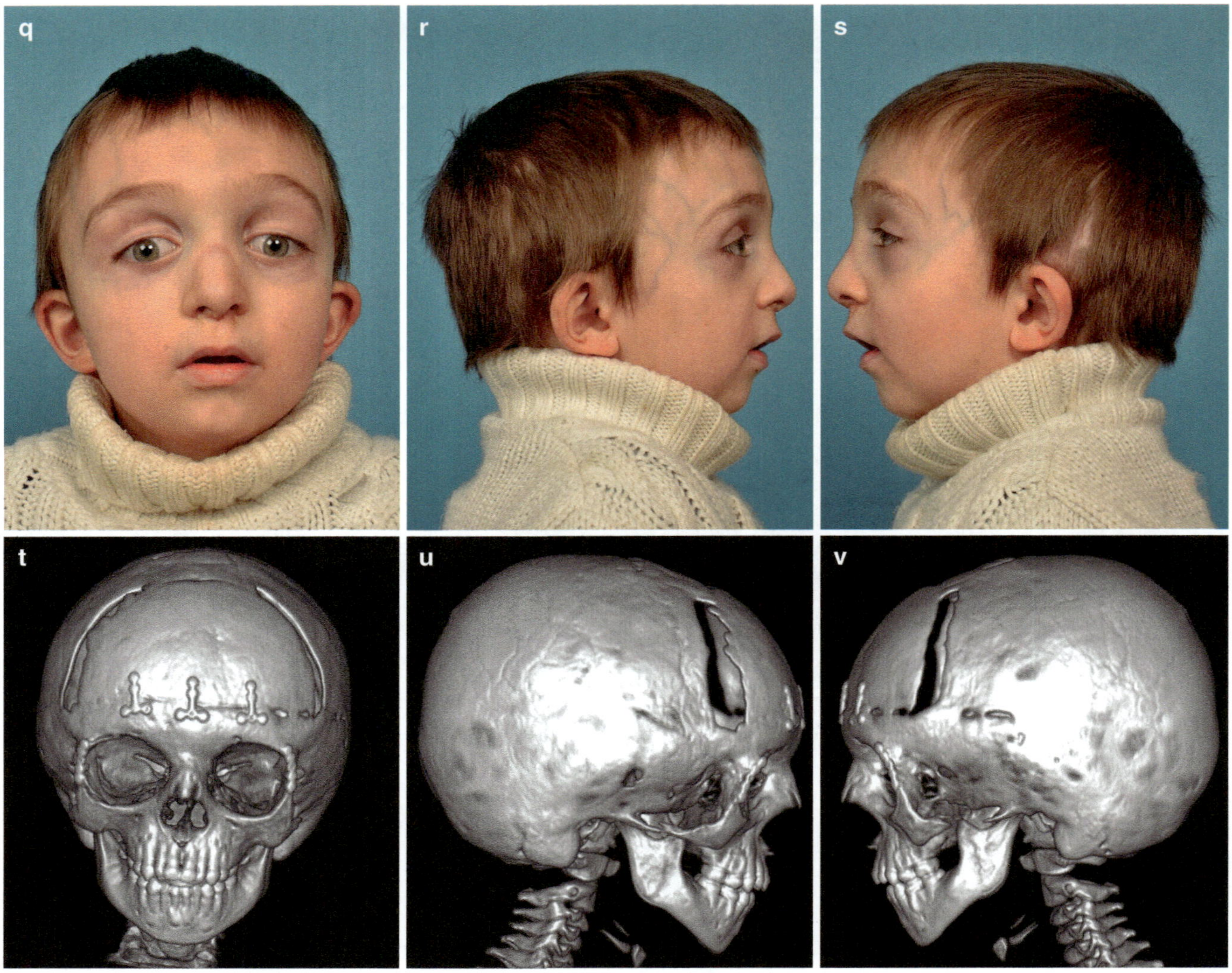

Fig. 10.3 (continued)

Fig. 10.4 (**a**) Management of a moderate form of Crouzon syndrome with a strategy involving early FFMBA, LF3 at adolescence and aesthetic improvements. (**b**, **c**) Clinical presentation at 3 years of age with mild exorbitism but OSA (IAH = 8/h). (**d**) MRI demonstrated the absence of obstruction to CSF flow. (**e**) Intraoperative view of FFMBA performed at 3 years of age. (**f**, **g**) Preoperative clinical presentation at 3 years of age. (**h**, **i**) One year after FFMBA at 4 years of age. (**j**, **k**) 5 years after FFMBA at 8 years of age. (**l**, **m**) Clinical presentation 11 years after FFMBA, at age 14 years, before secondary LF3. (**n**, **o**) CT scan at age 14 before LF3.Polysomnography demonstrated mild sleep ASOS (AHI = 8 per hour). (**p**, **q**) LF3 performed at 15 years of age with a rigid external device. (**r**, **s**) CT scan showing the osteotomies and the external traction. (**t**, **u**) At age 18 before rhinoplasty and orthognathic surgery. Polysomnography was normal (AHI = 0.2 per hour). (**v**, **w**) After rhinoplasty and orthognathic surgery involving genioplasty (cf. Fig. 13.8 for additional photographs of this patient)

10.1.2 Example №2 of Management Strategy in Crouzon Syndrome

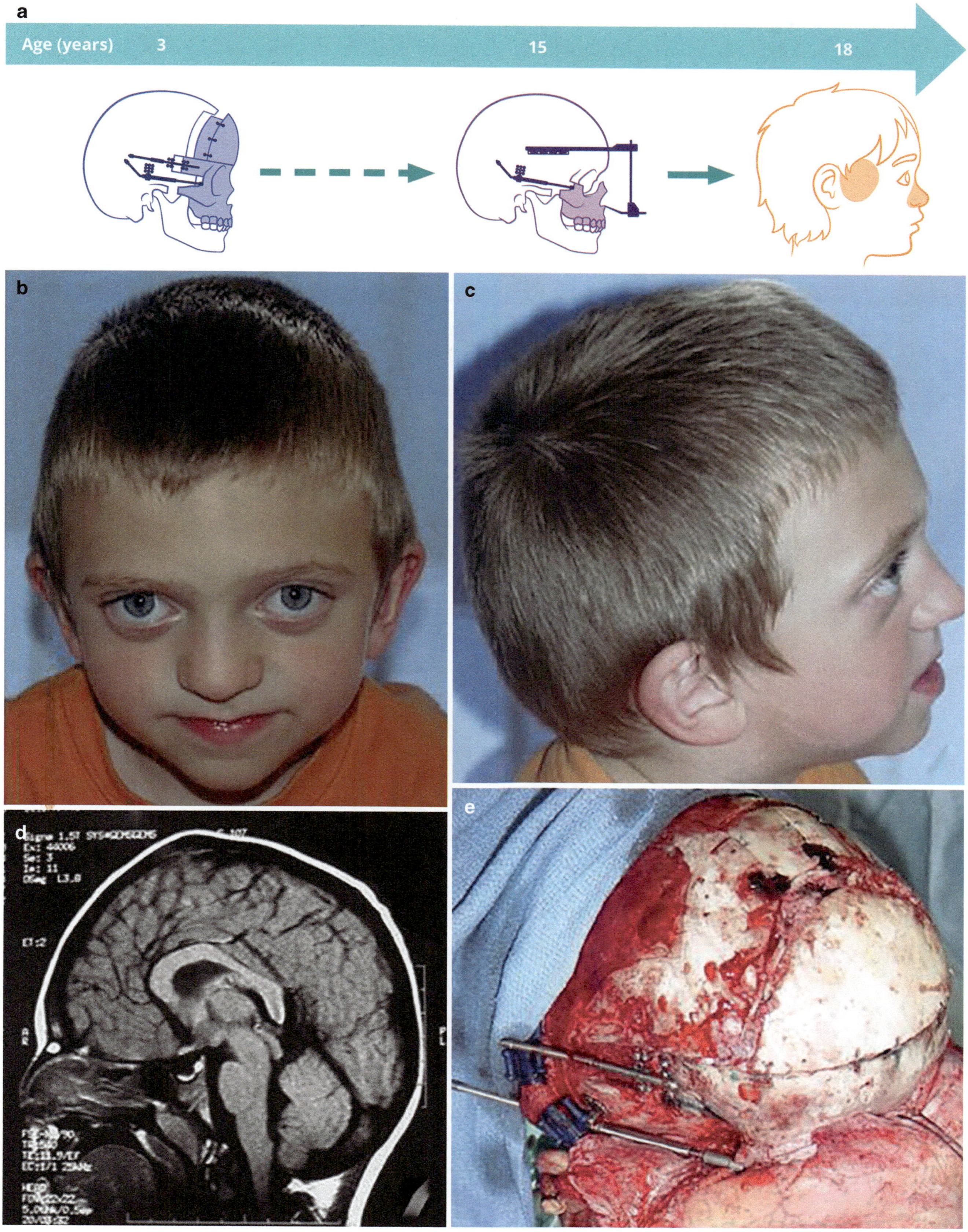

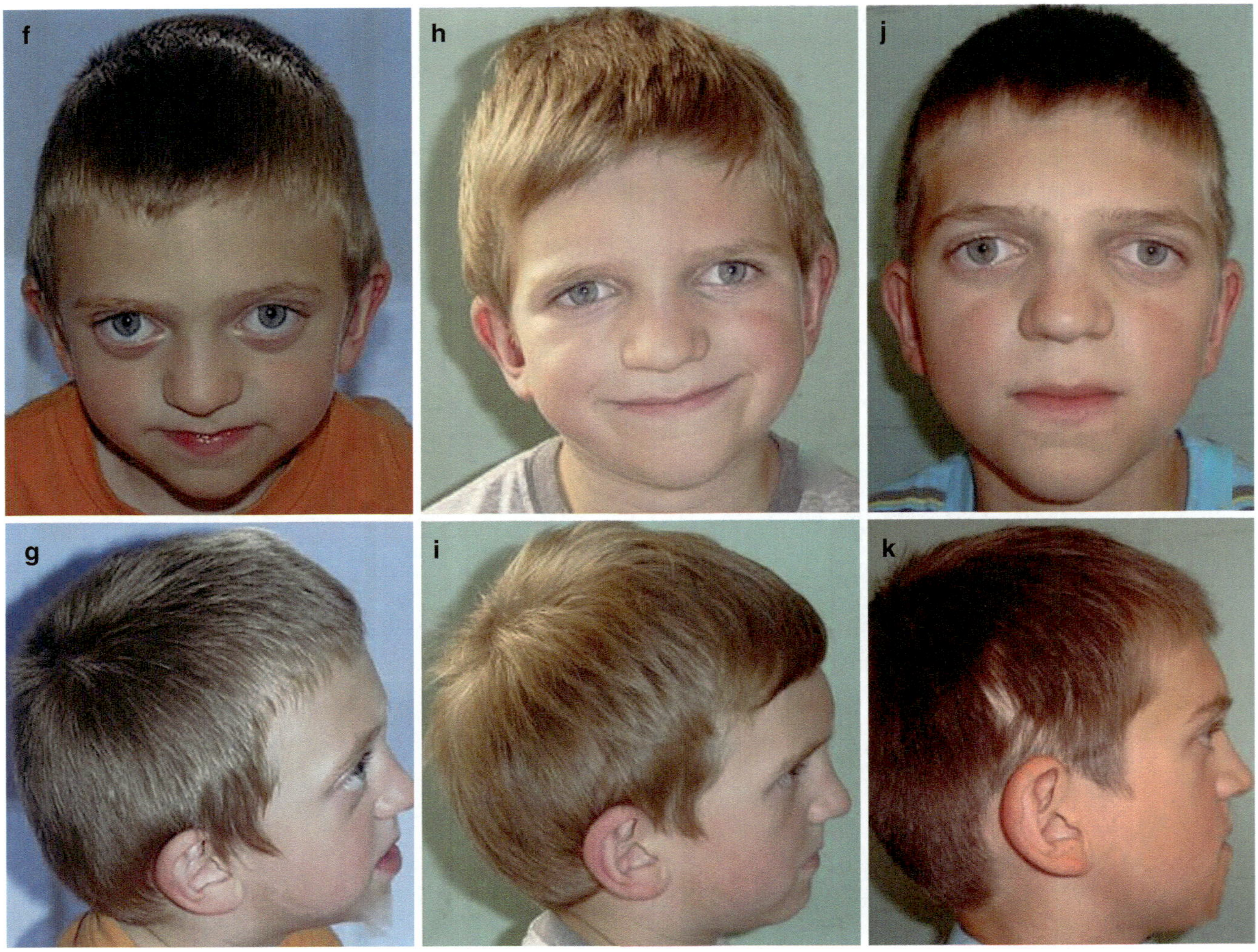

Fig. 10.4 (continued)

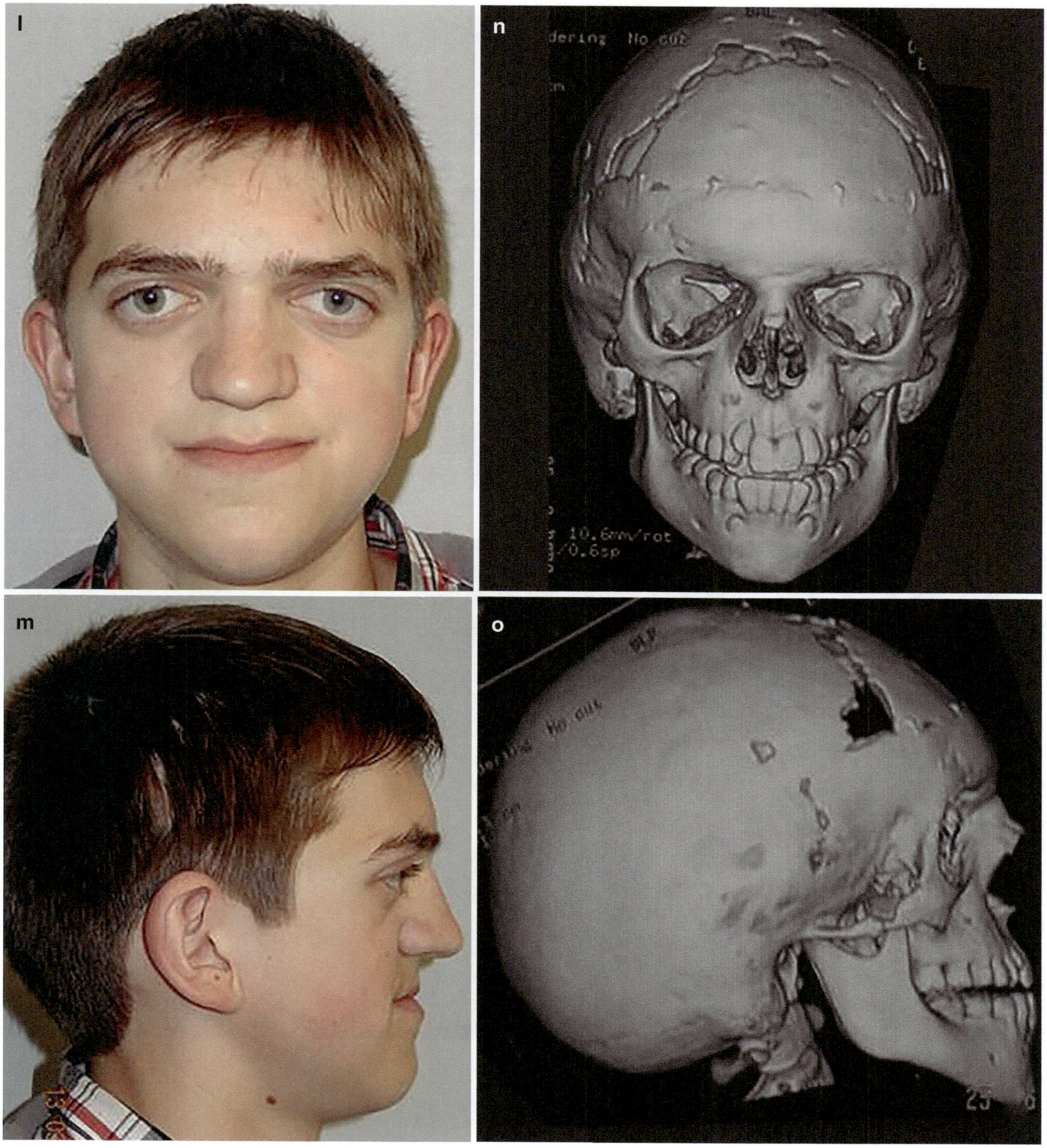

Fig. 10.4 (continued)

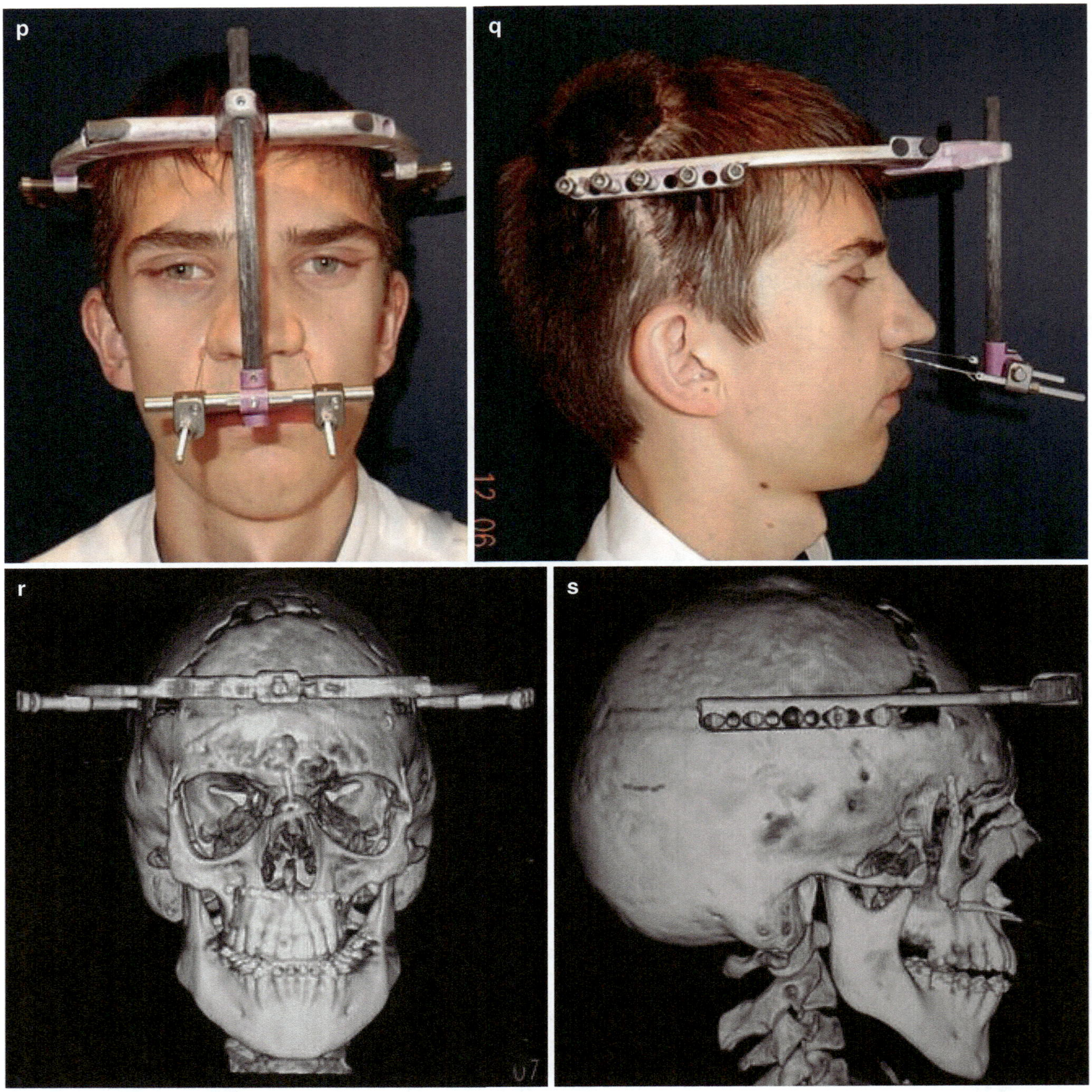

Fig. 10.4 (continued)

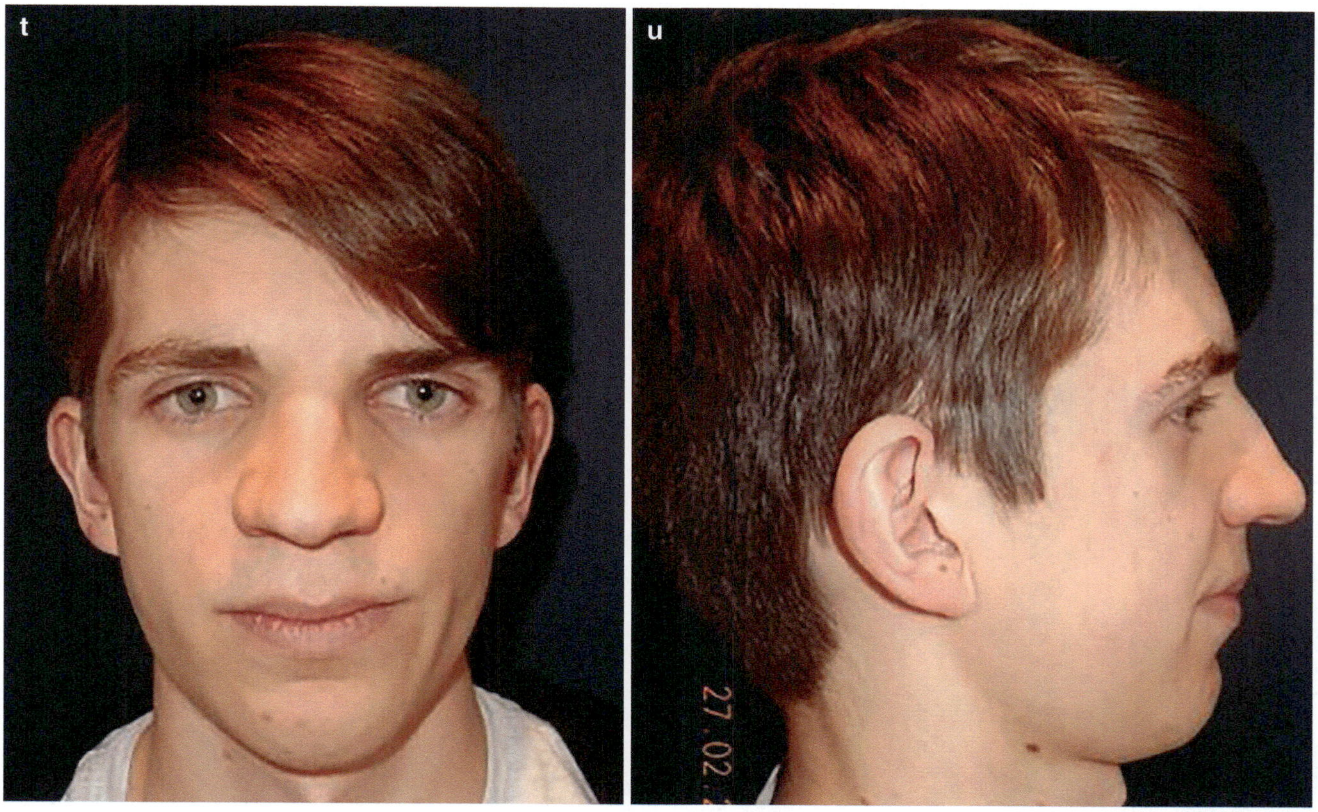

Fig. 10.4 (continued)

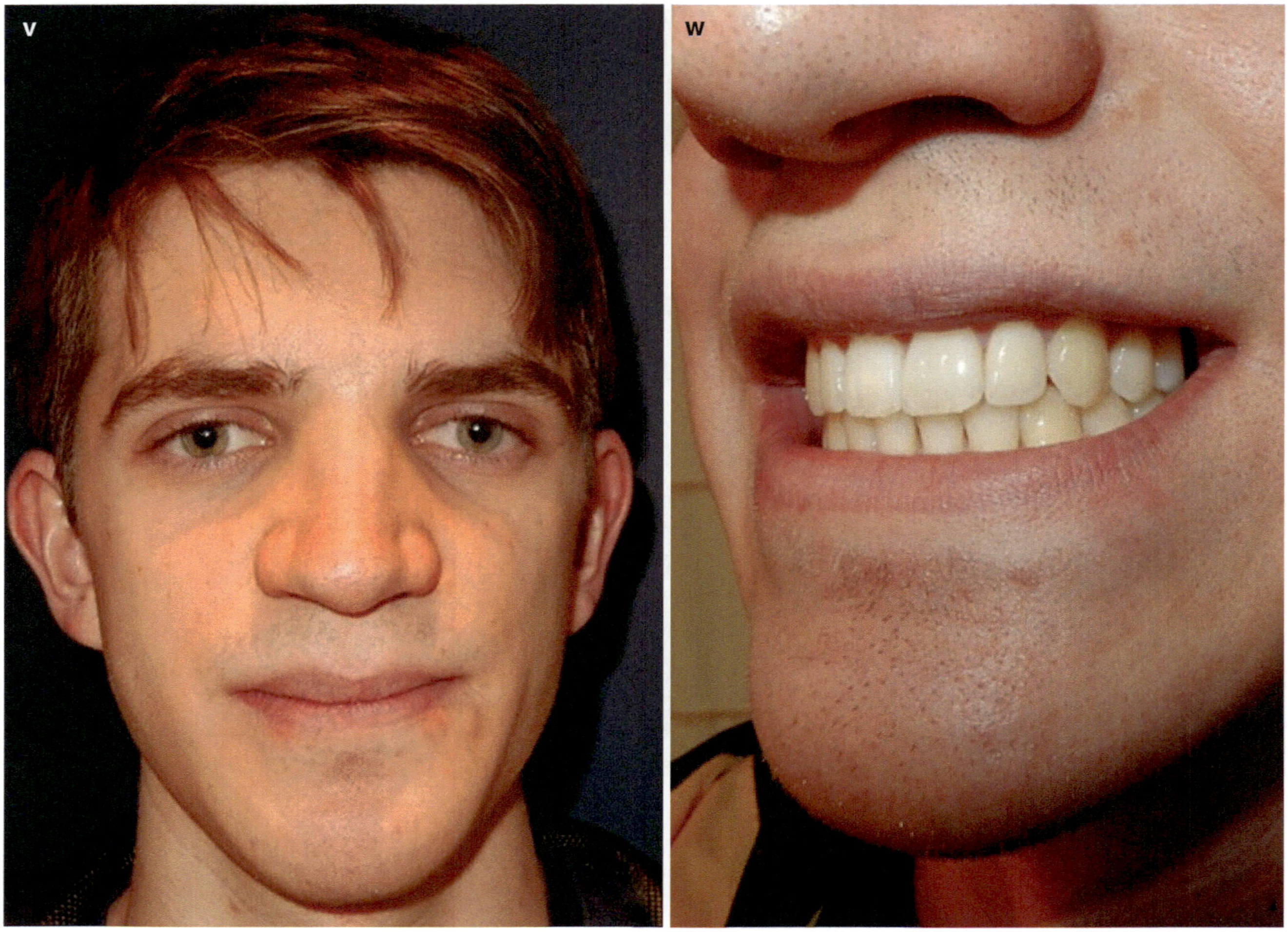

Fig. 10.4 (continued)

Fig. 10.5 (**a**) Management plan for a 15-year-old patient with Crouzon syndrome with previous FOA during infancy performed elsewhere. ©Cassandra Vion. (**b**, **c**, **d**) Clinical presentation at 15 years of age showing severe exorbitism due to maxillary hypoplasia and mild forehead retrusion. Occlusion is Angle class I. (**e**, **f**) CT scan at 16 years of age displaying coronal limited bony defects secondary to primary FOA. Polysomnography showed mild OSA (AHI = 6 per hour). (**g**, **h**) FFMBA performed at 16 years of age. (**i**, **j**) Initial presentation at 15 years of age before FFMBA. (**k**, **l**) Result 1 year after FFMBA demonstrating improvement of exorbitism and maxillary retrusion. Lateral canthal descent occurred despite intraoperative lateral canthopexies with overcorrection. Polysomnography was normalized (AHI = 1 per hour). (**m**, **n**) CT scan 1 year after FFMBA. Cf. Fig. 11.4. for subsequent aesthetic refinements to the chin and nose

10.1.3 Example №3 of Management Strategy in Crouzon Syndrome

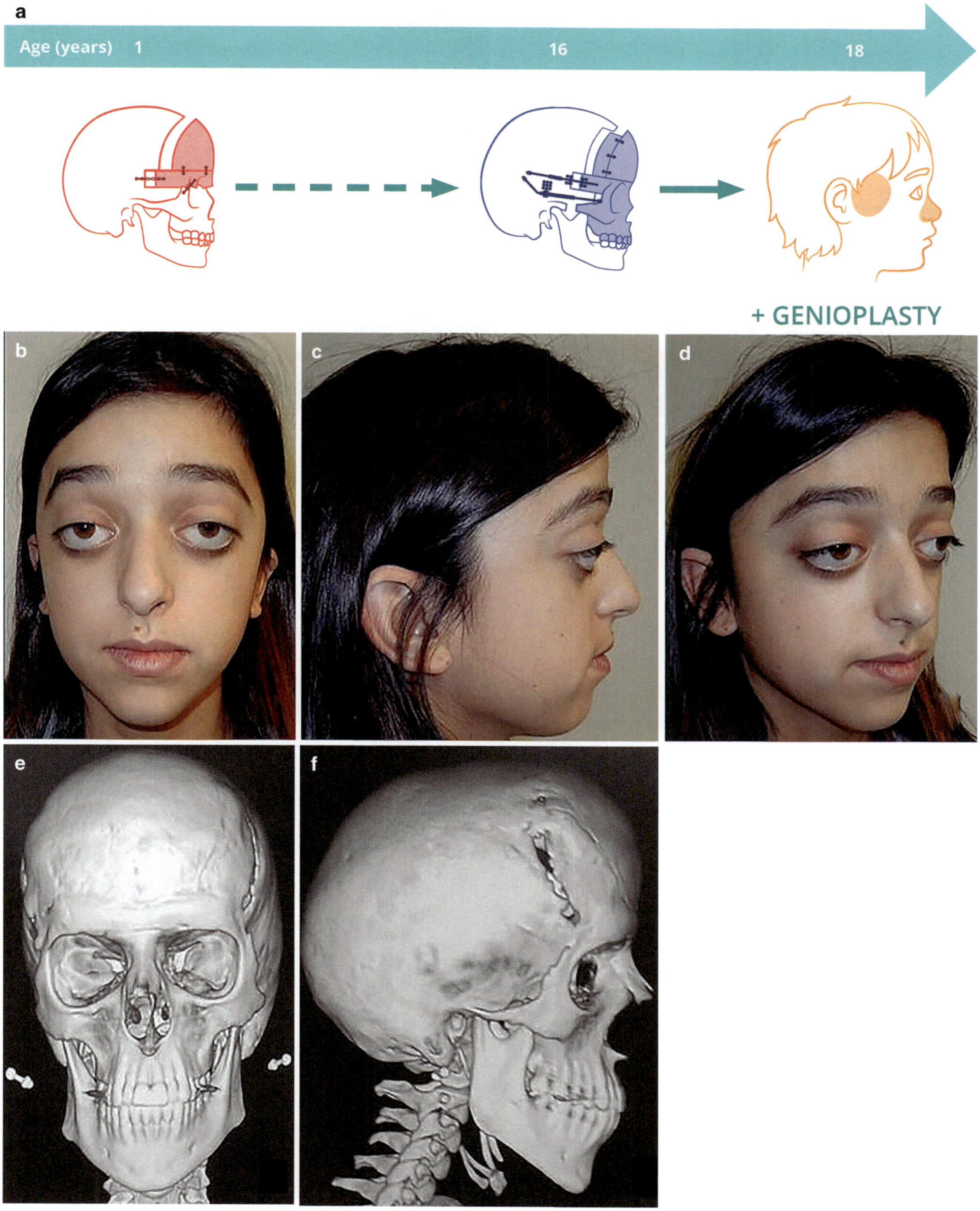

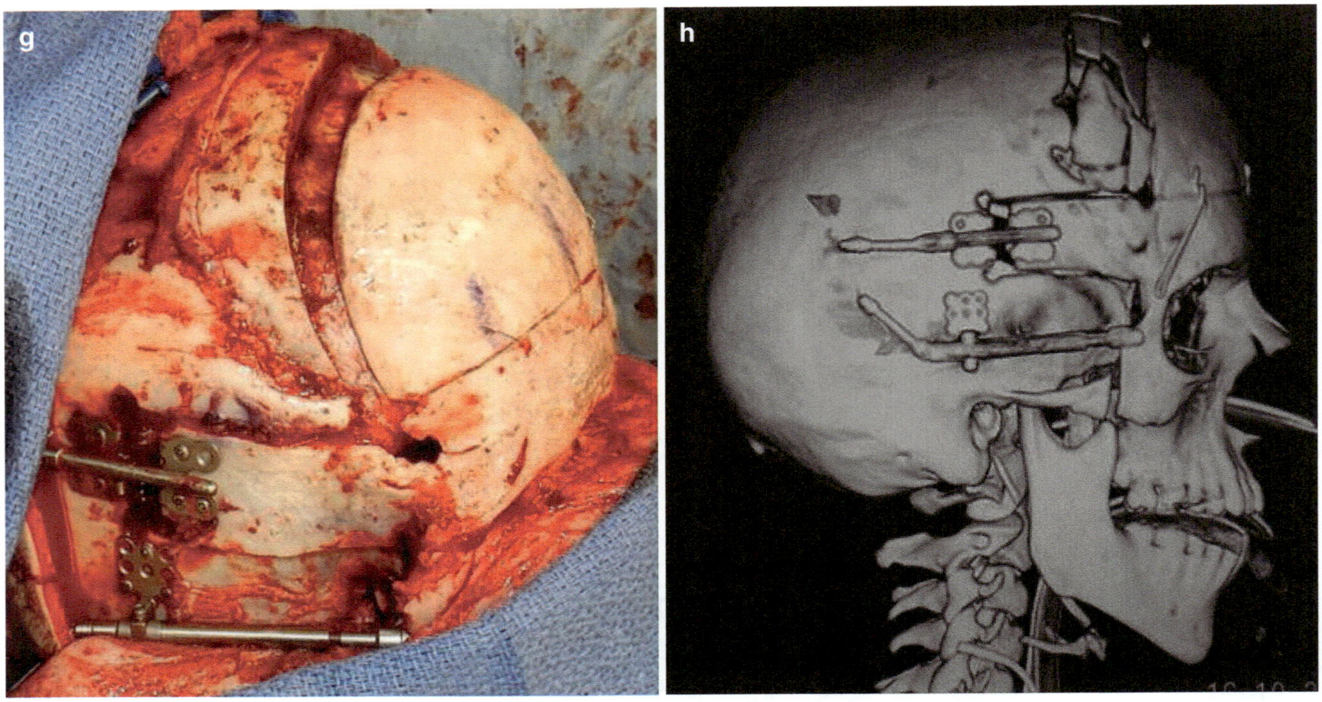

Fig. 10.5 (continued)

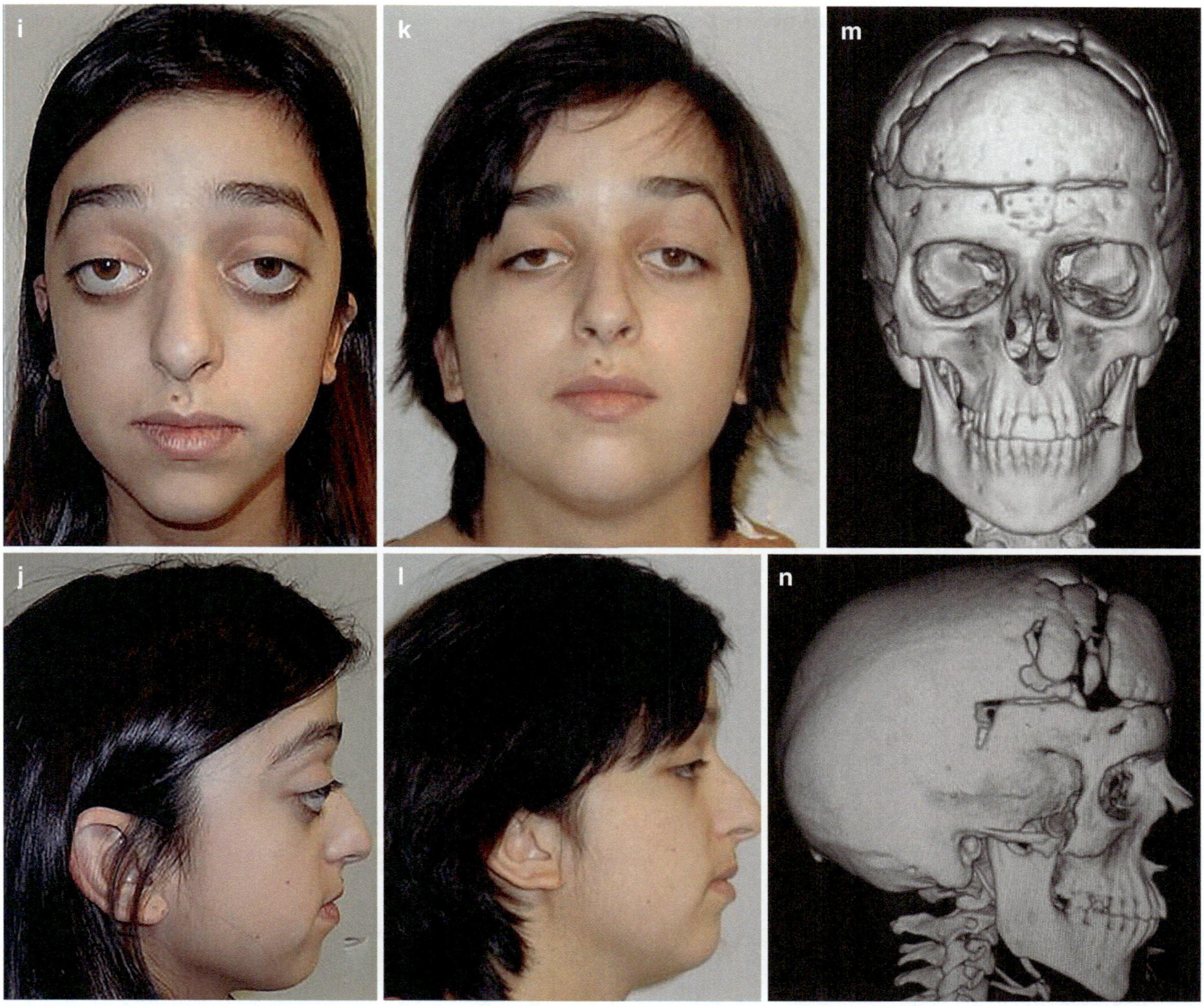

Fig. 10.5 (continued)

10.1.4 Example №4 of Management Strategy in Crouzon Syndrome

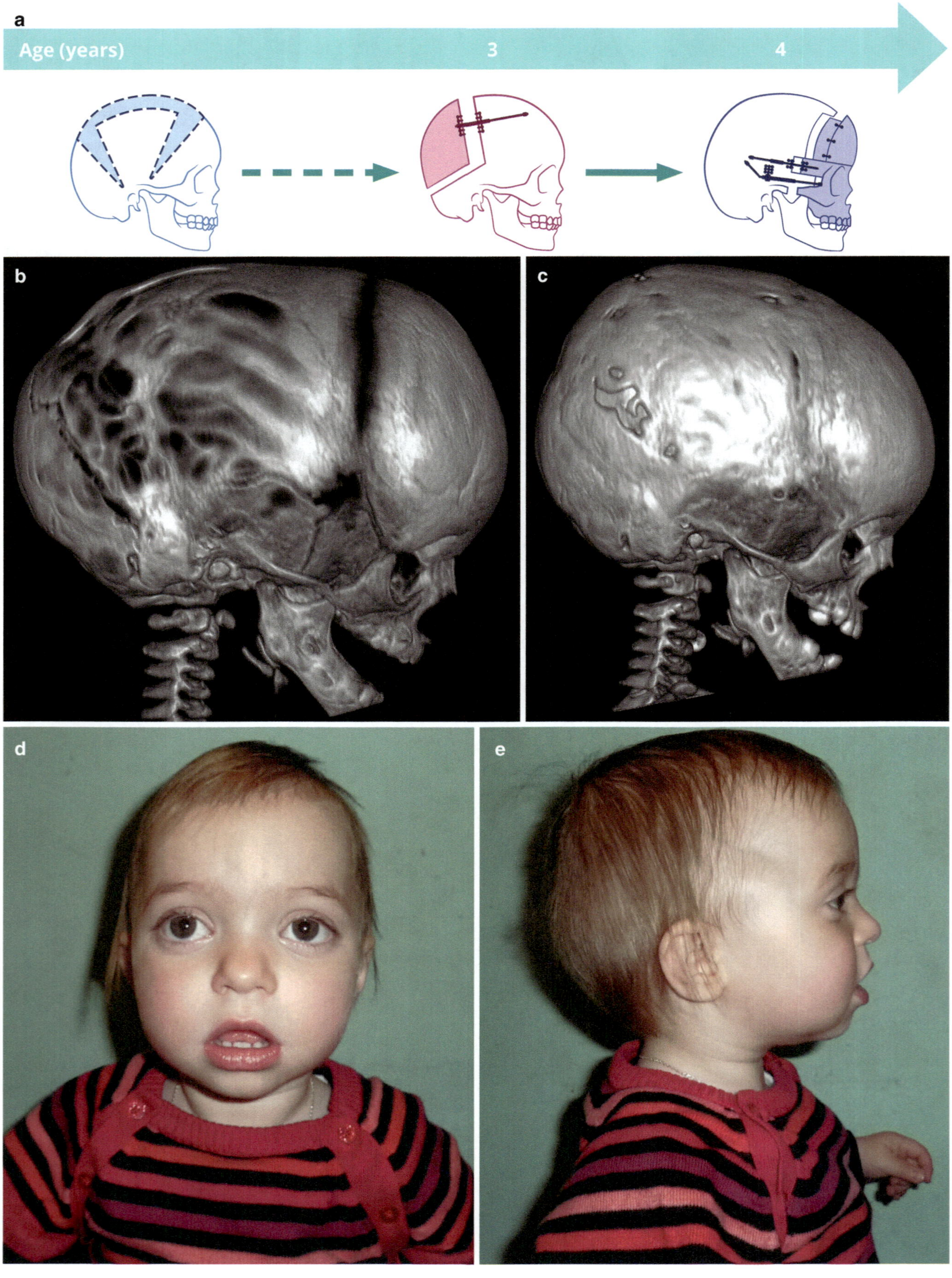

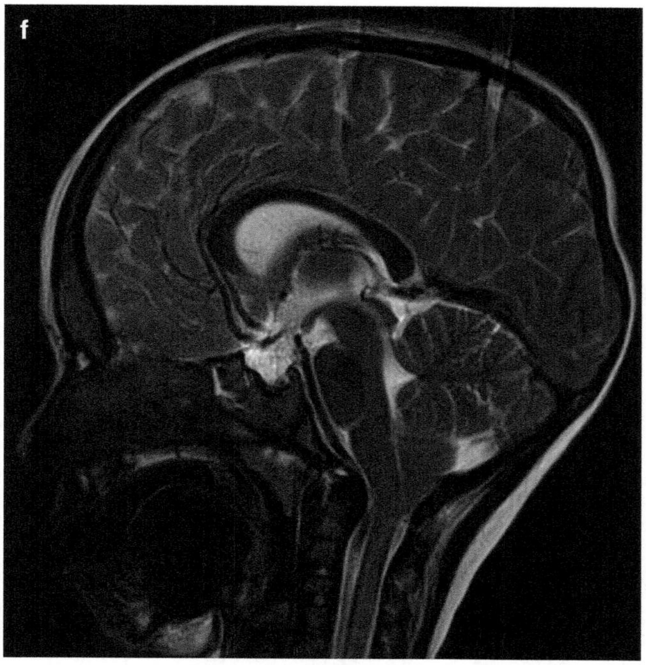

Fig. 10.6 (continued)

Fig. 10.6 (**a**) Management strategy in a patient with Crouzon syndrome involving calvarial remodeling, PVE, and subsequent FFMBA. ©Cassandra Vion. (**b**) The patient first presented with scaphocephaly due to initial sagittal craniosynostosis. She underwent H-craniectomy at age 5 months. The genetic workup was motivated by excessive copperbeating of the cranium. It revealed FGFR2 mutation. (**c**) Three-month-postoperative CT scan showing resolution of copperbeating (age 8 months). (**d**, **e**) Clinical photographs at 18 months of age. Anterior open bite is associated with nocturnal pacifier use. (**f**) At age 3 years, the systematic fundoscopy revealed papillary edema. Magnetic resonance imaging showed minor tonsillar herniation without obstruction. PVE was indicated to increase intracranial volume and relieve papilledema. (**g**, **h**, **i**) Clinical photographs at 42 months of age demonstrating mild midface hypoplasia. Moderate obstructive sleep apnea was diagnosed (Apnea-Hypopnea Index = 7 per hour). FFMBA was indicated to relieve respiratory symptoms. (**j**, **k**) Intraoperative view of the FFMBA performed at 43 months of age. (**l**) CT scan 3 weeks after FFMBA demonstrating the progress of distraction. (**m**) CT scan 6 weeks after FFMBA at the end of distraction. (**n**, **o**, **p**) Clinical presentation at age 6 years, 30 months after FFMBA. Polysomnography and fundoscopy confirm the resolution of obstructive sleep apnea and papilledema. Persistence of a residual anterior open bite. (**q**) CT scan at 6 years of age. (**r**) MRI confirms the improvement of cerebellar tonsillar herniation

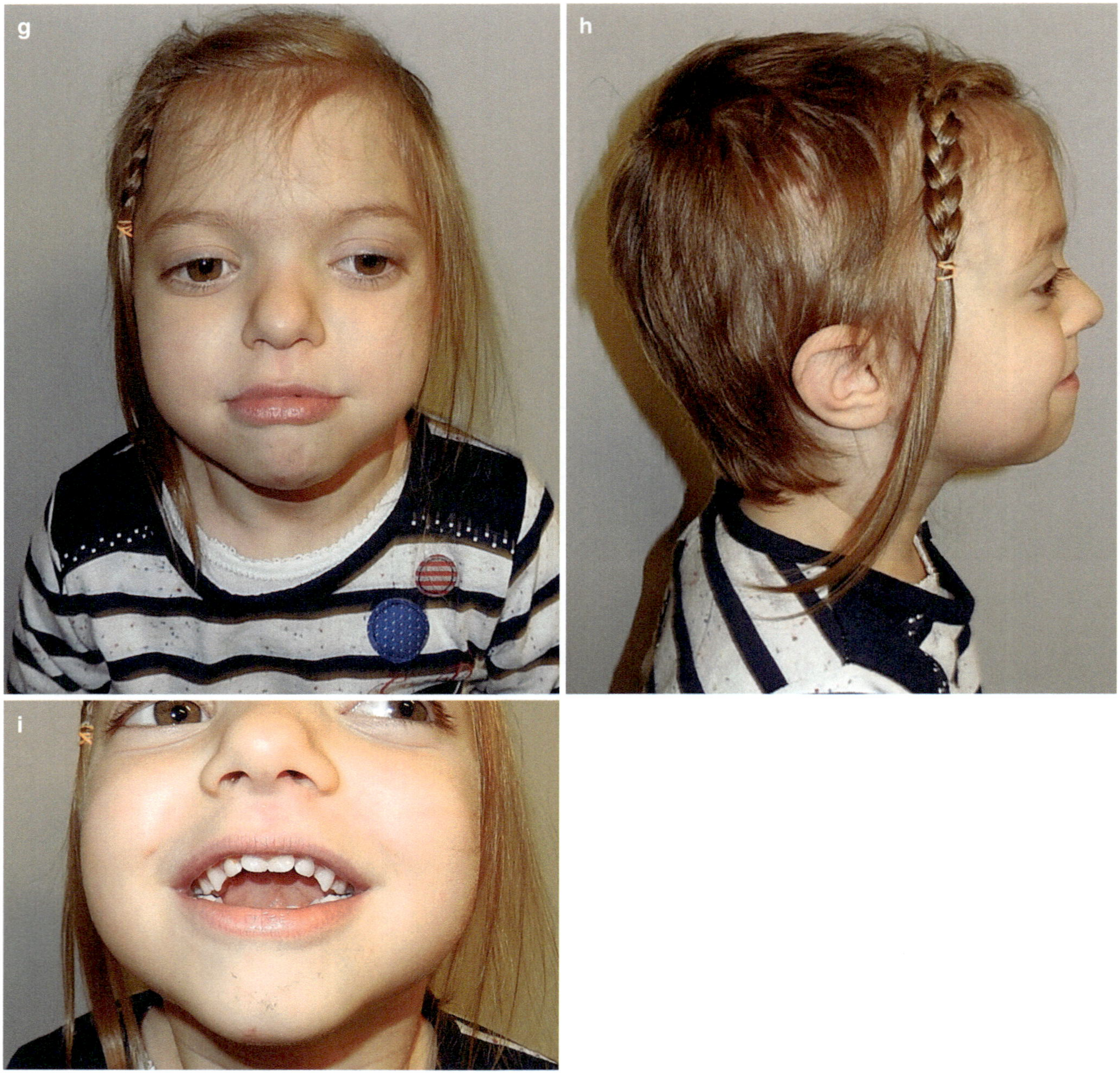

Fig. 10.6 (continued)

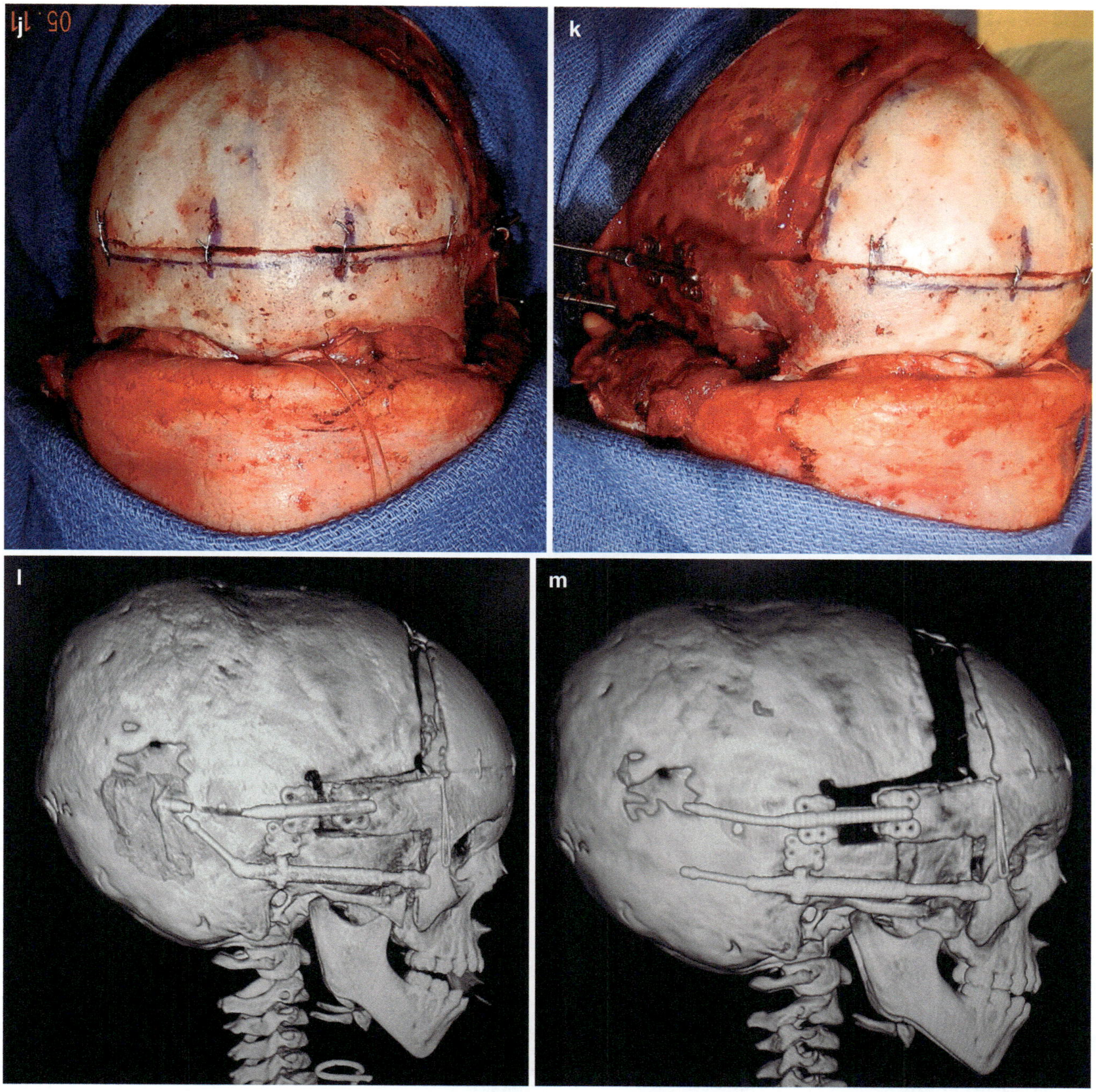

Fig. 10.6 (continued)

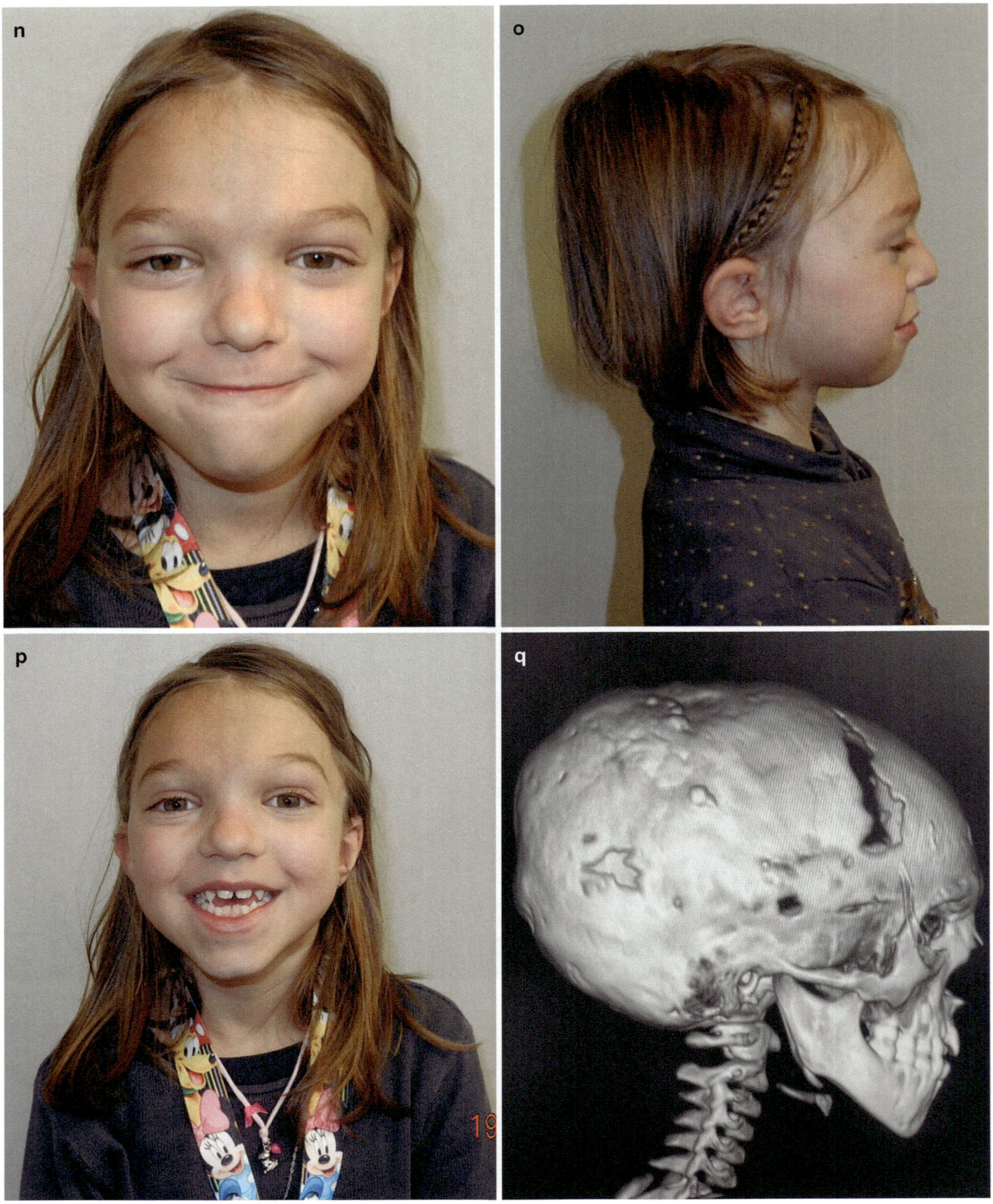

Fig. 10.6 (continued)

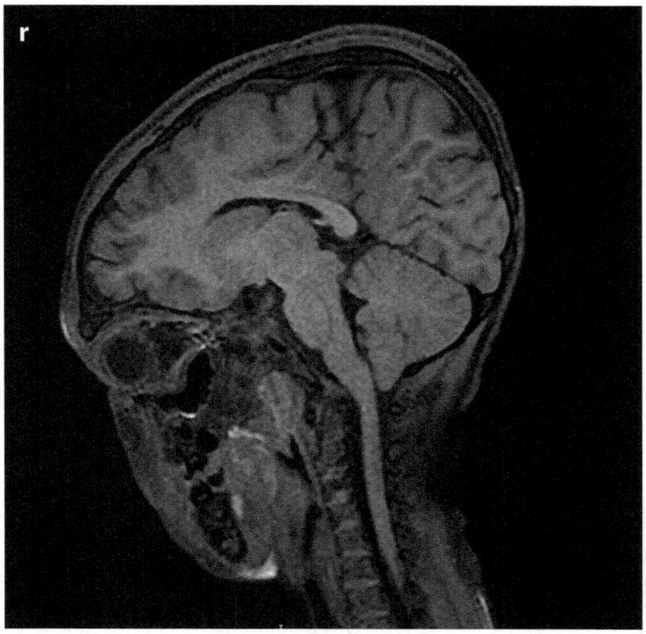

Fig. 10.6 (continued)

10.1.5 Example № 5 of Management Strategy in Crouzon Syndrome

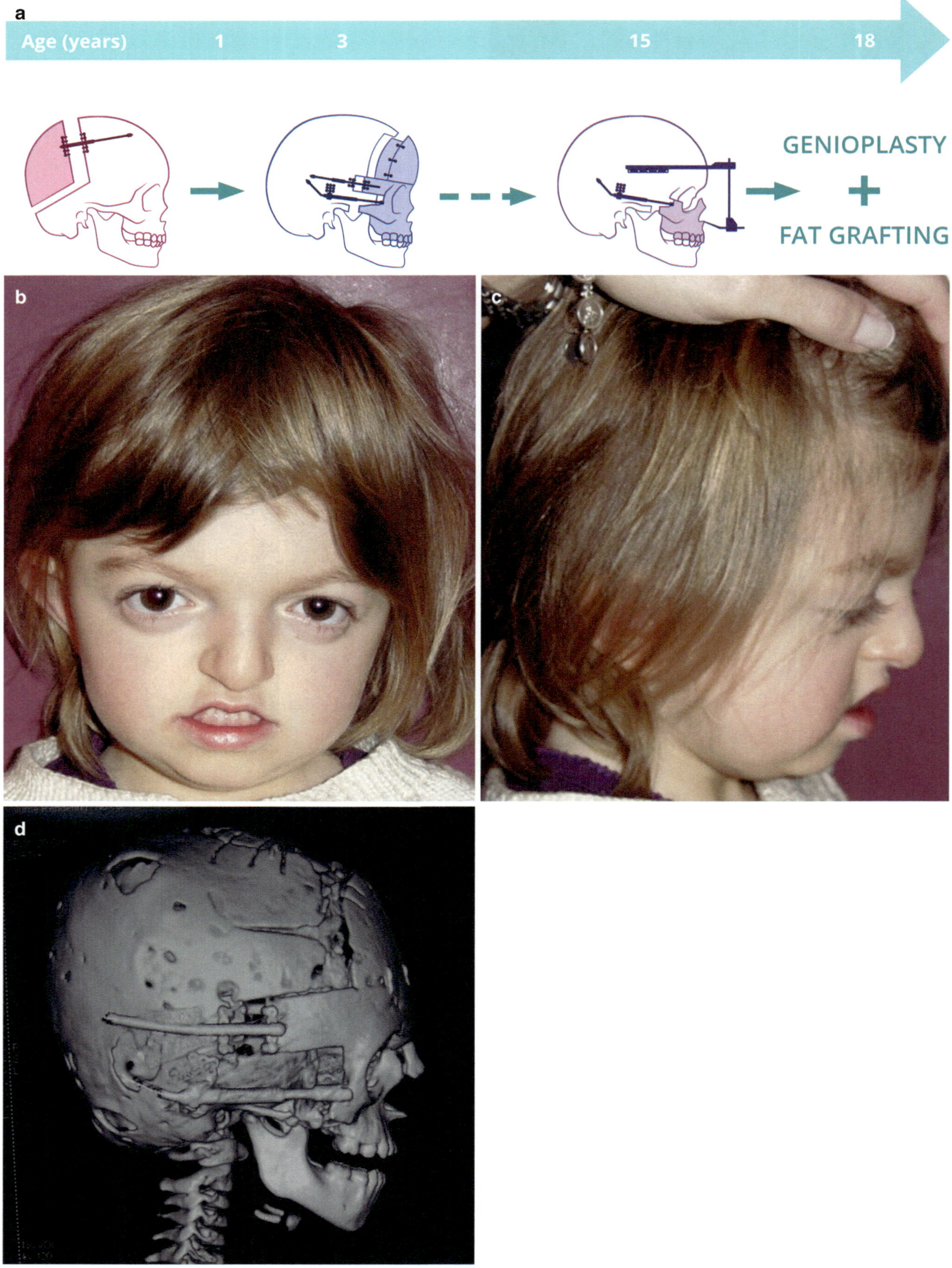

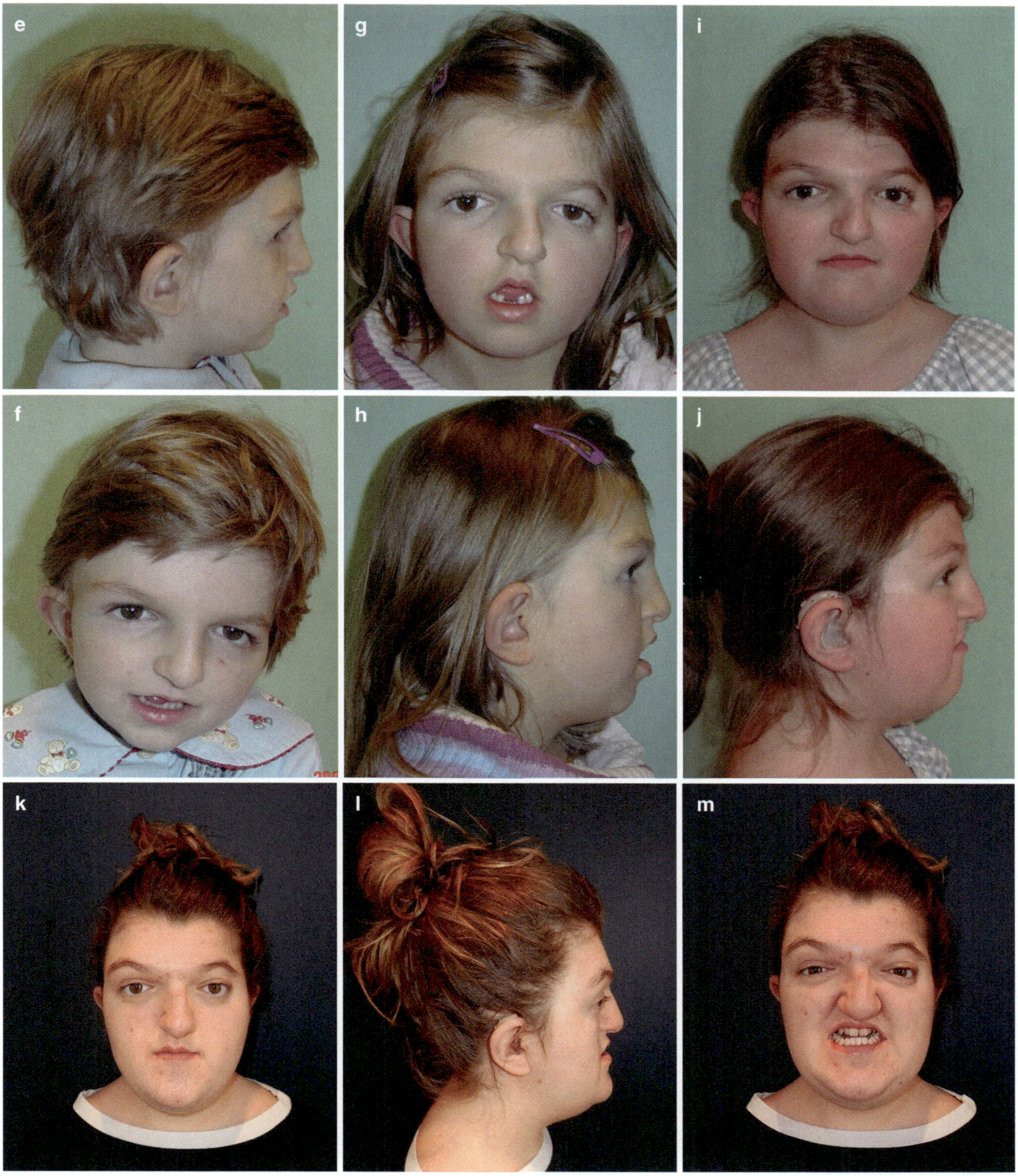

Fig. 10.7 (continued)

Fig. 10.7 (**a**) Management strategy in Crouzon syndrome involving PVE, FFMBA, LF3, and aesthetic procedures. ©Cassandra Vion. (**b**, **c**) At 3 years of age, after PVE performed at age 6 months. (**d**) FFMBA performed at age 3 years. (**e**, **f**) Morphological results at 4 years of age, 1 year after FFMBA. (**g**, **h**) Morphological results at 6 years of age, 3 years after FFMBA. (**i**, **j**) Morphological results at 10 years of age, 7 years after FFMBA. (**k**, **l**, **m**) Clinical presentation at 16 years of age, with midface hypoplasia indicating a LF3. (**n**) During the distraction phase of the LF3 at 16 years of age. (**o**, **p**) Morphological results 3 years after LF3, before orthognathic surgery and rhinoplasty (cf. Fig. 13.7)

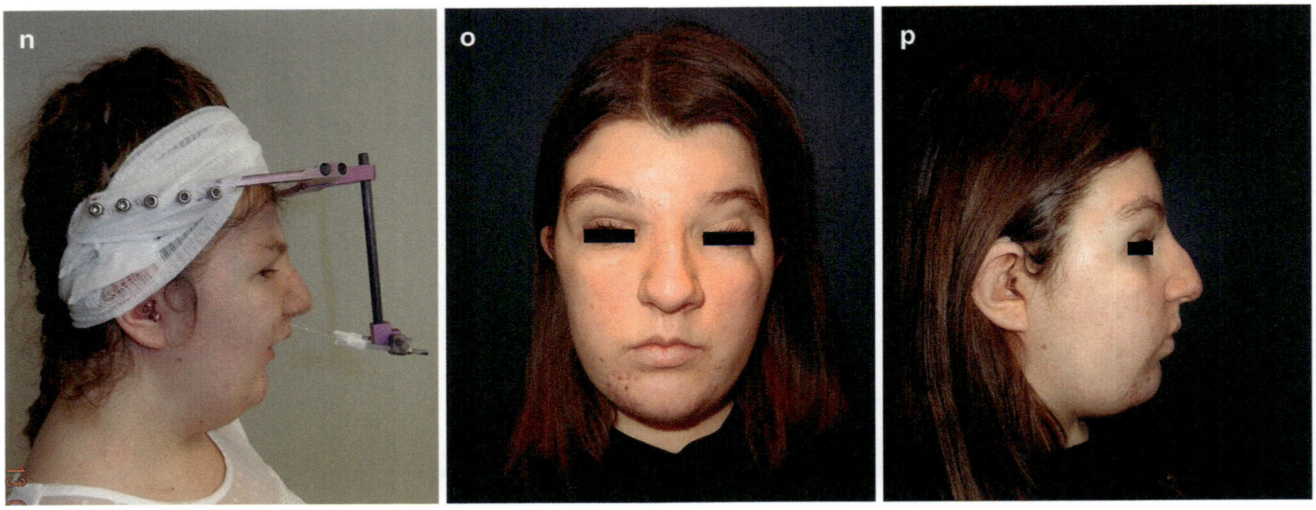

Fig. 10.7 (continued)

Fig. 10.8 (**a**) Management strategy for a patient with Crouzon syndrome presenting as scaphocephaly. ©Cassandra Vion. (**b**, **c**) Clinical presentation at 5 months of age. (**d**, **e**) CT scan demonstrating sagittal and partial bi-lambdoid craniosynostosis. (**f**, **g**) Morphological results 2 months after biparietal decompression performed at 5 months of age. (**h**, **i**, **j**) Clinical presentation at 3 years of age showing moderate midface hypoplasia. (**k**, **l**) Intraoperative view of the osteotomy lines of the FFMBA performed at 3 years of age. (**m-p**) FFMBA after distractor placement, before skin closure. (**q**, **r**, **s**) Morphological results, at 3 years and 4 months of age, 4 months after FFMBA showing overcorrection. (**t**, **u**) Clinical presentation at 13 years and 7 months of age, with progression of the midface hypoplasia. (**v**, **w**) CT scan confirmation of midface hypoplasia relapse at 12 years and 5 months of age (9 years after FFMBA). (**x**) Per-operative view of the LF3 performed at 14 years of age. (**y**, **z**) CT scan of the LF3 during the distraction period, with internal and external distractors. (**a'**, **b'**) Clinical presentation 1 year after the LF3, at 15 years of age

10.1.6 Example №6 of Management Strategy in Crouzon Syndrome

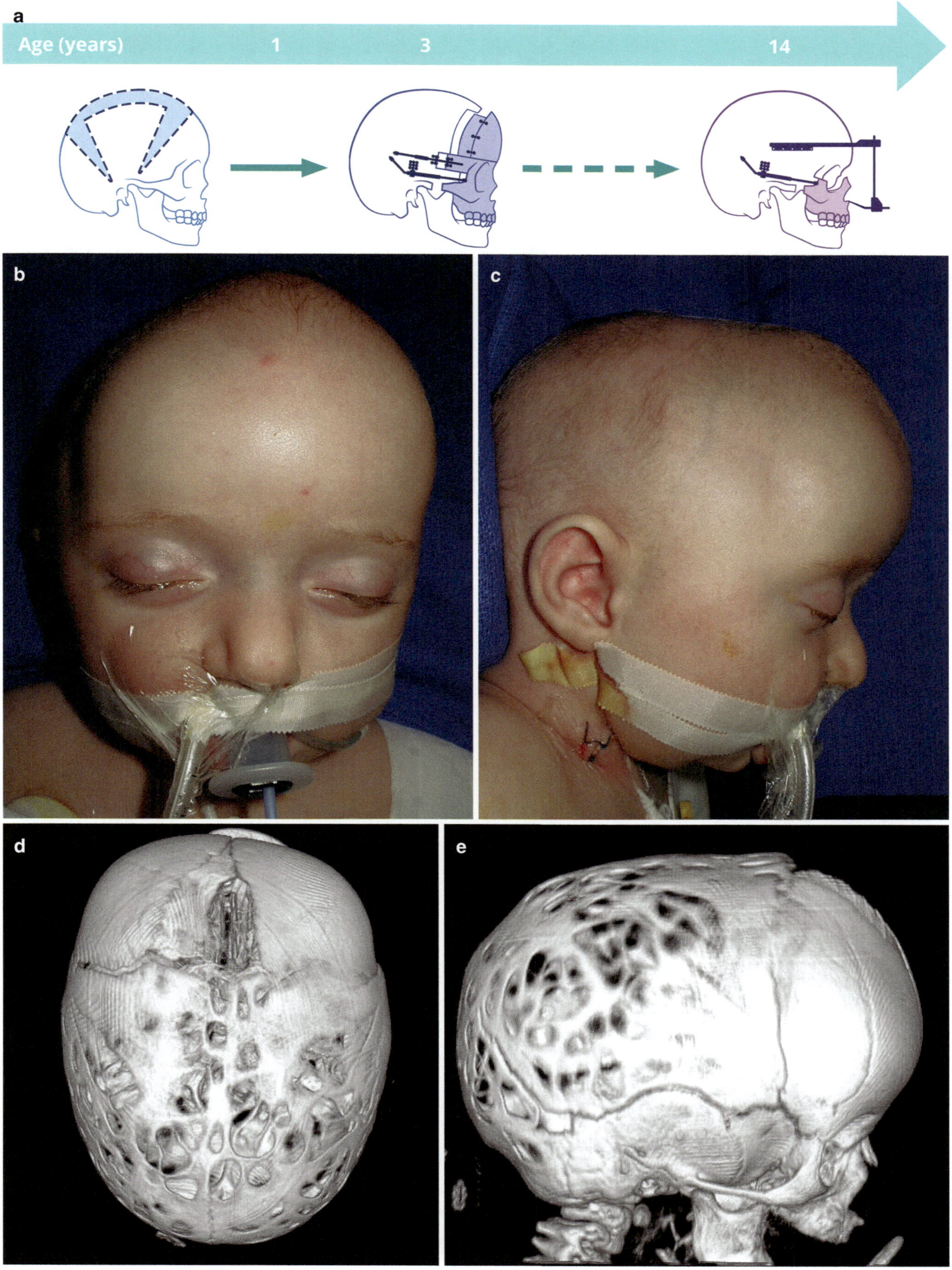

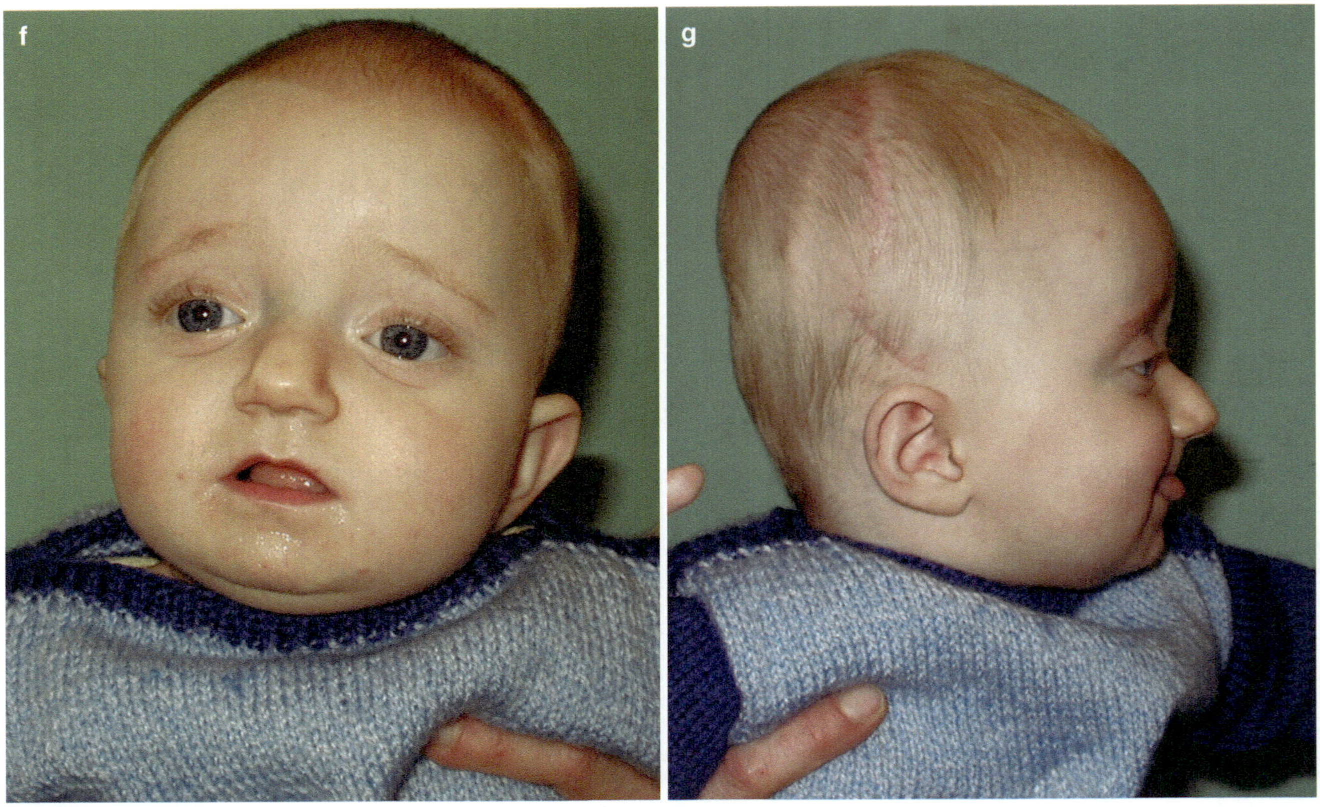

Fig. 10.8 (continued)

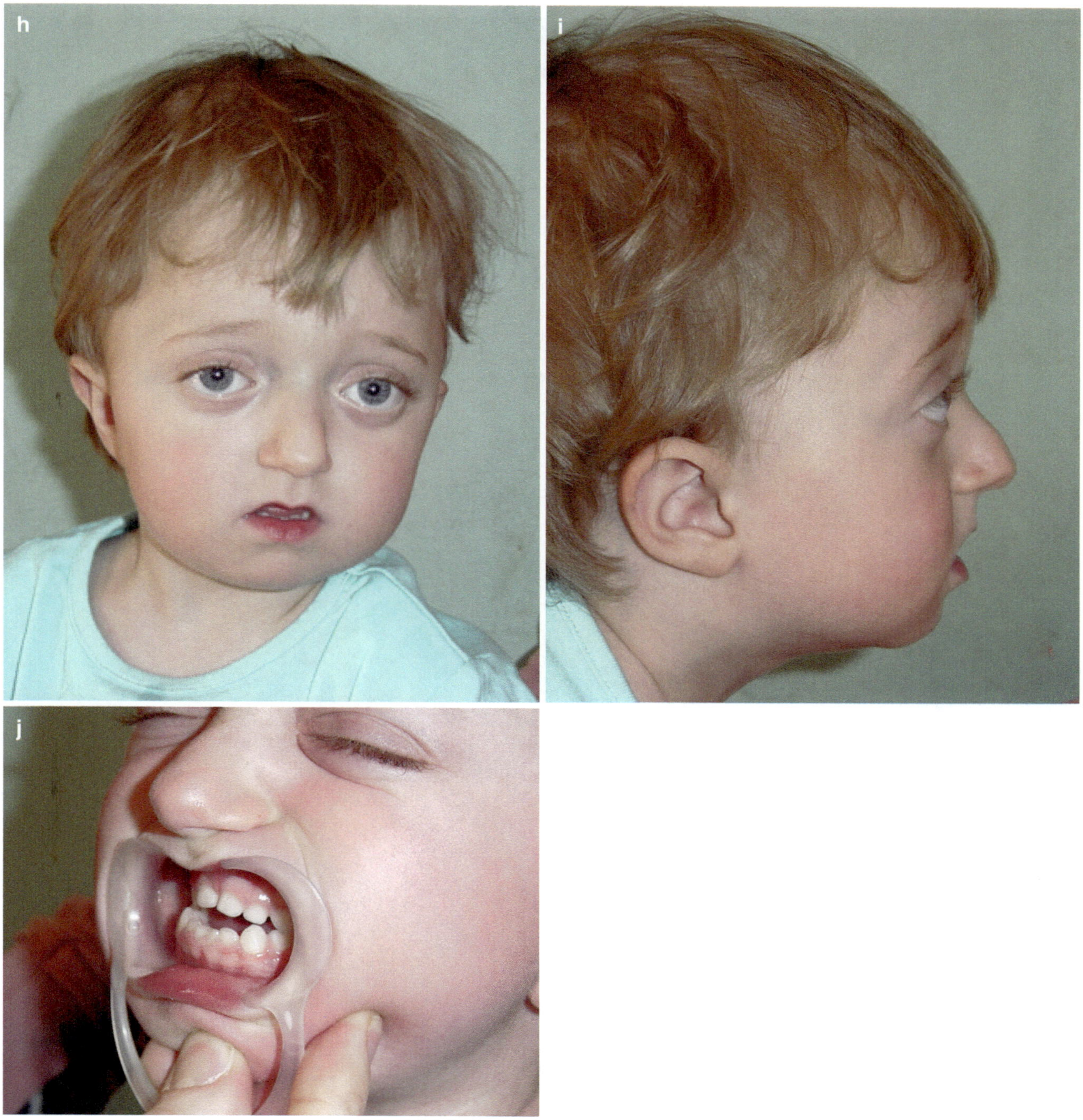

Fig. 10.8 (continued)

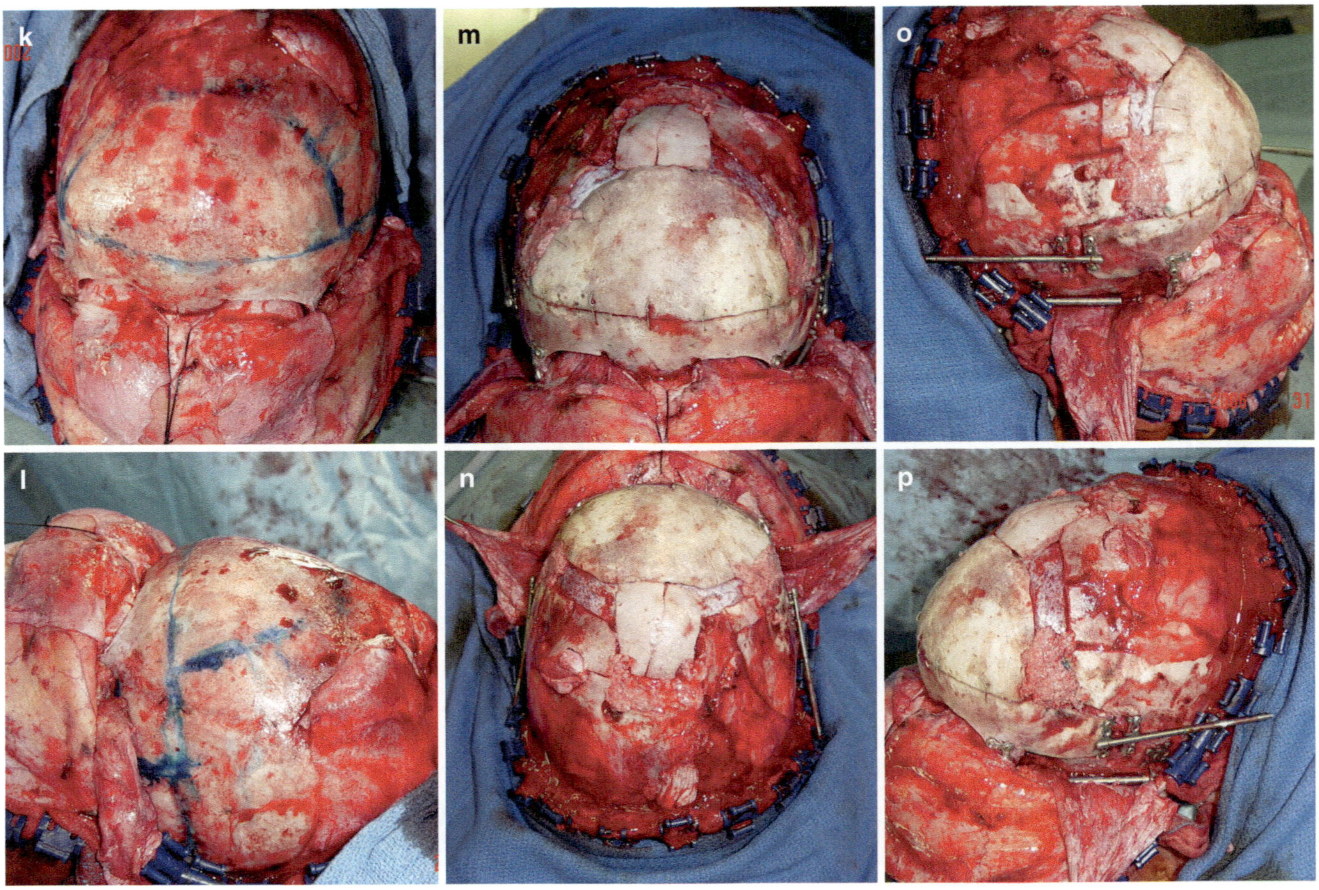

Fig. 10.8 (continued)

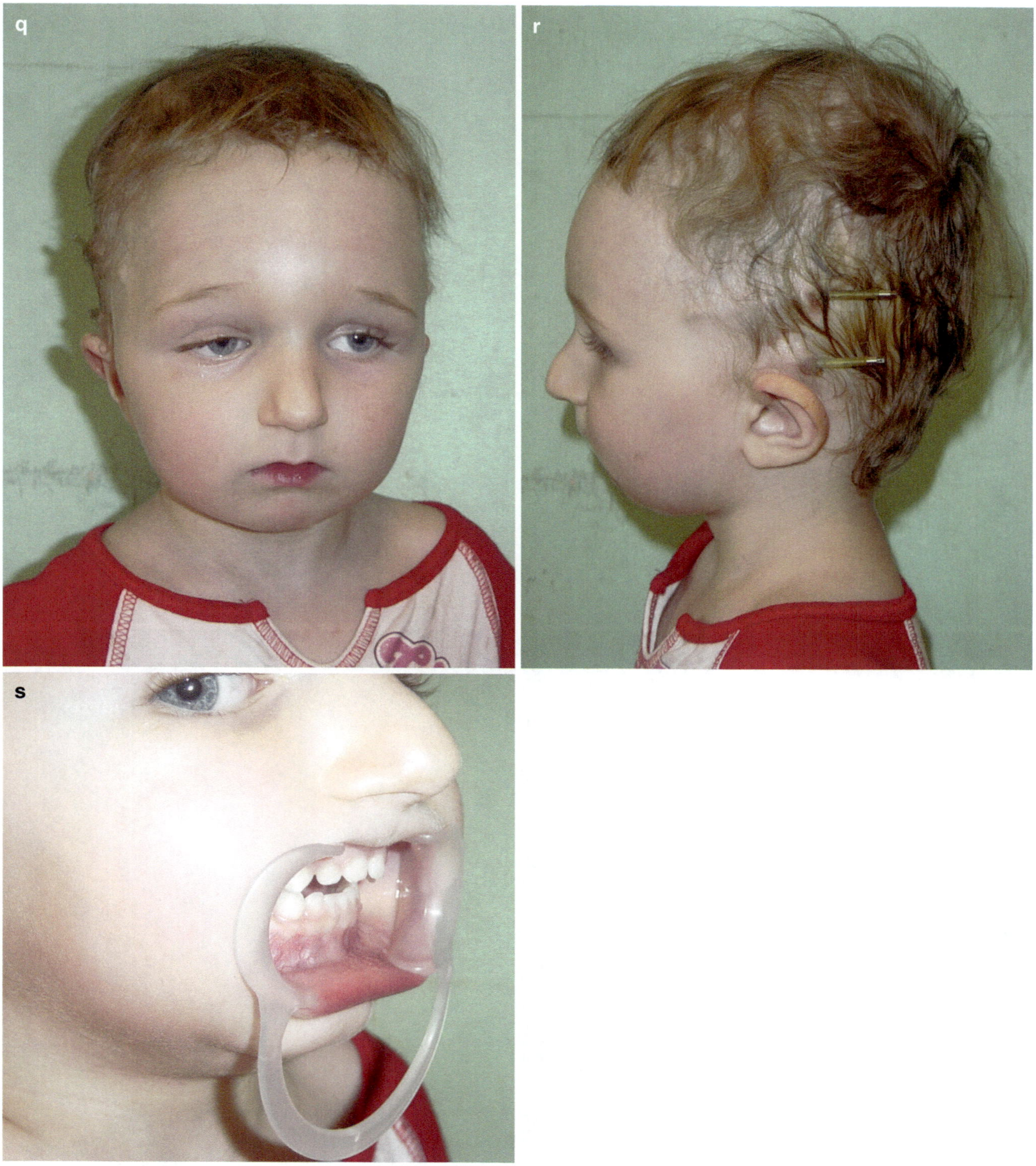

Fig. 10.8 (continued)

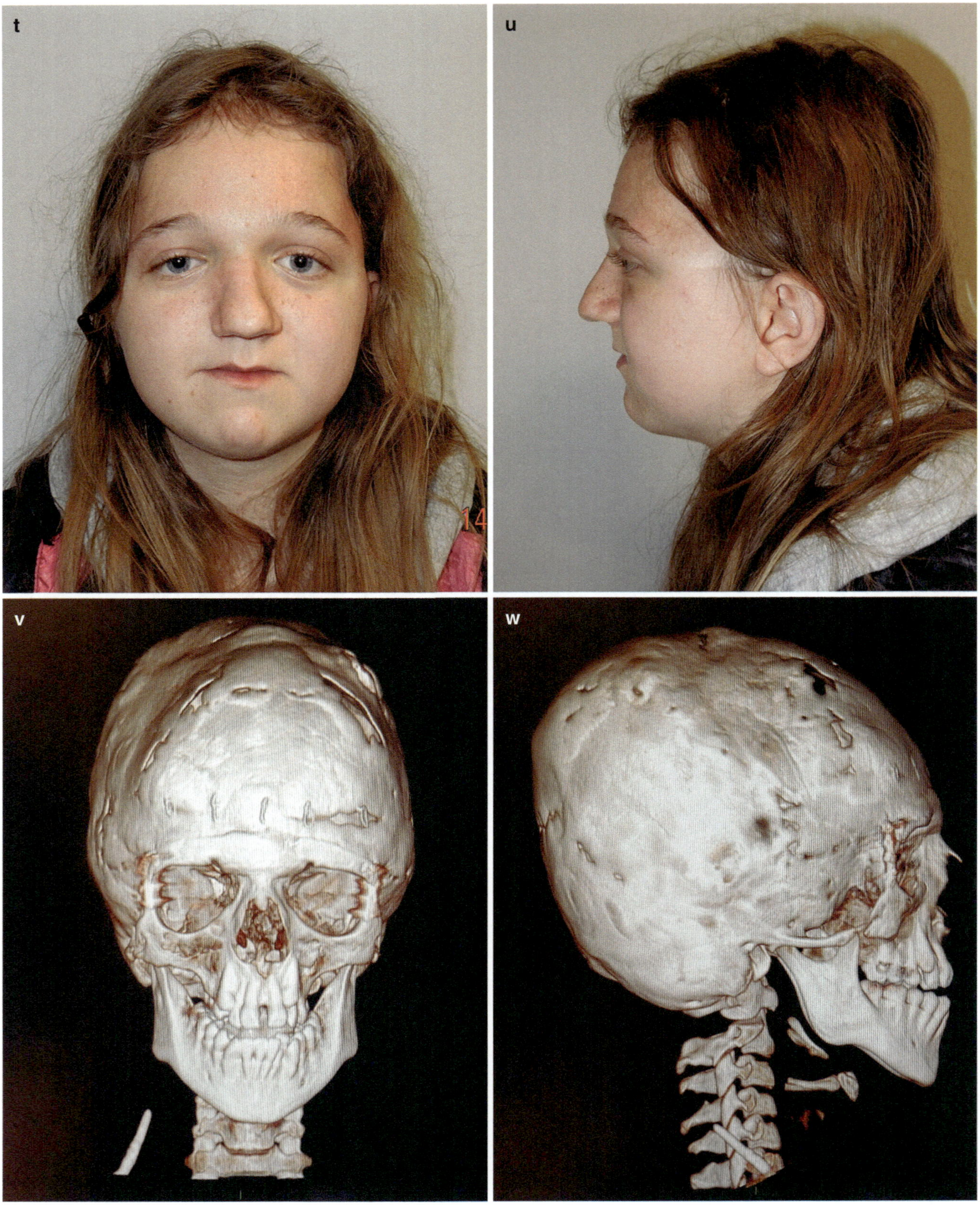

Fig. 10.8 (continued)

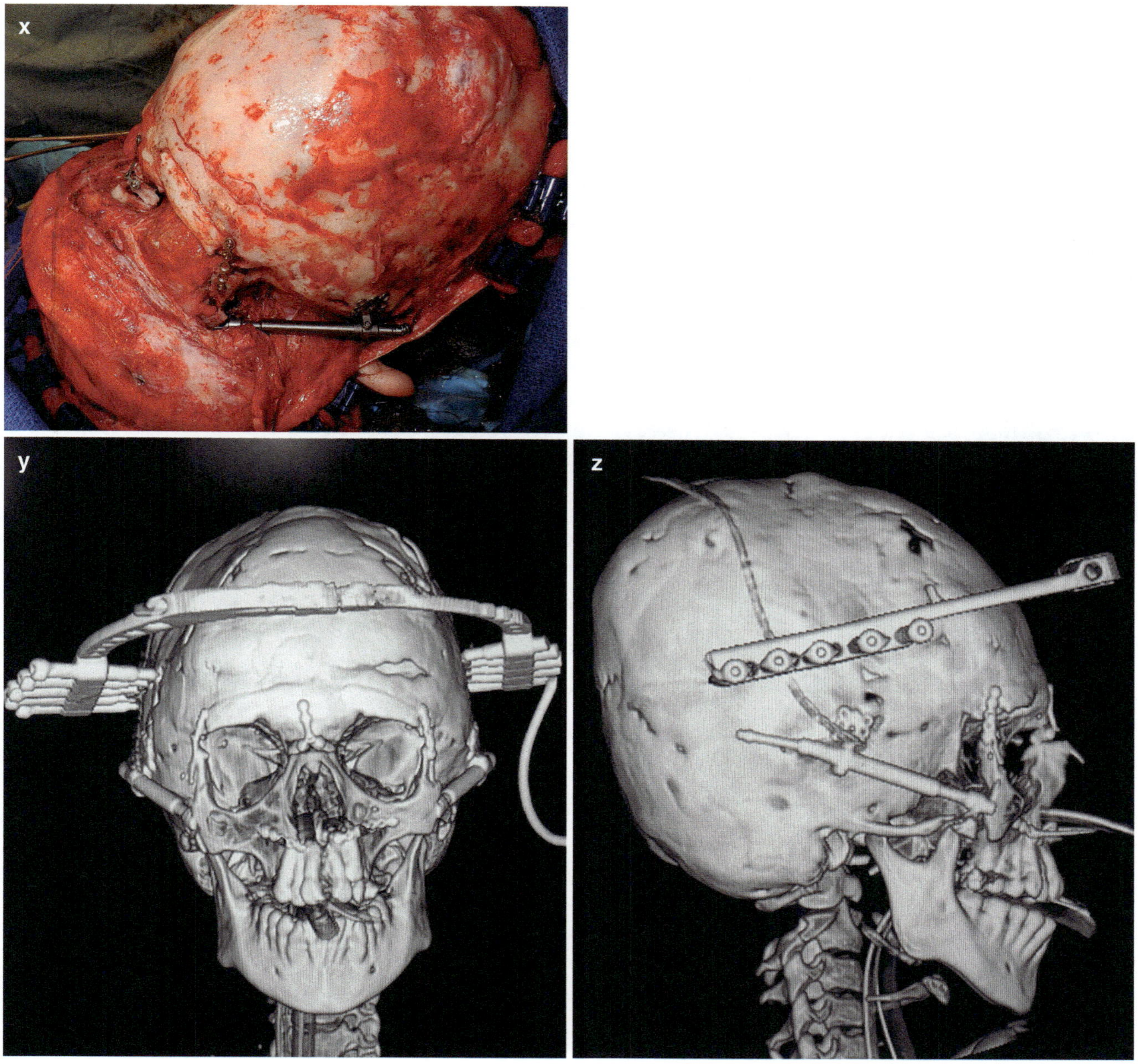

Fig. 10.8 (continued)

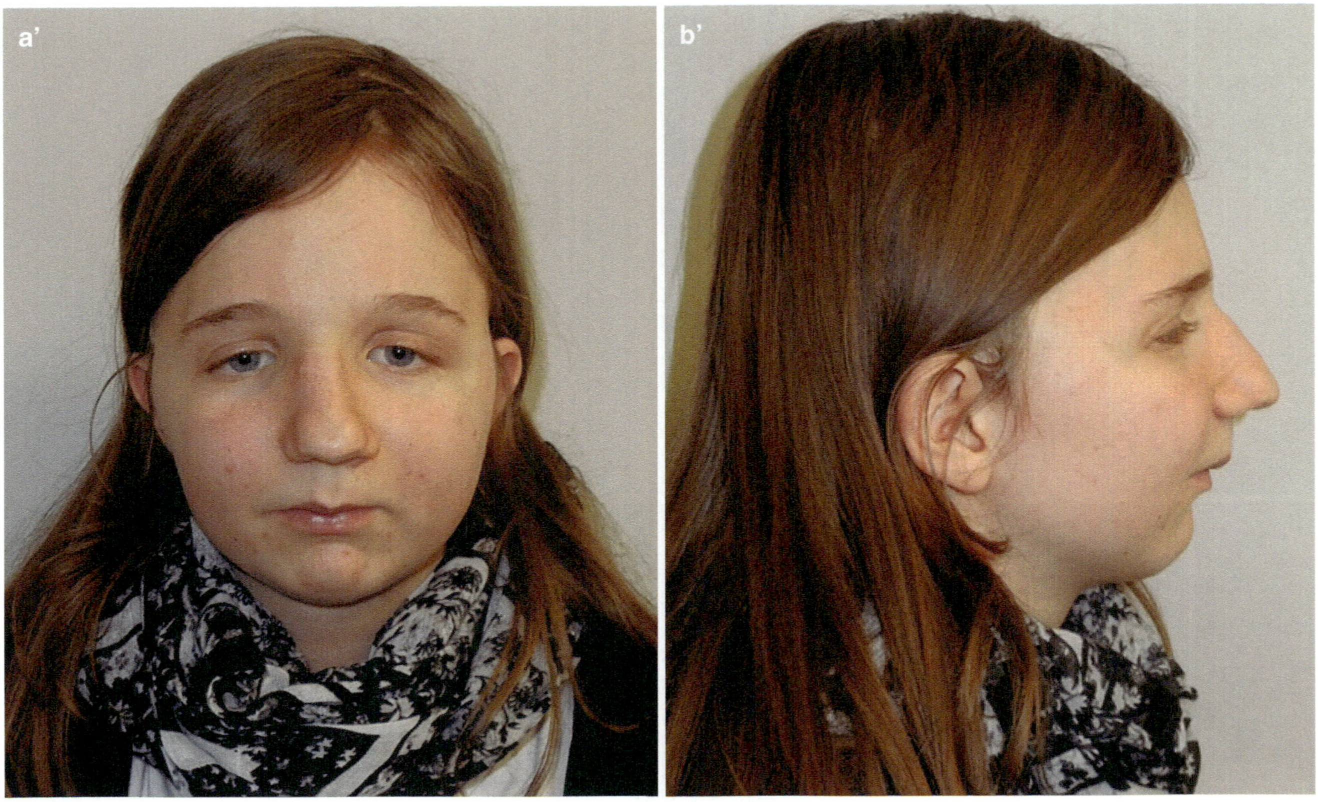

Fig. 10.8 (continued)

10.1.7 Example №7 of Management Strategy in Crouzon Syndrome

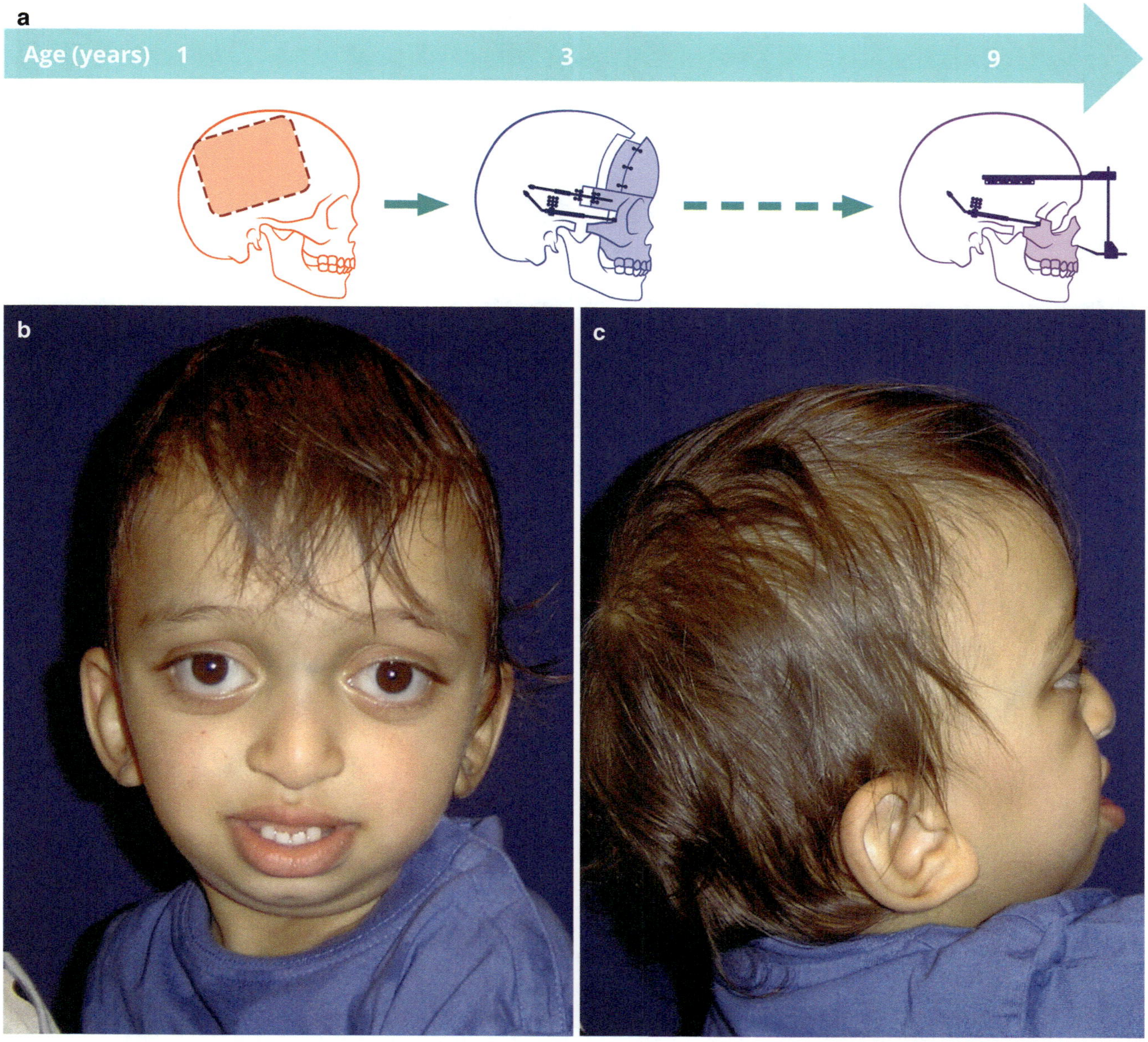

Fig. 10.9 (**a**) Management strategy for a patient with Crouzon syndrome initially presenting as scaphocephaly (Same patient as in Fig. 2.21). ©Cassandra Vion. (**b, c**) Initial clinical presentation at 18 months of age. (**d, e**) Bilateral parietal decompression for scaphocephaly correction. (**f, g**) Morphological results at 22 months of age, 4 months after initial bony flaps. (**h, i**) Clinical presentation at 27 months of age, showing the progression of midface hypoplasia. (**j, k, l**) Intraoperative views of the FFMBA performed at 33 months of age. (**m**) CT scan immediately after FFMBA showing the 4 internal distractors and the scars of the bilateral parietal flaps. (**n**) Dead space behind forehead advancement. (**o, p**) Clinical presentation at 45 months of age, 1 year after FFMBA, with progressive setting of midface hypoplasia. (**q, r**) Progression of midface hypoplasia at 7 years and 4 months of age (4 years and 7 months after FFMBA). (**s, t**) Progression of midface hypoplasia at 9 years and 3 months of age. (**u, v**) LF3 performed at 9 years and 6 months of age using internal and external distractions. (**w, x**) Morphological results at 12 years and 4 months of age, 34 months after LF3. (**y, z**) CT scan results showing correction of midface hypoplasia at 12 years and 4 months of age, 34 months after LF3

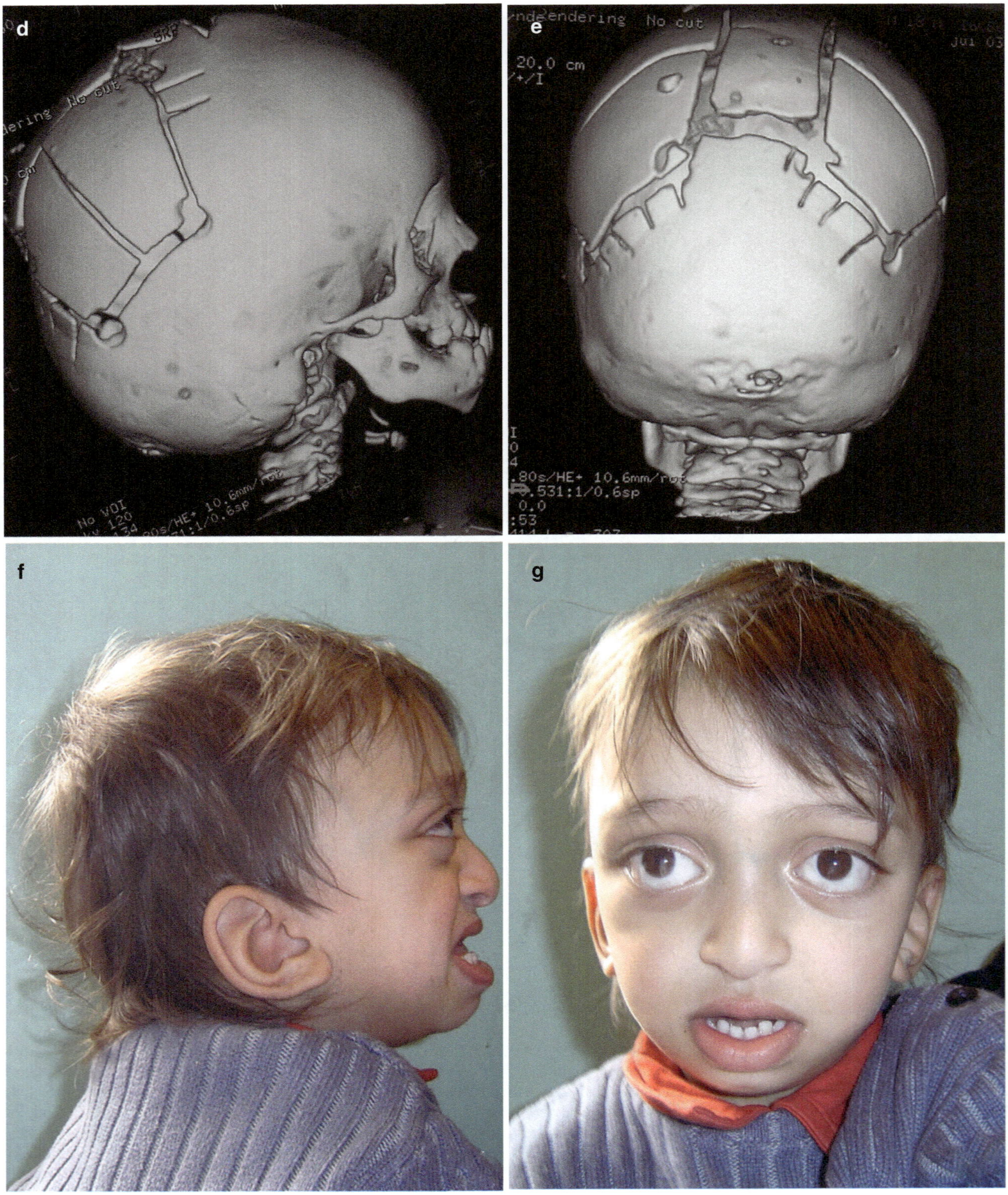

Fig. 10.9 (continued)

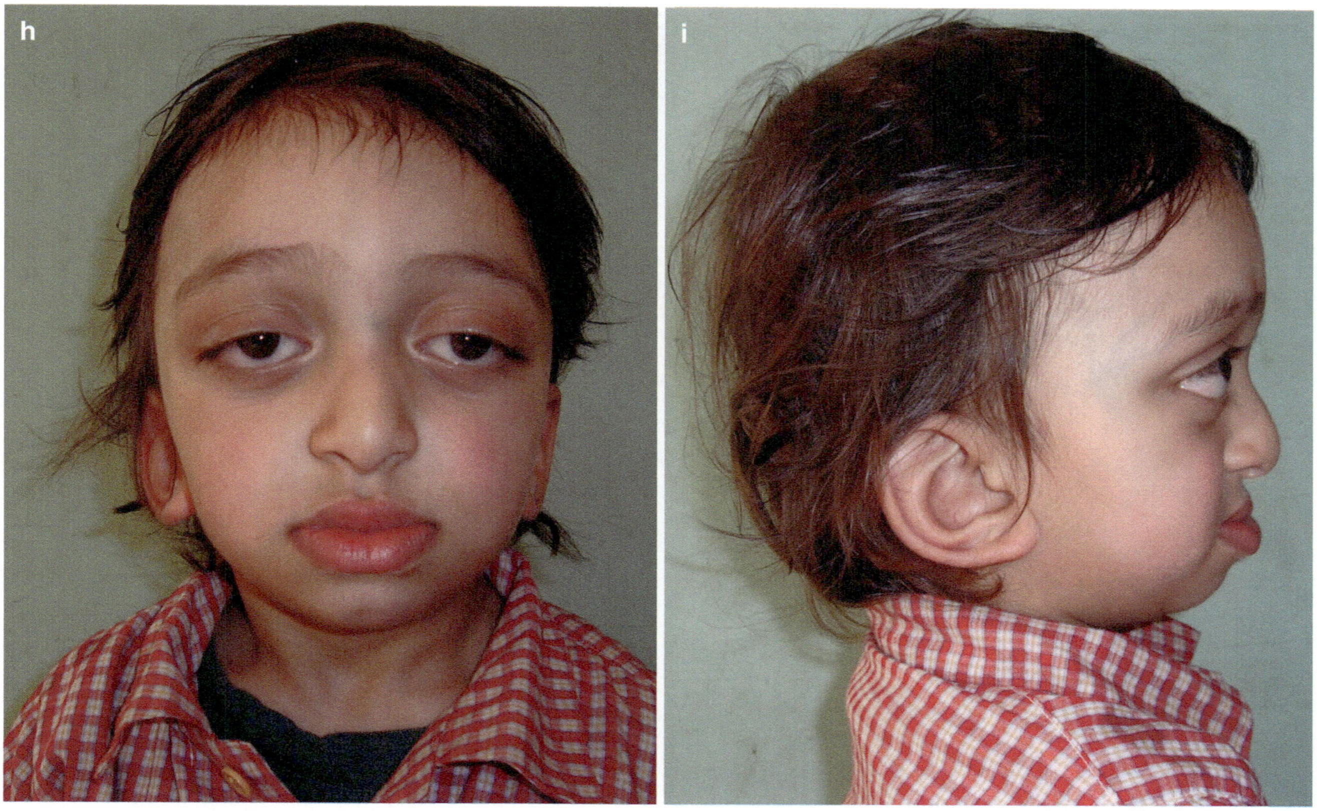

Fig. 10.9 (continued)

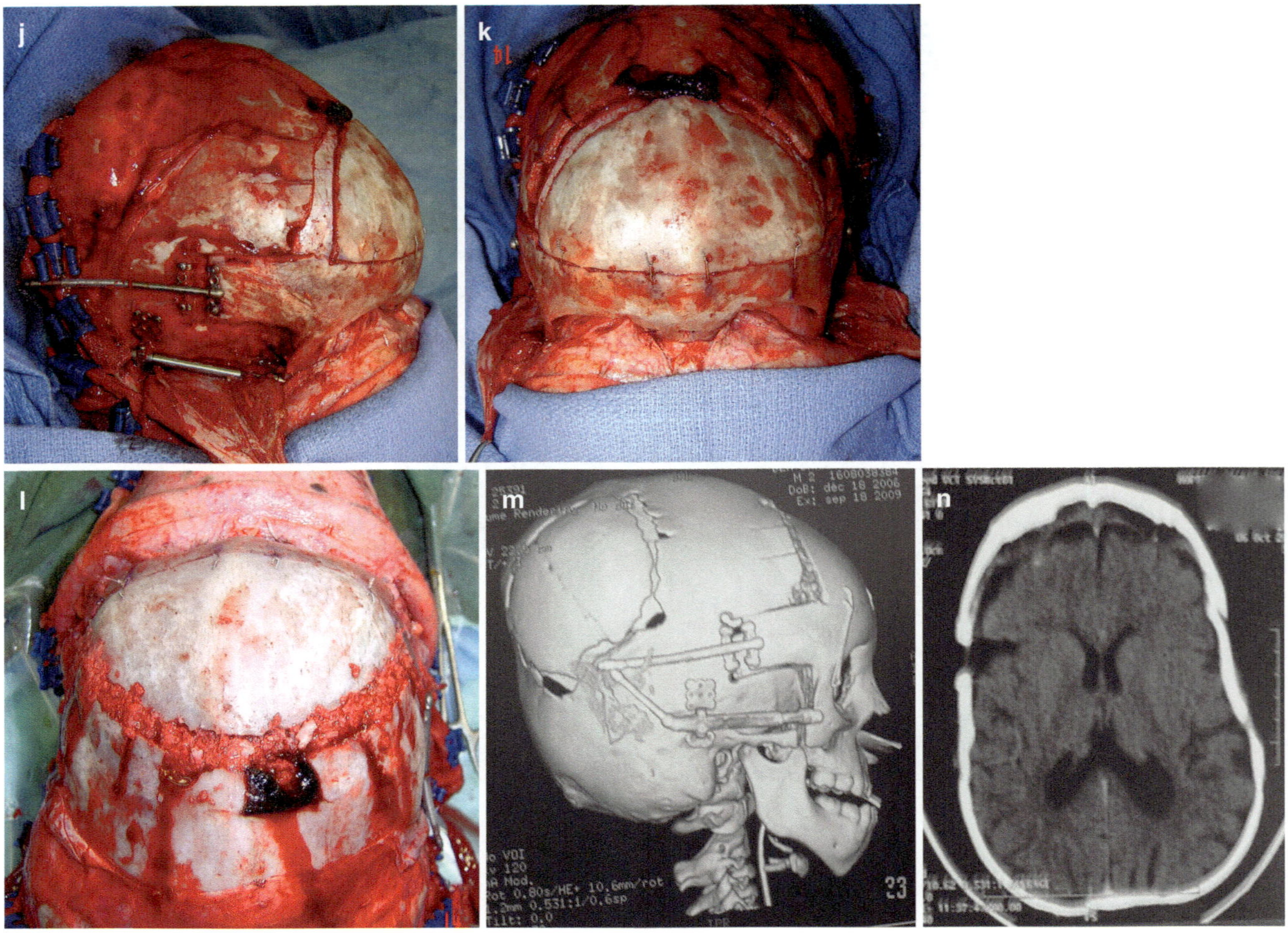

Fig. 10.9 (continued)

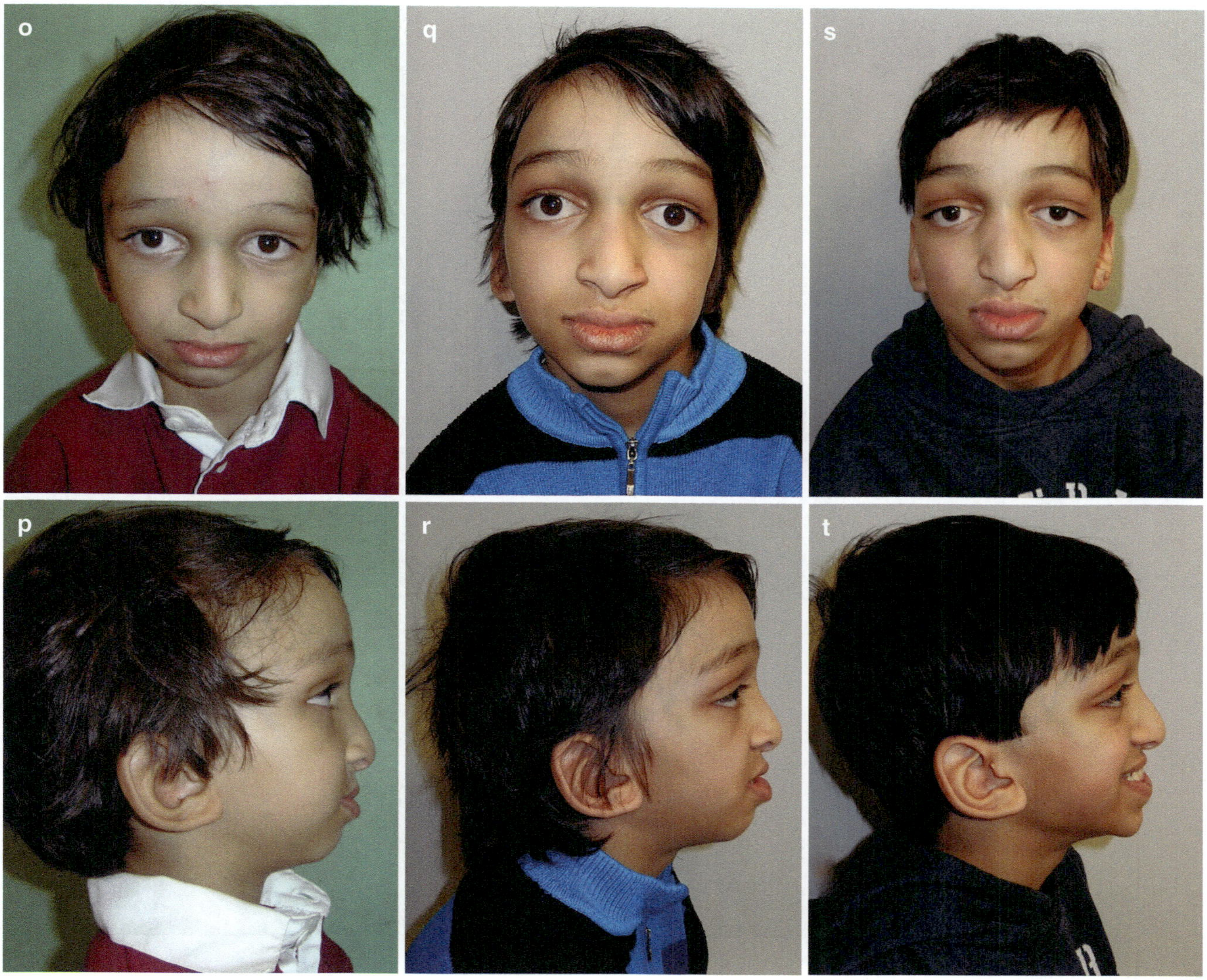

Fig. 10.9 (continued)

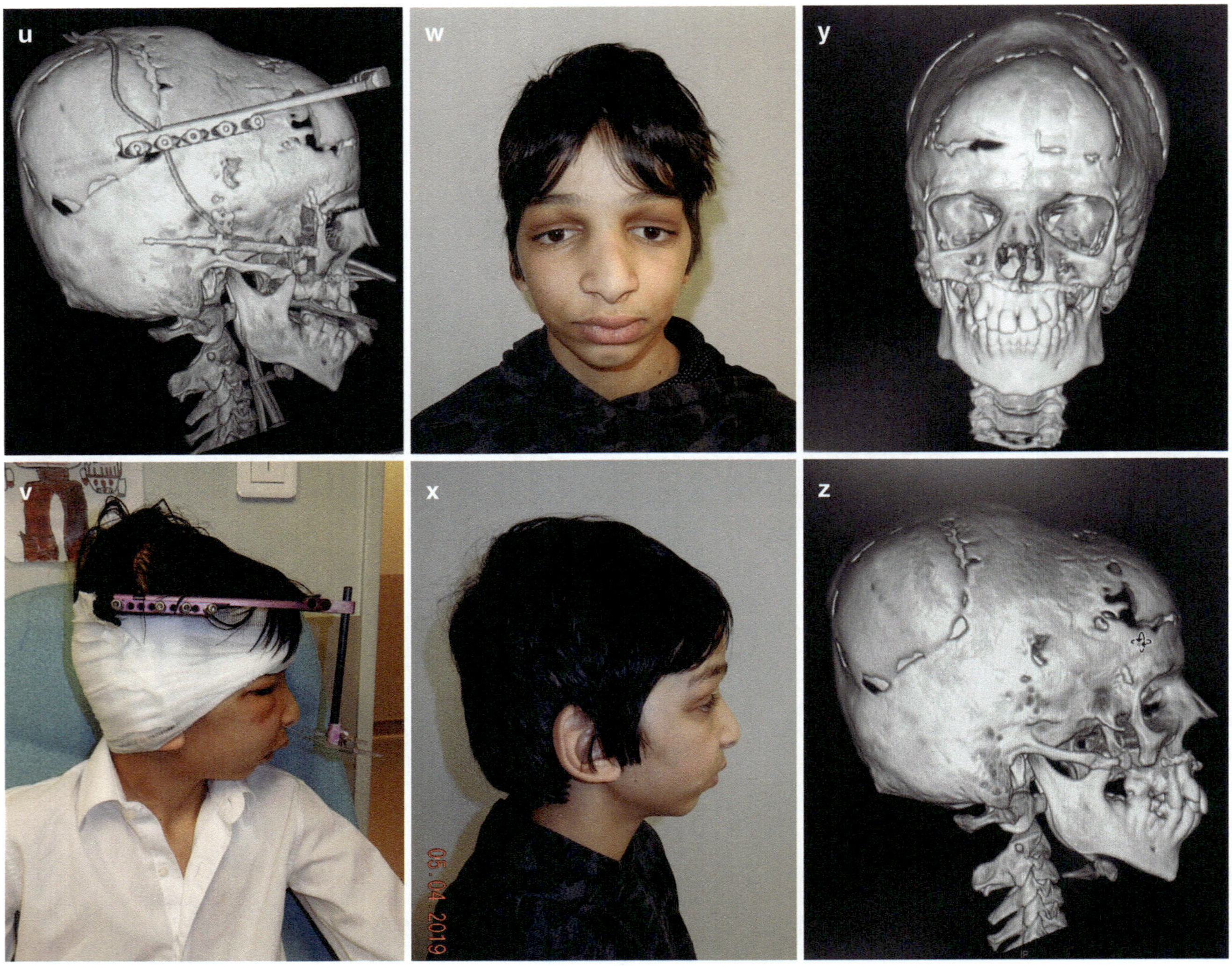

Fig. 10.9 (continued)

Fig. 10.10 (**a**) Management strategy for a patient with mild Crouzon syndrome presenting late, with exclusive FFMBA and aesthetic procedures. ©Cassandra Vion. (**b**) Initial presentation at 8 years and 6 months of age with severe obstructive sleep apnea (AHI = 90 per hour). Observe the discrepancy between the mildness of midface hypoplasia and the severity of OSA. (**d**) Intraoperative view of the FFMBA after distractor placement at age 9 years. (**e**, **f**) Clinical results at 10 years of age, 1 year after FFMBA. (**g**) Absence of midface hypoplasia at 12 years of age, 3 years after FFMBA. Polysomnography revealed persisting OSA (AHI = 26 per hour). This might be explained by the small mandible and residual laryngomalacia. Orthognathic surgery is indicated

10.1.8 Example №8 of Management Strategy in Crouzon Syndrome

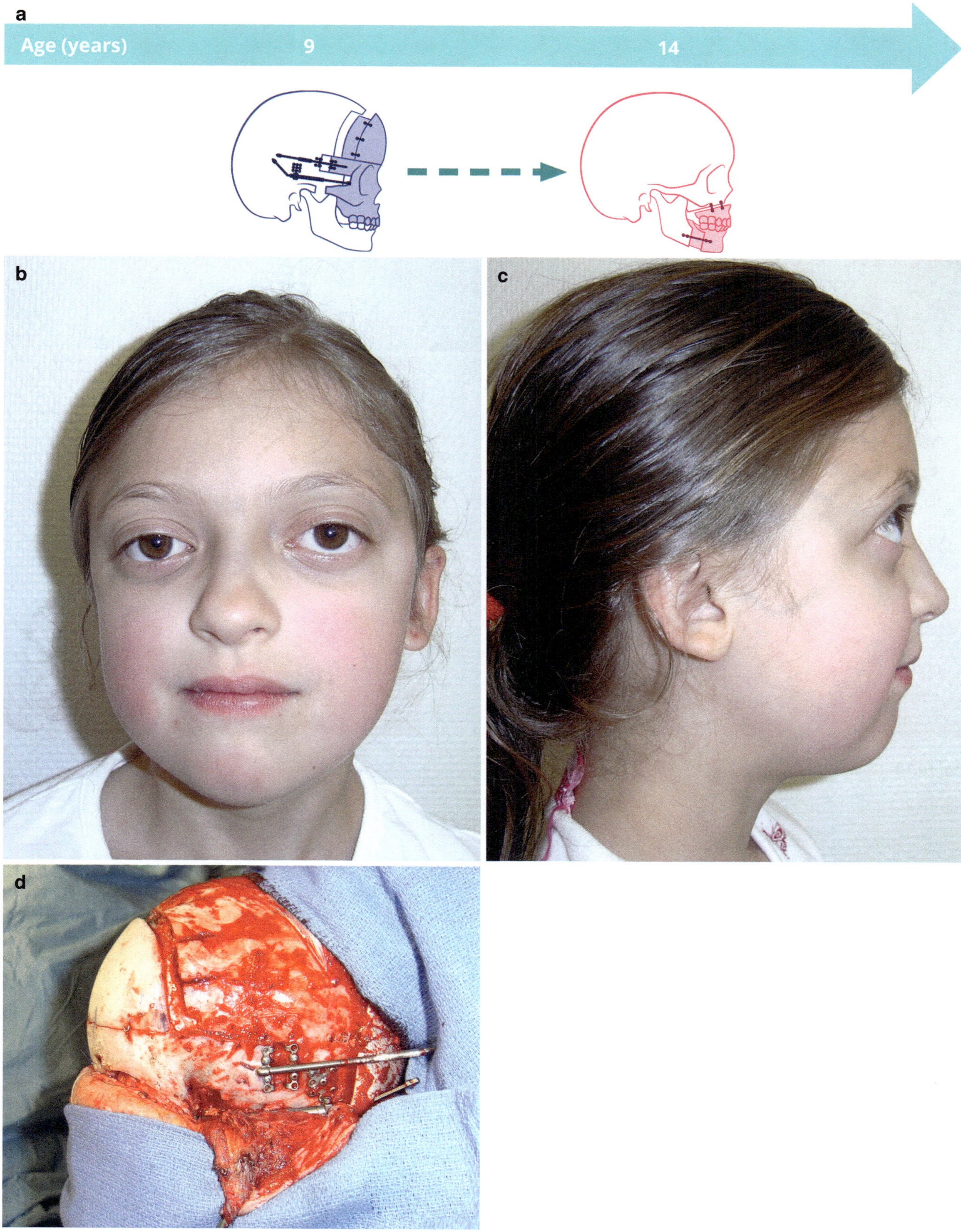

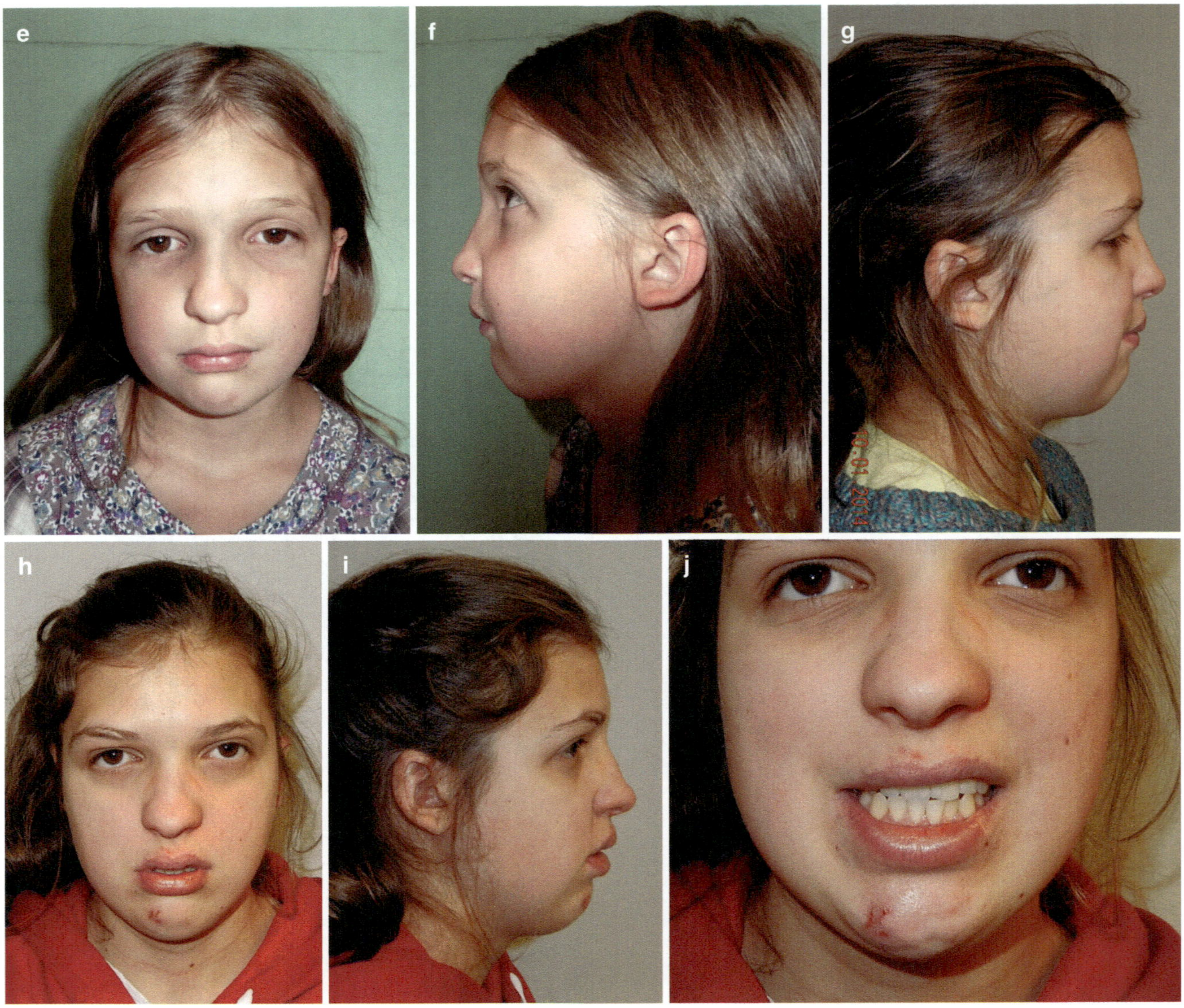

Fig. 10.10 (continued)

Fig. 10.11 (**a**) A Twenty-eight-month-old patient with Pfeiffer syndrome (FGFR2 p.Cys342Ser mutation) who had previously undergone PVE twice improving his tonsillar herniation at age 6 months and a Frisén stage 3 papilledema at age 11 months (Fig. 2.16). He has residual OSA despite considerable improvement after turbinectomy and adenoidectomy (AHI had decreased from 25 per hour to 7 per hour). Nocturnal noninvasive ventilation was not well tolerated and it seemed to worsen his maxillary retrusion and exorbitism. PVE, noninvasive ventilation, and ENT interventions were successfully employed to delay FFMBA as much as possible. The patient subsequently developed Frisén stage 2 papillary edema at age 28 months. FFMBA was indicated to simultaneously relieve intracranial hypertension, airway obstruction, and exorbitism. ©Cassandra Vion. (**b**, **c**, **d**) Preoperative clinical photographs at age 26 months before FFMBA. (**e**) Preoperative CT scan demonstrating severe maxillary retrusion and partial re-ossification of the previous PVE osteotomies. The temporal bone was intentionally spared for the distractors to come. (**f**) Black Bone MRI demonstrating mild tonsillar herniation without CSF obstruction. (**g**) Intraoperative photograph of FFMBA at age 28 months demonstrating the position of the internal distractors and the lateral orbital plate. (**h**, **i**) Two-day-postoperative CT scan demonstrating the position of the osteotomies and the hardware. (**j**, **k**) Nineteen-day-postoperative CT scan at the end of the activation phase of distraction demonstrating the achieved advancement. (**l**, **m**, **n**) Eighteen-month-postoperative photographs showing the resolution of exorbitism and maxillary retrusion at age 4 years. Polysomnography demonstrated the resolution of OSA (AHI was 2 per hour). (**o**, **p**, **q**) Eighteen-month-postoperative CT scan demonstrating satisfactory ossification of the osteotomies and Angle class I occlusion

10.2 Treatment Strategies in Pfeiffer Syndrome

For Pfeiffer syndromes, the necessity of very early monobloc was more frequent to address the severe exorbitism and the OSA.

10.2.1 Example №1 of Management Strategy in Pfeiffer Syndrome

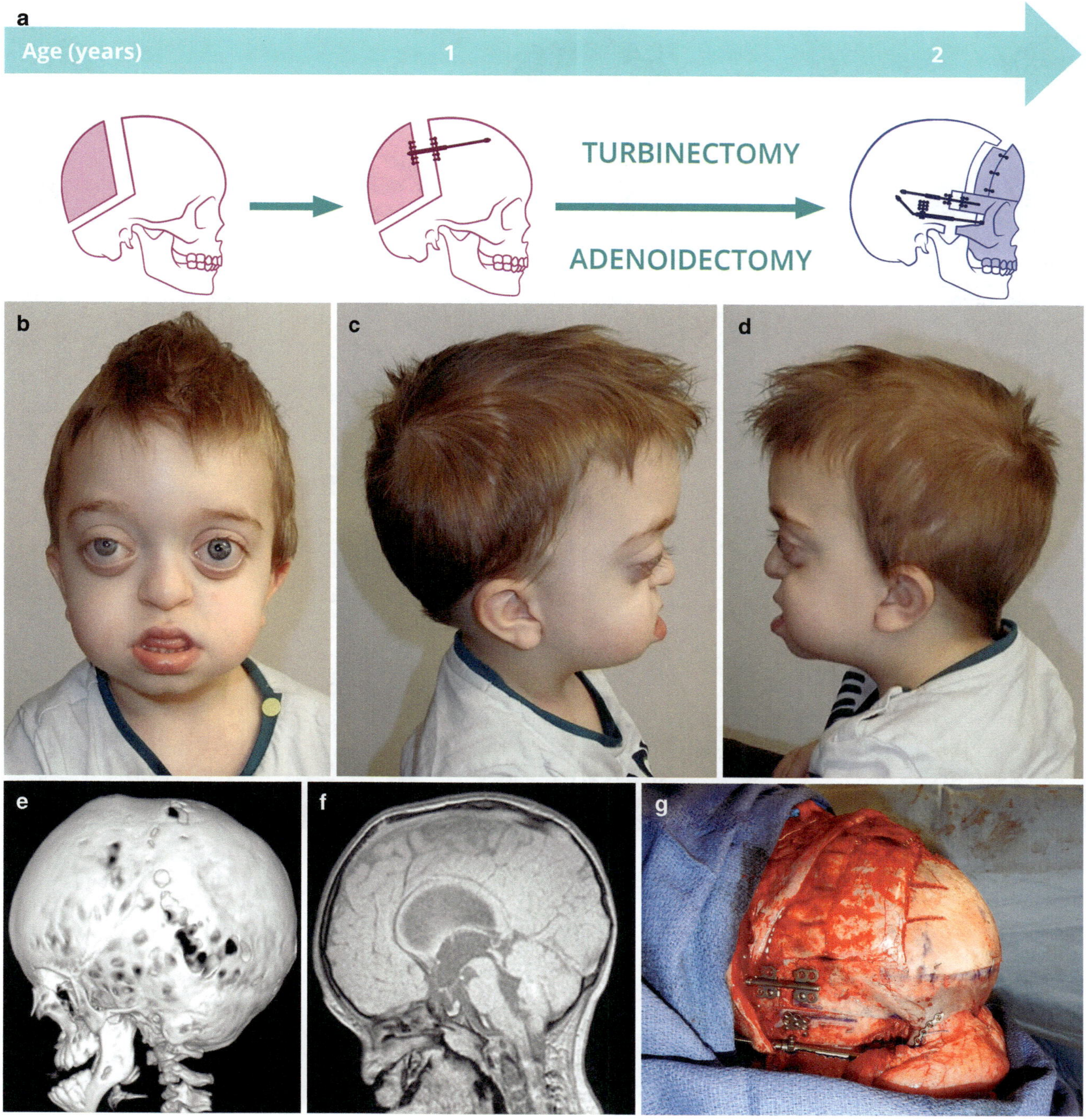

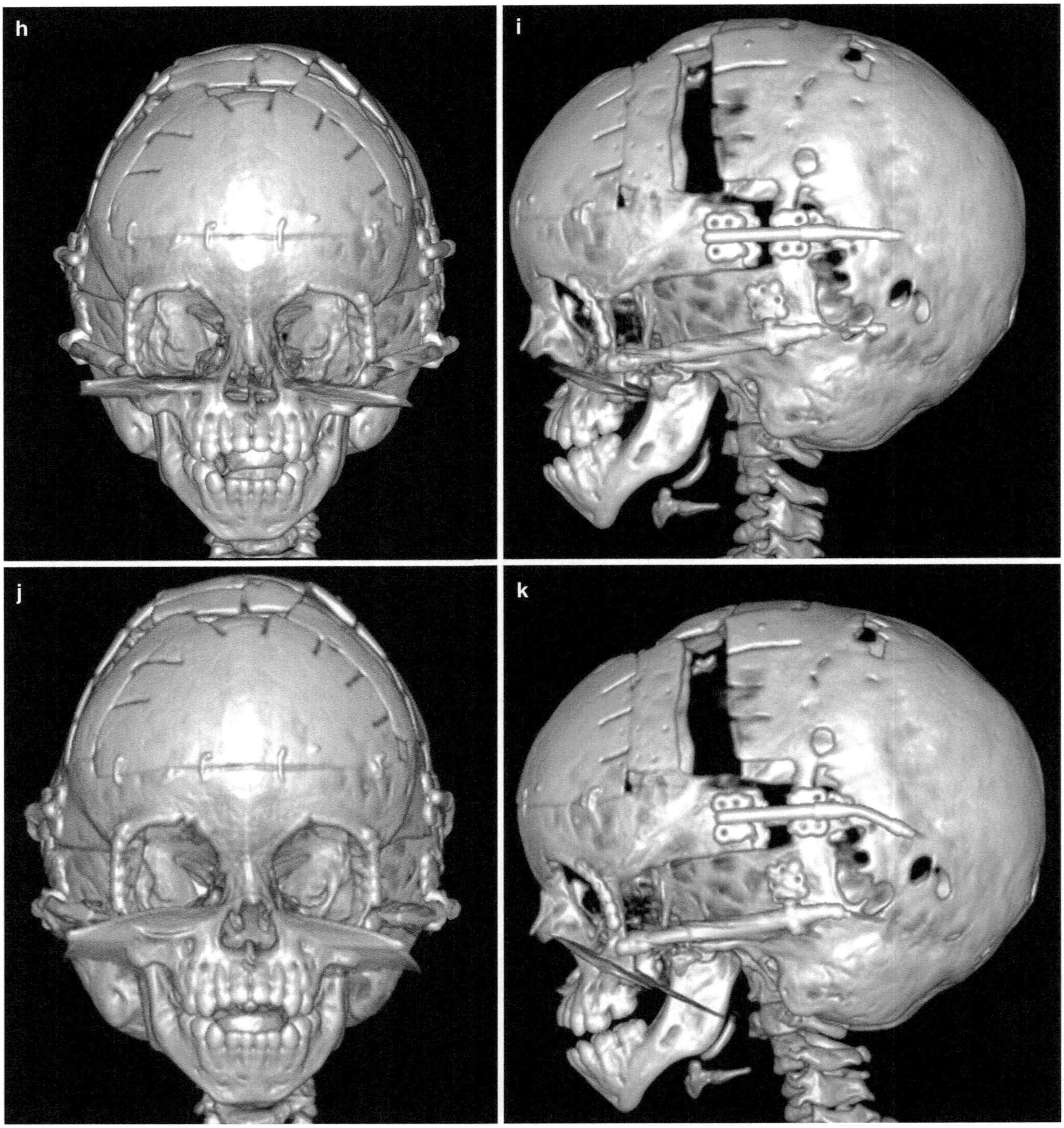

Fig. 10.11 (continued)

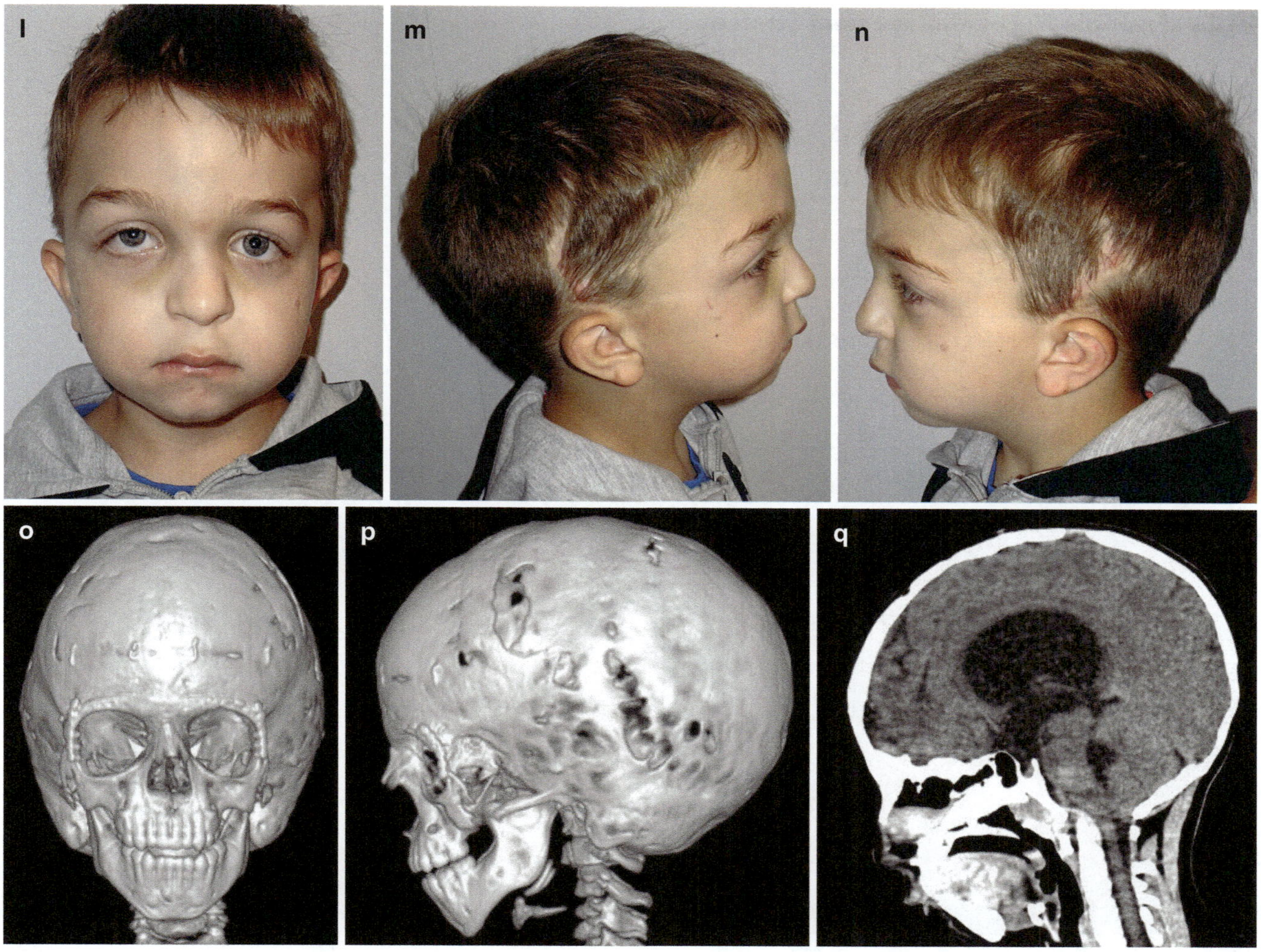

Fig. 10.11 (continued)

10.2.2 Example №2 of Management Strategy in Pfeiffer Syndrome

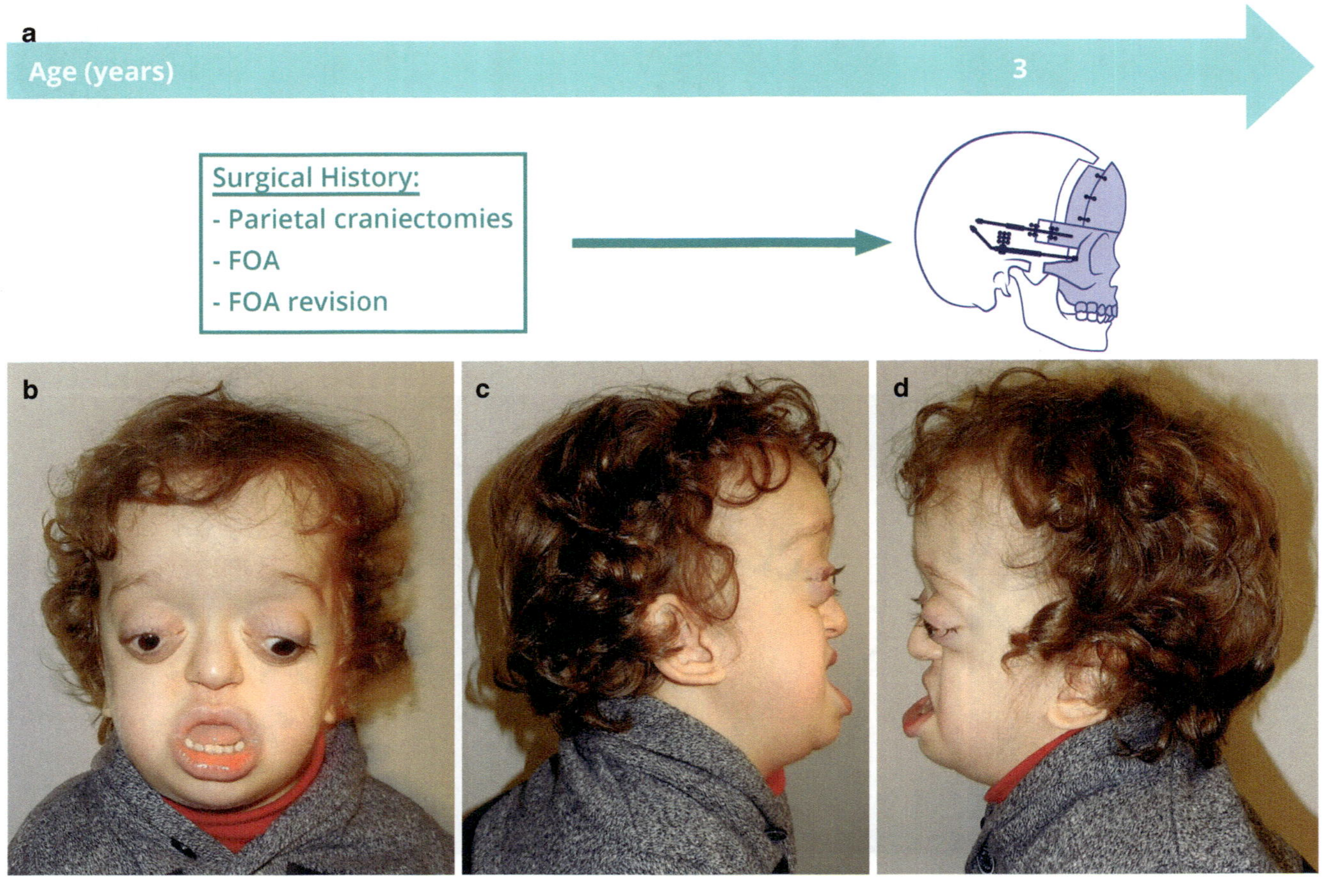

Fig. 10.12 (**a-d**) A 3-year-old patient with Pfeiffer syndrome was referred to our center from abroad. Medical history included feeding difficulties and OSA under CPAP since age 4 months. Surgical history included bilateral linear parietal craniectomies at age 5 months, FOA at age 12 months, and revision FOA with dural fistula repair at age 21 months because of fractured resorbable plates secondary to trauma. Notice the severe midface retrusion that was probably aggravated by CPAP. Severe exorbitism had required lateral and medial tarsorrhaphy for corneal protection. Fundoscopic examination revealed bilateral papilledema. FFMBA was indicated to decompress the brain, relieve respiratory symptoms, and protect the eyes. ©Cassandra Vion. (**d-i**) CT scan demonstrating severe maxillary retrusion, skull bone defects from previous surgeries, and crowding of the posterior fossa. (**j**) Intraoperative photograph showing the pericranial flaps and the osteotomy markings. External ventricular drainage (EVD) was performed before skin closure to control the highly likely postoperative CSF leakage due to multiple previous operations. Midline maxillary disjunction occurred during the separation of the fronto-facial complex from the skull base using Rowe forceps. Two hemi-facial 2.2-millimeter Kirschner wires were used to strengthen the horizontal zygomatico-maxillary buttress. Intraoperative advancement was performed for immediate brain decompression. The patient was extubated on postoperative day 3 and the EVD was removed on postoperative day 4. (**k, l, m**) Four-day-postoperative CT scan demonstrating the EVD, the osteotomies, the transfacial pin, the distractors, and the intraoperative advancement. (**n, o, p**) Two-week-postoperative CT scan demonstrating the fronto-facial advancement at the end of the activation phase. (**q, r**) Sagittal and axial views 2 weeks postoperatively showing the prefrontal dead space. The distractors were removed 3 months postoperatively and the lateral and medial tarsorrhaphies were simultaneously liberated. (**s, t, u**) Clinical results 5 months after FFMBA demonstrating the resolution of maxillary hypoplasia and exorbitism. OSA was resolved (AHI = 1.8 per hour). Feeding difficulties and papilledema were also resolved. (**v-z**) Five-month-postoperative CT scan demonstrating initial ossification of the distraction gap and dural advancement in the prefrontal dead space

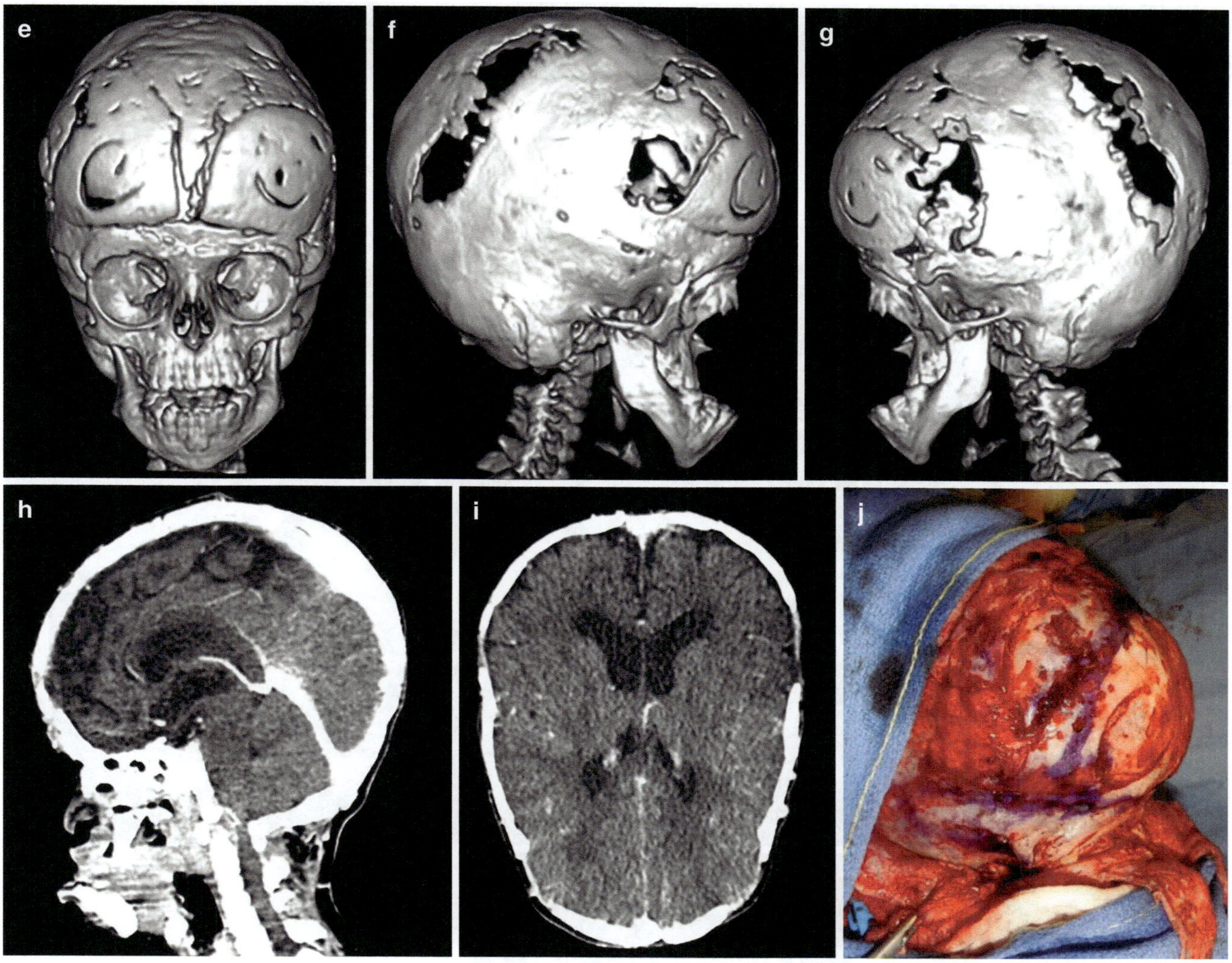

Fig. 10.12 (continued)

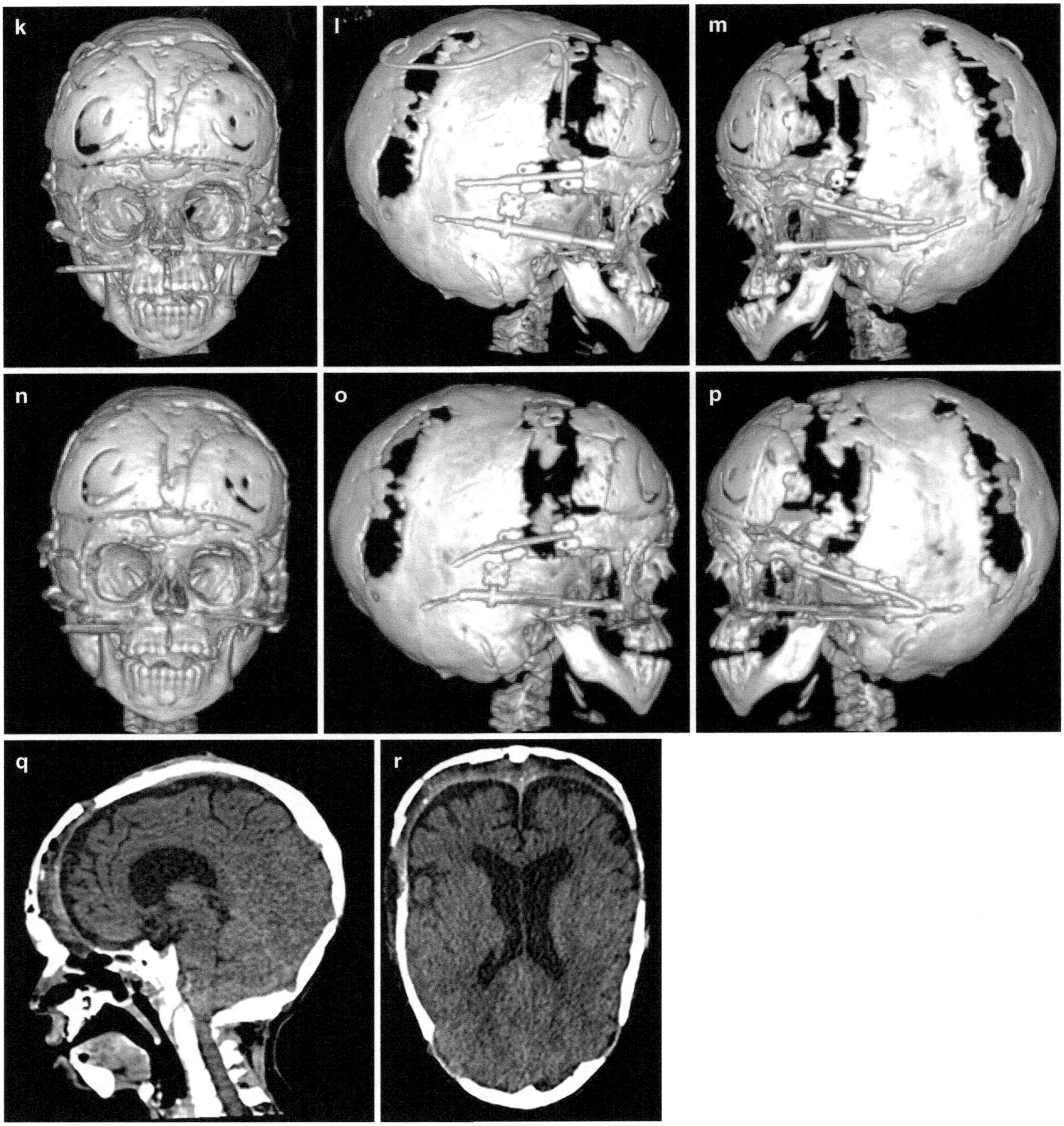

Fig. 10.12 (continued)

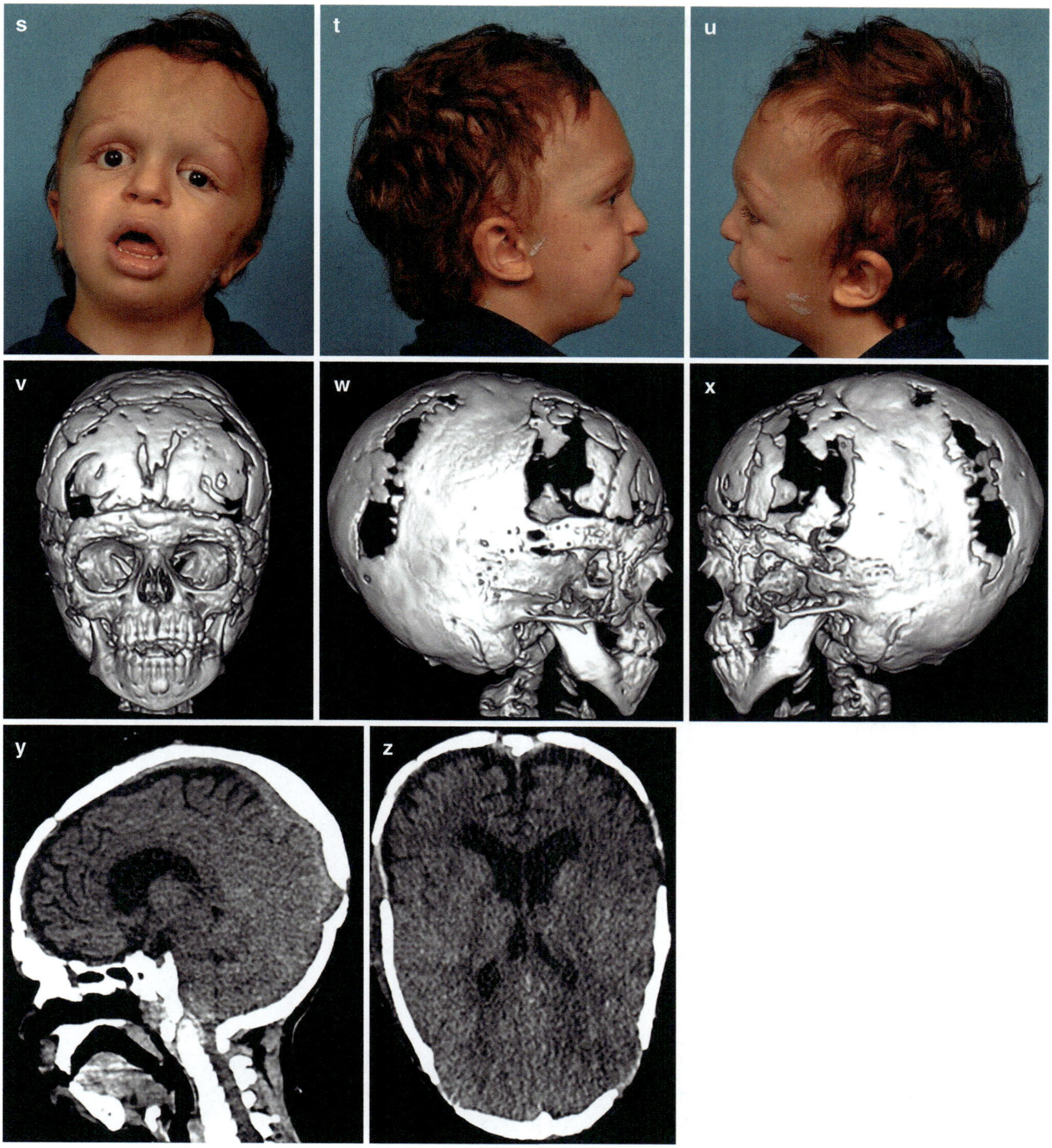

Fig. 10.12 (continued)

10.2.3 Example №3 of Management Strategy in Pfeiffer Syndrome

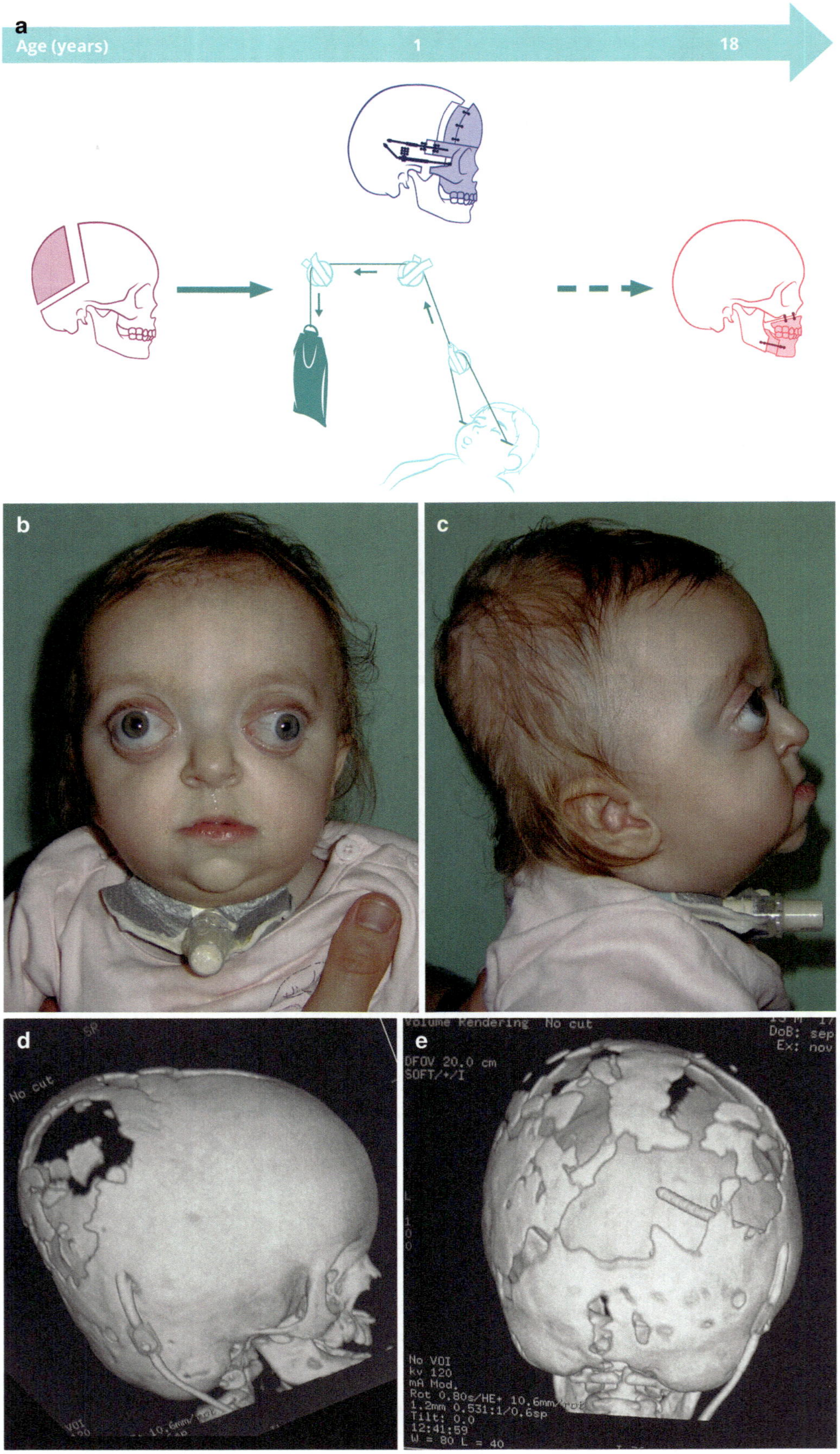

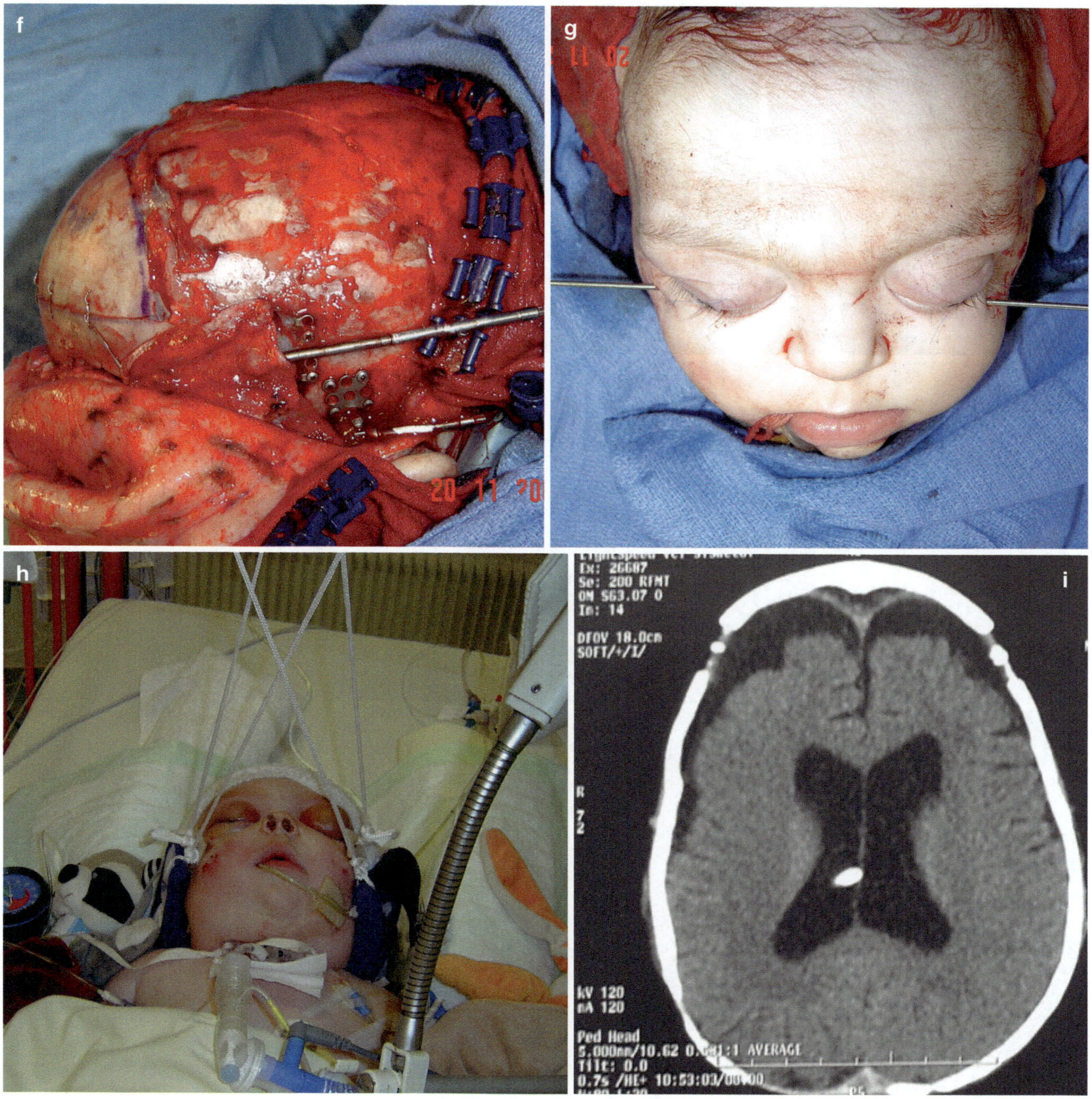

Fig. 10.13 (continued)

Fig. 10.13 (**a**) Management strategy for a patient with severe Pfeiffer syndrome (same patient as in Fig. 6.4). ©Cassandra Vion. (**b**, **c**) Fourteen-month-old girl with Pfeiffer syndrome initially managed in another center, where a PVE and a ventriculoperitoneal shunt had been performed. (**d**, **e**) Bony defects secondary to the PVE performed in another center and severe midface hypoplasia. (**f**) Intraoperative view of the very early FFMBA performed at 14 months of age. (**g**, **h**) Transfacial pin and external traction. (**i**) CT scan confirming the expansion of the dura mater filling the dead space behind the advanced forehead. (**j**, **k**, **l**) Major fronto-facial advancement with overcorrection after the end of the activation period of distraction osteogenesis. The midface gradually moves back postoperatively. (**m**, **n**) Age 17 months, 3 months post-FFMBA; (**o**, **p**) Age 29 months, 15 months post-FFMBA; (**q**, **r**) Age 31 months, 29 months post-FFMBA; (**s**, **t**) Age 5 years, 46 months post-FFMBA: at this point, the patient still displayed a slight overcorrection (Angle class II) with mandibular hypoplasia. (**u**, **v**, **w**) Age 5 years and 8 months, 4 years and 6 months post-FFMBA: the patient reached Angle class I occlusion with anterior open bite and bilateral crossbite. The growing patient subsequently developed Angle class III malocclusion without any obstructive sleep apnea on polysomnography (AHI = 0.2 per hour). (**x**, **y**) Age 6 years and 3 months, 5 years post-FFMBA; (**z**, **a'**) Age 6 years and 9 months, 5 years and 7 months post-FFMBA; (**b'**, **c'**) Age 8 years and 4 months, 7 years and 2 months post-FFMBA, palatal expansion underway; (**d'**, **e'**) Age 10 years and 8 months, 9 years and 6 months post-FFMBA: Angle class III malocclusion without respiratory involvement

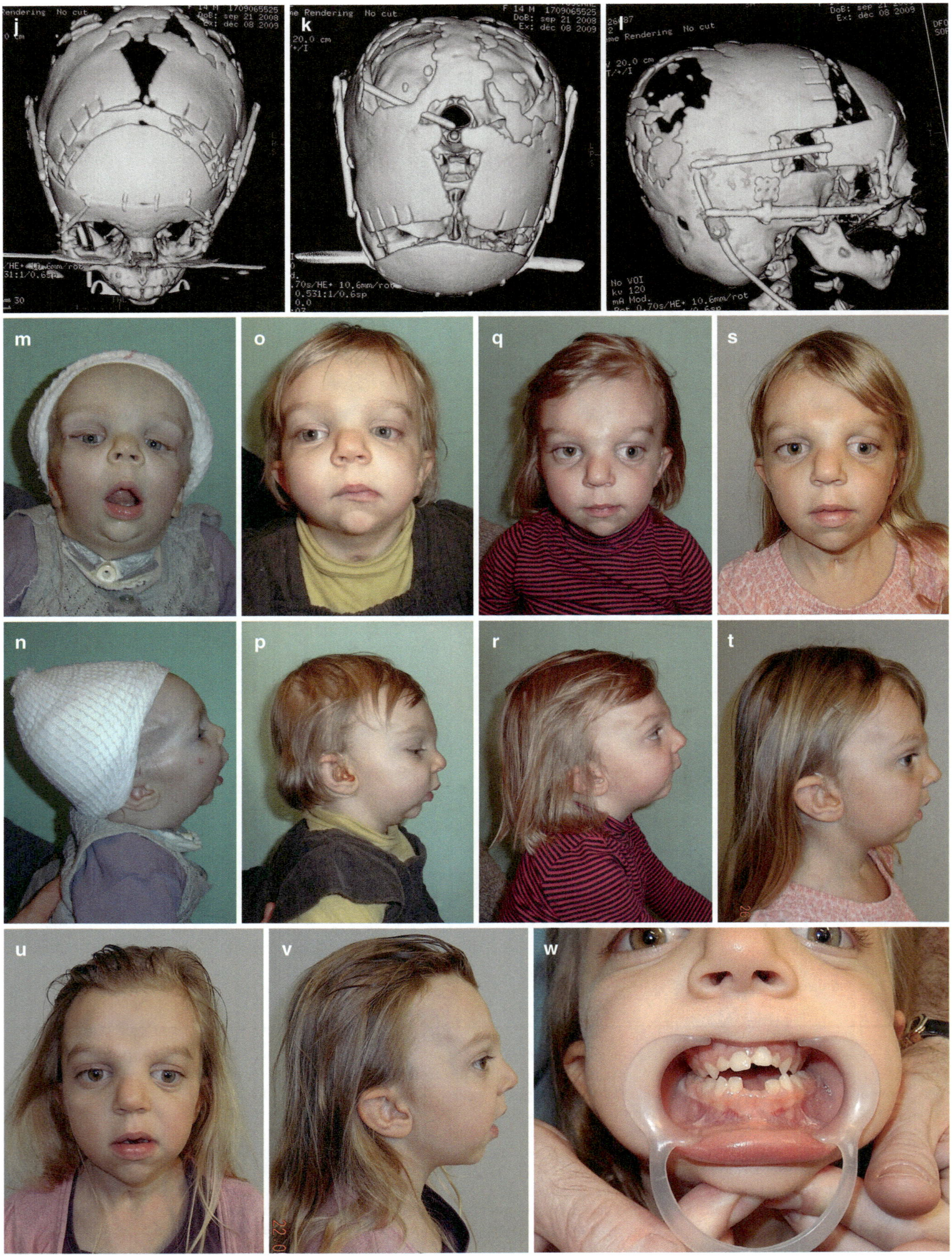

Fig. 10.13 (continued)

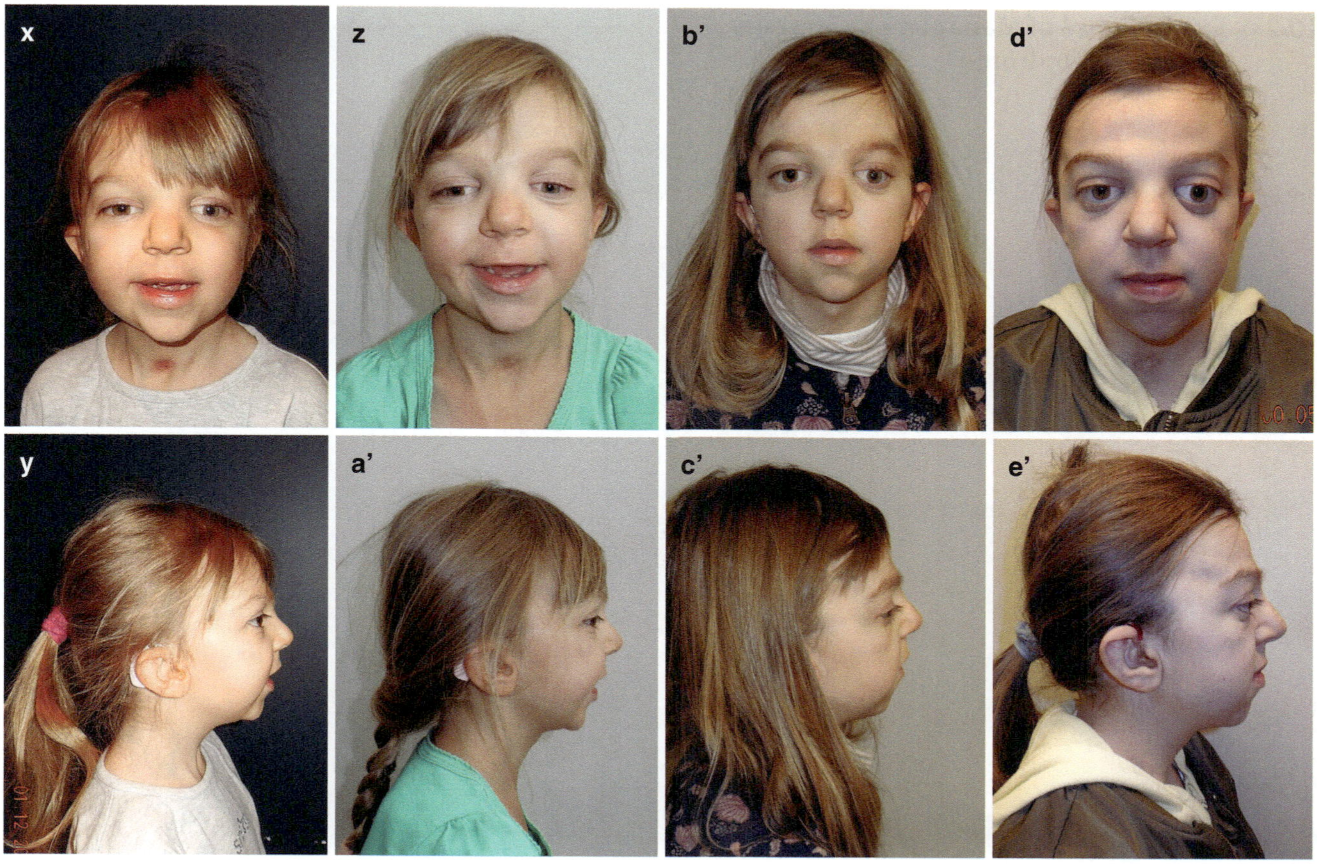

Fig. 10.13 (continued)

10.2.4 Example №4 of Management Strategy in Pfeiffer Syndrome

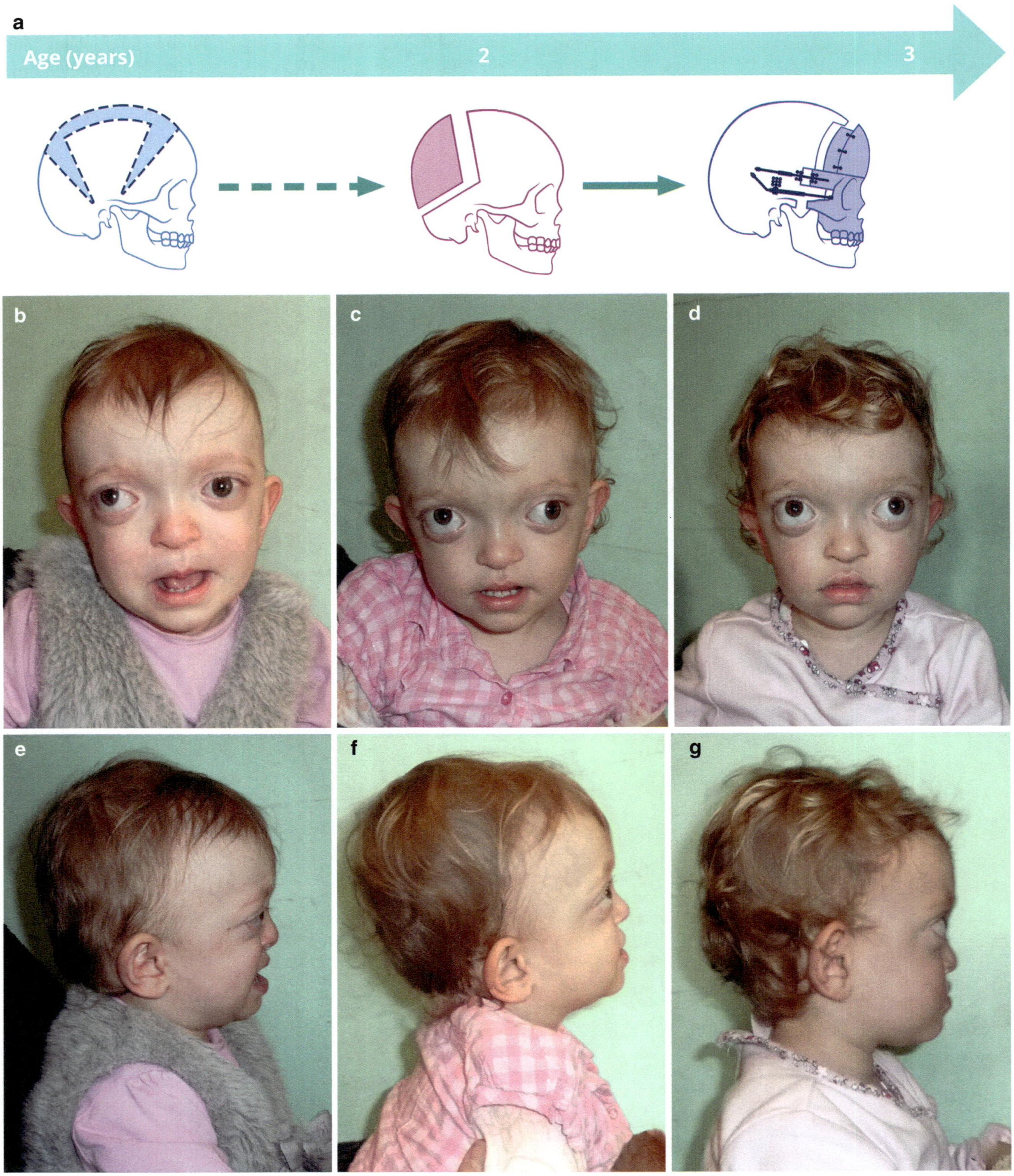

Fig. 10.14 (**a**) Management strategy for a girl with a moderate form of Pfeiffer syndrome initially presenting with sagittal craniosynostosis. H craniectomy was initially performed at age 5 months with adequate correction of the scaphocephalic shape. ©Cassandra Vion. (**b**, **c**) Preoperative pictures at 20 months of age show a normocephalic head with moderate exorbitism and midface hypoplasia. PVE was planned to delay the subsequent FFMBA. Two months later, papillary edema was detected on fundoscopy and brain-mediated PVE without distraction was urgently performed. (**d**, **e**) Morphological results at 2 years of age, 3 months after PVE without distraction. (**f**, **g**) Progression of midface hypoplasia at 28 months of age. (**h**) CT scan at 28 months of age before FFMBA. (i) Intraoperative view during FFMBA with the markings of the osteotomies. (**j**, **k**) Morphological results at 32 months, 3 months after FFMBA. (**l**, **m**, **n**) Clinical presentation at 8 years of age, 6 years after FFMBA, showing progressive midface hypoplasia. (**o**, **p**, **q**) Clinical presentation at 11 years of age, 9 years after FFMBA, demonstrating midface hypoplasia

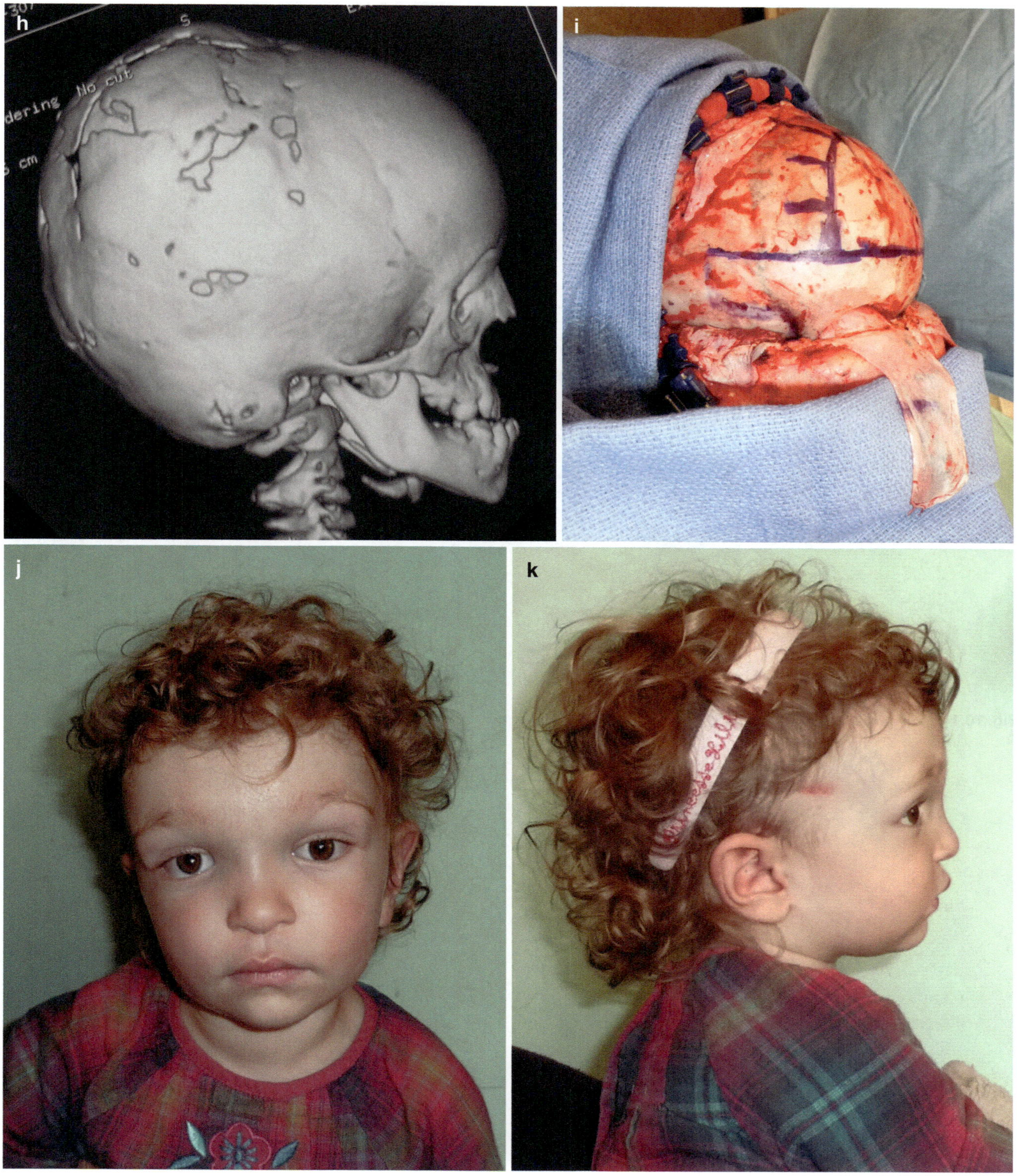

Fig. 10.14 (continued)

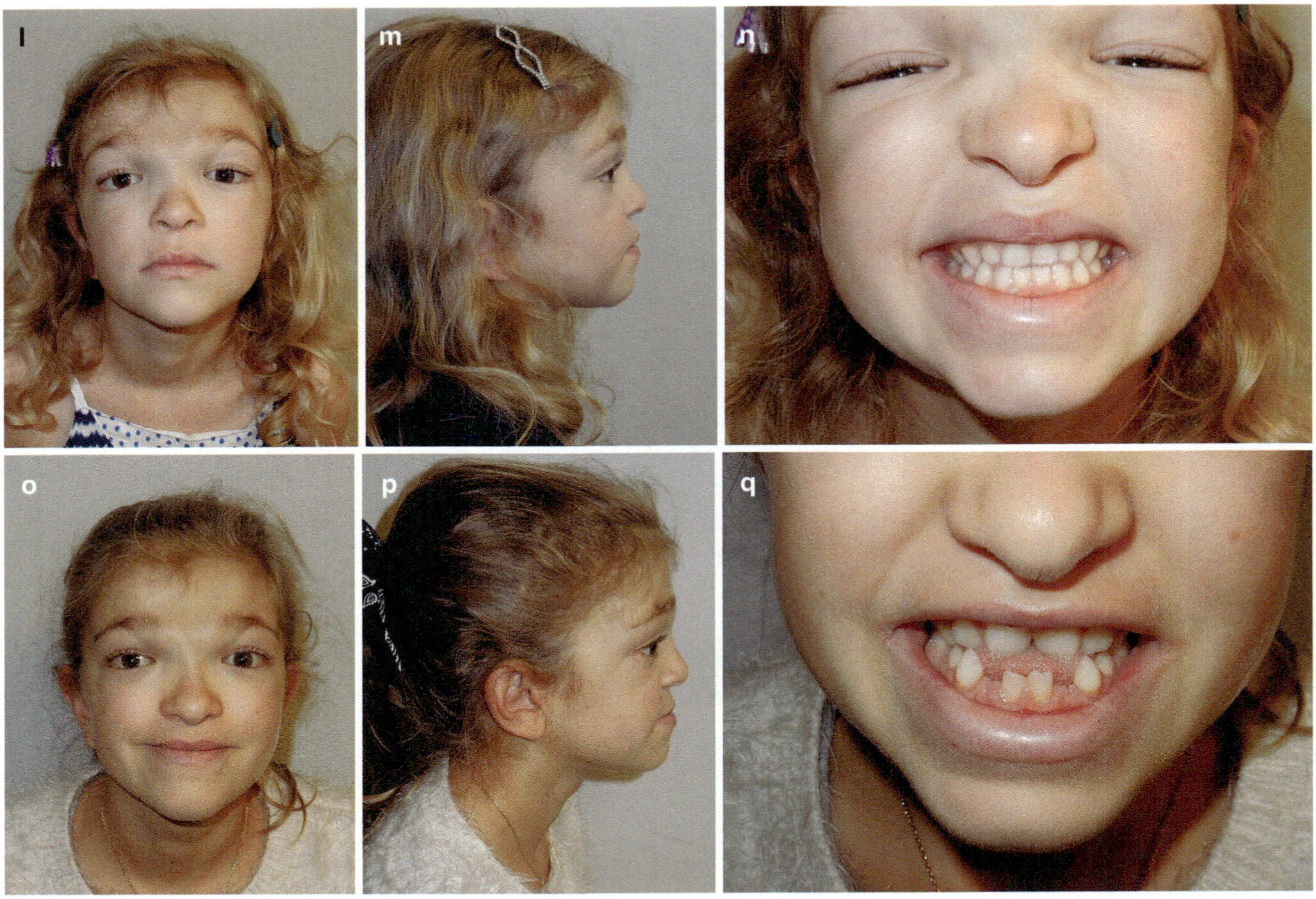

Fig. 10.14 (continued)

10.3 Treatment Strategies in Apert Syndrome

In Apert syndrome, the necessity of early FFMBA was less frequent and the alternative historical sequence remains valid because of delayed open frontal fontanella, absence of tonsillar herniation, and less severity of OSA.

10.3.1 Example №1 of Management Strategy in Apert Syndrome

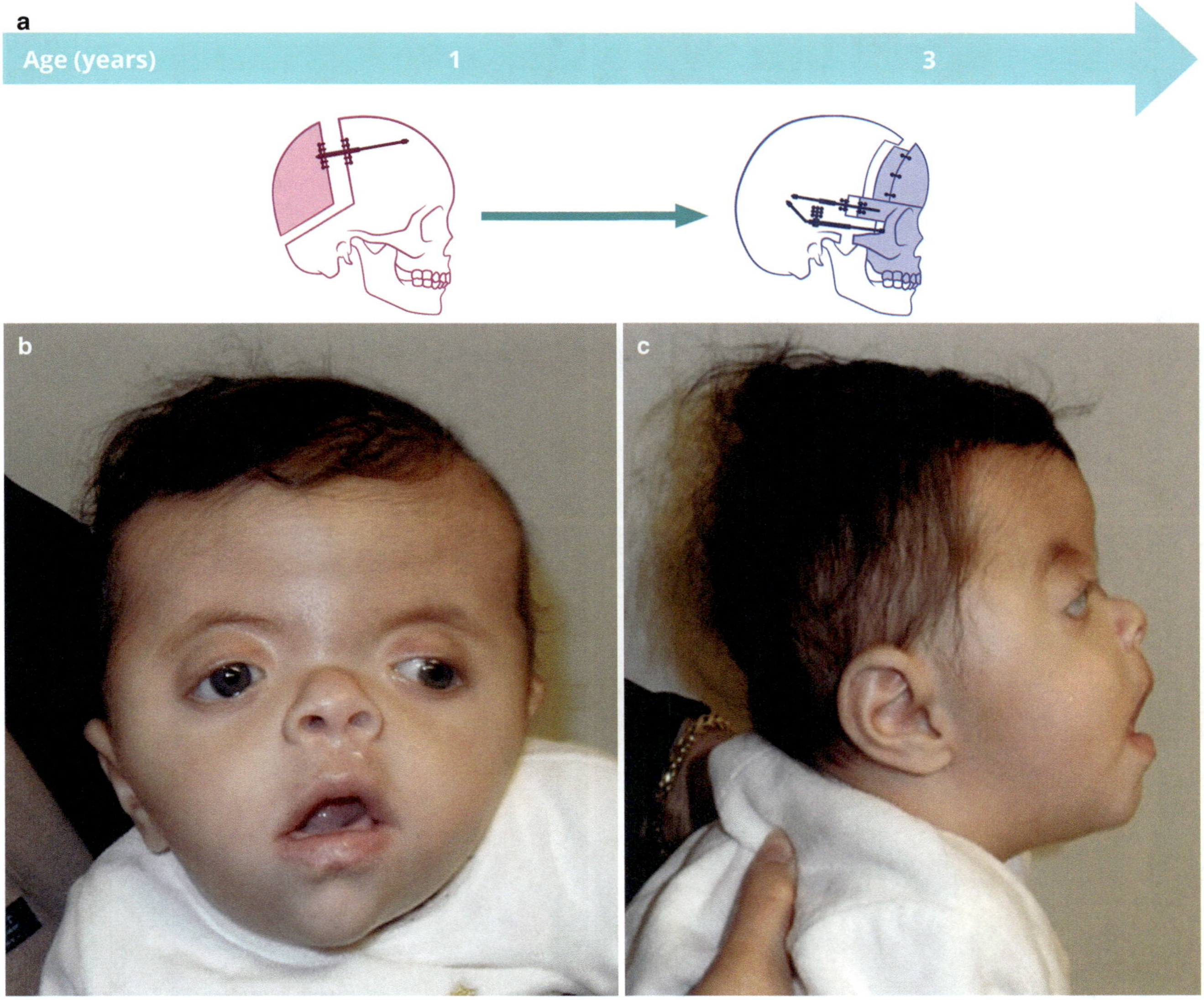

Fig. 10.15 (**a**, **b**, **c**) Four-month-old girl with Apert syndrome presenting with multiple syndactyly, cleft palate, and typical Apert facies: brachycephaly, hypertelorism, downslanting palpebral fissures, maxillary hypoplasia, V-shaped palate, and mild exorbitism. Breathing difficulties prompted an initial polysomnography at age 2 months that showed AHI at 3 per h. However, breathing difficulties worsened at age 4 months with recurring upper airway infections and inflection of the weight curve. Repeat polysomnography demonstrated severe OSA (AHI = 13 per hour). Continuous positive airway pressure was initiated and it was well tolerated with resumption of normal weight gain. ©Cassandra Vion. (**d**, **e**, **f**, **g**) CT scan at age 4 months demonstrating bicoronal craniosynostosis and widely open anterior fontanel and lambdoid sutures typical of Apert syndrome. The posterior fossa is also typically normal without tonsillar herniation. Typically, preventing turribrachycephaly would require PVE but the bone was too thin to support internal distractors at this age. (**h—m**) CT scan at age 9 months demonstrating thicker skull bone than the previous scan. The skull is now slightly turribrachycephalic. PVE with distractors was indicated. (**n**, **o**,**p**) Preoperative photographs at age 9 months before PVE with distraction. (**q**, **r**, **s**) Consecutive CT scans after PVE with distraction at postoperative day 2, postoperative day 12, and at 1 year, respectively. (**t**, **u**) Clinical photographs at age 3 years. CPAP ceased to be well tolerated. Polysomnography revealed mild OSA (AHI = 5.2 per h). Dental rehabilitation was performed in preparation for FFMBA. Notice the moderate exorbitism. (**v**) Intraoperative photograph during FFMBA at age 3 years. (**w**, **x**) Two-day-postoperative CT scan demonstrating the osteotomy lines and intraoperative advancement of the fronto-facial complex. (**y**) Three-week-postoperative CT scan at the end of the activation phase of distraction demonstrating overcorrection and Angle class II malocclusion. (**z**, **a'**, **b'**) Three-week-postoperative photographs at the end of the activation phase of distraction demonstrating the resolution of exorbitism and maxillary hypoplasia

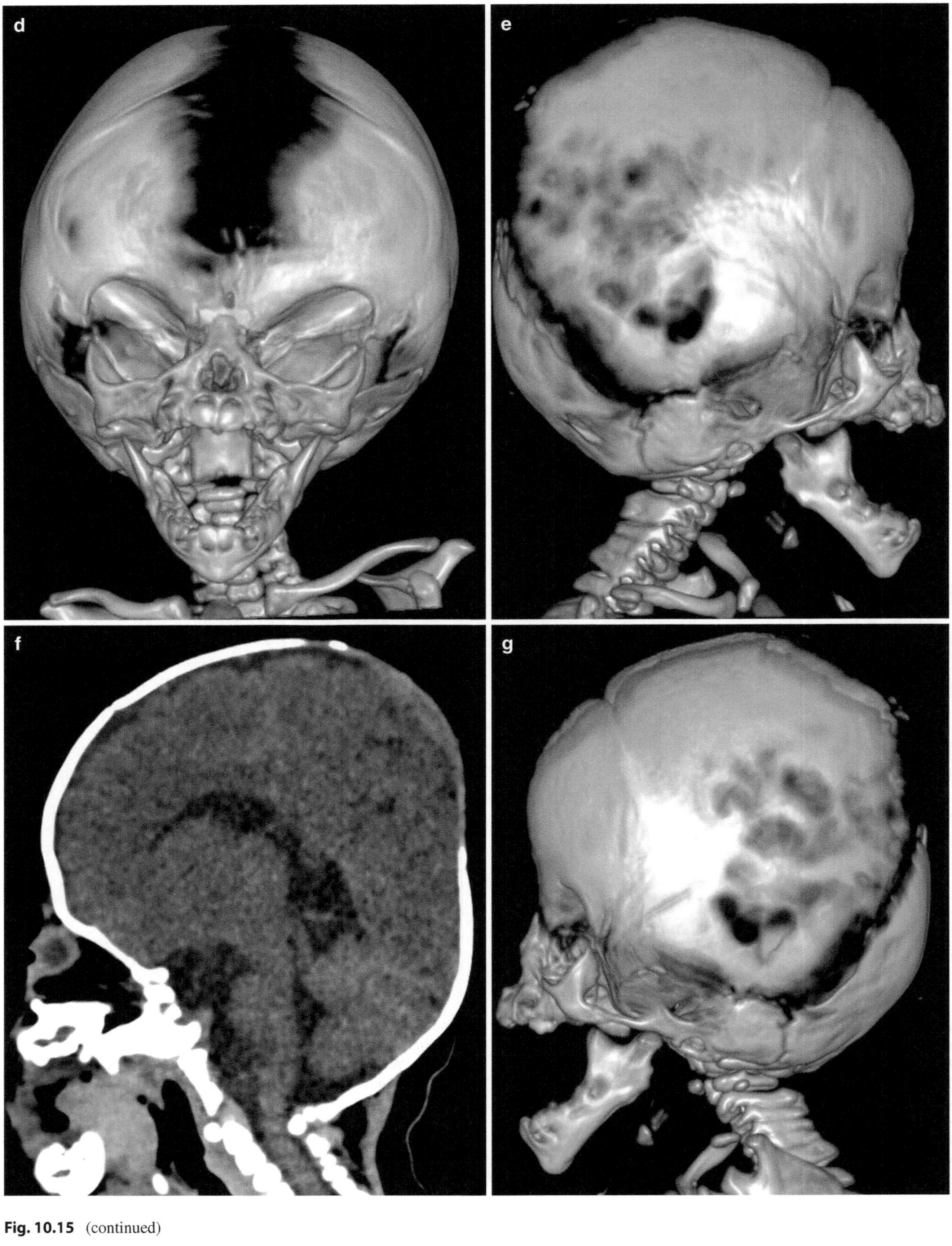

Fig. 10.15 (continued)

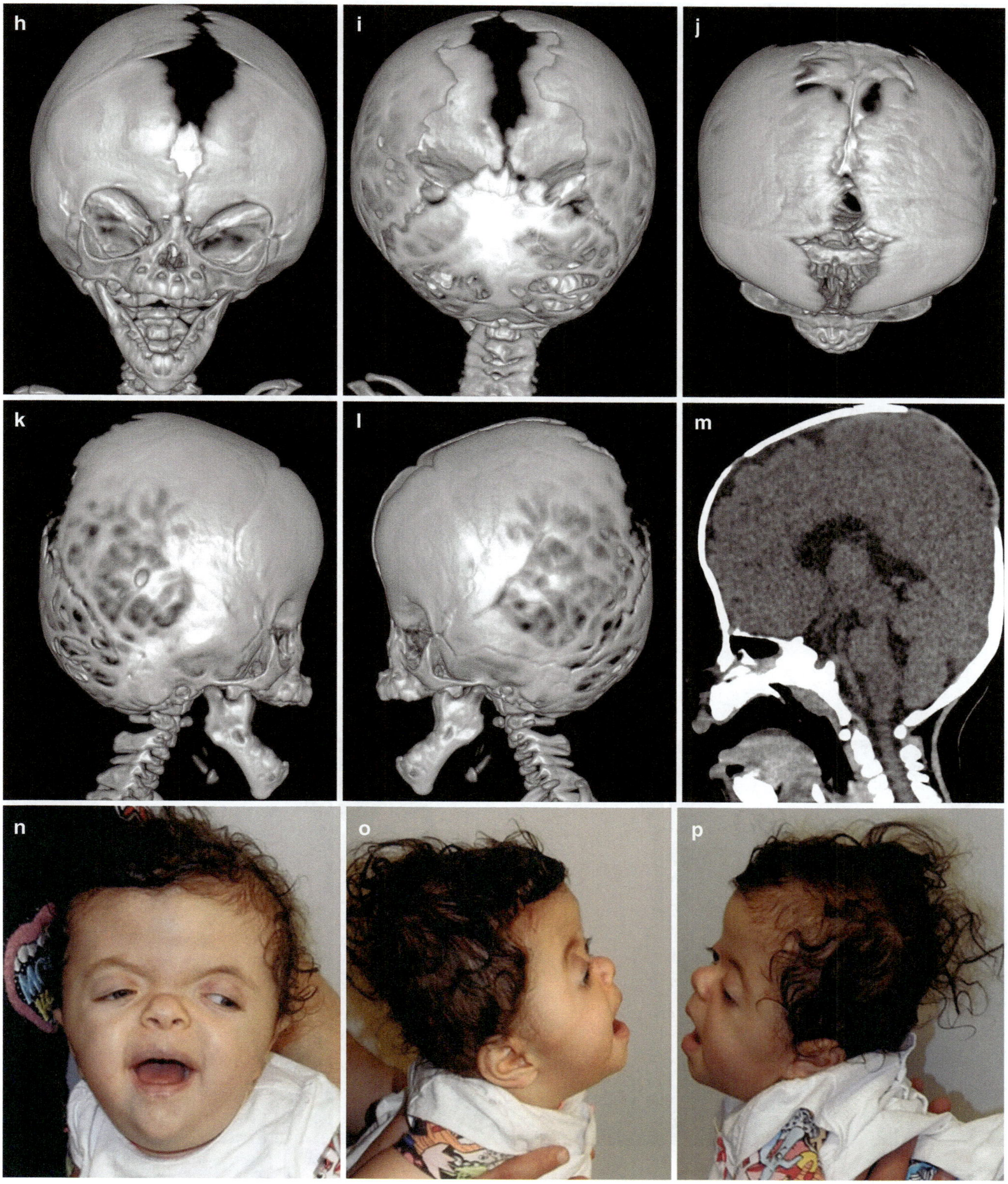

Fig. 10.15 (continued)

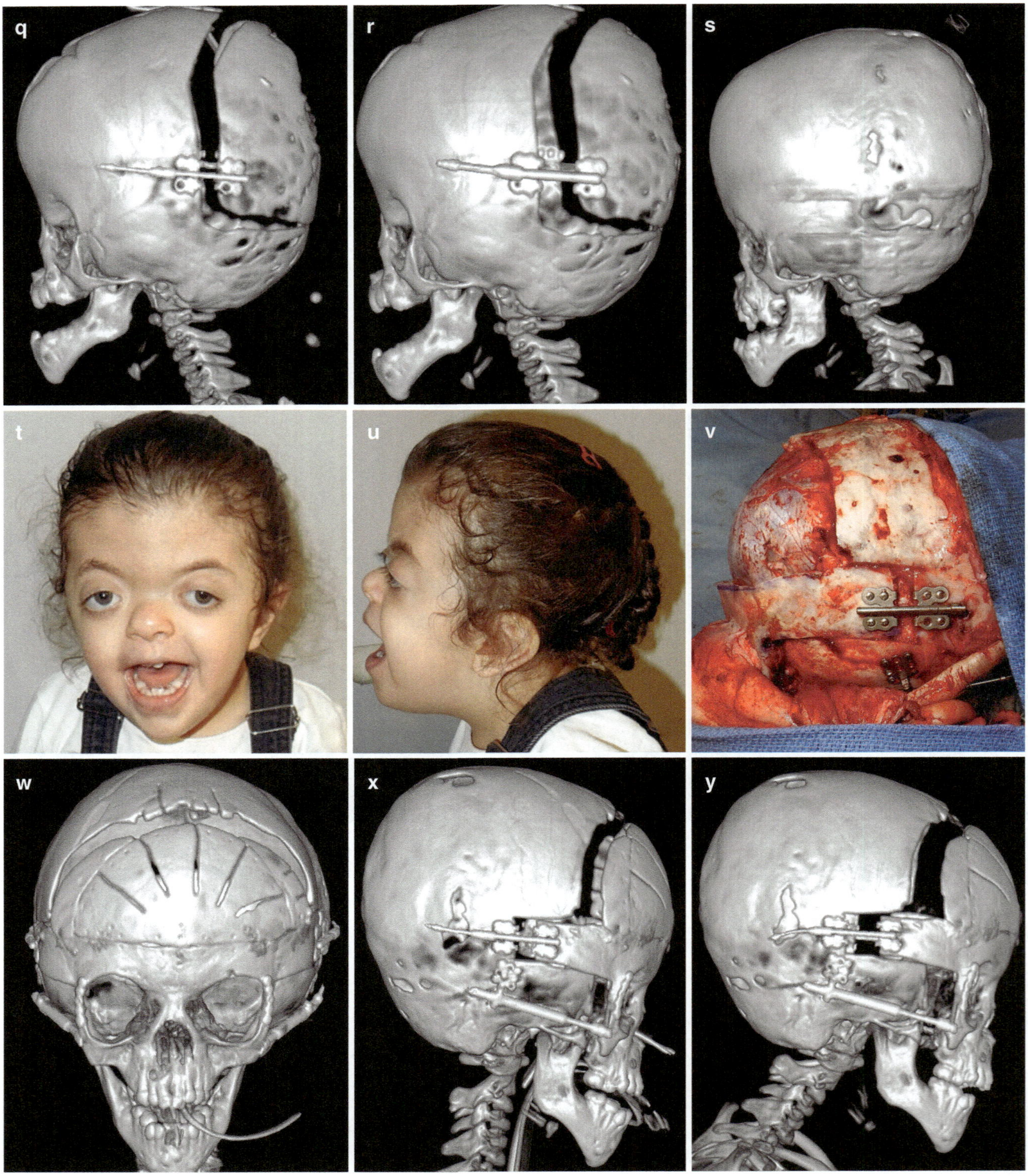

Fig. 10.15 (continued)

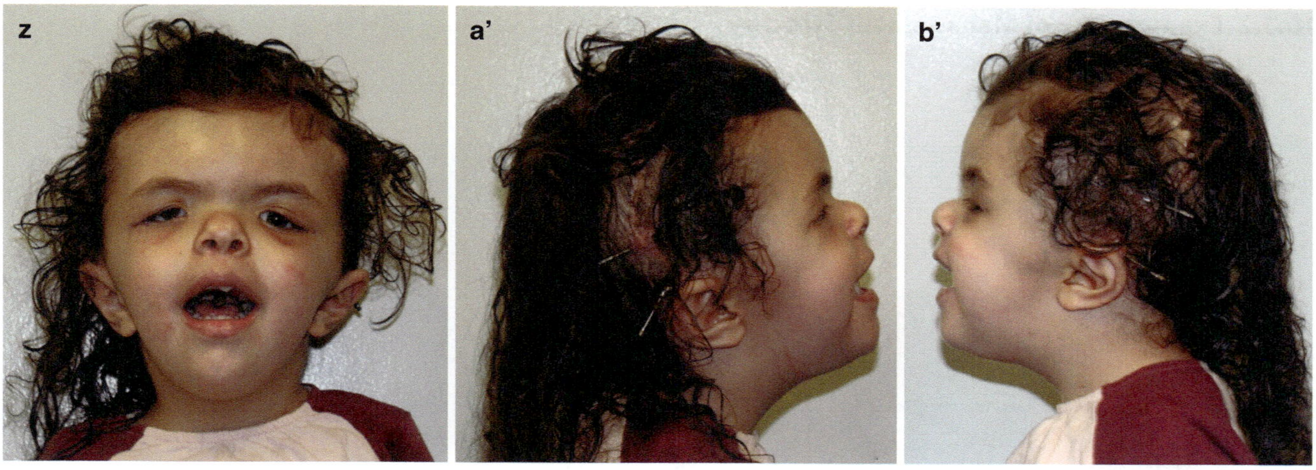

Fig. 10.15 (continued)

10.3.2 Example №2 of Management Strategy in Apert Syndrome

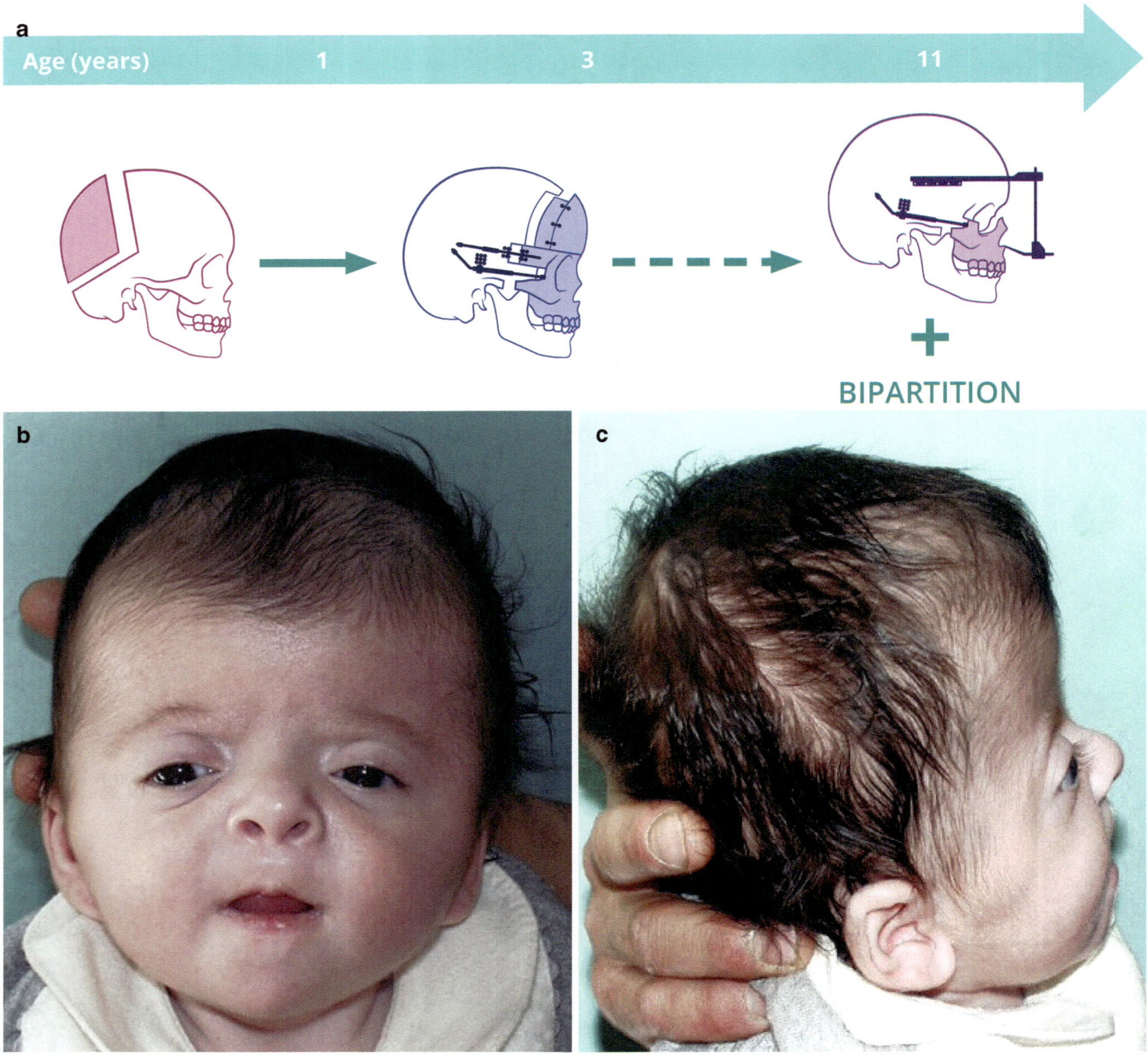

Fig. 10.16 (**a**) Management strategy in a patient with Apert syndrome (same patient as in Fig. 2.3). (**b, c**) Initial clinical presentation at 1 month of age. ©Cassandra Vion. (**d, e**) PVE without distraction at age 4 months using the historical tongue and groove technique without distraction (abandoned because of unnecessary morbidity risk, replaced by distraction). (**f**) Large undermining of the occipital and posterior parietal bone (Photograph taken on a back table). (**g**) The posterior skull bones are advanced posteriorly and stabilized with absorbable sutures. (**h, i**) Morphological result at 7 months, 3 months after PVE. (**j, k**) Clinical presentation at 2 years of age showing maxillary retrusion with Angle class III malocclusion and moderate exorbitism. Severe obstructive sleep apnea was diagnosed (AHI was 34 per hour). FFMBA was indicated. (**l**) Per-operative view of the FFMBA performed at 2 years and 5 months of age. (**m, n**) CT scans during the distraction period after FFMBA. (**o, p**) Four-month-postoperative pictures demonstrating maxillary and forehead advancement with overcorrection (Angle class II malocclusion). Resolution of exorbitism and improvement of obstructive sleep apnea (AHI was reduced to 6 per hour). (**q, r**) Clinical photographs at age 3 years and 4 months demonstrating stability of the fronto-facial advancement 1 year postoperatively. (**s**) One-year-postoperative CT scan showing ossification of the temporal, zygomatic and coronal osteotomies, and overcorrection of the maxillary advancement. (**t, u, v**) Clinical photographs at age 5 years (2.5 years after FFMBA) demonstrating edge-to-edge occlusion and a narrow high-arched palate. No relapse at the orbital level. (**w, x, y**) Clinical photographs at age 7 years (4.5 years after FFMBA) showing class III malocclusion and bilateral crossbite. (**z**) CT scan at age 7 years showing class III malocclusion. Obstructive sleep apnea was episodically aggravated by hypertrophic tonsils (AHI = 12 per h). Tonsillectomy and laser turbinoplasty were performed. (**a', b', c'**) Clinical photographs at age 10 years showing class III malocclusion with characteristic hypertelorbitism and downslanting palpebral fissures. AHI was reduced to 2 per hour. (**d', e'**) Secondary LF3 with bipartition and external distraction was performed at age 11 years and 5 months, 9 years after FFMBA. (**f', g'**) Clinical photographs 4 months after the Le Fort III demonstrating midface advancement with overcorrection. Hypertelorbitism and downslanting of palpebral fissures were also improved. Polysomnography demonstrated complete resolution of obstructive sleep apnea (AHI was reduced to one per hour)

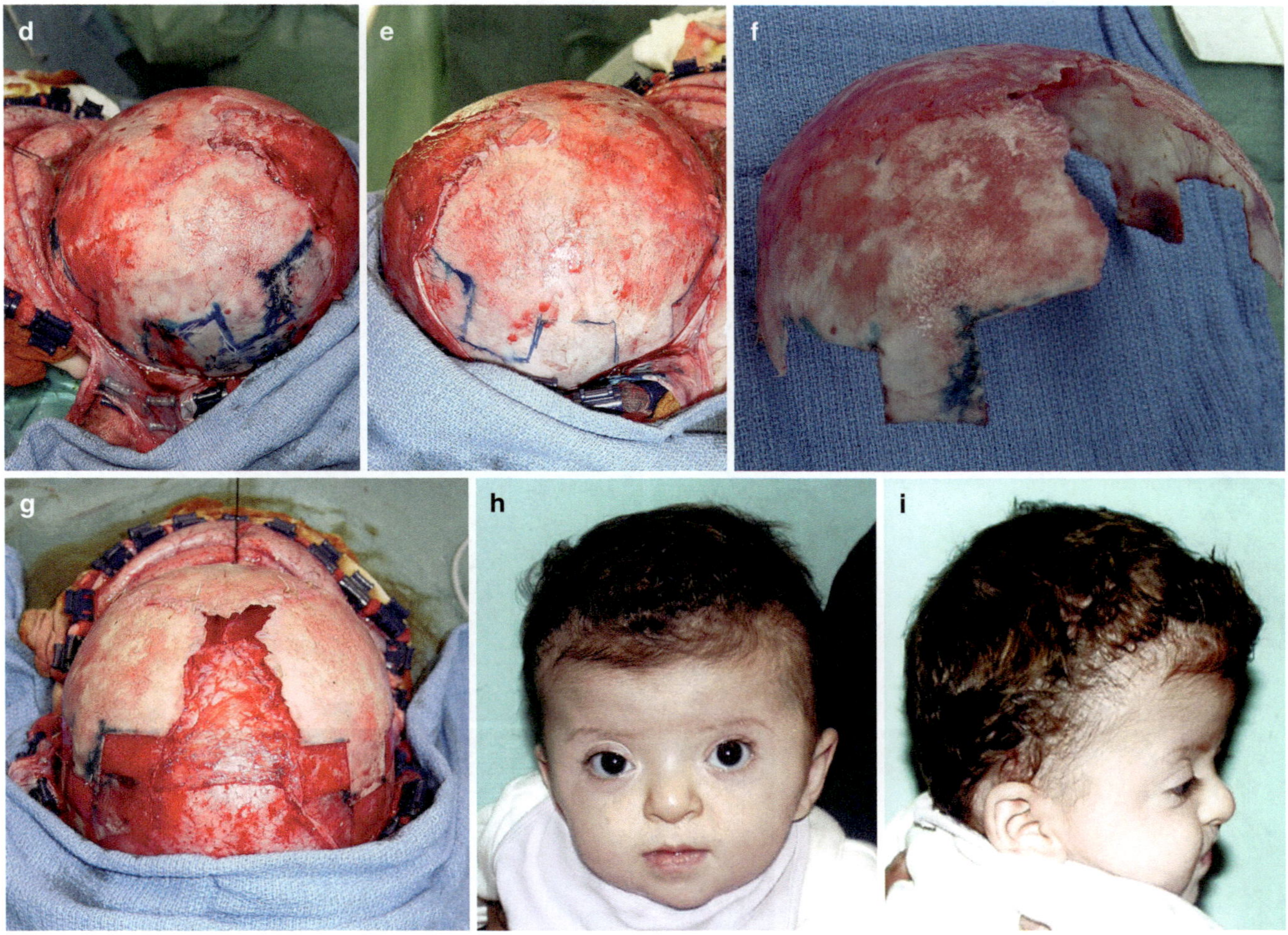

Fig. 10.16 (continued)

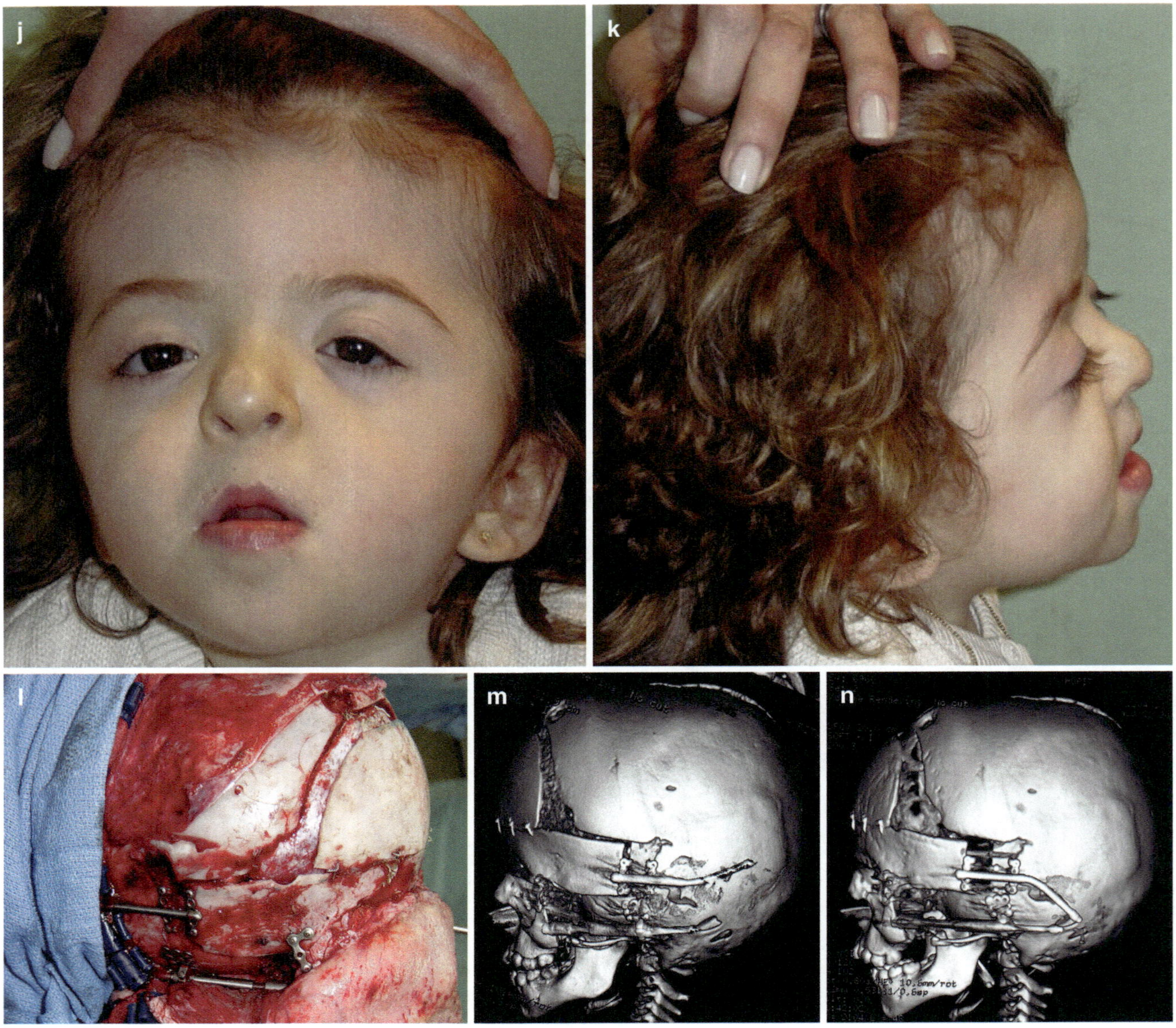

Fig. 10.16 (continued)

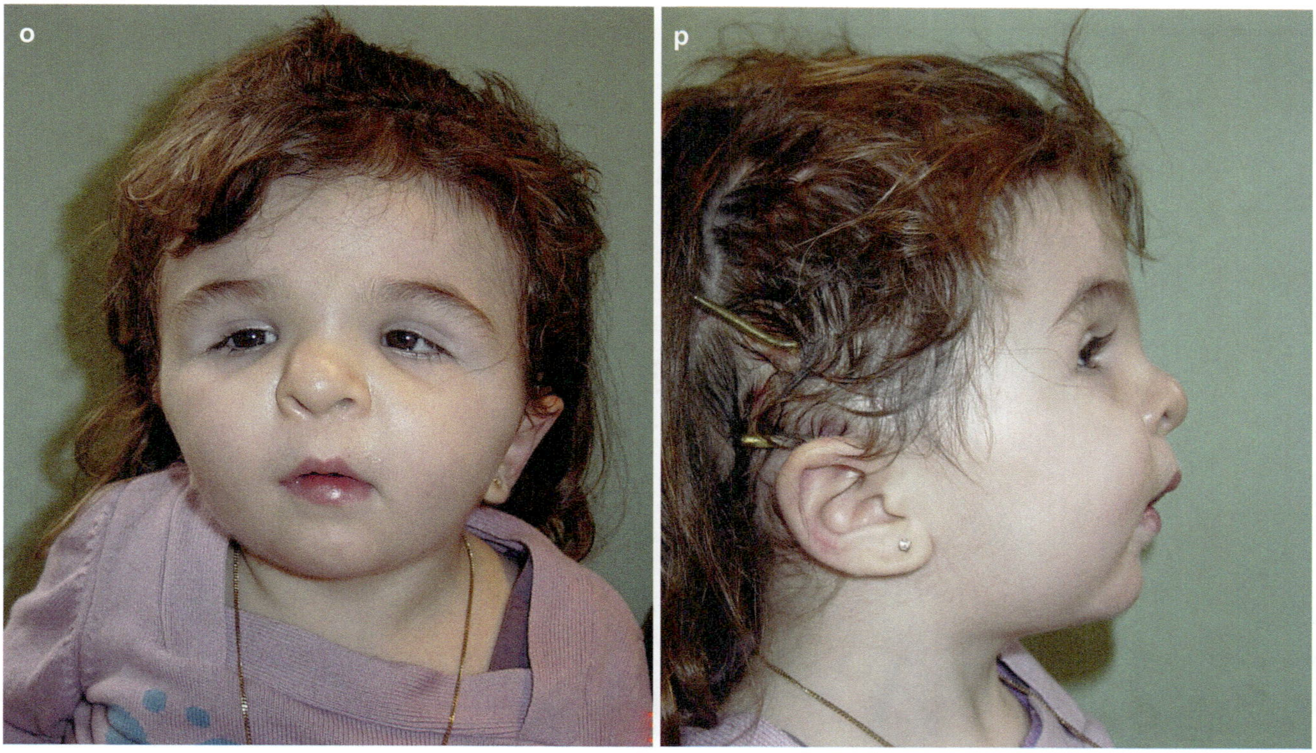

Fig. 10.16 (continued)

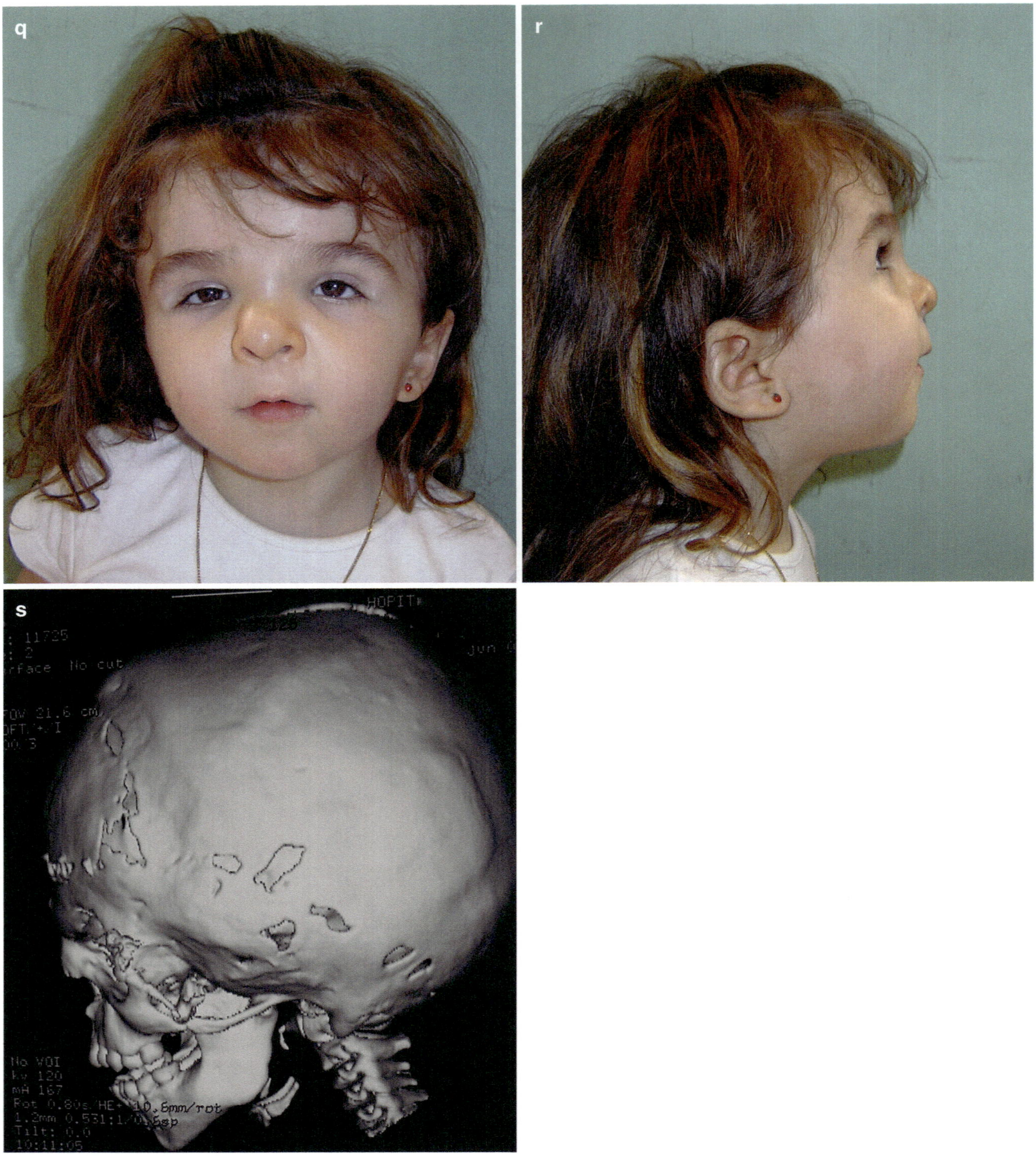

Fig. 10.16 (continued)

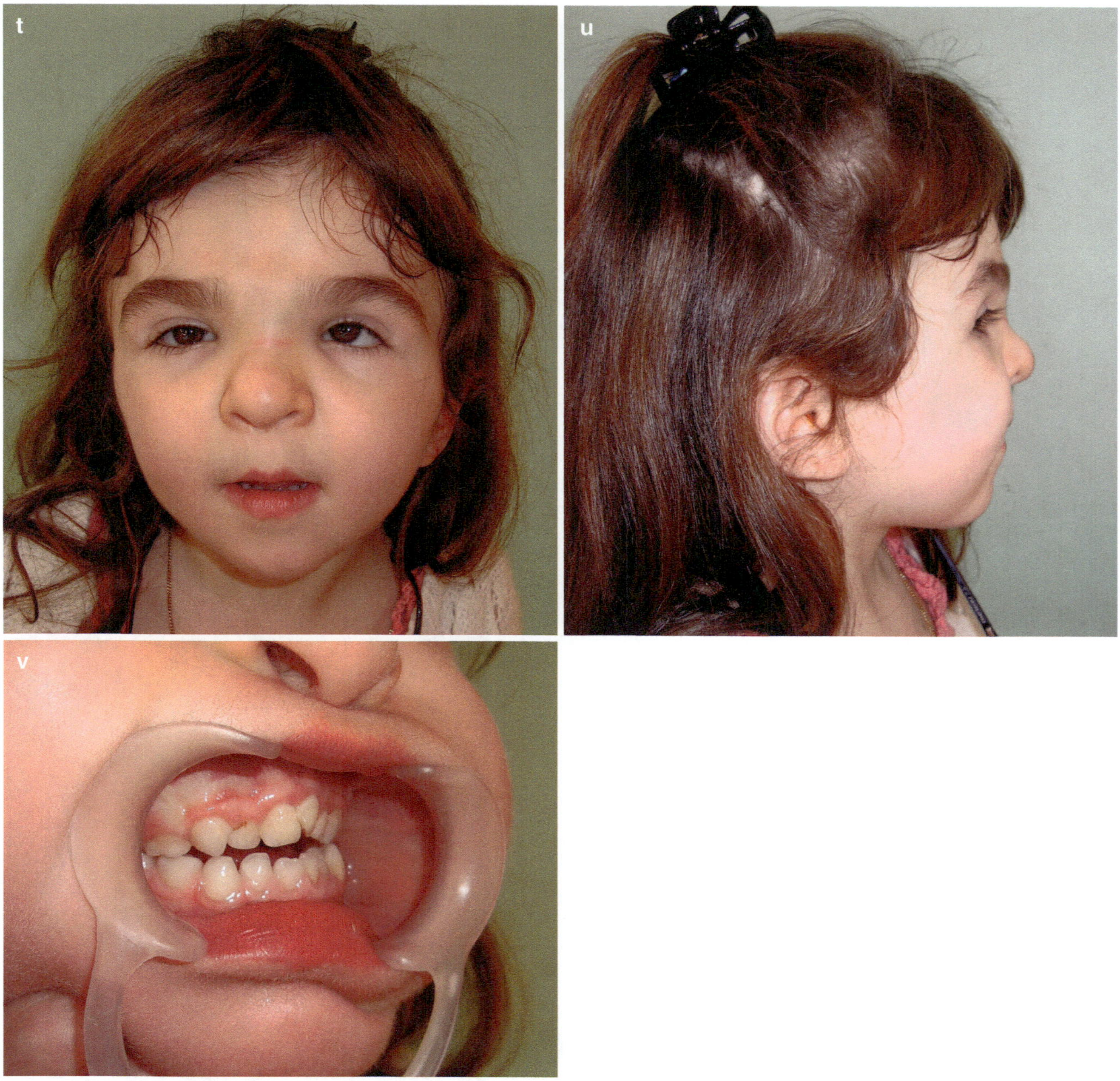

Fig. 10.16 (continued)

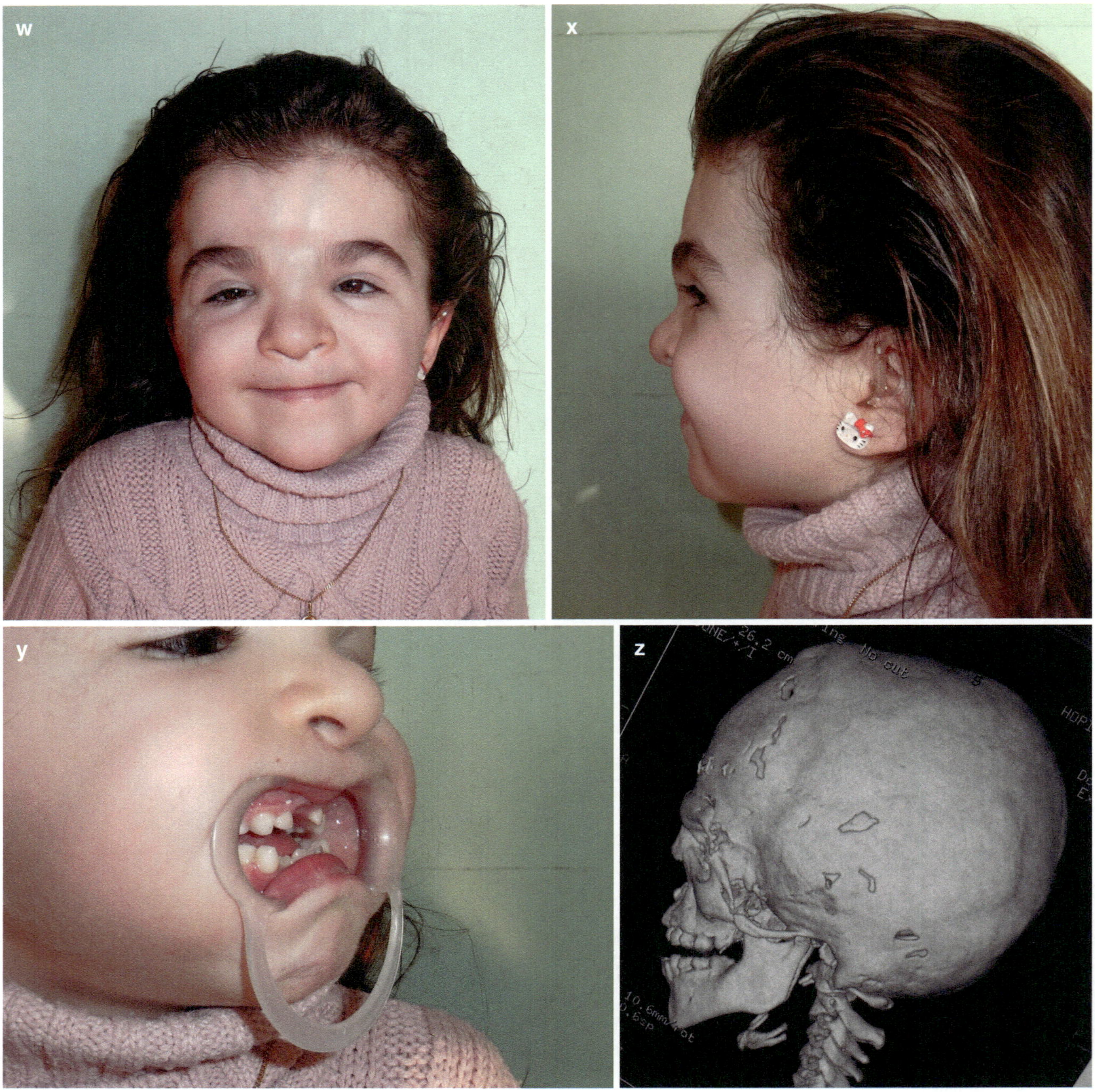

Fig. 10.16 (continued)

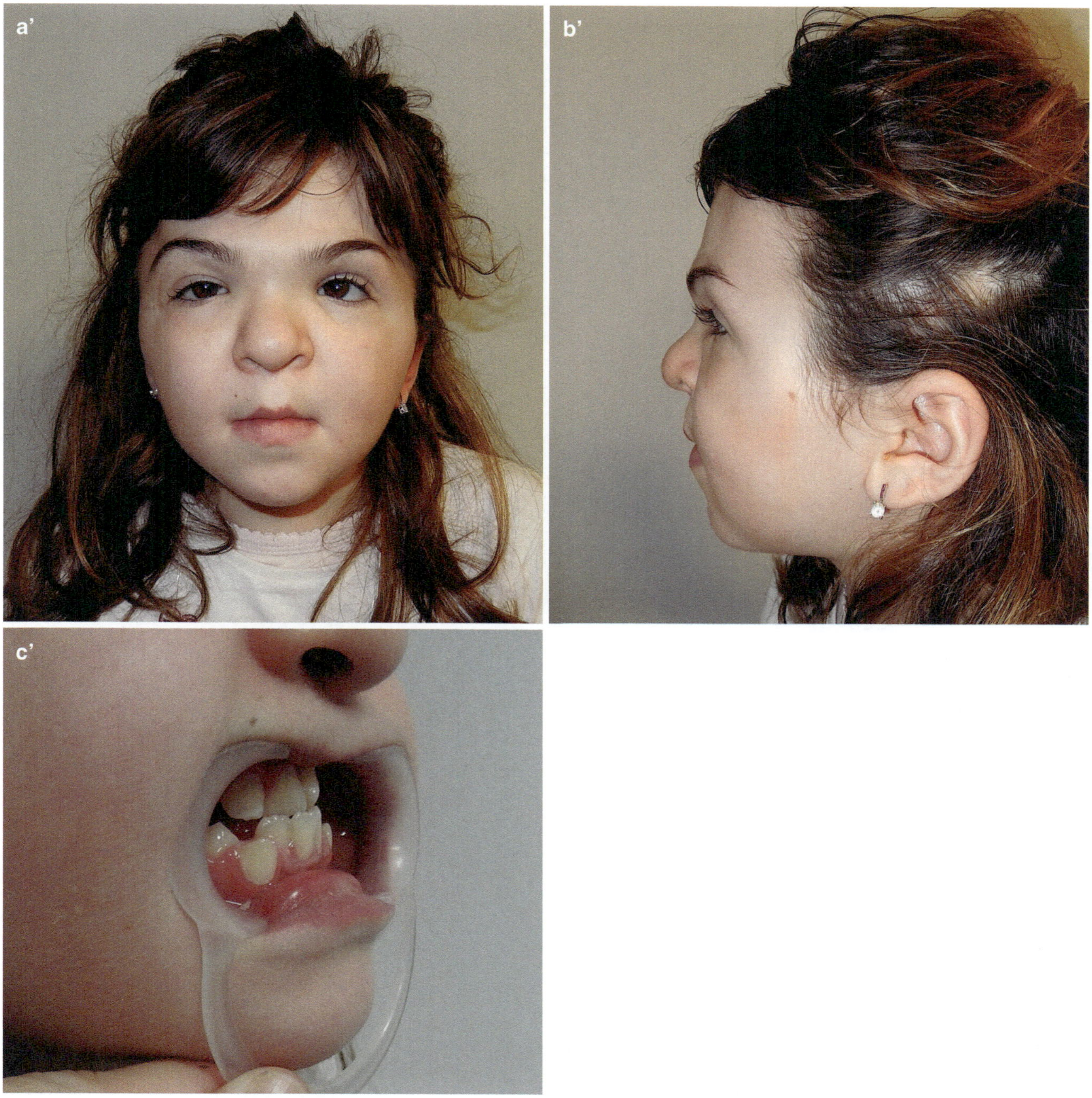

Fig. 10.16 (continued)

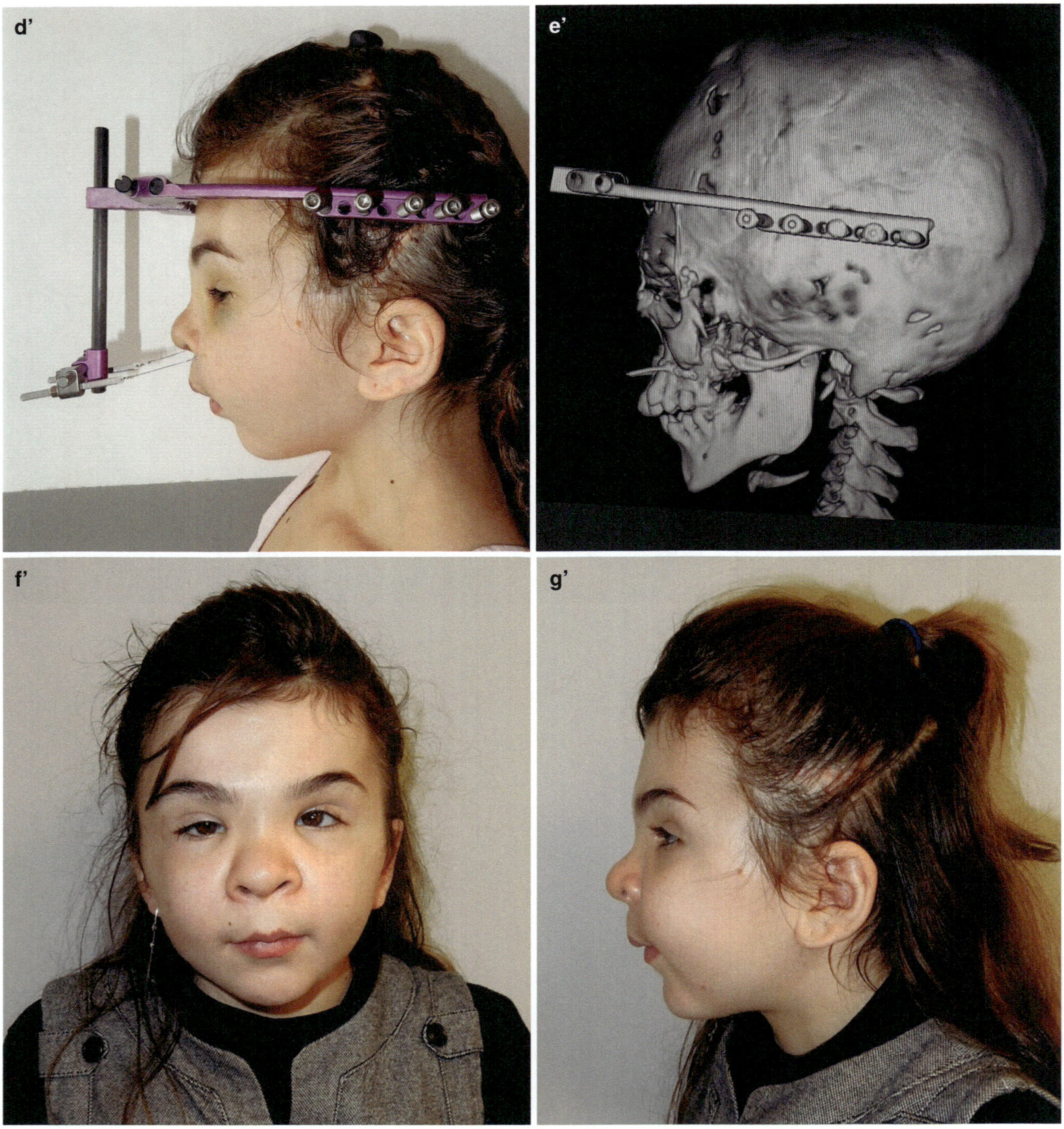

Fig. 10.16 (continued)

10.3.3 Example №3 of Management Strategy in Apert Syndrome

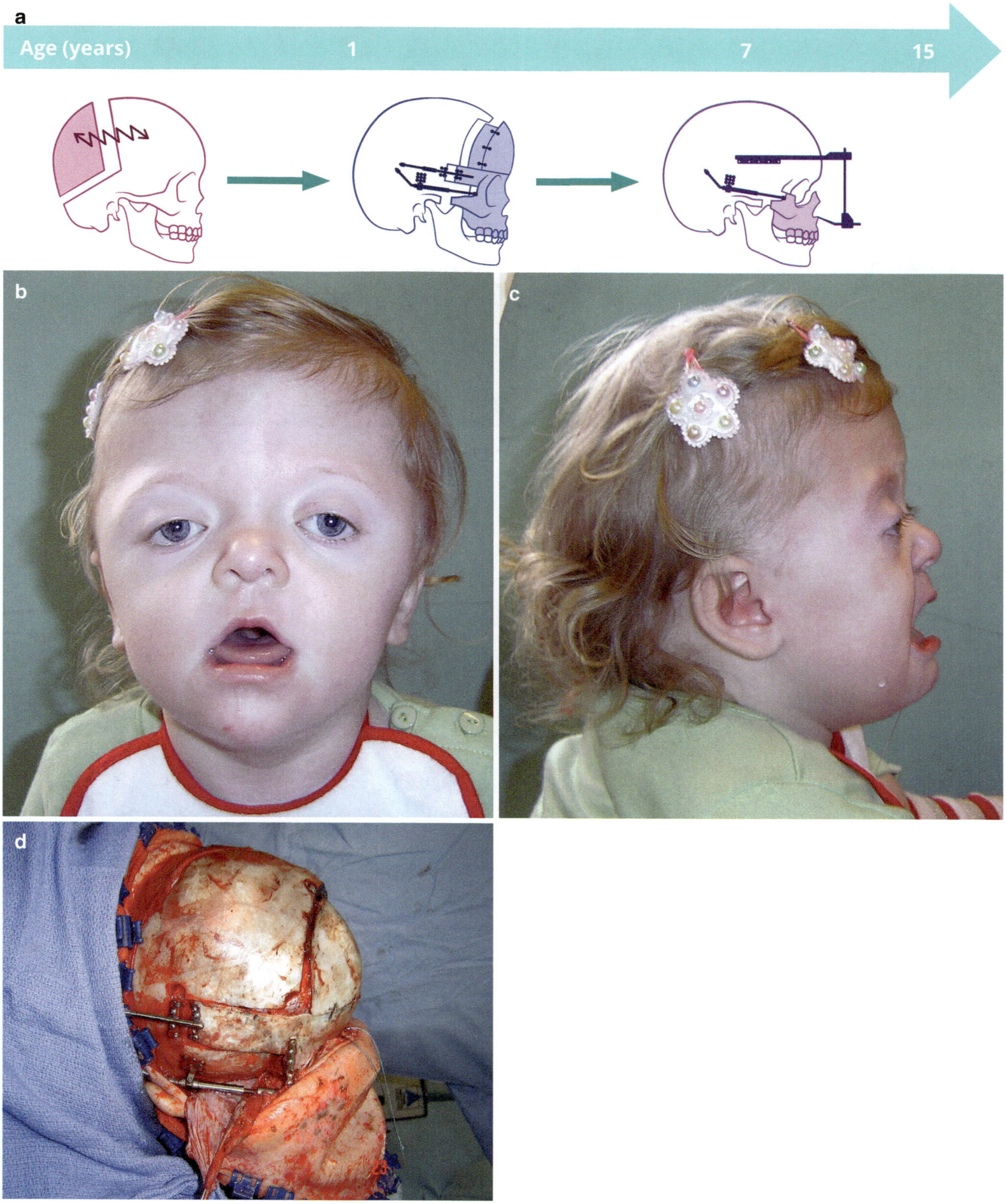

Fig. 10.17 (**a**, **b**, **c**) Nineteen-month-old patient with Apert syndrome, 1 year after trans-lambdoid spring insertion (same patient as in Fig. 2.12). Polysomnography revealed severe OSA (AHI = 21 per hour). FFMBA was indicated to improve breathing. ©Cassandra Vion. (**d**) Intraoperative photograph during FFMBA performed at age 21 months. (**e**, **f**) Clinical photographs at 4 years of age, 2 years after FFMBA. (**g-j**). Clinical photographs at 8 years of age, 6 years after FFMBA. (**k**, **l**) Secondary LF3 performed at 8 years of age with moderate overcorrection, 6 years after FFMBA. (**m-p**) Results 7 years after LF3, at 15 years of age, showing partial relapse of the midface hypoplasia with Angle class III malocclusion. Polysomnography was normal (AHI = 3 per h). Orthognathic surgery is indicated

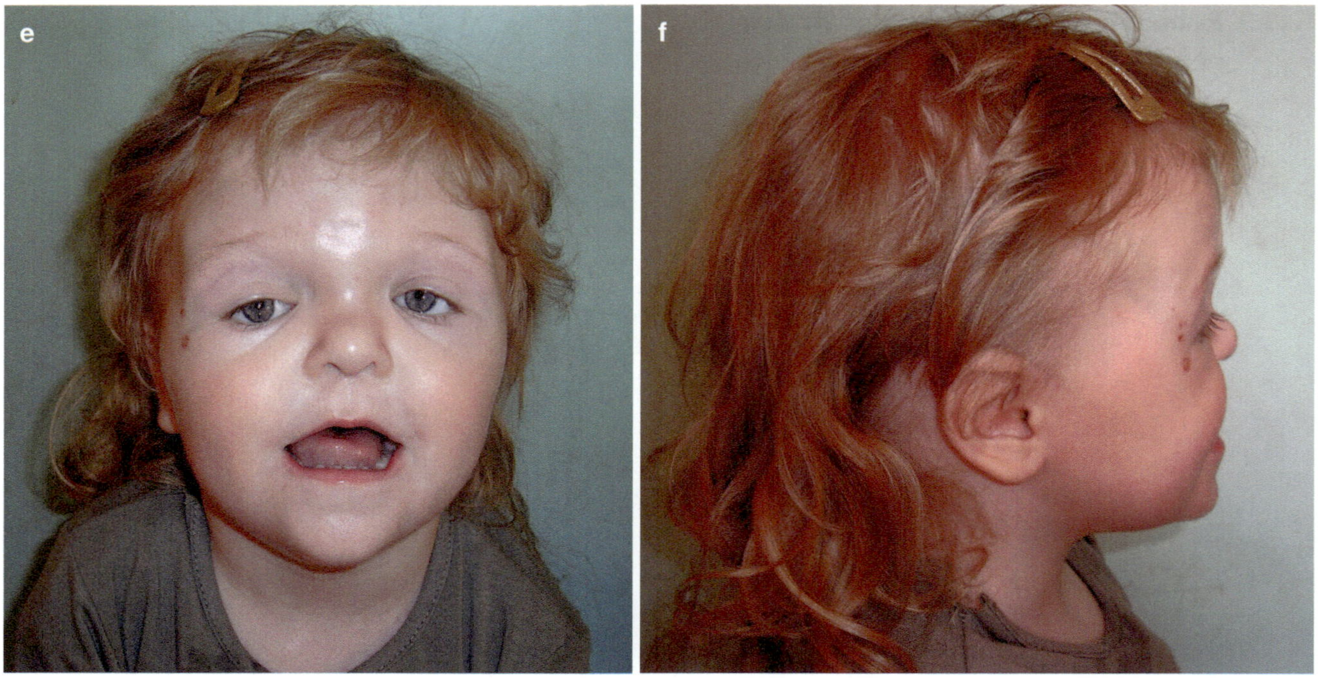

Fig. 10.17 (continued)

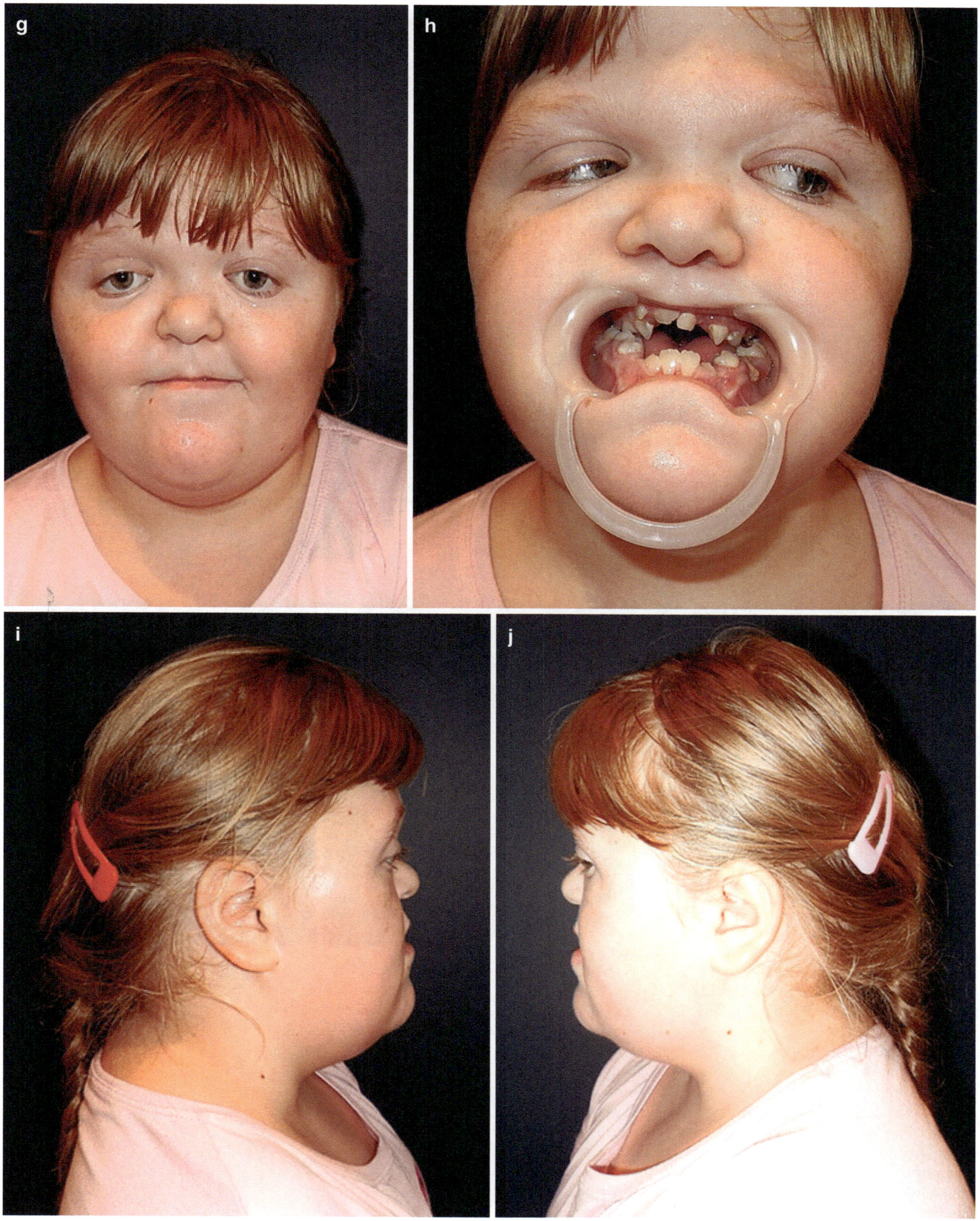

Fig. 10.17 (continued)

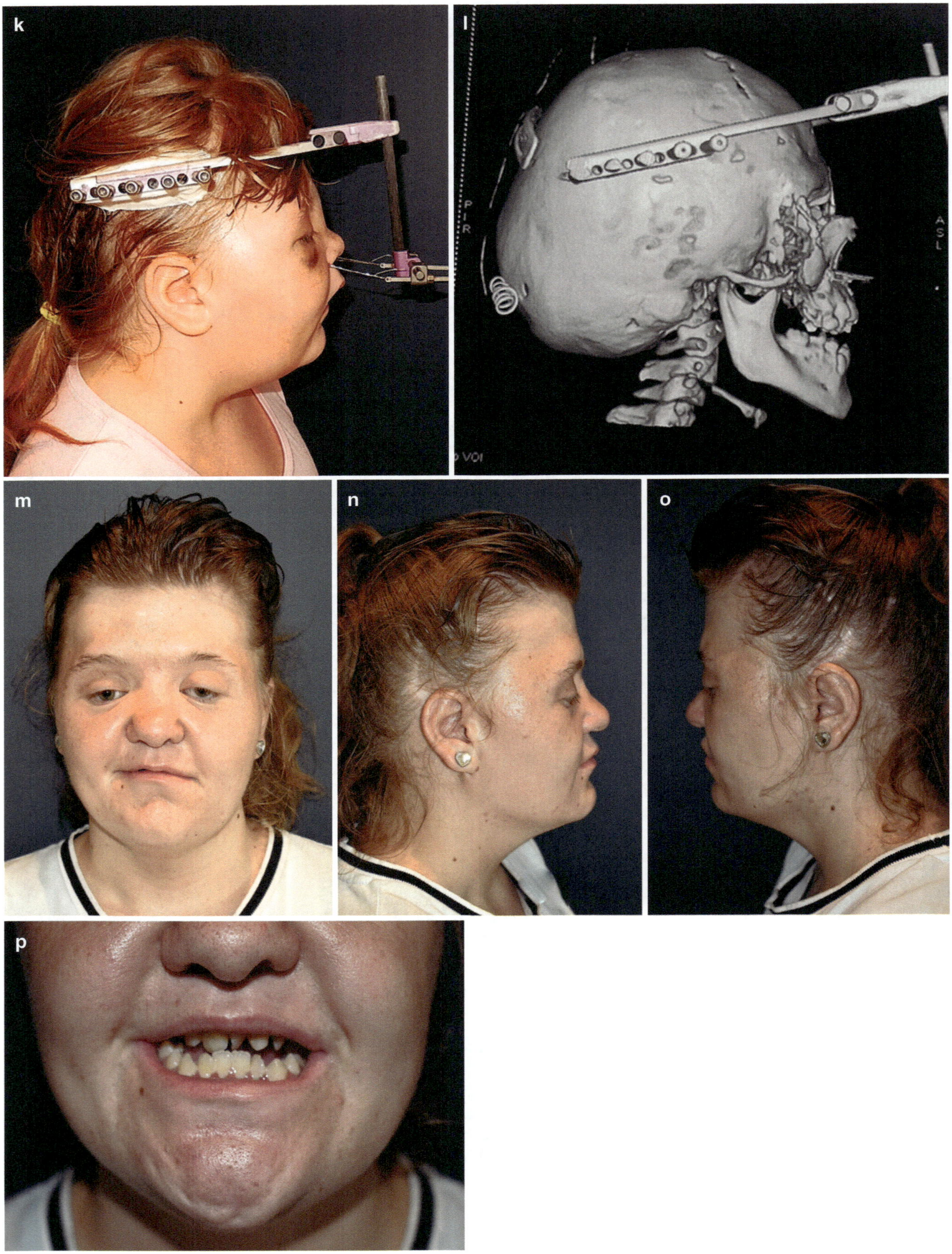

Fig. 10.17 (continued)

References

1. Cinalli G, Renier D, Sebag G, et al. Chronic tonsillar herniation in Crouzon's and Apert's syndromes: the role of premature synostosis of the lambdoid suture. J Neurosurg. 1995 Oct;83(4):575–82.
2. Nowinski D, Di Rocco F, Renier D, et al. Posterior cranial vault expansion in the treatment of craniosynostosis. Comparison of current techniques. Childs Nerv Syst. 2012 Sep;28(9):1537–44.
3. Arnaud E, Marchac A, Jeblaoui Y, et al. Spring-assisted posterior skull expansion without osteotomies. Childs Nerv Syst. 2012 Sep;28(9):1545–9.
4. Swanson JW, Samra F, Bauder A, et al. An algorithm for managing syndromic Craniosynostosis using posterior vault distraction osteogenesis. Plast Reconstr Surg. 2016 May;137(5):829e–41e.
5. Florisson JMG, Barmpalios G, Lequin M, et al. Venous hypertension in syndromic and complex craniosynostosis: the abnormal anatomy of the jugular foramen and collaterals. J Craniomaxillofac Surg. 2015 Apr;43(3):312–8.
6. Jeevan DS, Anlsow P, Jayamohan J. Abnormal venous drainage in syndromic craniosynostosis and the role of CT venography. Childs Nerv Syst. 2008 Dec;24(12):1413–20.
7. Cornelissen MJ, de Goederen R, Doerga P, et al. Pilot study of intracranial venous physiology in craniosynostosis. J Neurosurg Pediatr. 2018 Jun;21(6):626–31.
8. Ghali GZ, Zaki Ghali MG, Ghali EZ, et al. Intracranial venous hypertension in craniosynostosis: mechanistic underpinnings and therapeutic implications. World Neurosurg. 2018 Aug;6
9. Arnaud E, Di Rocco F. Faciocraniosynostosis: monobloc frontofacial osteotomy replacing the two-stage strategy? Childs Nerv Syst. 2012 Sep;28(9):1557–64.
10. Arnaud E, Paternoster G, James S, et al. Craniofacial strategy for syndromic craniosynostosis. Ann Chir Plast Esthet. 2016 Oct;61(5):408–19.
11. Choi M, Flores RL, Havlik RJ. Volumetric analysis of anterior versus posterior cranial vault expansion in patients with syndromic craniosynostosis. J Craniofac Surg. 2012 Mar;23(2):455–8.
12. Derderian CA, Wink JD, McGrath JL, et al. Volumetric changes in cranial vault expansion: comparison of fronto-orbital advancement and posterior cranial vault distraction osteogenesis. Plast Reconstr Surg. 2015 Jun;135(6):1665–72.
13. Noordzij N, Brouwer R, van der Horst C. Incomplete Reossification after Craniosynostosis surgery. J Craniofac Surg. 2016 Jan;27(1):e105–8.
14. Thenier-Villa JL, Sanromán-Álvarez P, Miranda-Lloret P, et al. Incomplete reossification after craniosynostosis surgery-incidence and analysis of risk factors: a clinical-radiological assessment study. J Neurosurg Pediatr. 2018;22(2):120–7.
15. Bouaoud J, Hennocq Q, Paternoster G, et al. Excessive ossification of the bandeau in Crouzon and Apert syndromes. J Craniomaxillofac Surg. 2020 Apr;48(4):376–82.
16. Morice A, Paternoster G, Ostertag A, et al. Anterior Skull Base and Pericranial flap ossification after Frontofacial Monobloc advancement. Plast Reconstr Surg. 2018;141(2):437–45.
17. Kaban LB, Conover M, Mulliken JB. Midface position after Le fort III advancement: a long-term follow-up study. Cleft Palate J. 1986 Dec;23(Suppl 1):75–7.
18. Ishii K, Kaloust S, Ousterhout DK, et al. Airway changes after Le fort III osteotomy in craniosynostosis syndromes. J Craniofac Surg. 1996;7(5):363–70. discussion P-371
19. Mathijssen I, Arnaud E, Marchac D, et al. Respiratory outcome of midface advancement with distraction: a comparison between Le fort III and frontofacial monobloc. J Craniofac Surg. 2006 Jul;17(4):642–4.
20. Wall SA, Butler L, Byren J, et al. Combined internal and external Le fort III distraction osteogenesis--the "elusive vector". J Craniofac Surg. 2009 Sep;20(Suppl 2):1806–8.

11 Aesthetic Refinements in Faciocraniosynostosis Surgery

1. Aesthetic refinements are mandatory to achieve a good morphological outcome and are often requested between adolescence and adulthood.
2. All major osteotomies (FFMBA, LF3) improve the aesthetic status but the result deteriorates until completion of growth.
3. Aesthetic improvements are mainly obtained with soft tissue surgery, rhinoplasty being usually as the last step.

It is exceptional for a syndromic child to reach adulthood without expressing the need for cosmetic improvement. Aesthetic refinements in faciocraniosynostoses are usually requested around adolescence or later [1]. There is no usual protocol or predefined sequence of interventions but rather a variable set of ancillary procedures that may—or may not—be undertaken.

If an orthognathic procedure is necessary, usually after 14 years of age, it is preferable to have it performed before the other aesthetic procedures, particularly the rhinoplasty.

The non-exhaustive list of possible improvements includes the following:

- Bicoronal scar revision
- Burring of frontal/calvarial irregularities
- Frontal sinus reduction (particularly in Apert syndrome)
- Lateral/medial canthopexies
- Fat grafting in the temporal and zygomatic regions
- Genioplasty (advancement type)
- Rhinoseptoplasty (especially after LF3, which disrupts the nasal dorsum)

11.1 Bicoronal Scar Revision

Bicoronal scar widening often occurs bitemporally. Hypertrophic scarring is less frequently encountered. Both conditions may generate a demand for aesthetic scar improvement around adolescence or later in adulthood. Scar revision may or may not achieve improvement as the scalp has thick dermis; patient information is crucial to manage expectations. In general, it is possible to achieve a 50% width reduction in the majority of cases.

11.2 Burring of Frontal/Calvarial Irregularities

Bony irregularities of the forehead or of the hair-bearing region are frequently palpable in operated patients. If they are not visible, surgery is not justified. However, when they cause visible deformity or asymmetry with an aesthetic demand, surgery is indicated using the preexisting bicoronal approach to flatten the bony lumps using a surgical bur (Fig. 11.1).

E. Arnaud et al., *Frontofacial Monobloc Advancement with Internal Distraction*, https://doi.org/10.1007/978-3-031-07574-2_11

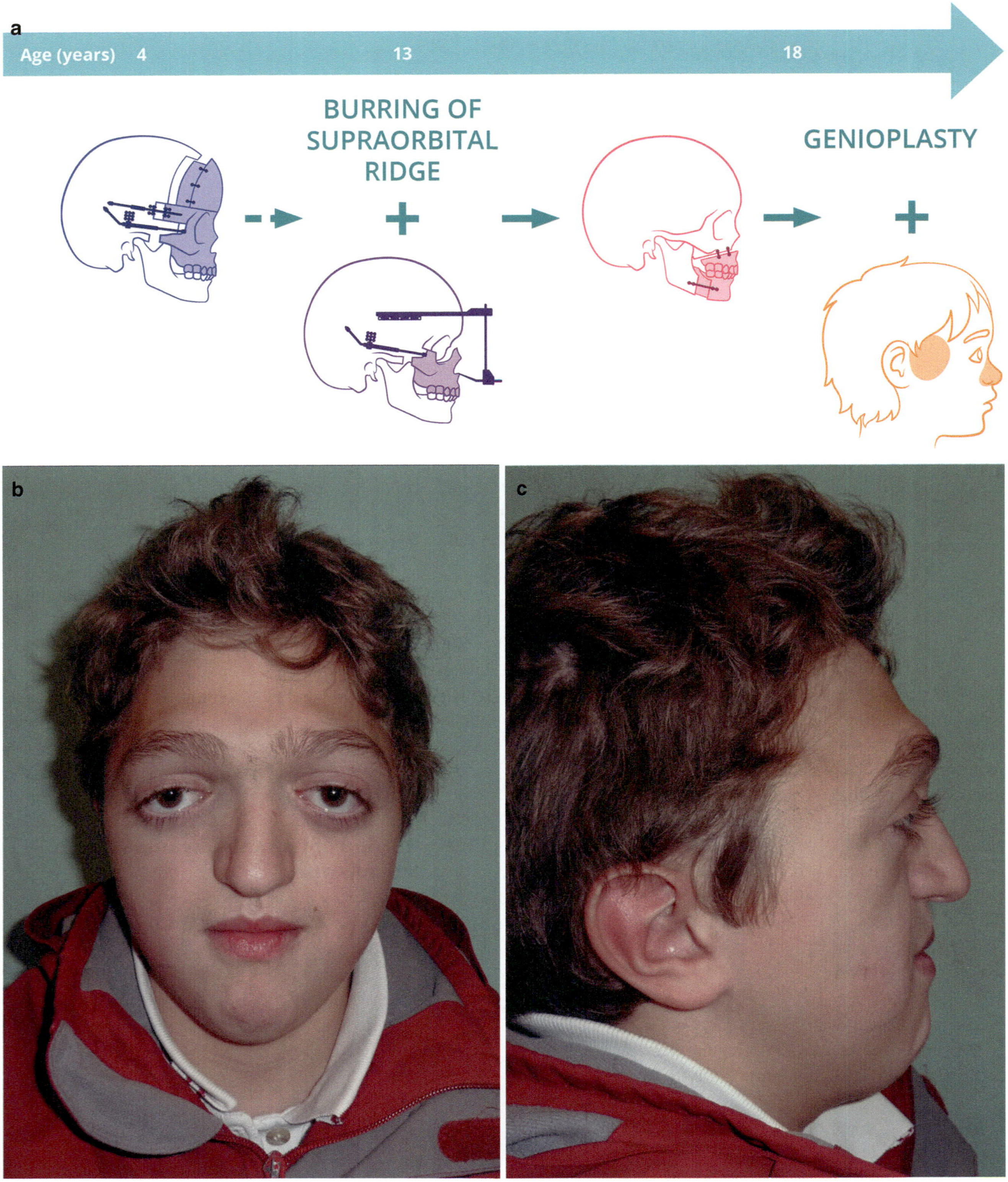

Fig. 11.1 (**a**, **b**, **c**) Patient with Crouzon syndrome at 14 years of age. Hypertrophic ossification of the supraorbital ridge. FFMBA had been performed at age 3 © Cassandra Vion. (**d**, **e**, **f**) Intraoperative views showing the burring of the supraorbital ridge and an onlay bone graft at the level of the nasion during the LF3 procedure. (**g, h**) Result after 2 years, at 16 years of age

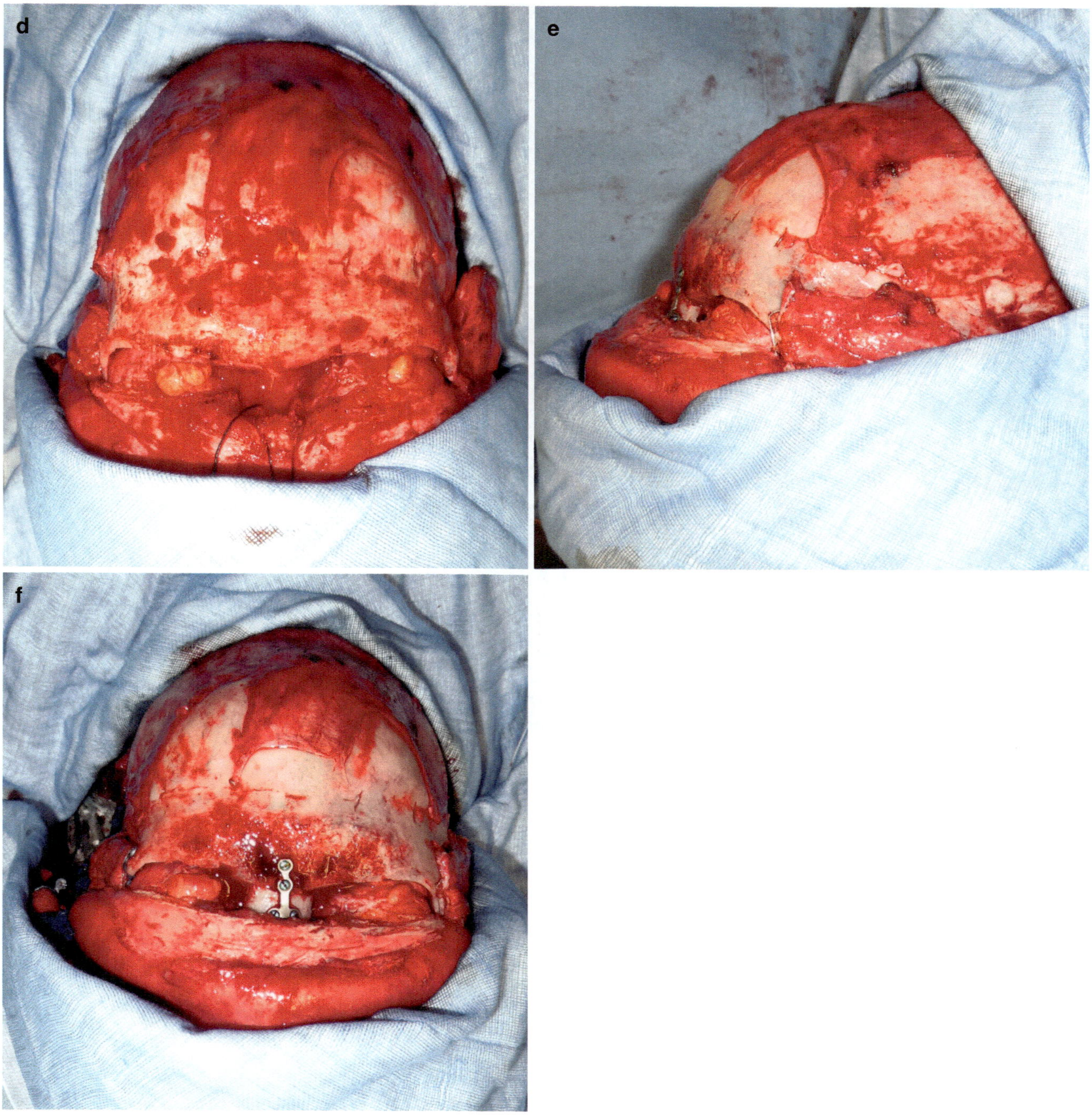

Fig. 11.1 (continued)

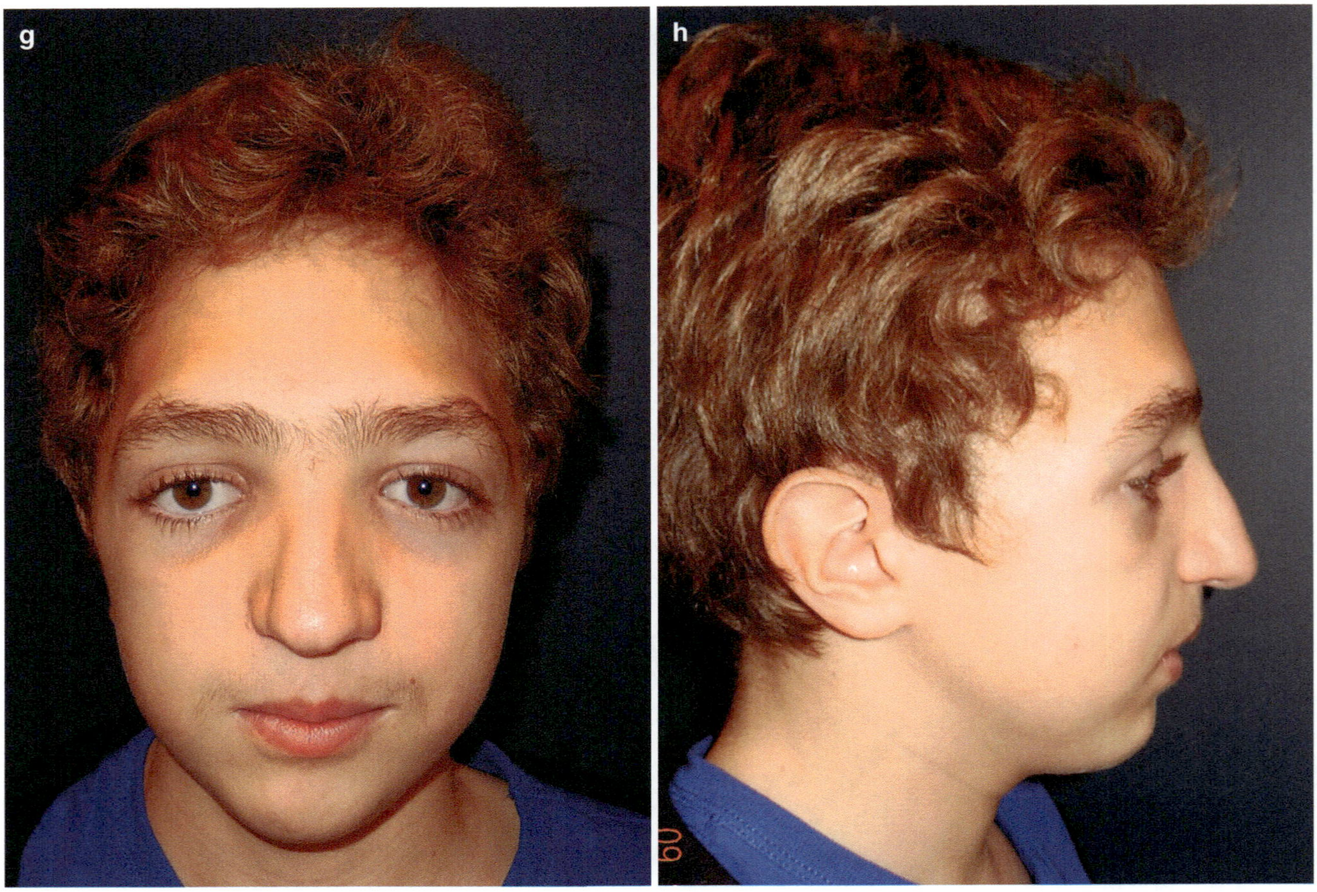

Fig. 11.1 (continued)

11.3 Frontal Sinus Reduction (Particularly in Apert Syndrome)

The supraorbital ridge may become hypertrophic and/or overprojecting after fronto-facial monobloc advancement. The hypertrophy is either purely bony or associated to an overpneumatized frontal sinus. The enlarged frontal sinus is frequently encountered in Apert syndrome: the mechanism may be related to the FFMBA which preserves the vascularization of the supraorbital ridge and/or to the absence of raised intracranial pressure.

The consequences are strictly aesthetic: the overprojecting glabellar region and supraorbital ridge cause masculinization of the face in women and a rough appearance in men. The treatment is surgical through the preexisting bicoronal scar. The forehead bone is exposed. The reciprocating saw is used to carefully harvest an oval-shaped bony cap spanning the glabella and both supraorbital regions. The underlying bone projection is then reduced uniformly with a surgical bur. The frontal sinus is usually widely exposed in the process. It is abundantly irrigated with normal saline to avoid debris blocking sinus drainage at the level of the frontal ostium. Care is taken to avoid excessive widening of the sinus opening causing the bony cap to fall into the sinus cavity. The bony cap is thinned using the surgical bur and it is ultimately repositioned using titanium microplates and screws. In case of strictly bony thickening, it is simply burred to an acceptable level (Fig. 11.2).

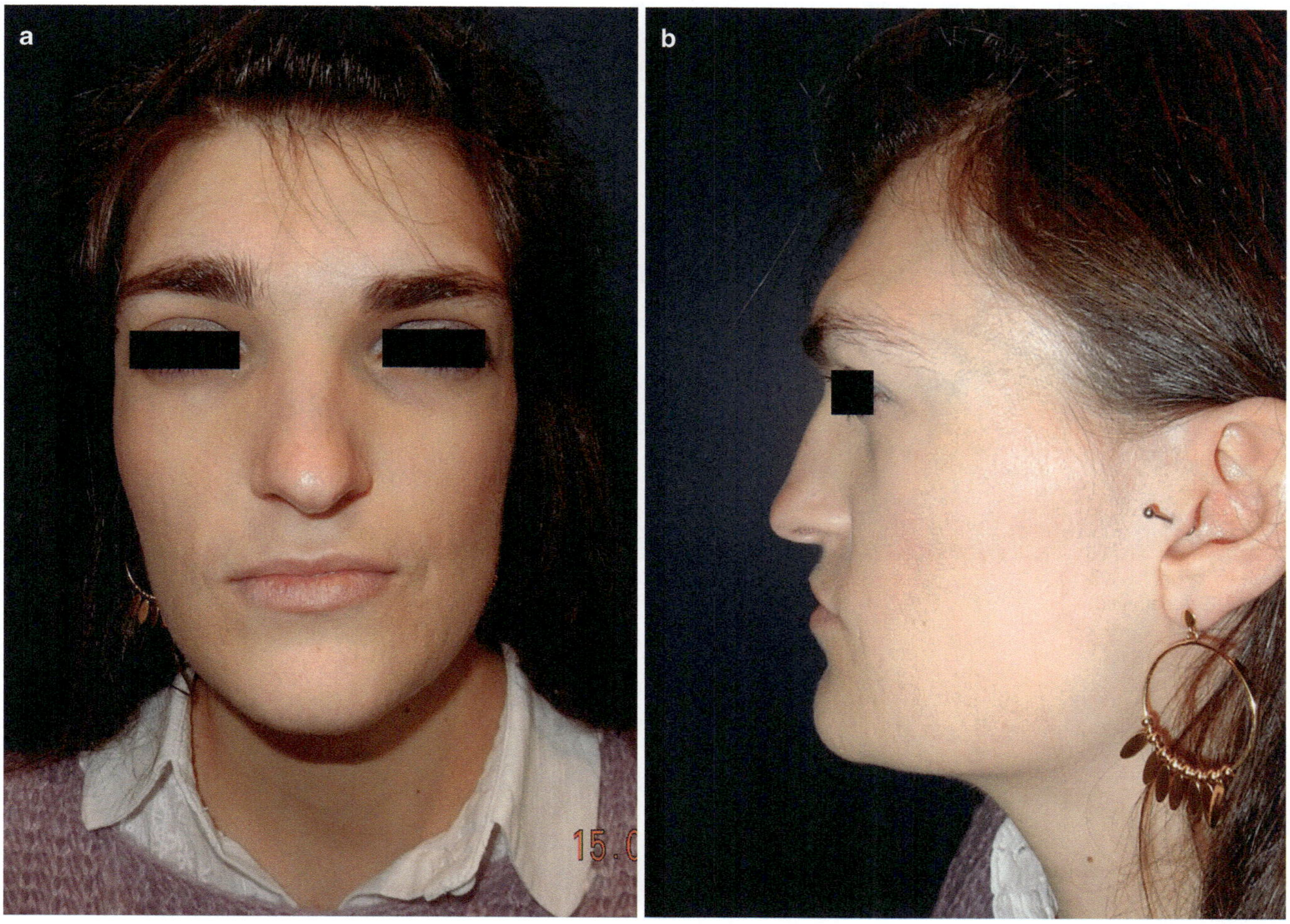

Fig. 11.2 (**a**, **b**) Patient with very moderate Crouzon syndrome at 20 years of age. FOA had been performed at 2 years of age. (**c**, **d**) Harvest of an oval-shaped cap along the surface of the supraorbital rim. (**e**) Fixation of the cap after thinning using titanium microplates. At the same time, fat grafting in zygomatic region has been performed. (**f**, **g**) Result after 1 year

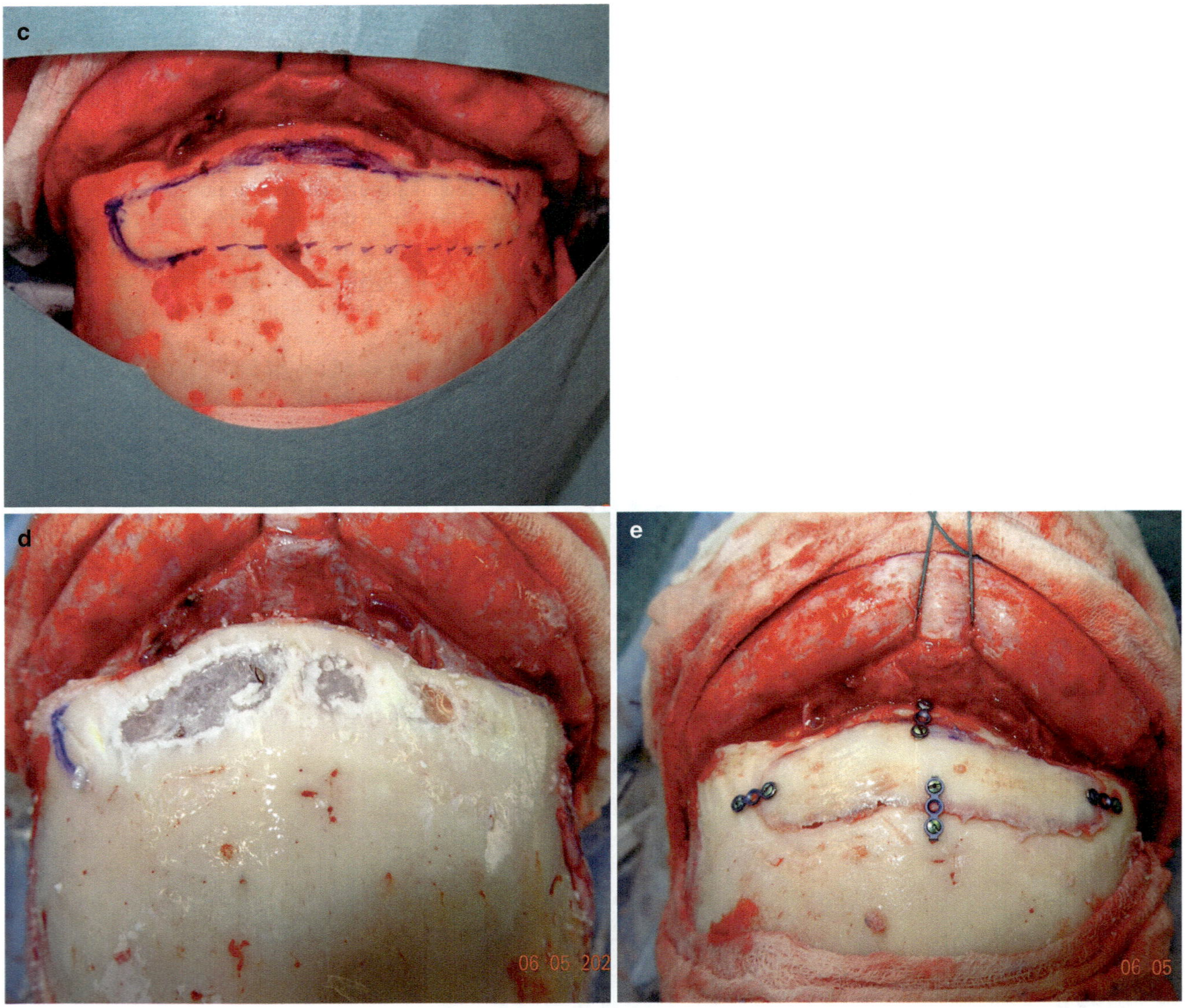

Fig. 11.2 (continued)

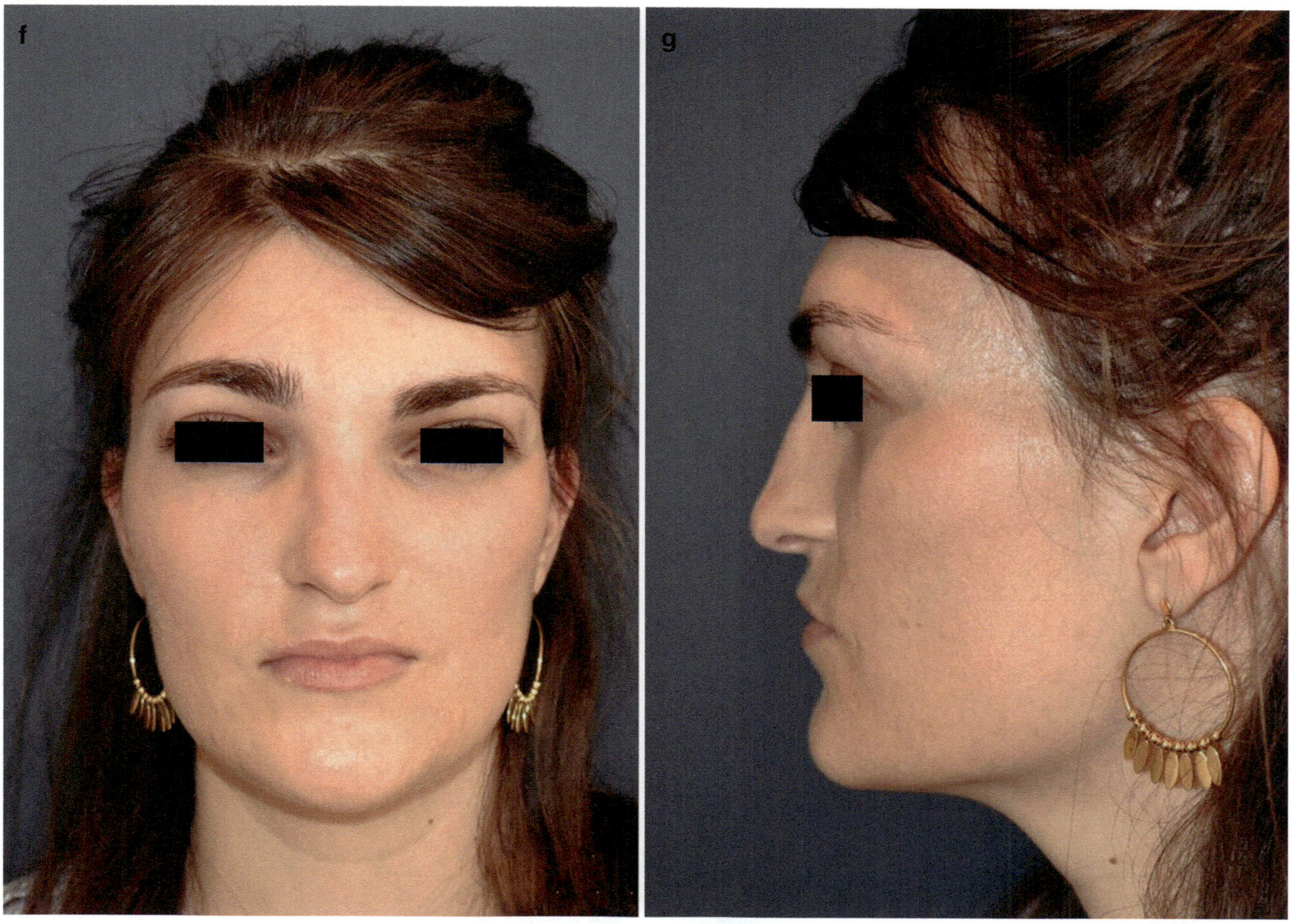

Fig. 11.2 (continued)

11.4 Lateral Canthopexy

FCST patients frequently present antimongoloid slanting of the palpebral fissures. The lateral canthal descent is either related to the disease itself (Apert syndrome) or to the subperiosteal undermining causing soft tissues to sag. This inferior displacement could be caused by gravity and/or by the inelastic maxillary periosteal downward traction during maxillary distraction.

The indication for lateral canthopexy can be curative in patients who display antimongoloid slanting of the palpebral fissures, or prophylactic during FFMBA or LF3 to prevent this type of deformity [2].

Technically, the lateral canthopexy should not charge the lateral canthus itself. In contrast with the sturdy medial canthal tendon, the lateral canthus typically has a much looser soft tissue structure. This precludes the possibility of a direct suspension suture as it would cut through the tissues under long-term traction. It is rather the lateral edge of the lower-lid tarsal plate that is sutured. Its dense connective tissue provides better tensile strength.

In a prophylactic setting during FFMBA and LF3 (bicoronal approach), the suspension suture is either anchored to bone or to a titanium plate using a non-resorbable non-braided suture (3–0 Surgical steel, FS-2 needle, ETHICON™, San Lorenzo, Puerto Rico, USA) with on-demand horizontal periosteal discharge incisions inferiorly (Fig. 11.3).

When the suspension is performed in a curative setting, a subciliary approach is used in the lateral third of the lower lid with a horizontal back-cut through a lateral canthal rhytid. The lateral edge of the inferior tarsus is then suspended to the lateral orbital periosteum using 5–0 Polypropylene suture.

The tension applied in a lateral canthopexy is slightly more important than the desired effect to account for postoperative tissue distension. A useful landmark is the inferior border of the pupil which should not be obstructed by the raised lower lid to avoid interference with the visual field. Similarly, it is contraindicated (relative contraindication) to perform concomitantly a lateral and a medial canthopexy on the same orbit.

Complications of lateral canthopexy include relapse and extrusion of the suture material.

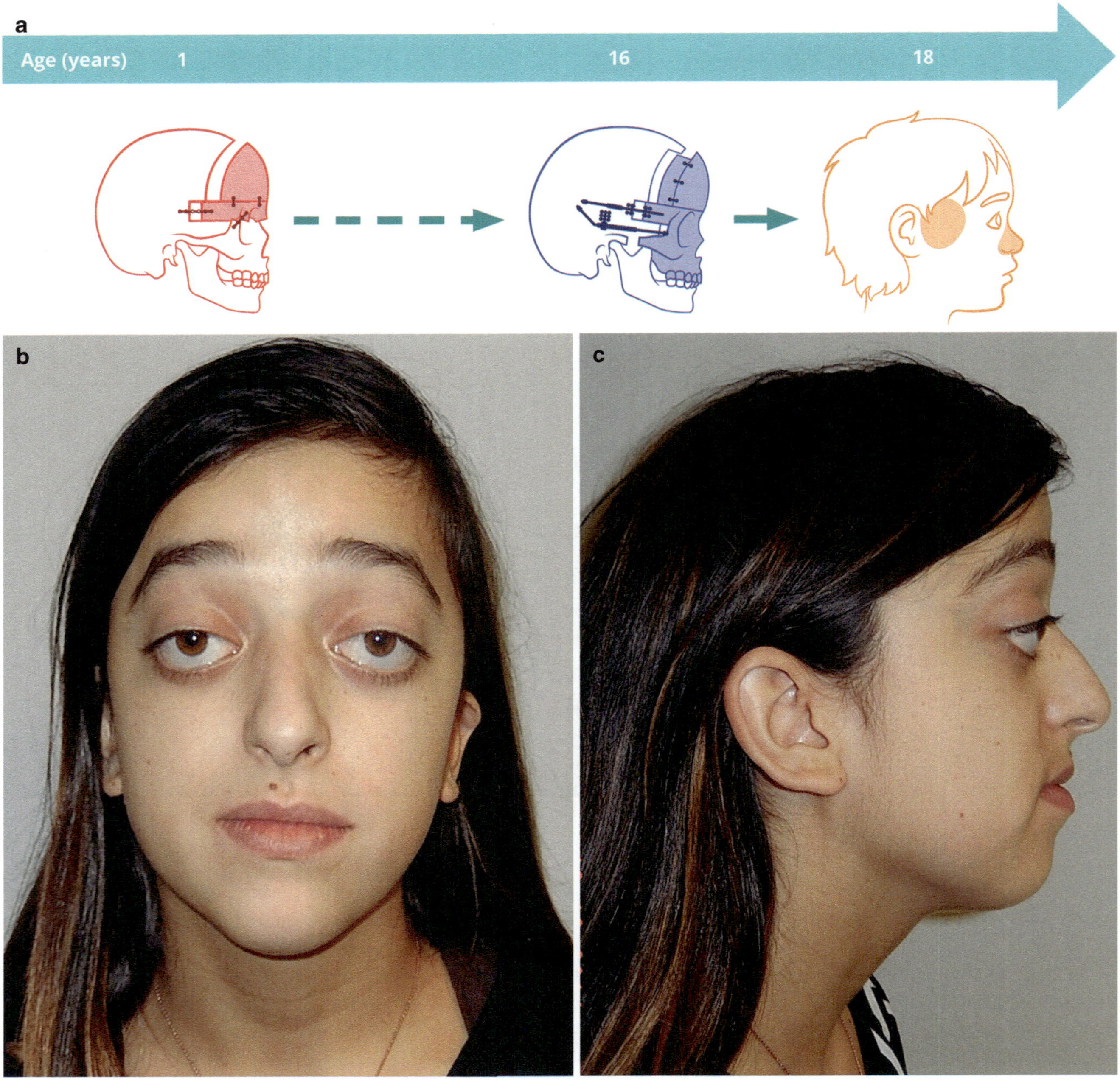

Fig. 11.3 (**a**, **b**, **c**) Patient with Crouzon syndrome at 15 years of age before FFMBA (corresponding to Fig. 11.4 (a-f)) © Cassandra Vion. (**d**, **e**) FFMBA performed at 15 years of age with lateral canthopexies using stainless steel sutures. (**f**, **g**) Immediate postoperative result with overcorrection. (**h**) Partial relapse of canthal tilt and inferior palpebral retraction 12 months after FFMBA, at 16 years of age. (**i**, **j**) Result 2 years after FFMBA, at 17 years of age, showing partial relapse. (**k**, **l**) One year after bilateral canthopexy, genioplasty, and rhinoplasty, and 5 years after FFMBA

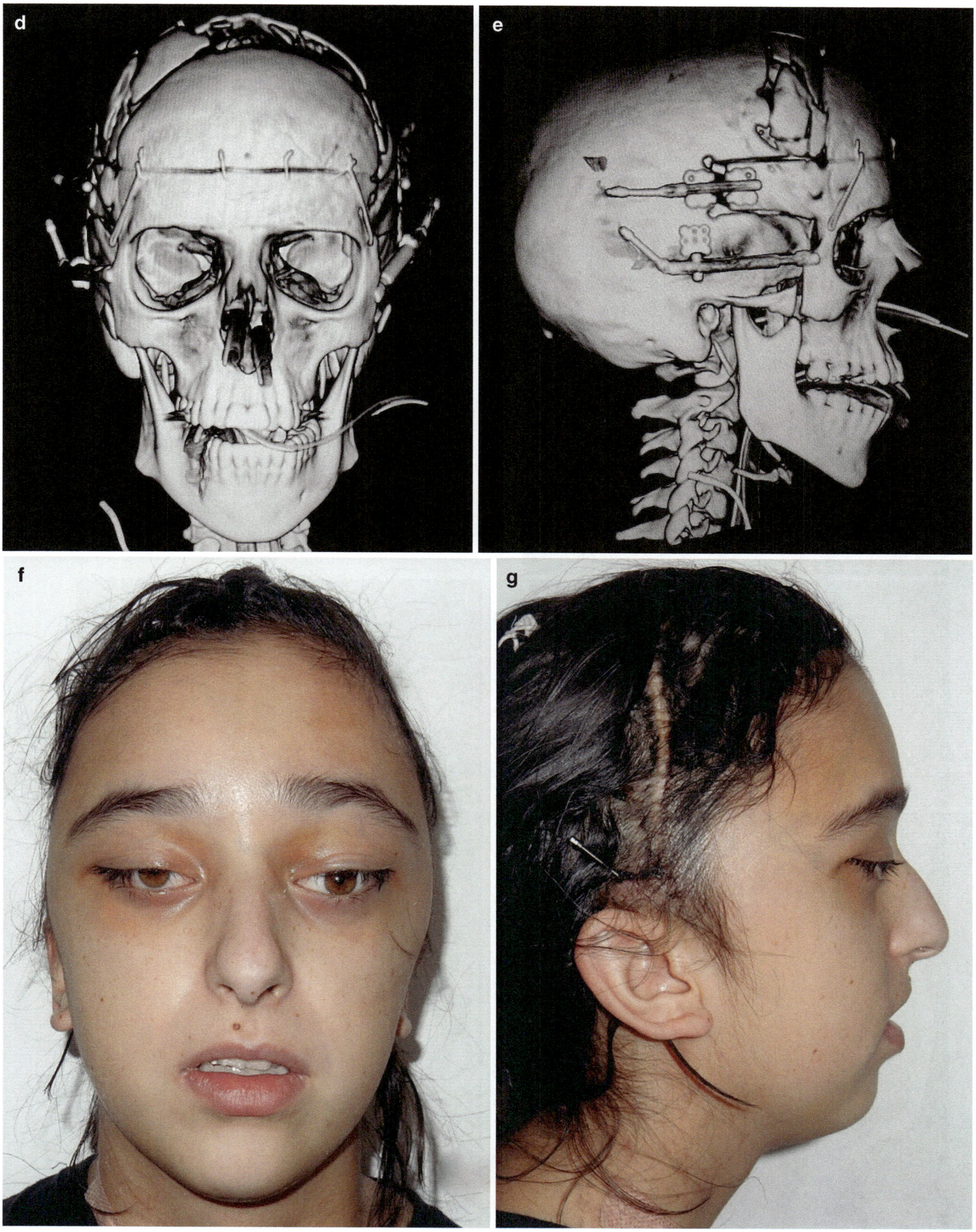

Fig. 11.3 (continued)

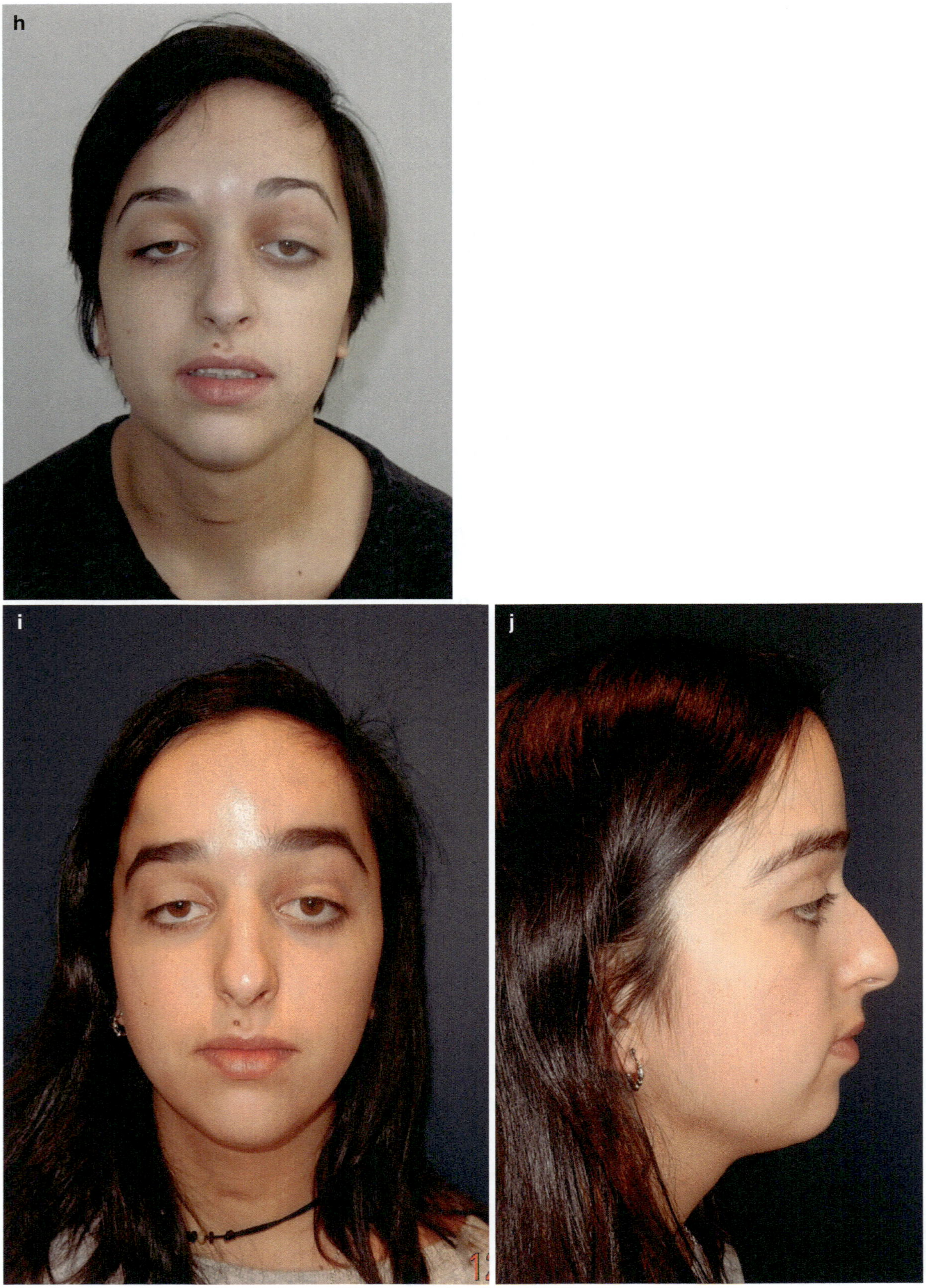

Fig. 11.3 (continued)

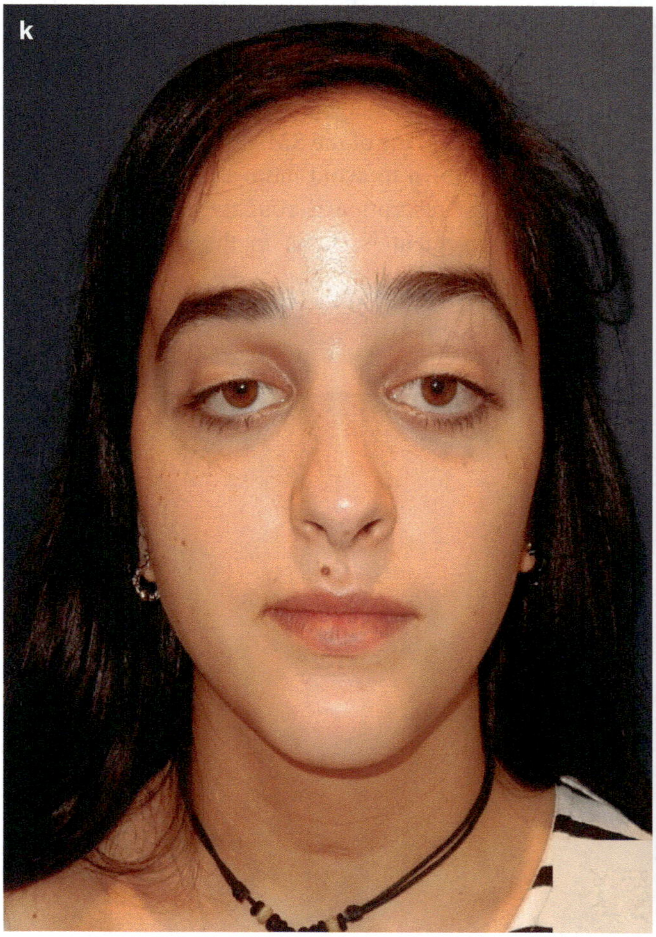

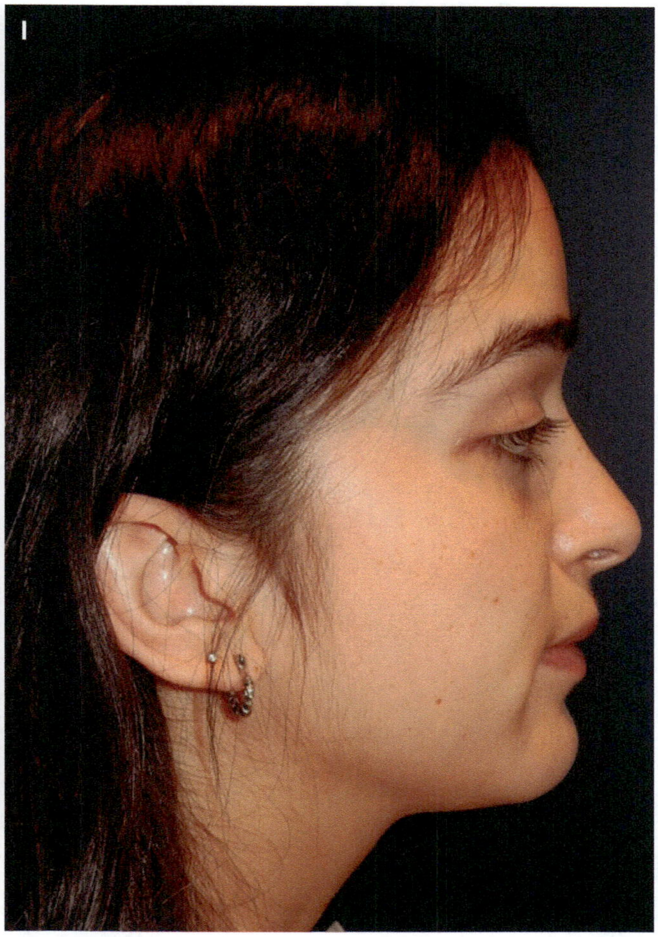

Fig. 11.3 (continued)

11.5 Medial Canthopexy

The main objective of medial canthopexy in faciocraniostenotic patients is to reduce the intercanthal distance. It is indicated in patients with hypertelorism and telecanthus. The most common indication is Apert syndrome where it is usually performed during bipartition and medial rotation of the Le Fort III segment.

Stainless steel wires are used transnasally to medialize the medial canthi. When performed bilaterally, the canthopexy wires may be tied together transnasally. Otherwise, the wire is anchored contralaterally around either a bone graft or a twisted locking wire.

11.6 Fat Grafting in the Temporal and Zygomatic Regions

Fat is usually aspirated manually in the periumbilical region or from the inner thigh using a superwet technique and a 3-mm cannula. Usually, the harvested fat is processed on a back table while other ancillary procedures are performed on the face (most commonly genioplasty and rhinoplasty). Centrifugation is limited to 1 min at 3000 revolutions per minute. Fat manipulation avoids direct exposure to air. One-milliliter syringes are filled with the prepared fat and counted. Stab puncture wounds are then used to introduce a 16-gauge cannula in the subcutaneous plane and/or in the plane of the SMAS. Fat is injected as the cannula is withdrawn to avoid intravascular fat migration. Postoperative fat resorption is roughly around 50%. The aesthetic improvement is stable in the long term [3, 4] (Figs. 11.2 and 11.4).

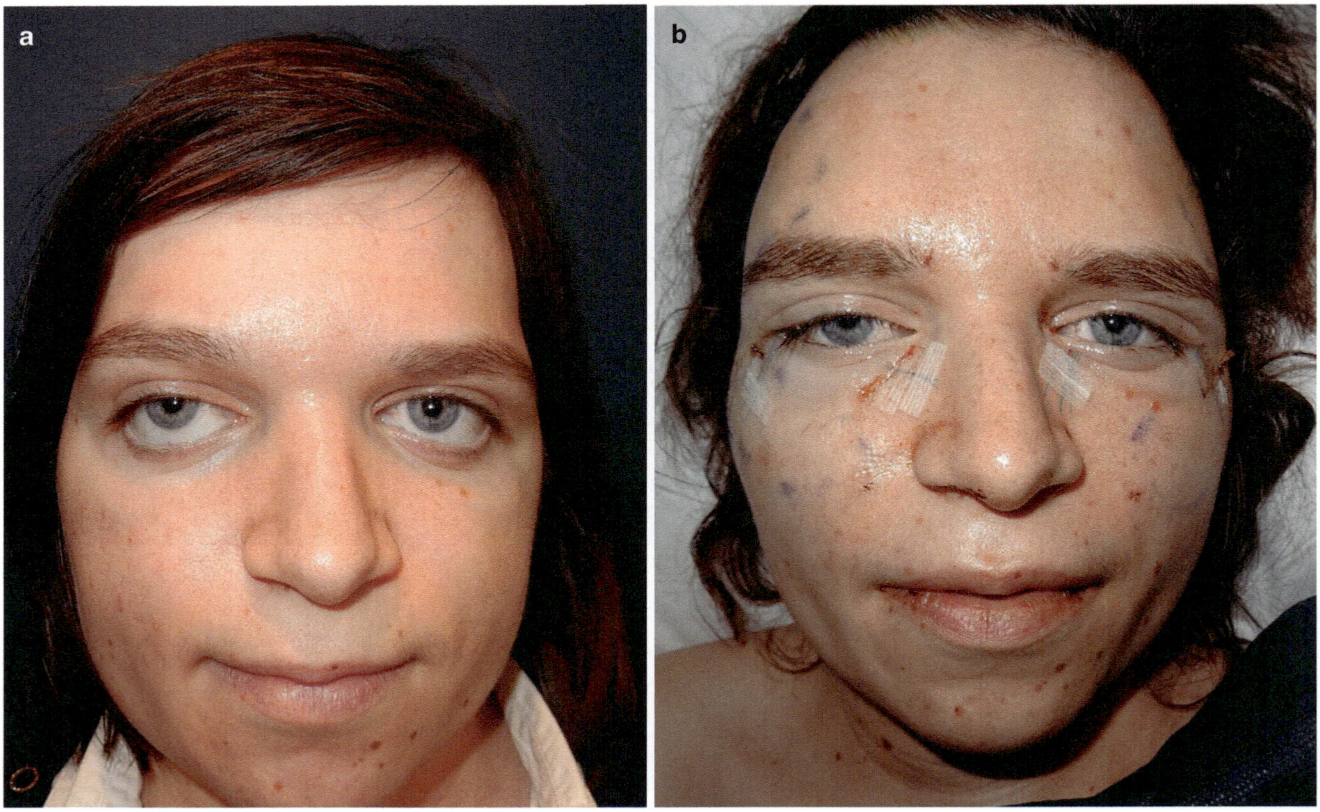

Fig. 11.4 (**a**, **b**) Patient with Crouzon syndrome aged 18 years with autologous fat transfer in the temporal and zygomatic regions. (**c**) Result after fat transfer and oral mucosa grafts of the lower eyelids

11.7 Genioplasty (Advancement Type)

Children with FCST may develop mandibular retrusion with retrogenia due to overcorrection when a LF3 is performed. Orthognathic surgery usually addresses the mandibular malposition but genioplasty remains necessary in many cases for optimal projection. The inferior vestibular surgical approach is classically used with horizontal suprabasilar osteotomy, advancement, and osteosynthesis with locking plates and/or lag screws [5] (Fig. 11.5).

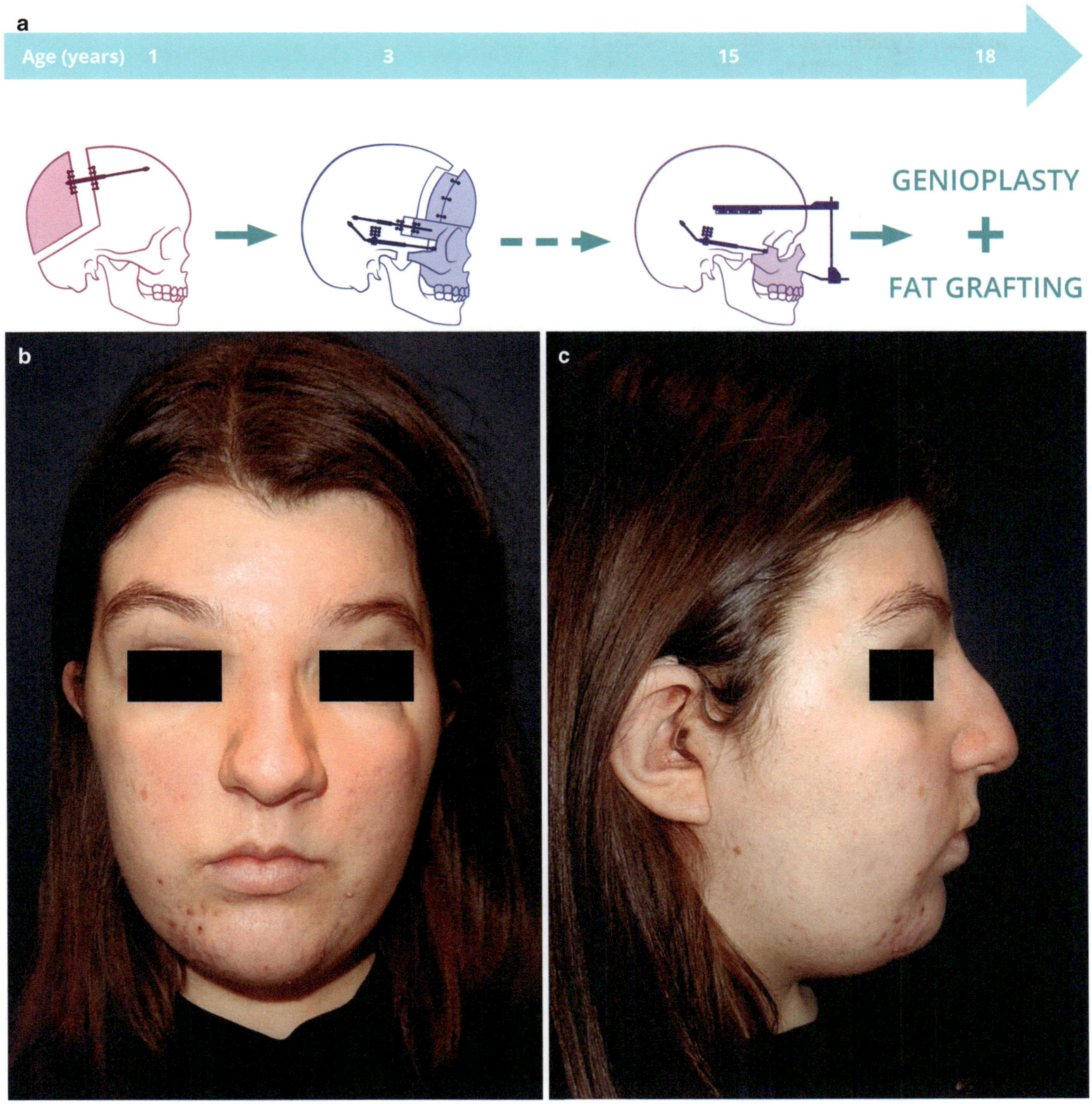

Fig. 11.5 (**a**, **b**) Patient with Crouzon syndrome aged 18 years, 15 years after FFMBA and 3 years after LF3, presenting with chin retrusion (same patient as in Fig. 10.7). © Cassandra Vion. (**c**) Per-operative with of the chin osteotomy and osteosynthesis after advancement. (**d**, **e**) Postoperative results at 19 years of age, 12 months after genioplasty, rhinoplasty, and fat grafting

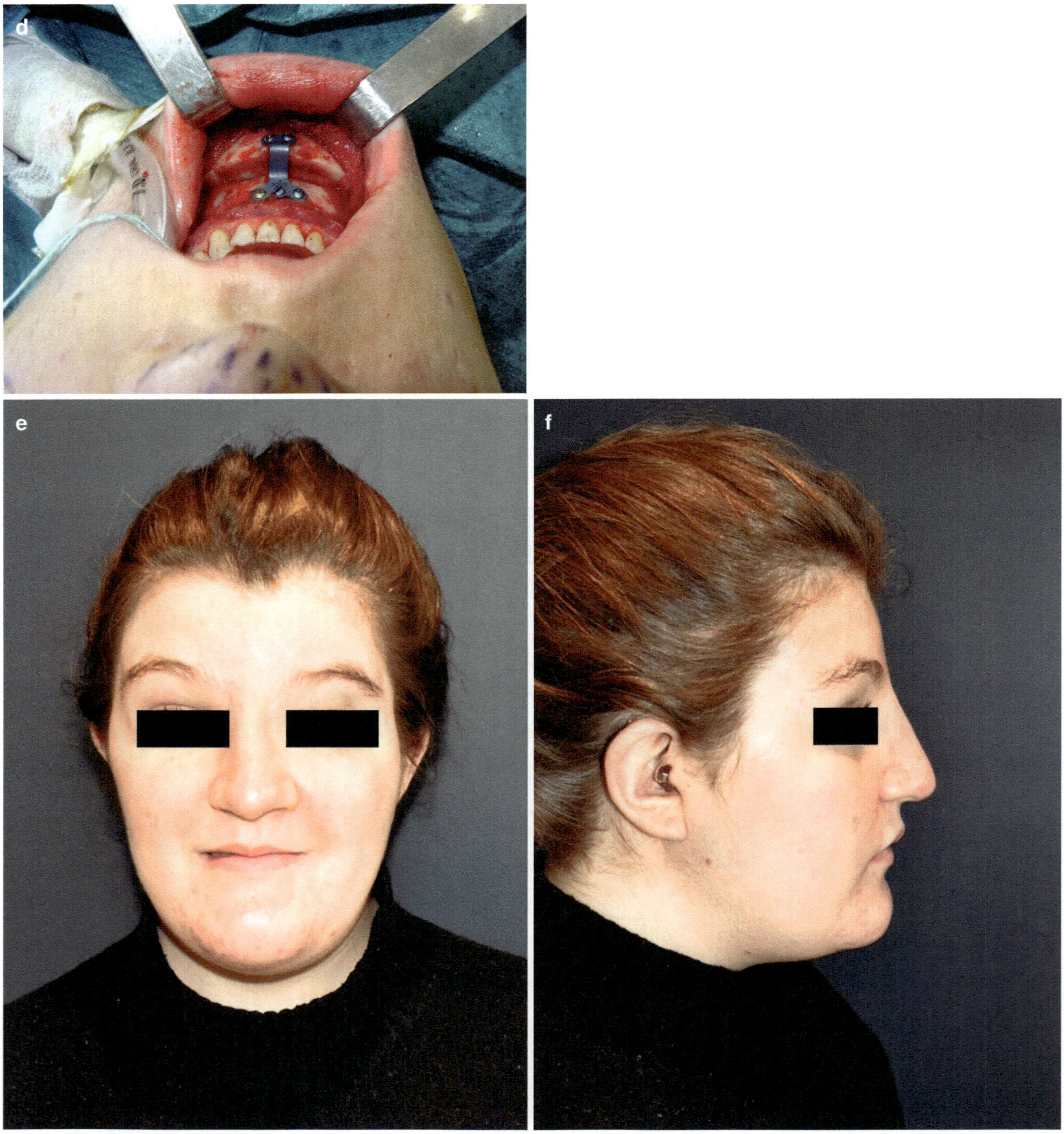

Fig. 11.5 (continued)

11.8 Rhinoseptoplasty (Especially after LF3)

Rhinoseptoplasty is usually the last procedure to be performed on the child's face. It is commonly described as the cherry on the cake thanks to the significant aesthetic improvement and the relatively minimal downtime compared to the much more invasive previous facial advancements. The nasal septum is characteristically deviated after FFMBA and LF3. It commonly presents a longitudinal fibrous fracture that corresponds to the transnasal osteotomy line. Unless necessary, it is prudent to avoid dissecting the septal cartilage through this fibrous barrier to preserve mucosal integrity. The dorsal hump is separated and removed as usual, regardless of an eventual glabellar titanium plate that was previously inserted during Le Fort III facial advancement [1] (see Rhinoplasties results after FFMBA in Fig. 11.3 and after FFMBA and LF3 in Figs. 11.5 and 11.6).

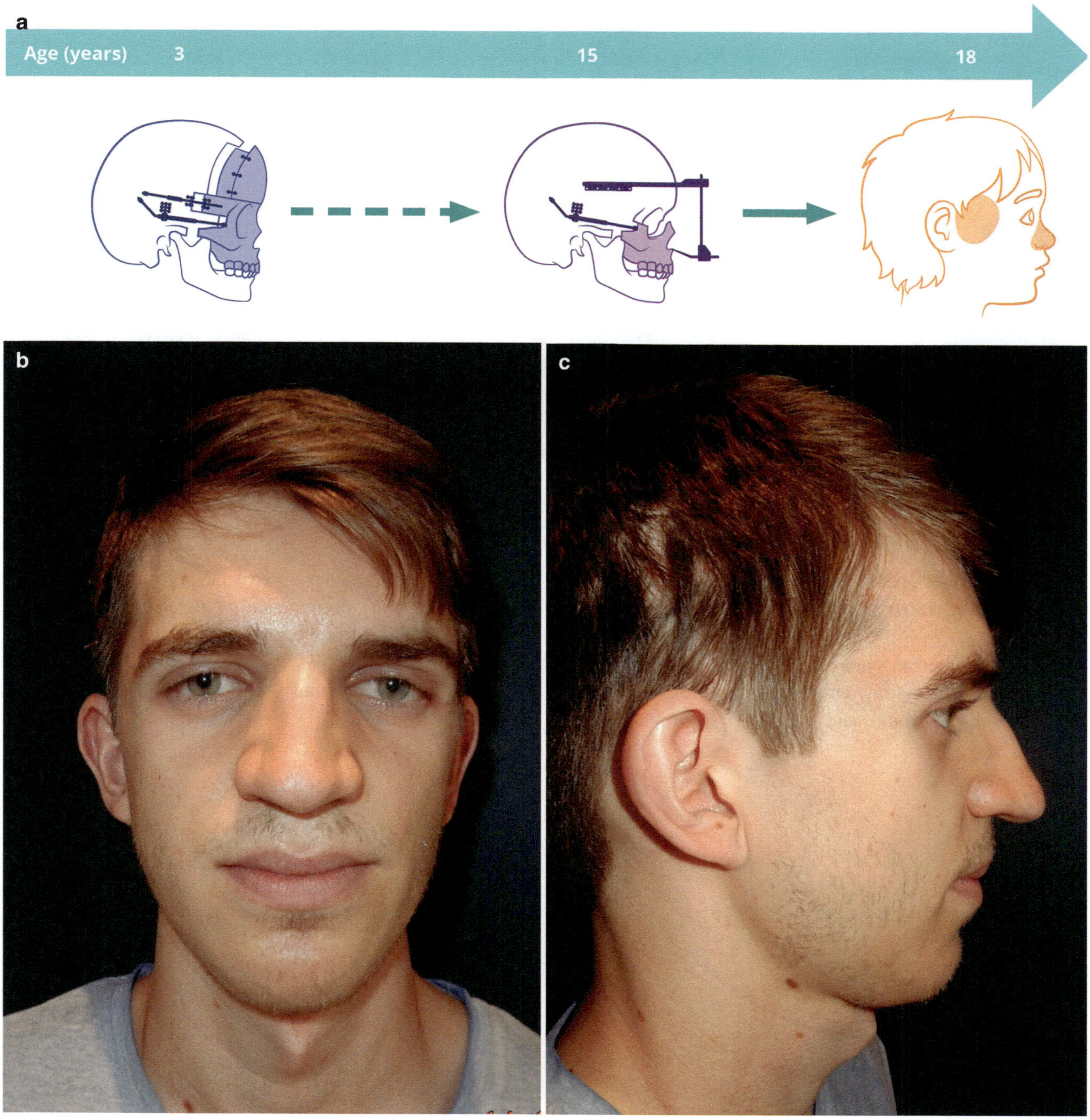

Fig. 11.6 (**a**, **b**, **c**) Crouzon syndrome aged 18 years after LF3 performed 3 years before (corresponding to Fig. 11.3) © Cassandra Vion. (**d**,**e**) Clinical view at 19, after genioplasty and rhinoplasty

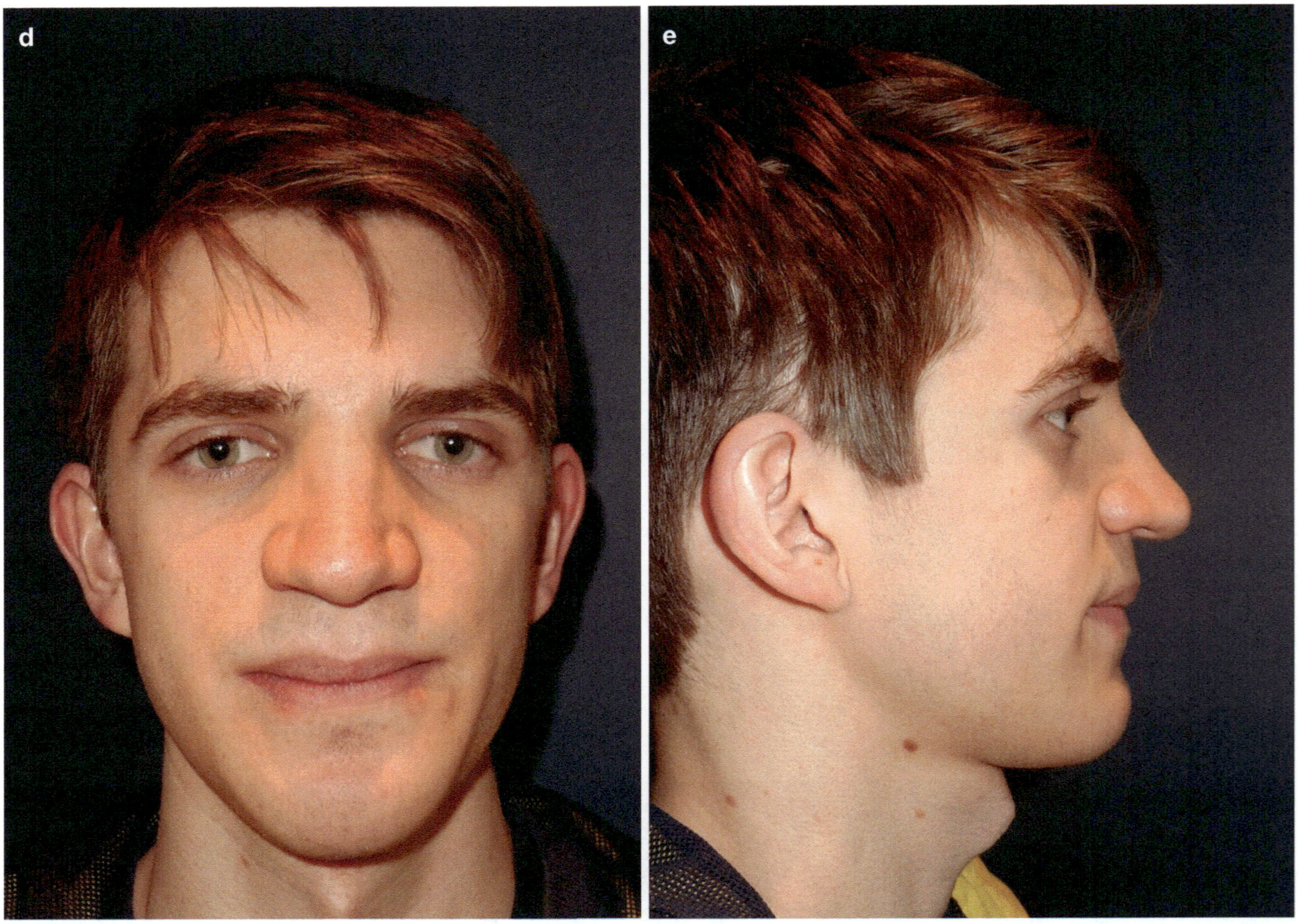

Fig. 11.6 (continued)

11.9 Specific Aesthetic Refinements in Crouzon Syndrome

Patients with Crouzon syndrome who have undergone facial advancement with distraction typically require fat grafting to the forehead, periorbital, and malar regions around adolescence to correct facial asymmetry and add soft tissue projection over the bony prominences. Lateral canthopexies are commonly required at this age as well. A septorhinoplasty is most often performed at skeletal maturity, especially in patients who had previously undergone Le Fort III facial advancement.

11.10 Specific Aesthetic Refinements in Apert Syndrome

In some Apert patients, particularly after FFMBA, excessive ossification or hyperpneumatization occurs at the level of the supraorbital bar. The mechanism underlying this phenomenon is unknown. It might be explained by the persistence of the vascularization of the bone during and after the distraction, and a simultaneous decrease in intracranial pressure. Correction requires revisiting the bicoronal incision and it is usually an opportunity to burr other cranial irregularities (Fig. 11.7).

Medial canthopexy is also very common in Apert syndrome. Successful acne treatment is warranted before any surgery is performed in adolescents with Apert syndrome, in order to control infection risks. Figure 11.8 shows a 15-year-old Apert patient with controlled acne before and after LF3.

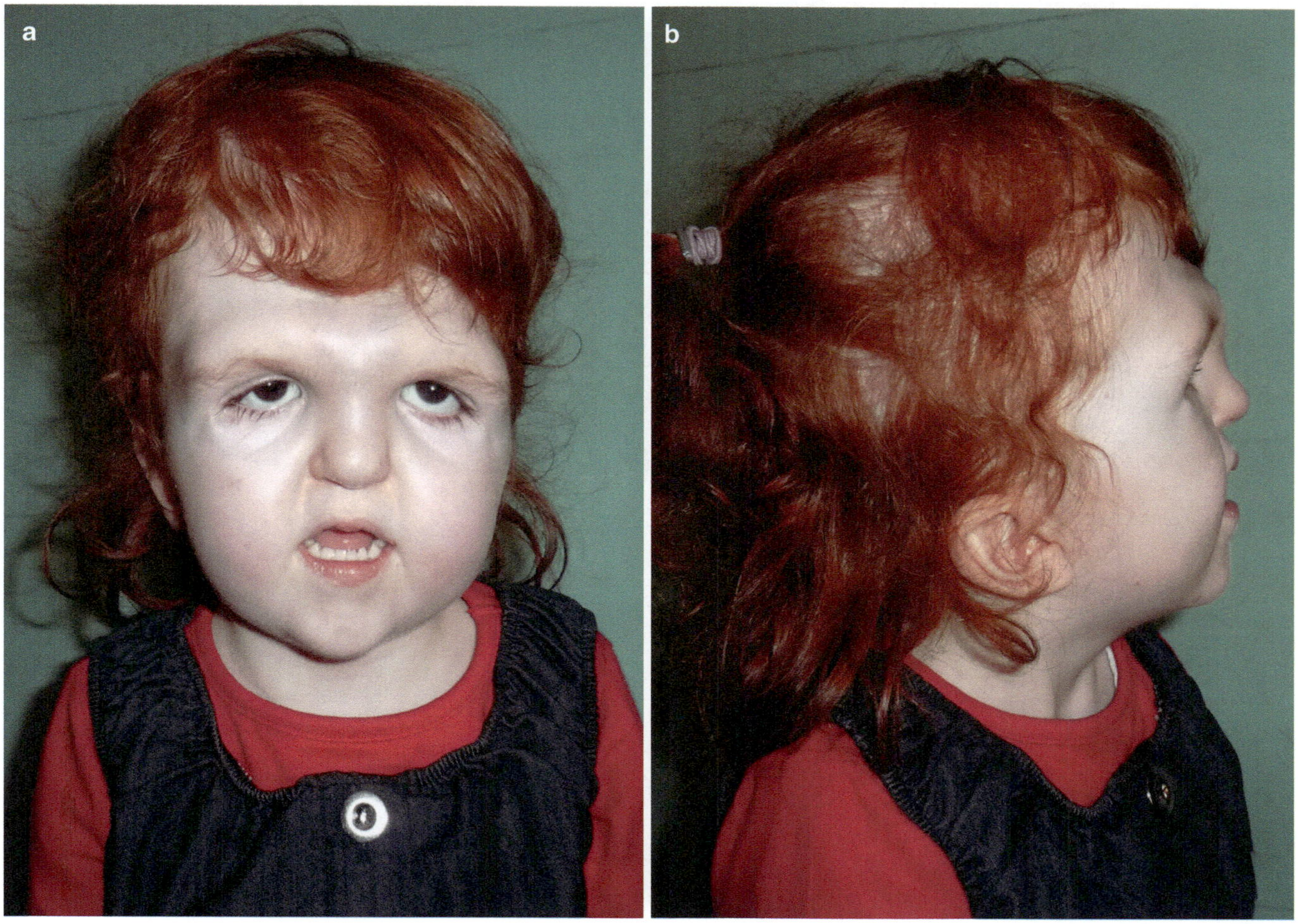

Fig. 11.7 (**a**, **b**) Patient with Apert syndrome at 6 years of age, 4 years after FFMBA, showing excessive projection of the supraorbital bar. (**c**, **d**) Per-operative view showing the bulging of the supraorbital bar. (**e**) Longitudinal osteotomy of the supraorbital bar. (**f**, **g**) Supraorbital bar after osteotomy showing that the bulging was mostly the result of frontal sinus hyperpneumatization. (**h**-**k**) Fixation of the supraorbital bar using miniplates after volume reduction

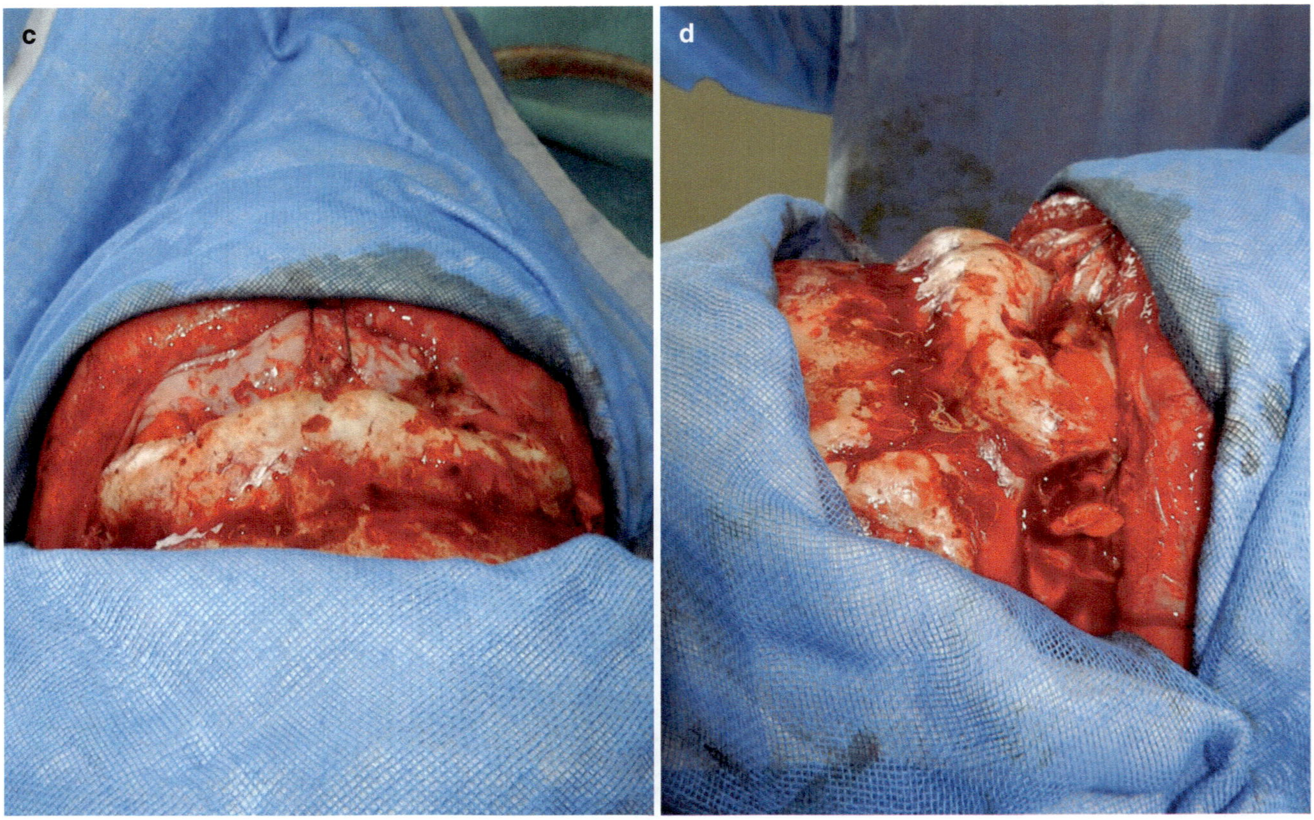

Fig. 11.7 (continued)

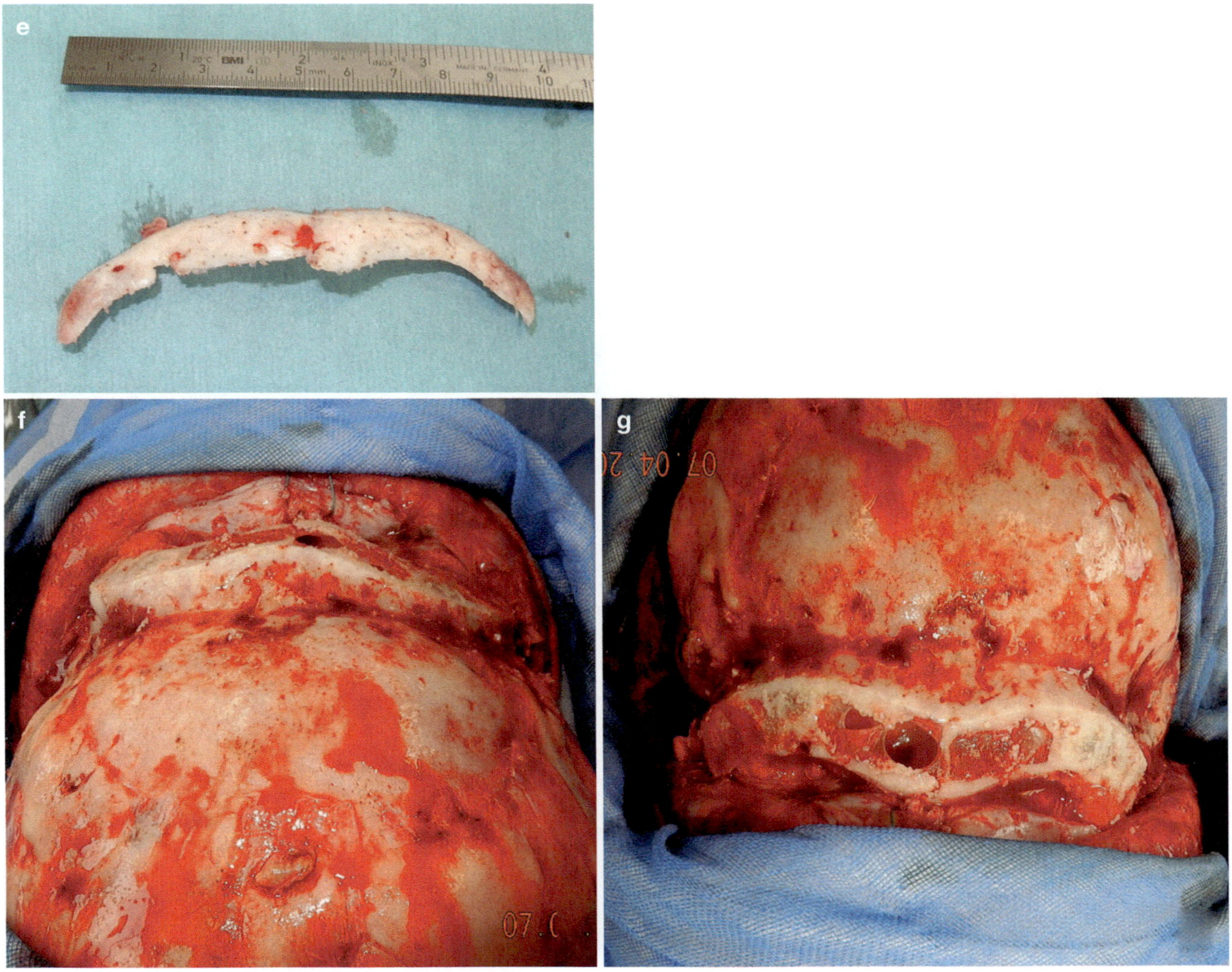

Fig. 11.7 (continued)

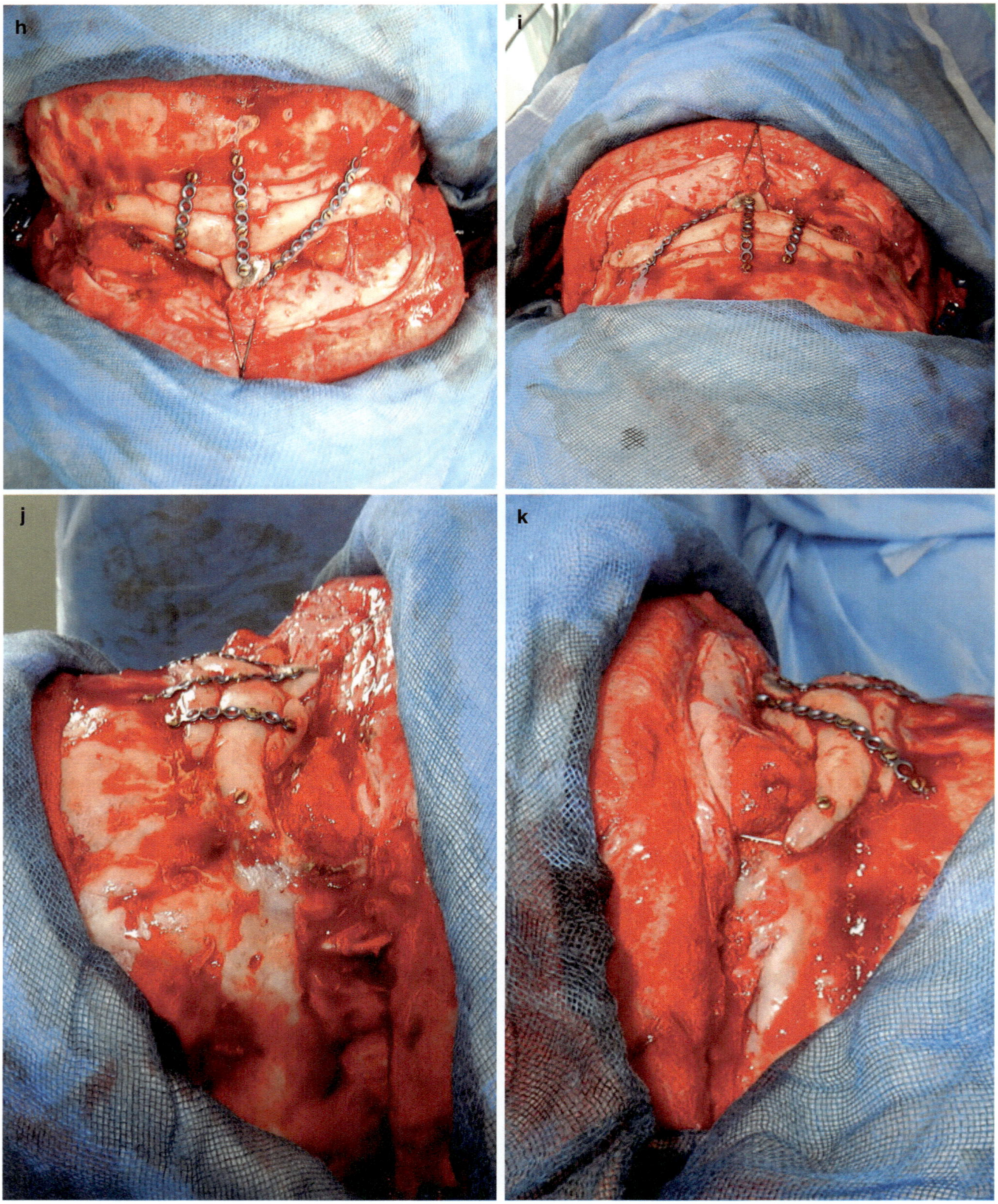

Fig. 11.7 (continued)

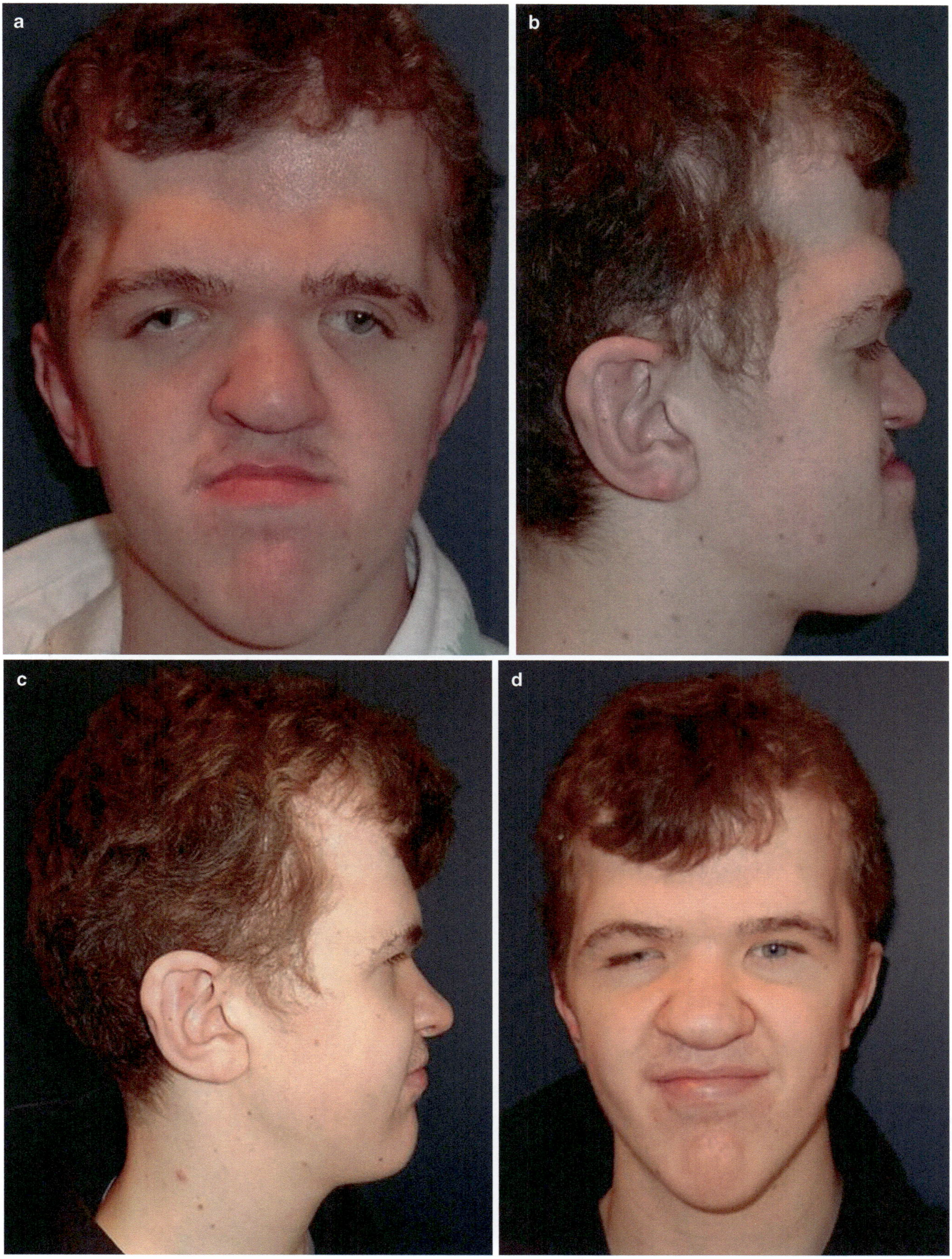

Fig. 11.8 (**a**, **b**) Patient with Apert syndrome at 15 years of age before LF3. (**c**, **d**) At 16 years of age after LF3 (including bipartition and medial canthopexy), frontal sinus remodeling, and nasal bone graft

References

1. Arnaud E, Haber SE, Paternoster G, et al. Secondary surgeries in craniosynostosis and faciocraniosynostosis. Ann Chir Plast Esthet. 2019 Nov;64(5–6):494–505.
2. Chetty V, Haber SE, Khonsari RH, et al. Improvement of periorbital appearance in Apert syndrome after subcranial Le fort III with bipartition and distraction. J Craniofacial Surg. 2020 May;31(3):711–5.
3. Cervelli D, Tambasco D, Grussu F, et al. Fat grafting as adjunct refinement procedure in craniosynostosis management. J Craniofac Surg. 2013 Mar;24(2):691–2.
4. Fahradyan A, Goel P, Williams M, et al. Temporal fat grafting in children with craniofacial anomalies. Ann Plast Surg. 2020 Nov;85(5):505–10.
5. Ousterhout DK, Vargervik K. Aesthetic improvement resulting from craniofacial surgery in craniosynostosis syndromes. J Craniomaxillofac Surg. 1987 Aug;15(4):189–97.

12 Conclusions

The management of faciocraniosynostosis is best undertaken by a multidisciplinary team that allies multiple competences (Fig. 12.1). A significant caseload is required to increase experience in rare diseases and to build cohorts.

In his original publications in the late 1960s, Paul Tessier advocated the need for a specialized craniofacial center for every 25 million persons (this excludes the treatment of cleft lip and palate abnormalities the prevalence of which is much higher, and therefore requires more centers). The rarity of faciocraniosynostoses (less than 1/20.000 births) and the complexity of care restrict de facto the number of eligible centers capable of treating these conditions. These centers are currently connected through rare disease networks such as the European Rare Disease Network (https://www.orpha.net/consor/cgi-bin/Clinics_ERN.php?lng=EN), which basically accredits one reference group per European country (ERN CRANIO). Before that, the International Society of Craniofacial Surgery (ISCFS, www.iscfs.org) has advocated and promoted the formation of craniofacial groups worldwide since 1983.

While all kinds of surgical procedures have been extensively used in most centers, the FFMBA remains considered at higher risk, and this atlas book tries to popularize this extensive procedure, which remains one of the most complete osteotomies ever designed. The routine use of all types of osteodistractors has lowered significantly the risks, making it safe in almost all surgical hands.

We still lack more comprehension on the diversity of the forms and severities of all the *FGFR* mutations to be more predictive in terms of outcomes. We also lack more comprehensive studies on the mental outcomes and quality of life (QOL) of our patients, who, in a vast majority of cases attain satisfactory aesthetic outcomes through a series of many procedures. Particular complexity of treatment in severe Pfeiffer cases still remains challenging even in the most experienced teams. We are fortunate in the craniofacial unit of Hôpital Necker-Enfants Malades, that since 1976 a huge cohort has been built. The current team continues on the track (Fig. 12.2), by pursuing clinical work and research within the newly founded Craniofacial Growth and Form laboratory, that brings together fundamental scientists, engineers and surgeons (growthnform.com).

Acknowledgments and Disclosure The authors declare having no financial disclosure: since the conception of the distractors that carry his name, Eric Arnaud has renounced any royalty from KLS Martin Group.

The study about respiration improvement of FFMBA was authorized through an ethical committee and was scientifically promoted under the "Protocole Hospitalier de Recherche Clinique" (PHRC—CRANIORESP) by Assistance Publique—Hôpitaux de Paris through the assistance of Raphaël Serreau and Caroline Élie (Départment de Recherche Clinique, Hôpital Necker-Enfants Malades, Paris, France).

E. Arnaud et al., *Frontofacial Monobloc Advancement with Internal Distraction*, https://doi.org/10.1007/978-3-031-07574-2_12

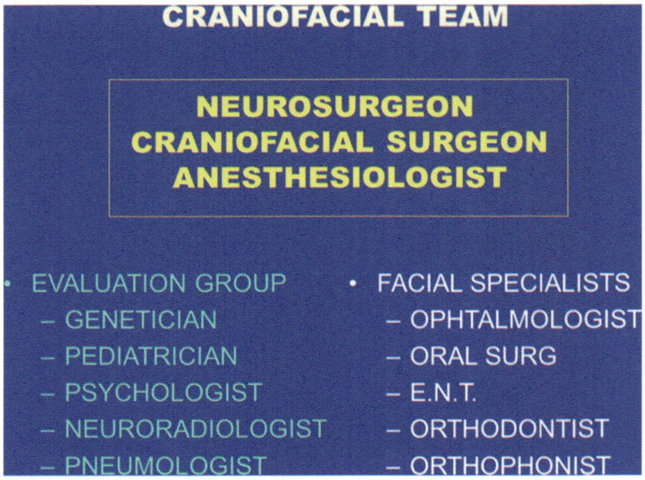

Fig. 12.1 Structure of a multidisciplinary craniofacial team it is more than ever emphasized that a multidisciplinary approach remains one of the key factors to treat those syndromic conditions

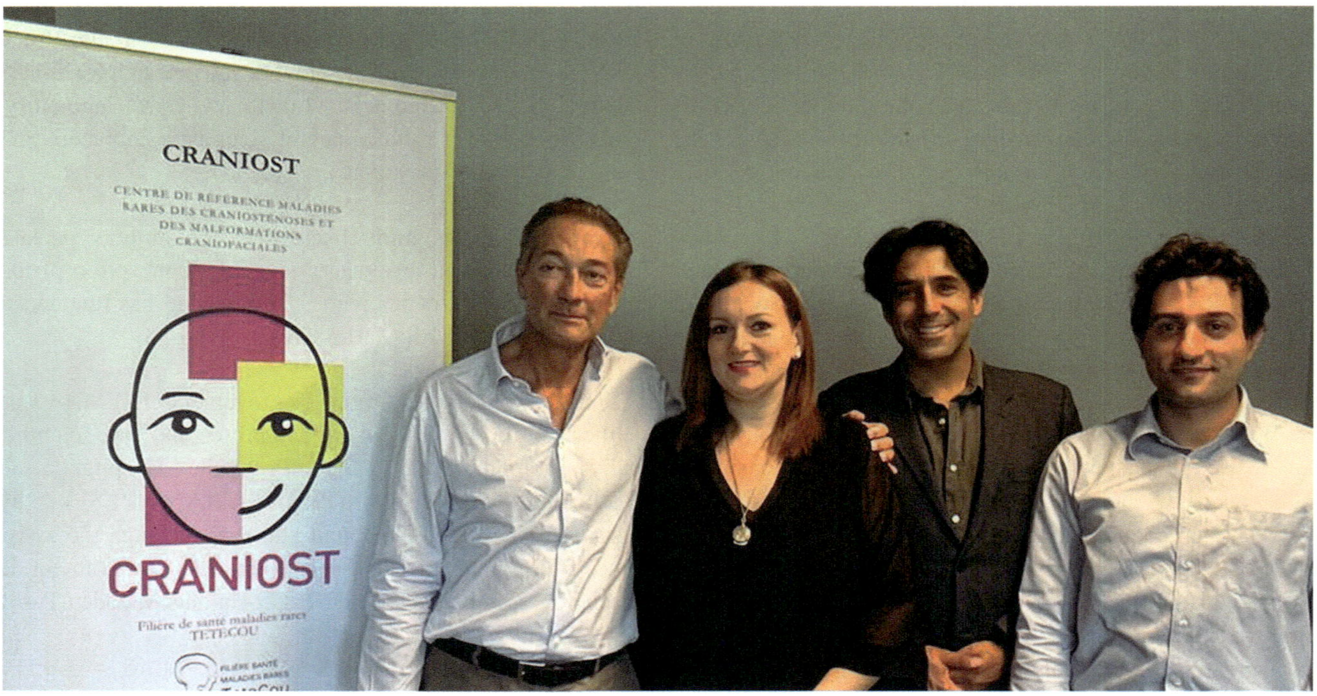

Fig. 12.2 *Craniofacial core team in Hôpital Necker-Enfants Malades* (from left to right: Eric Arnaud, Giovanna Paternoster, Roman Khonsari, Samer Haber)

GPSR Compliance

The European Union's (EU) General Product Safety Regulation (GPSR) is a set of rules that requires consumer products to be safe and our obligations to ensure this.

If you have any concerns about our products, you can contact us on ProductSafety@springernature.com

In case Publisher is established outside the EU, the EU authorized representative is:

Springer Nature Customer Service Center GmbH
Europaplatz 3
69115 Heidelberg, Germany

Batch number: 10731524

Printed by Printforce, the Netherlands